The Handbook of the Neurobiology of Eating Disorders

The Handbook of the Neurobiology of Eating Disorders

Edited by

CHRISTINA E. WIERENGA

JOANNA E. STEINGLASS

OXFORD
UNIVERSITY PRESS

OXFORD
UNIVERSITY PRESS

Oxford University Press is a department of the University of Oxford.
It furthers the University's objective of excellence in research, scholarship,
and education by publishing worldwide. Oxford is a registered trade mark of
Oxford University Press in the UK and in certain other countries.

Published in the United States of America by Oxford University Press
198 Madison Avenue, New York, NY 10016, United States of America.

CIP data is on file at the Library of Congress

ISBN 9780197675182

DOI: 10.1093/9780197675212.001.0001

Printed by Marquis Book Printing, Canada

The manufacturer's authorized representative in the EU for product safety is
Oxford University Press España S.A., Parque Empresarial San Fernando de Henares,
Avenida de Castilla, 2 – 28830 Madrid (www.oup.es/en).

MIX
Paper | Supporting responsible forestry
FSC® C103567

Contents

PART V EMERGING TOPICS

List of Figures

List of Tables

Acknowledgments

We set out with the goal of creating a book that would be a comprehensive resource on the neurobiology of eating disorders and, more importantly to us, would invite discourse within the field. While we recognize that it is natural to primarily pursue and view science through one's own lens, we hoped to inspire the consideration of multiple viewpoints. As we started planning for this book, we (Christina and Joanna) read and discussed *Think Again: The Power of Knowing What you Don't Know*, by Adam Grant, PhD—we had our own mini-book club! Dr. Grant's book provided the inspiration and framework for the Alternative Perspectives section of each chapter, to explicitly encourage readers to reconsider existing conceptualizations of eating disorders and to integrate data from different perspectives. We would like to thank Dr. Grant for encouraging us to embrace what we don't know and to appreciate the excitement in shifting our perspectives and rethinking what we thought we knew.

Any compilation of this nature comes about only through the dedication of the contributing authors—we are tremendously grateful to all our esteemed colleagues who gave this work so much thought and effort. We are also thankful to Caroline Touzeau for all her help keeping us on task.

Christina Wierenga would like to acknowledge the career-changing mentorship of Dr. Walter Kaye, who encouraged her to relearn by introducing her to the neurobiology of eating disorders, and the many trainees and patients over the years who have continued to help her rethink, and who have inspired this work. And, of course, to her family of thinkers, who have eagerly embraced curiosity, learning, and unlearning.

Joanna Steinglass wishes to acknowledge the truly extraordinary mentorship of Dr. Tim Walsh, who first taught her to think in terms of what we know and don't know, and Dr. Evelyn Attia, whose indefatigable support is the secret sauce in her career. And, of course, her husband, Dr. David Alfandre, who has always had an eye for alternative perspectives and makes outside-the-box thinking seem easy.

Grant, A. (2021). *Think again: The power of knowing what you don't know.* Viking Press.

List of Contributors

Mohamed Abdulkadir, PhD, is a Postdoctoral researcher at the National Centre for Register-based Research, Aarhus University, Denmark. https://orcid.org/0000-0002-6080-257X

Stefana Aicoboaie is a Research Assistant and PhD Student, Center for Eating and Feeding Disorders Research, Mental Health Center Ballerup, Copenhagen University Hospital, Mental Health Services Copenhagen, Copenhagen, Denmark. https://orcid.org/0009-0006-7732-2907

Ines Aitsahalia is a PhD Student, Center for Theoretical Neuroscience, Columbia University, New York, NY, US. https://orcid.org/0009-0006-5838-2146

Laura A. Berner, PhD, is an Associate Professor of Psychiatry, Icahn School of Medicine at Mount Sinai, New York, NY, US. https://orcid.org/0000-0002-1430-8028

Valentina Cardi, PhD, DClinPsychol is an Associate Professor of Clinical Psychology at the University of Padova, Italy and Clinical Psychologist at the University Hospital in Padova, Italy. She is also a Visiting Senior Lecturer at the Dept. of Psychological Medicine, King's College London (London, UK). https://orcid.org/0000-0002-7763-7099

Valentina Cazzato, PhD, is an Associate Professor of Cognitive Neuroscience, Department of Cognitive Sciences, Psychology, Education, and Cultural Studies (COSPECS), University of Messina, Messina, Italy, and Honorary Visiting Research Fellow, School of Psychology, Liverpool John Moores University, Liverpool, UK. https://orcid.org/0000-0001-9826-7798

Maia A. Chester, BA, is a PhD Student in Clinical Health Psychology, Department of Psychology, University of Miami, Miami, FL, US. https://orcid.org/0000-0002-9858-7174

Emily M. Choquette, PhD, is an Associate Investigator, Laureate Institute for Brain Research, Tulsa, OK, US. https://orcid.org/0000-0002-8265-6833

Philippe De Vloo, MD, PhD, is an Assistant Professor, KU Leuven, Belgium, and Neurosurgeon, University Hospitals Leuven, Belgium. https://orcid.org/0000-0003-3280-6503

Alexandra G. DiFeliceantonio, PhD, is an Assistant Professor, Fralin Biomedical Research Institute, VTC, Roanoke, VA, US, and Assistant Professor, Department of Human Nutrition, Foods, and Exercise, Virginia Tech, Blacksburg, VA, US. https://orcid.org/0000-0002-7155-6060

Stella Dong, BA, is a Research Coordinator and a Masters' Student, Department of Computer Science, Columbia University, New York, NY, US. https://orcid.org/0009-0006-9517-0441

Stephanie Dulawa, PhD, is a Professor of Psychiatry, University of California San Diego, San Diego, CA, US. https://orcid.org/0000-0003-1281-782X

Jamie D. Feusner, MD, is a Professor of Psychiatry, University of Toronto, Canada and Senior Scientist, Centre for Addiction and Mental Health, Toronto, Canada. https://orcid.org/0000-0002-0391-345X

Karin Foerde, PhD, is an Assistant Professor, Department of Psychology, Brain and Cognition, University of Amsterdam, Netherlands. https://orcid.org/0000-0002-5804-9312

Guido Klaus Wilhelm Frank, MD, is a Professor of Psychiatry, University of California San Diego, San Diego, CA, US. https://orcid.org/0000-0002-6590-3441

Maxwell Frank, BS, is a Research Coordinator, Department of Psychiatry, University of Wisconsin Madison, WI, US.

Deborah R. Glasofer, PhD, is an Associate Professor of Clinical Medical Psychology (in Psychiatry), Columbia University Irving Medical Center/New York State Psychiatric Institute, New York, NY, US. https://orcid.org/0000-0001-7434-8630

Sasha Gorrell, PhD, is an Assistant Professor, Department of Psychiatry and Behavioral Sciences, University of California, San Francisco, San Francisco, CA, US. https://orcid.org/0000-0002-8861-8547

Angela Guarda, MD, is the Stephen and Jean Robinson Professor of Eating Disorders, Professor of Psychiatry and Behavioral Sciences, Johns Hopkins University School of Medicine, Baltimore, MD, US, and Director, Johns Hopkins Eating Disorders Program, Johns Hopkins Medicine, Baltimore, MD, US. https://orcid.org/0000-0003-1355-729X

Natalie Gukasyan, MD, is an Assistant Professor, Department of Psychiatry, Columbia University Medical Center/New York State Psychiatric Institute, New York, NY, US. https://orcid.org/0000-0003-3567-1421

Kelsey Hagan, PhD, is an Assistant Professor of Psychiatry, Virginia Commonwealth University, Richmond, VA, US. https://orcid.org/0000-0001-5723-3591

Amy Harrison, PhD, DClinPsy, Psychology and Human Development, University College London, London, UK. https://orcid.org/0000-0002-3771-9735

Ann Haynos, PhD, is an Assistant Professor of Psychology, Virginia Commonwealth University, Richmond, VA, US. https://orcid.org/0000-0002-2548-1731

Samantha Hilbert is a Research Data Analyst, School of Medicine, Johns Hopkins University, Baltimore, MD, US.

Laura Hill, PhD, is an Adjunct Associate Clinical Professor of Psychiatry and Behavioral Health, The Ohio State University, OH, US.

Hans Wijbrand Hoek, MD, PhD, is an Adjunct Professor of Epidemiology, Columbia University Mailman School of Public Health, New York, NY, US, and Professor of Psychiatry, University of Groningen, University Medical Center Groningen, Groningen, Netherlands and Psychiatrist, Parnassia Psychiatric Institute, The Hague, Netherlands. https://orcid.org/0000-0001-6353-5465

Laura Holsen, PhD, is a Psychologist, Division of Women's Health, Department of Medicine, Brigham and Women's Hospital, Boston, MA, US, Associate Professor of Psychiatry, Department of Psychiatry, Harvard Medical School, Boston, MA, US, Research Psychologist, Department of Psychiatry, Brigham and Women's Hospital, Boston, MA, US, and Director of Research Training, Connors Center for Women's Health, Brigham and Women's Hospital, Boston, MA, US. https://orcid.org/0000-0003-1292-7789

William M. Howe, PhD, is an Assistant Professor, School of Neuroscience, Virginia Tech, Blacksburg, VA, US. https://orcid.org/0000-0003-0433-6591

Kiyohito Iigaya, PhD, is an Assistant Professor of Neurobiology, Department of Psychiatry, Columbia University Irving Medical Center, New York, NY, US, and Research Scientist, New York State Psychiatric Institute, New York, NY, US. https://orcid.org/0000-0002-4748-8432

Adanya D. Johnson, BS, is a Clinical Research Coordinator, Department of Psychology, Virginia Commonwealth University, Richmond, VA, US. https://orcid.org/0000-0001-5314-4532

Walter H. Kaye, MD, is an Emeritus Distinguished Professor, University of California San Diego, San Diego, CA, US. https://orcid.org/0000-0002-4478-4906

Pamela Keel, PhD, is a Distinguished Research Professor, Department of Psychology, Florida State University, Tallahassee, FL, US. https://orcid.org/0000-0001-6542-5147

Sahib Khalsa, MD, PhD, is an Associate Professor in the Department of Psychiatry and Biobehavioral Sciences, Semel Institute for Neuroscience and Human Behavior, David Geffen School of Medicine, University of California at Los Angeles, CA, US, and Affiliate Investigator at Laureate Institute for Brain Research, Tulsa, OK, US. https://orcid.org/0000-0003-2124-8585

Millie C. Kirchberg, BS, is a Medical Student, University of California, San Diego, CA, US.

Stephanie Knatz Peck, PhD, is an Associate Clinical Professor of Psychiatry at the University of California San Diego, San Diego, CA, US. https://orcid.org/0000-0001-9421-9158

Natalia Lawrence, BSc, PhD, is an Associate Professor in Psychology, Psychology Department, Faculty of Health and Life Sciences, University of Exeter, UK. https://orcid.org/0000-0003-1969-6637

Elizabeth A. Lawson, MD, MMSc, is Associate Professor of Medicine at Harvard Medical School and Director, Interdisciplinary Oxytocin Research Program in the Neuroendocrine Unit at Massachusetts General Hospital, Boston, MA, US. https://orcid.org/0000-0001-8619-3349

Nir Lipsman, MD, PhD, is the Harquail Chair in Neuromodulation, Chief of Hurvitz Brain Sciences Program and Neurosurgeon at Sunnybrook Health Sciences Center, Toronto, Ontario, CA. https://orcid.org/0000-0002-4820-3056

Siyi Lou, BA, MA, is a Research Associate, New York University, New York, NY, US. https://orcid.org/0009-0005-3794-4165

Andres Lozano, OC, MD, PhD, FRSCS, FRSC, FCAHS, is a University Professor and Alan & Susan Hudson Cornerstone Chair in Neurosurgery, Division of Neurosurgery, University Health Network, University of Toronto, Toronto, Canada. https://orcid.org/0000-0001-8257-3694

Carrie J. McAdams, MD, PhD, is an Associate Professor of Psychiatry, University of Texas at Southwestern Medical School, Dallas, TX, US. https://orcid.org/0000-0002-4768-6703

Stephanie Miles, BA, BPsych (Hons), PhD, is a Research Fellow, Centre for Youth Mental Health, The University of Melbourne, Australia and Research Fellow, Orygen, Melbourne, Australia. https://orcid.org/0000-0001-8190-894X

Susan Murray, PhD, is a Supervising Psychologist, Princeton Center for Eating Disorders, Penn Medicine Princeton Medical Center Plainsboro, NJ, US. https://https://orcid.org/0000-0002-3246-0357

Andrea Phillipou, BSc, BSc (Hons), PhD, is an Associate Professor and Principal Research Fellow in Eating Disorders, Centre for Youth Mental Health, The University of Melbourne, Australia, and Head, Eating Disorders, Orygen, Melbourne, Australia. https://orcid.org/0000-0003-1009-6619

Lauren Pictor holds a BA from the Department of Psychological Sciences, Auburn University, AL, US.

Jessica L. Qiu, BA, is a Clinical Research Coordinator, Department of Psychiatry, Icahn School of Medicine at Mount Sinai, New York, NY, US.

Blair R. K. Shevlin, PhD, is a Postdoctoral Fellow, Icahn School of Medicine at Mount Sinai, New York, NY, US. https://orcid.org/0000-0002-5420-0046

Katherine Schaumberg, PhD, is an Assistant Professor, Department of Psychology, University of Texas at Austin, Austin, TX, US. https://orcid.org/0000-0003-3193-2233

Jochen Seitz, MD, is a Professor of Child and Adolescent Psychiatry, Psychosomatics, and Psychotherapie, LVR-University Hospital, Essen, University of Duisburg-Essen, Germany. https://orcid.org/0000-0002-0110-7980

Pradyumna Sepúlveda, PhD, is a Postdoctoral Researcher at Department of Psychiatry, Vagelos College of Physicians and Surgeons, Columbia University Irving Medical Center, New York, NY, US, and Fellow of The Italian Academy for Advanced Studies, Columbia University, New York, NY, US. https://orcid.org/0000-0003-0159-6777

Joanna E. Steinglass, MD, is a Professor of Psychiatry, Columbia University Irving Medical Center and New York State Psychiatric Institute, New York, NY, US. https://orcid.org/0000-0001-8434-8212

Annabel Susanin, BA, is a PhD student, Psychology Department, St. John's University, Queens, NY, US. https://orcid.org/0000-0003-1917-4409

Jet D. Termorshuizen, PhD. Department of Medical Epidemiology and Biostatistics, Karolinska Institutet, Stockholm, Sweden. https://orcid.org/0000-0002-5912-3975

Jennifer J. Thomas, PhD, is a Professor of Psychology, Department of Psychiatry, Harvard Medical School, Boston, MA, US and Co-Director, Eating Disorders Clinical and Research Program, Massachusetts General Hospital, Boston, MA, US. https://orcid.org/0000-0003-2601-581X

C. Alix Timko, PhD, is an Associate Professor of Psychology, Perelman School of Medicine, University of Pennsylvania, Philadelphia, PA, US, and Department of Child and Adolescent Psychiatry and Behavioral Science, Children's Hospital of Philadelphia, Philadelphia, PA, US. https://orcid.org/0000-0002-2927-7527

Stefanie Trinh, PhD, is at the Institute of Neuroanatomy, Uniklinik RWTH Aachen, Germany. https://orcid.org/0000-0001-5719-5265

Kira G. Venables, BA, is a Clinical Research Coordinator, Department of Psychology, Virginia Commonwealth University, Richmond, VA, US. https://orcid.org/0009-0001-3713-928X

Elske Vrieze, PhD, DM, is a Professor of Psychiatry, Department of Neuroscience, KU Leuven, Leuven, Belgium. https://orcid.org/0000-0001-7766-9245

B. Timothy Walsh, MD, is a Professor of Psychiatry, Columbia University Irving Medical Center, New York, NY, US. https://orcid.org/0000-0001-8626-5859

Christina E. Wierenga, PhD, is a Professor of Psychiatry, University of California San Diego, San Diego, CA, US. https://orcid.org/0000-0002-4843-1809

Diana L. Williams, PhD, is a Kravis Professor of Integrated Sciences: Neuroscience, Kravis Department of Integrated Sciences, Claremont McKenna College, CA, US. https://orcid.org/0000-0002-3548-7440

D. Blake Woodside, MD, MSc, FRCPC, is an Adjunct Professor, Department of Psychiatry, University of Toronto, Toronto, Canada. https://orcid.org/0000-0001-6833-3264

Zeynep Yilmaz, PhD, is a Senior Researcher, National Centre for Register-based Research, Aarhus University, Denmark and Associate Professor, Department of Biomedicine, Aarhus University, Denmark. https://orcid.org/0000-0002-8145-1596

Nancy Zucker, PhD, is a Professor of Psychiatry and Behavioral Sciences and Psychology and Neuroscience, Duke University, Durham, NC, US. https://orcid.org/0000-0003-2278-5008

Introduction

Christina E. Wierenga and Joanna E. Steinglass

Introduction

During the last decades, research into the causes and characteristics of eating disorders has undergone a momentous transformation with the recognition that eating disorders, like all psychiatric illnesses, have a neurobiological basis. This shift results from astounding advances in basic science, including brain imaging and molecular genetics, which have led to breakthroughs in understanding of the biological underpinnings of complex behaviors and traits. While this is true across psychiatry, advances in understanding ingestive behavior and cognitive and computational neuroscience related to reward processing, interoception, decision-making, and emotional function have had particular relevance for eating disorders. Today, neurobiological research examines genetic, metabolic, neuroendocrine, neurocognitive, and neurocircuit-based contributors to the onset and maintenance of eating disorders. New approaches to treatment and innovative forms of intervention are being developed based on these insights from basic research.

This Handbook captures these exciting developments in a single volume. Each section reviews what is known and what remains unknown across the biobehavioral mechanisms of eating disorders. Differences of opinion about many aspects of mechanisms of eating disorders abound. This debate is an important component of advancing and testing ideas, making this an exciting time for discovery in eating disorders. The eating disorders field encompasses a rich scientific discourse with a range of perspectives—sometimes conflicting—on the key elements of etiology and clinical expression. The Editors have come together to create this book specifically because of differences in perspectives between our work. Later in the Introduction, we use these differences to briefly debate our own competing hypotheses. In so doing, we apply skepticism to our own ideas to demonstrate the approach encouraged by this Handbook.

Philosophers dating back to Aristotle have defended the merits of argumentation to arrive at truth. Recent conflict-focused research has shown that debates about ideas and opinions are linked to greater creativity and better solutions (de Wit et al., 2012). Debate is commonly seen through the questioning of other people's arguments. Yet, applying skepticism to our own opinions and being willing

Christina E. Wierenga and Joanna E. Steinglass, *Introduction*. In: *The Handbook of the Neurobiology of Eating Disorders*. Edited by: Christina E. Wierenga and Joanna E. Steinglass, Oxford University Press. © Oxford University Press (2025). DOI: 10.1093/9780197675212.003.0001 to change our minds is also key to advancing knowledge. In fact, the principles of the scientific method, the foundation of science dating back as early as the 1600s, rely on inquiry, skepticism, and evidence-based explanations: this empirical approach to discovery occurs through asking questions, making careful observations, applying skepticism to observations to prevent cognitive assumptions or bias from distorting interpretation, using inductive reasoning to formulate hypotheses, experimentally testing the deductions drawn from the hypotheses, and refining (or rejecting) the hypotheses based on the experimental findings. These principles have been fruitful. With the accelerating growth of research and published studies in eating disorders, we now have an opportunity to apply these principles to evaluate the science, recognize the limits of our understanding, and reconsider and update our views based on new evidence in the service of acquiring a more accurate, data-driven understanding of eating disorders.

The Buddhist parable of the blind scholars and the elephant offers a cautionary tale for the dangers of debate stemming from bias or limited information. According to legend, several blind scholars were positioned around an elephant and asked to describe it. Not surprisingly, each person observes the elephant to be something different based on their vantage point (e.g., the person standing next the trunk views the elephant to be like a snake, the person next to the tail judges the elephant to be like a rope, the person next to the ear characterizes the elephant as a fan). The scholars commence to argue among each other. A wise sage happened to hear the argument, stopped and asked them "What is the matter?" They said, "We cannot agree to what the elephant is like." The wise sage, who happened to be able to see, calmly said, "Each one of you is correct; and each one of you is wrong." The sage continued, "each of you only had a partial view of the animal. If you put your partial views together, you will get an idea of what an elephant looks like." The parable's function is to call attention to a lack of objectivity and the need for consideration of other approaches and perspectives when trying to understand the nature of things. Of course, it's important to recognize that not all perspectives are equally valid, and even valid arguments are not necessarily equally sound. The elephant represents some absolute reality (e.g., causes and characteristics of eating disorders) and the scholars (i.e., scientists) represent different approaches to understanding this reality. All the scholars have correctly described their piece of reality but ultimately fail if they see their reality as the only truth.

This Handbook aims not only to assemble scientific information from a range of areas of neurobiology of eating disorders but also to promote discourse and encourage integration of perspectives. Eating disorders are associated with dangerous and costly medical morbidity, high rates of comorbid psychopathology, significant psychosocial impairment, substantial economic burden, and the highest mortality rate of any psychiatric disorder. There is an urgent need to improve understanding of these serious disorders. By highlighting the controversies in the field, we aim to clarify the distinctions between what is known from the data and what is not yet known, to drive further discovery toward the common goal of improving understanding and treatment of eating disorders.

One scientific difference that emerges is in the framework, or orientation, of programs of research. Some of the chapters in this book will address basic neurocognitive processes and how they may differ in populations with eating disorders. Other chapters will address manifest symptoms of eating disorders and examine the neurobiological underpinnings. Addressing basic processes (e.g., neuropsychological functioning, reward processing) can be considered a "bottom-up" approach, by starting with the foundations of neuroscience of behavior and assessing functioning in patient populations. Addressing symptoms (e.g., restrictive eating) can arguably be described as a "top-down" approach, by starting with the observable and examining the underlying determinants. Considering one perspective "bottom" and the other "top" is somewhat arbitrary. McArthur's Universal Corrective Map of the World (1979) places the Southern Hemisphere at the top, and it may be a useful exercise to note how this changes worldviews. Nonetheless, for this book we will adopt the directional view with basic processes as the bottom, to maintain consistency.

There are advantages and disadvantages inherent in each approach, of course. Bottom-up approaches have the advantage of starting with well characterized neural circuits (for example) and identifying differences that may be implicated as predisposing, precipitating, and perpetuating factors in eating disorders. These circuits can prove to be accessible targets for therapeutic interventions. On the other hand, the bottom-up approach does not always yield connections with clinical manifestations of illness, calling into question their relevance in the etiology or maintenance of the disorder. Top-down approaches can have the advantage of ecological validity and clinical relevance. On the other hand, the top-down approach can be limited by focusing on a single set of symptoms and may overlook associated disturbances. Furthermore, the idea of a clear distinction between bottom-up and top-down approaches is false—most science includes features of both. These two perspectives might be expected to eventually meet in the middle, with complementary findings that identify neurobiological disturbances in eating disorders. Nonetheless, the framework can be useful for discussion. This Handbook is organized around this framework to facilitate the contributing authors' discussion and integration of perspectives.

Each chapter also includes a section on Alternate Perspectives. The authors have used these sections to fully discuss the limitations within the work presented, or to consider how the question itself might benefit from being approached differently. We see these discussions as critical to this book, and valuable for shaping thinking for students, trainees, and all those joining the scientific community.

As Editors of this Handbook, we have identified a topic of discourse in which our perspectives differ: the neural mechanisms of food restriction in anorexia nervosa (AN). This topic is considered in more depth in several chapters in this book. Here, we present our own debate regarding mechanisms of food restriction that can serve as a model for the types of conversations we hope this book will foster.

Food restriction can be approached from the bottom-up lens. Animal models of consummatory behavior have identified approach and avoidance motivation mechanisms and research studies have examined whether these are abnormal in AN (Christina Wierenga [CW] and others). These animal models have delineated basic reward mechanisms that guide approaching food and anxiety-related mechanisms that guide avoidance of harm. Differences in brain response to pleasant taste, a primary reward, suggest that individuals with AN experience less reward signaling from food in reward and incentive-motivation circuits including the ventral striatum and insula, especially when hungry (Kaye et al., 2020). In addition, individuals with AN who have higher scores on a measure of trait harm avoidance have lower reward response to pleasant taste in the dorsal caudate, a region associated with cognitive control. The theoretical model, based on the animal and basic science literature of appetitive and inhibitory drives, suggests that food restriction can result from decreased intrinsic hedonic drive and increased anxiety. Neural findings in patients with AN are consistent with this model, suggesting anxiety and inhibition may influence reward processing, leading to food avoidance mediated by dorsal caudate. If food restriction results from a combination of decreased food reward sensitivity or motivation and anxiety, treatments that leverage external motivators and use anxiety-management strategies may be effective in compensating for these biologically driven deficits. A treatment approach based on this model is described in Part 4, Chapter 19 (CW and colleagues).

Food restriction can be approached from a top-down lens. Limiting intake below the body's needs involves a series of maladaptive decisions about what to eat. Studies have examined the neural correlates of food choice in patients with AN (Joanna Steinglass [JS] and colleagues). Numerous behavioral studies have demonstrated that individuals with AN consistently limit the intake of high-fat foods. Studying the neural circuits associated with these decisions has shown that dorsal striatum (specifically, anterior caudate) and related cortical regions are associated with food choices among patients with AN but not among healthy controls (Foerde et al., 2015). The theoretical model posits that the decision to limit intake of high-fat foods begins as a goal-oriented choice. Individualized rewards, whether internal or external, serve to reinforce this behavior and, over time, this becomes habitual. The dorsal striatum is involved in habit learning and habit behavior in translational and cognitive neuroscience such that the neural findings are consistent with the model. Identifying the behavioral and neural processes that guide food restriction leads to treatment development focused on habits, such as habit-reversal based treatments, and to neuromodulatory approaches targeting dorsal striatum and associated circuits. These treatment approaches are described in Part 4, Chapter 18 (JS and colleagues) and Chapter 21.

Both programs of research address the question, "what are the neural mechanisms of food restriction in AN?" Yet there are differences in theoretical background and in study methods that lead in different directions. To move the science forward, it is helpful to first acknowledge the common ground (Rackham, 2007), where both the Editors of this Handbook interpret these data similarly. One, food that is understood to be palatable in healthy populations is not treated as a primary reward by patients with AN. Two, there are alterations in reward systems in AN that may be a mechanism of pathological restrictive eating. Three, food restriction is a complex behavior. Even describing the primary process as "taste" overlooks that taste includes complex processing of reward, which is likely disturbed in AN, combined with complex decision-making disturbances. Four, the dorsal striatum recurrently appears as a region critically involved in dietary restriction in AN. Finding common ground can be a launching-off point for effective debate (Grant, 2021). As will be described, we each interpret the role of the dorsal striatum in food restriction differently.

CW remains skeptical that the dorsal striatum engagement during the food choice task necessarily indicates habit involvement for several reasons. One, the tests of decision-making about food did not test habitual behavior directly. Two, the dorsal caudate has numerous functions aside from cue-driven behavior. The dorsal caudate activation during the food choice task may reflect avoidance of high-fat food options related to anxiety rather than habit-based selection. There are data suggesting that the dorsal caudate is involved in balancing risk and reward, in making decisions under conflict, and in avoidance learning (Ilango et al., 2014; LeBlanc et al., 2020). Three, using a food choice task creates a set of binary choices, which is an oversimplified version of the types of decisions made around food in real-life, thereby potentially undermining the validity of the neural findings.

JS remains skeptical that patients with AN have fundamental disturbances in taste/taste processing for several reasons. One, the data indicate that the participants do not distinguish the sweet bolus from the water bolus in the neural tasks, suggesting that the findings may not be related to taste, per se. Related to this, reduced ventral striatal response to small boluses of sugary water may not translate to actual eating behavior disturbances. In the food choice task, there were no differences between patients and controls in ventral reward system engagement related to eating. A set of studies (non-imaging) asked participants to make some taste discrimination assessments (i.e., to identify the high-fat and low-fat versions of foods) and these did not find group differences (Schebendach et al., 2014). Two, most of the basic neuroendocrine correlates of appetitive and inhibitory drive for food are as expected in a starved individual. This suggests that the disturbances are in cortical processing, and may not be abnormal at more basic levels. Three, studying how the brain processes food is predicated on an assumption that pleasure is the primary motivator to eat and neglects cognitive or learning influences (e.g., association between food and the feared negative consequence of weight gain).

Having established both common ground and scientific differences, the following key points emerge:

1. First, each scientific approach has validity. Studying tastants serves as a way to elicit brain response to a primary reward reinforcer, and there are ample data from a larger body of work that have shown a range of reward deficits in AN. Performance on high-fat food trials (i.e., tendency to select the trial-unique high-fat food item over the reference item) has been shown repeatedly to correlate with actual calorie and fat intake in a meal, suggesting that while a task is necessarily a simplification of behavior, the approach is well-validated.
2. Second, while one cannot infer habitual behavior based on neural activity, the a priori prediction from the habit model was supported. Yet, avoidance learning and inhibitory processes depend on the same circuitry that is involved in habit formation. Both explanations of the function of the dorsal caudate during food restriction may have merit.
3. Third, the context of the experiment influences the interpretation. Using taste tasks to focus on disturbances in subcortical reward processing in AN limits the evaluation of associated interoceptive and cognitive processes (e.g., learning, inhibitory control, decision making) involved in eating behavior, which are important influences. As discussed, if the choice processes are considered from the lens of avoidance of high-fat foods, alternative hypotheses about the functional role of caudate engagement emerge that are worthy of investigation.

In keeping with the value of healthy debate to advance knowledge rather than change someone's mind (Grant, 2021), the open-minded and rigorous consideration of areas of disagreement does not necessarily lead to consensus. Rather, each program of scientific inquiry is strengthened. For a bottom-up approach, CW notes that the finding that patients with AN have altered decision making that corresponds to greater engagement of habit circuity begins to characterize *how* decision-making is altered. Updated research in the reward deficit model of AN may consider how altered reward processing, including reinforcement learning from rewarding and aversive outcomes, influences reliance on habit when making decisions about what food to eat in AN. For a top-down approach, JS notes that the finding that patients with AN find food less rewarding than their healthy peers is robust. One cannot assume that patients and healthy peers are considering food outcomes similarly, and assessment of restrictive eating—and other symptoms—needs to account for this group difference. Additionally, the role of anxiety in food-based decisions needs to be considered. Thus, updated research in the habit model of food restriction may need to integrate assessment of diminished reward responsiveness and heightened anxiety driving eating in AN.

Examining each of these models in depth—rather than voting to agree or disagree—leads to a rich and diverse characterization of a complex psychiatric disorder. Viewing these alternative perspectives through the lens of discovery and what is yet to be learned yields new questions about how the processes are interrelated. In other words, taste response as a basic biological function (bottom-up) may influence or bias the learning system toward one behavior, like a vulnerability to develop habits quickly, and away from others (like resource-heavy goal-directed behavior). Or perhaps these functions are implicated in AN but to varying degrees in different people, raising the question of whether AN is more heterogeneous than previously thought. As we demonstrated here, we can present scientific discoveries that have emerged from differing approaches and consider how these findings might influence each path forward.

The Handbook is organized in five parts. Part 1 opens the book by providing broad overviews of models, neurobiological systems, and methods relevant to eating disorders. Parts 2 and 3 address brain–behavior relationships in eating disorders from two different perspectives, taking a bottom-up systems-driven perspective in Part 2 and a top-down conceptually driven perspective in Part 3. Here we consider "bottom up" to include basic processes studied in the neuroscience of behavior fields and "top down" to refer to beginning with the manifest symptom and examining the underlying neuroscience. Part 4 brings together research and clinical practice to highlight recent advances in neurobiologically informed treatments. Lastly, Part 5 offers a look forward by introducing some emerging topics with growing empirical evidence and interest in the field.

This book invites discourse and aims to engender curiosity about differences in vantage points, methods, approaches, and interpretations. Our major goal is to provide a comprehensive overview of the interface between theories, clinical observations, and data, with a view to answering the central questions: what are the underlying mechanisms of eating disorders and how can we use this information to develop more effective treatments? To this end, we invite the readers to practice the following directive from Walt Whitman when approaching this Handbook: "Be curious, not judgmental."

References

de Wit, F. R., Greer, L. L., & Jehn, K. A. (2012). The paradox of intragroup conflict: A meta-analysis. *Journal of Applied Psychology, 97*(2), 360–390. https://doi.org/10.1037/a0024844

Foerde, K., Steinglass, J., Shohamy, D., & Walsh, B. (2015). Neural mechanisms supporting maladaptive food choices in anorexia nervosa. *Nature Neuroscience, 18*(11), 1571–1573. https://doi.org/10.1038/nn.4136

Grant, A. (2021). *Think again: The power of knowing what you don't know.* Viking Press.

Ilango, A., Shumake, J., Wetzel, W., & Ohl, F. W. (2014). Contribution of emotional and motivational neurocircuitry to cue-signaled active avoidance learning. *Frontiers in Behavioral Neuroscience, 8*, 372. https://doi.org/10.3389/fnbeh.2014.00372

Kaye, W., Wierenga, C., Bischoff-Grethe, A., Berner, L., Ely, A., Bailer, U., Paulus, M., & Fudge, J. (2020). Neural insensitivity to the effects of hunger in women remitted from anorexia nervosa. *American Journal of Psychiatry, 177*(7), 601–610. https://doi.org/10.1176/appi.ajp.2019.19030261

LeBlanc, K. H., London, T. D., Szczot, I., Bocarsly, M. E., Friend, D. M., Nguyen, K. P., Mengesha, M. M., Rubinstein, M., Alvarez, V. A., & Kravitz, A. V. (2020). Striatopallidal neurons control avoidance behavior in exploratory tasks. *Molecular Psychiatry*, *25*(2), 491–505. https://doi.org/10.1038/s41380-018-0051-3

Rackham, N. (Ed.). (2007). *The behavior of successful negotiators*. McGraw-Hill.

Schebendach, J. E., Klein, D. A., Mayer, L. E., Devlin, M. J., Attia, E., & Walsh, B. T. (2014). Assessment of fat taste in individuals with and without anorexia nervosa. *International Journal of Eating Disorders*, *47*(2), 215–218. https://doi.org/10.1002/eat.22226

PART I
OVERVIEWS

1

Overview of the Classification and Epidemiology of Eating Disorders

B. Timothy Walsh and Hans W. Hoek

Introduction

The two most widely used systems for the classification of eating disorders are (1) the *Diagnostic and Statistical Manual of Mental Disorders, Fifth Edition* (DSM-5) from the American Psychiatric Association, published in 2013 (APA, 2013)—the text was updated in the DSM-5-TR, published in 2022, but only a single, minor change was made to the criteria for one of the eating disorders—and (2) the *International Classification of Diseases, 11th Revision* (ICD-11) from the World Health Organization, officially adopted in 2019 (WHO, 2022). Both the DSM-5 and the ICD-11 recognize six eating disorders: anorexia nervosa, bulimia nervosa, binge-eating disorder, avoidant/restrictive food intake disorder, pica, and rumination disorder. The diagnostic criteria for the disorders in DSM-5 and ICD-11 are almost identical; the few differences are noted in what follows.

State of the Science in Eating Disorders

History

Anorexia nervosa is the earliest-recognized eating disorder. It was well-characterized and named in the 1860s and 1870s by Dr. Charles Lasègue in France, who referred to it as *anorexia hysterique*, and by Sir William Gull in England, who coined the term anorexia nervosa. Anorexia nervosa is briefly referred to in both the DSM-I (1952) and the DSM-II (1968), but as was typical of those editions, no specific diagnostic criteria are provided. The publication of the DSM-III in 1980 represented a major transformation in the approach to psychiatric diagnosis. For over 200 disorders, the DSM-III provided specific criteria and made no assumptions regarding etiology. Four eating disorders were included—anorexia nervosa, bulimia *[sic]*, pica, rumination disorder of infancy—and a residual disorder, atypical eating disorder. Although the DSM-III was developed in parallel with the ICD-9, the latter did not include criteria and, in general, was not as detailed

B. Timothy Walsh and Hans W. Hoek, *Overview of the Classification and Epidemiology of Eating Disorders*.
In: *The Handbook of the Neurobiology of Eating Disorders*. Edited by: Christina E. Wierenga and Joanna E. Steinglass,
Oxford University Press. © Oxford University Press (2025). DOI: 10.1093/9780197675212.003.0002

as the DSM-III. Such concerns extended to other areas of medicine leading to the development of the ICD-9-CM (for clinical modification) in 1979 which included all the DSM-III eating disorder categories.

A significant revision to the DSM-III was published in 1987 (DSM-IIIR) (APA, 1987). The eating disorders remained largely unchanged although the name "bulimia" was replaced by "bulimia nervosa" and the criteria for that disorder required that the individual regularly engaged in inappropriate compensatory behavior, such as self-induced vomiting.

The DSM-IV, published in 1994, made several important changes to the categorization of eating disorders (APA, 1994). First, eating disorders were placed in their own section but included only anorexia nervosa and bulimia nervosa plus a residual category, eating disorder not otherwise specified. Pica and rumination disorder remained in the section on disorders usually first diagnosed in infancy, childhood, or adolescence, and a new disorder, feeding disorder of infancy or early childhood, was added to that section. Second, in the years leading up to the publication of the DSM-IV studies on binge-eating disorder had begun, but the committee overseeing the development of the DSM-IV believed there were insufficient data on the nature of binge-eating disorder to permit its official recognition. Therefore, draft criteria for binge-eating disorder were included in an appendix of the DSM-IV, providing criteria sets for further study. The development of the DSM-IV was closely linked to that of the ICD-10 which was published in 1992, and anorexia nervosa and bulimia nervosa were described similarly in both. Although a text revision of the DSM-IV (DSM-IV-TR) was published in 2000, it made no changes to the diagnostic criteria for eating disorders.

The DSM-5 was published in 2013 and it included a number of important changes both in its broad approach and to the eating disorders section (APA, 2013). The organization of sections was changed with the elimination of the section on "Disorders Usually First Diagnosed in Infancy, Childhood, or Adolescence," but with disorders usually recognized early in life described early in the manual and disorders typically developing late in life at the end. The removal of the section on disorders usually first diagnosed in infancy, childhood, or adolescence led to pica, rumination disorder, and avoidant/restrictive food intake disorder (re-conceptualized from feeding disorder of infancy or early childhood) being included in the section on eating disorders and the name of that section being changed to "Feeding and Eating Disorders." Noting that mental disorders often occur over a spectrum, a number of the disorders included dimensions of severity, including several of the eating disorders. In addition, recognizing the shift to digital technology, this edition of the DSM was signified by an Arabic numeral ("5"), not the traditional Roman numeral ("V"), in hopes that this would afford room for incremental changes (e.g., "5.1"). A text revision was published in 2022 (DSM-5-TR), but it made only a single, small change to the criteria for eating disorders, specifically to those for avoidant/restrictive food intake disorder, as will be discussed.

Strong efforts were made to harmonize the DSM-5 with the ICD-11 (2019) so that the descriptions of eating disorders in both systems are extremely similar and diagnostic agreement is extremely high (Quadflieg et al., 2023).

Anorexia nervosa

As previously noted, the syndrome of anorexia nervosa was clearly described late in the 19th century. The criteria in the subsequent editions of the DSM and the ICD have changed somewhat over time, but the fundamental conceptualization of anorexia nervosa has not. The key features of the diagnostic criteria in the DSM-5 and in the ICD-11 are a restriction of food intake leading to a body weight that is significantly below expected for the individual's developmental stage, an extreme fear of weight gain or persistent behavior that interferes with weight gain, and an overconcern with body shape and weight. Both the DSM-5 and the ICD-11 note two subtypes of anorexia nervosa: the binge eating/purging subtype describes presentations in which the individual, in addition to restricting calorie intake, also engages in frequent episodes of binge eating or purging behavior; the restricting subtype describes presentations in which the individual does not engage in such behaviors.

Anorexia nervosa is associated with numerous physiological disturbances secondary to low body weight, and, historically, amenorrhea was a diagnostic criterion. However, in the development of the DSM-5 criteria, it was noted that the key characteristics of the disorder were occasionally seen among women still reporting menstrual activity and that the requirement for amenorrhea was waived for women on birth control medication or postmenopausal women and for men, leading to the recommendation that this criterion be dropped.

Looking ahead, one of the major questions about the diagnostic criteria for eating disorders relates to what was termed "atypical anorexia nervosa" in the DSM-5. This term was applied to an example in the section on "Other Specified Feeding or Eating Disorders," described as:

> All of the criteria for anorexia nervosa are met, except that despite significant weight loss, the individual's weight is within or above the normal range.

In the last decade, an increasing number of publications on atypical anorexia nervosa have appeared, likely reflecting an increasing number of individuals presenting for care. The current evidence suggests that atypical anorexia nervosa occurs at least as frequently as does "typical" anorexia nervosa (Harrop et al., 2021), and that individuals with atypical anorexia experience the same or even greater levels of concerns regarding shape and weight, similar levels of anxiety and depression, and are at risk for many of the physiological disturbances characteristic of anorexia nervosa (Walsh et al., 2023). However, little information is available about the course, outcome, or treatment response of individuals with atypical anorexia nervosa. These observations raise questions regarding whether the definition of anorexia nervosa in the DSM-5 should be expanded to include what is now termed "atypical anorexia nervosa." Notably, the ICD-11 has subcategories of anorexia nervosa entitled "anorexia nervosa with significantly low body weight," "anorexia nervosa with dangerously low body weight," and "anorexia nervosa in recovery with normal body weight." Perhaps atypical anorexia nervosa could be captured in another subcategory. However, until more information about atypical anorexia becomes available, it may be premature to make such changes.

Bulimia nervosa

The core characteristics of bulimia nervosa, binge eating followed by purging, especially via self-induced vomiting, were described in antiquity in a number of medical texts (Tsagkaris et al., 2022). However, the disorder came to prominence only in the 1960s and 1970s as clinicians specializing in eating disorders began to see an increasing number of young women with the syndrome. In 1979, the British psychiatrist Gerald Russell described a series of 30 patients presenting with recurrent episodes of binge eating and purging, and he labeled the syndrome bulimia nervosa (Russell, 1979). "Bulimia" was included in the DSM-III. The diagnostic criteria required recurrent episodes of binge eating and several additional behavioral characteristics; purging was noted as one of these characteristics but was not required. In the DSM-IV, the criteria were changed in several important ways. A binge was defined on the basis of two features: the consumption of an objectively large amount of food in a discrete period of time and a sense of loss of control during the eating episode. Purging ("inappropriate compensatory behavior") was specifically required. And the binge eating and purging were required to occur at least twice weekly over the previous three months. A single minor change was made in the DSM-5; the frequency criterion was reduced to at least once weekly for the previous three months.

The ICD-11 criteria for bulimia nervosa are virtually identical to those of the DSM-5, with one important exception. Binge episodes are characterized by a sense of loss of control and eating "notably more or differently than usual." The consumption of an objectively large amount of food is not required. It is not yet known whether individuals who meet the ICD-11 criteria differ significantly from those who meet the DSM-5 criteria in clinical or community samples.

Binge-eating disorder

A syndrome of binge eating without subsequent purging associated with obesity was clearly described by the American psychiatrist Albert Stunkard in 1959 (Stunkard, 1959). But it was not until the DSM-IV was under development that criteria were drafted for what was then termed binge-eating disorder. The criteria required recurrent binge eating, defined identically as for bulimia nervosa, at least three indicators of loss of control, and marked distress about the binge eating; binge episodes were required to occur on at least two days, on average, over the previous six months. Although there was interest in formally recognizing what was termed "binge-eating disorder" in the DSM-IV, it was eventually decided that insufficient information was available about the characteristics, complications, course, and outcome, and the criteria were therefore provided in an appendix on "Criteria Sets and Axes Provided for Further Study."

By the time the DSM-5 was under development, about 15 years later, a very large literature, including almost 1,000 papers, had emerged. This literature testified to the high level of interest in binge-eating disorder of clinicians and investigators and described objective disturbances in eating among individuals with binge-eating disorder, association with substantial psychological distress, and responsiveness to a range of specific interventions. On the basis of this literature, binge-eating disorder was officially recognized in the DSM-5. The single change from the draft criteria included in the DSM-IV was a change in the minimum required average frequency of binge episodes to at least once a week over the previous three months, identical to that for bulimia nervosa.

As for bulimia nervosa, the ICD-11 criteria for binge-eating disorder are virtually identical to those of DSM-5, with the important exception that the definition of a binge does not require the consumption of an objectively large amount of food.

Avoidant/restrictive food intake disorder

Two important observations that emerged during the development of the DSM-5 were (1) the DSM-IV category of "feeding disorder of infancy or early childhood" was rarely used by clinicians and was the subject of almost no research, and (2) there was a large group of individuals, mostly young people, who did not have anorexia nervosa but who engaged in persistent and serious patterns of food restriction, a pattern of behavior not captured by any of the DSM-IV categories. For these reasons, feeding disorder of infancy or early childhood was re-characterized as avoidant/restrictive food intake disorder. The criteria for this disorder require persistent avoidance or restriction of food intake associated with weight loss, nutritional deficiency, dependence on nutritional caloric supplements, or with substantial psychosocial impairment. In addition, individuals do not endorse the concerns regarding shape and weight characteristic of anorexia nervosa. This reconceptualization appears to have met a significant need, with almost 500 citations to the disorder in PubMed in the 10 years since the publication of the DSM-5.

The definition of avoidant restrictive food intake disorder in ICD-11 is virtually identical to that in DSM-5.

Pica and rumination disorder

Pica refers to the persistent eating of non-food substances and rumination disorder to the repeated regurgitation of already swallowed food. As noted earlier, these disorders entered the section on "Feeding and Eating Disorders" when the DSM-IV section "Disorders Usually First Diagnosed in Infancy, Childhood, or Adolescence" was eliminated. The only significant change to the criteria in the DSM-5 was to make it clear that, although these disorders often appear in children, they can also be seen among adults. The definitions in the DSM-5 and the ICD-11 are virtually identical.

An Alternative Perspective

Research Domain Criteria (RDoC)

The diagnostic criteria for mental disorders embodied in the DSM-5 and in the ICD-11 provide a "top-down" view of these disorders. They are widely used in practice and in research and have documented clinical utility. Diagnoses can be assigned reliably, greatly facilitating communication among clinicians and between clinicians and patients. Disorders are defined based on current and past signs and symptoms and are distinguished by having different courses, complications, and treatment responses, underscoring their utility. For example, bulimia nervosa is quite responsive to treatment with cognitive behavioral therapy (CBT) and with antidepressants, but anorexia nervosa is not. However, a major problem with the current diagnostic systems is that they have not opened a path to understanding, in any detail, the neurobiology underlying mental disorders. Exactly how a genetic predisposition coupled with environmental, psychological, and physiological stressors leads to the development of a specific disorder, such as binge eating-disorder, is unknown. In fact, it is likely that different individuals with the same DSM-5 disorder have differing underlying psychobiological abnormalities, making the development of biomarkers virtually impossible and severely handicapping the development of new and more effective treatments as has happened in other fields of medicine, such as for cardiovascular disease and cancer.

These concerns prompted the National Institute of Mental Health (NIMH) to propose a "bottom-up" approach—the Research Domain Criteria (RDoC) (Cuthbert & Insel, 2013; Insel et al., 2010). This framework conceptualizes mental disorders as brain disorders, involving abnormalities in neural circuits. It posits that these abnormalities can be identified by examining circuits known to underlie basic behavioral phenomena, such as fear and defense, reward, and working memory. A key goal of the RDoC is to develop measures of these phenomena and to examine them, not in a single disorder, but across individuals with a wide range of presenting symptoms to identify cross-cutting underlying abnormalities.

It is likely that the RDoC proposal has significantly impacted current research on eating disorders. For example, Schaefer and Steinglass (Schaefer & Steinglass, 2021) noted an increase in publications on reward-related processes among individuals with eating disorders and refinements in how the RDoC organizes such constructs. The emerging data point to disturbances in reward learning across the eating disorders, which may also characterize co-morbid conditions such as anxiety and depression. However, as yet, this line of research has not clarified how disturbances in different reward processes may operate during different stages of illness development or what differences and similarities in reward processes characterize eating and related disorders. For example, although deficits in reinforcement learning have been reported in anorexia nervosa, it is not clear how such deficits are related to the core behavioral disturbances of this disorder. To date, RDoC-based research has not led to suggestions to modify the existing DSM-5/ICD-11 classification system.

Epidemiology of Eating Disorders

Epidemiological studies aim to provide estimates of the frequency of disorders at a point or over an interval in time and of the number of new cases appearing in a population or presenting for treatment. The high level of agreement between the DSM-5 and ICD-11 criteria provides a solid foundation for epidemiological studies. However, it is important to note several limitations. First, the frequency of eating disorders in the general population is quite low and many individuals with eating disorders do not seek out care because of shame regarding their condition and/or a lack of recognition of a need for help. These issues make studies of the general population challenging and expensive. An alternate strategy is the use of case registries or studies based on the review of medical records. However, these methods will inevitably yield an underestimate of the actual frequency in the population because a significant number of individuals do not seek care and barriers to accessing care are often considerable. A second challenge to assessing the frequency of eating disorders in the community is that diagnoses are made solely on the basis of interviews, and different interviews (e.g., the Structured Clinical Interview for the DSM, the Eating Disorder Examination) may yield different estimates. Third, changes in estimates of frequencies may not represent true increases, but an increased awareness of eating disorders in the lay and professional communities.

Epidemiological studies assess two critical metrics: (1) the incidence of a disorder, defined as the number of new cases over a specified interval, usually one year. The incidence of eating disorders is typically reported as the number of new cases per 100,000 persons per year (100,000 person-years); (2) the prevalence of a disorder, or the proportion of the population with a disorder at a specific point in time or over an interval of time, akin to a "head count."

The most frequently assessed intervals are over a year and over an individual's lifetime. Information is summarized on incidence and prevalence separately in what follows.

Incidence of anorexia nervosa

Estimates of the incidence of anorexia nervosa vary widely, depending on the population studied (e.g., general population, outpatient clinics), the diagnostic criteria (e.g., ICD-8, ICD-9, DSM-III), and the method of ascertainment (e.g., diagnostic interview, health care records). For many years, incidence rates of anorexia nervosa have been based on detected cases in hospital records and case registers of inpatients and outpatients in mental health care facilities. Although different strategies have been used in these studies, the results suggest an increase in the incidence of anorexia nervosa between 1930 and 1970. Since the 1970s and into the 21st century, the incidence of anorexia nervosa in mental health care facilities in The Netherlands has been stable at around five per 100,000 total population per year (Hoek, 2016). Studies in general practices present incidence rates at the earliest stage of detection within the healthcare system. A long-running study of patients presenting to Dutch primary care doctors has reported a fairly stable incidence of anorexia nervosa, 6.0 to 8.4 per 100,000 person-years between 1985 and 2019 (van Eeden et al., 2023). Although the overall incidence rate of anorexia nervosa is considerably stable, the incidence of anorexia nervosa among 10- to 14-year-old girls increased significantly over four decades. Both biological and sociocultural factors, for example, earlier pubertal timing and most likely the high impact of social media, might explain this (van Eeden et al., 2023).

Recent population-based studies among the high-risk group of adolescent girls and young women (usually around 15 to 25 years) reported rates ranging from 100 up to even 580 per 100,000 person-years. The highest of these was from a study of twins using DSM-5 criteria; it is possible that the somewhat broader criteria of the DSM-5 (versus the DSM-III) and shared genetic and environment risk factors of twins contributed to this relatively high estimate. These population-based estimates are substantially higher than those based on primary care and healthcare facilities, reflecting not only that young females are the high-risk group, but also the well-established fact that only a fraction of individuals with anorexia nervosa receive medical care.

Prevalence of anorexia nervosa

Many studies have measured the lifetime and point prevalence of anorexia nervosa in the general population, especially among young female populations, using a range of assessment instruments, diagnostic criteria, and methods (e.g.,face-to-face interview, paper-and-pencil questionnaire) leading to a relatively wide range of estimated rates. Lifetime prevalence rates range from 0.1% to 3.6% among females and 0% to 0.3% in males. Studies using DSM-5 criteria have generally reported higher prevalence rates, reflecting the somewhat broader criteria than earlier criteria sets. Point prevalence rates using DSM-5 criteria range from 0.2% to 1.3% among females; few point prevalence estimates are available for males but are considerably lower than for females.

The prevalence of anorexia nervosa is very low (< 0.1%) in Africa and Latin America and among Hispanics/Latinos in the United States compared with the rates in Western countries, but also compared to at least some Asian countries, such as China and Japan (Hoek, 2016).

Incidence of bulimia nervosa

Only a few studies have assessed the incidence of bulimia nervosa. A population-based study of Finnish female twins ages 10 to 20 years reported an incidence of 100 cases per 100,000 person-years (Silen et al., 2020). A lower rate (ranging from 20.5 to 22.0 per 100,000 person-years) was found among similarly aged females in a Dutch primary care study, reflecting the small proportion of cases presenting to primary care (Smink et al., 2016). The rates among males are substantially lower. This Dutch primary care study documented a significant decline in the incidence of bulimia nervosa, from 8.7 to 3.2 per 100,000 person-years between 1985 to 1989 and 2015 to 2019 (van Eeden et al., 2023). An English primary care study and a Norwegian study of secondary care reported similar findings (van Eeden et al., 2021). The reasons for this decline are unknown, but it has been speculated that it may be an indirect reflection of the increase in overweight/obesity and a decrease in the social pressure to lose weight (Smink et al., 2016). In a changing weight landscape, where a fuller-figured body is the norm, there might be less pressure to aggressively counteract the effects of binge eating by means of purging. The declining rates of bulimia nervosa over time run parallel to the recognition of binge-eating disorder as a "new" eating disorder diagnosis.

Prevalence of bulimia nervosa

The lifetime prevalence of bulimia nervosa is estimated to be 0.3% to 4.6% among females and 0.1% to 1.3% among males. In self-report studies, point prevalence rates range from 0.5% to 8.7% among females (van Eeden et al., 2021). While anorexia nervosa is a rare disorder in some parts of the world (as previously discussed), bulimia nervosa and, especially, binge-eating disorder appear to be common mental disorders in, for example, Latin America and among Hispanics/Latinos in the United States (Hernandez et al., 2022).

Prevalence of binge-eating disorder

There is virtually no information on the incidence of binge-eating disorder or its change over time. According to the DSM-5, binge-eating disorder is currently estimated to affect 1.5% of women and 0.3% of men worldwide (Keski-Rahkonen, 2021). In adolescence, binge-eating disorder is even more prevalent, but often transient. The estimated point prevalence of binge-eating disorder for young women is 0.6% to 4.1% and for young men 0.2% to 1.2% (Silen & Keski-Rahkonen, 2022).

The prevalence of eating disorders among older persons

Most epidemiological studies on eating disorders are conducted among young females. However, recent studies find that, among older (40 to 80 years) persons, the prevalence rates with full diagnoses of eating disorders based on the DSM-IV or the DSM-5 criteria are between 2.1% and 7.7% for women and less than 1% for men. These studies show that the prevalence of eating disorders decreases by age, but the prevalence rate does note reach zero, even in very old age. What puberty is for eating disorders in adolescence is menopausal transition for midlife. Women who reported substantial menopausal symptoms showed more eating pathology compared to those with low symptoms during menopausal transition (Mangweth-Matzek et al., 2023).

Implications

The two leading systems providing criteria for the diagnosis of eating disorders, the DSM-5 and the ICD-11, describe the same six disorders in very similar terms and, in general, are not controversial. One emerging question is whether what is currently termed "atypical anorexia nervosa" in the DSM-5 should be incorporated into an expanded definition of anorexia nervosa. Although the DSM-5/ICD-11 definitions of eating disorders have clear clinical utility, progress in understanding the underlying pathophysiology is limited and no reliable biomarkers have been developed; these problems characterize the current definitions of virtually all mental disorders. The RDoC has been proposed to encourage the exploration of abnormalities in neural systems that cut across existing diagnoses and has prompted novel investigations of individuals with eating disorders; however, studies so far have not yielded clinically impactful results.

Studies of the epidemiology of eating disorders are challenging for a number of reasons, including the fact that eating disorders are relatively uncommon. The incidence of anorexia nervosa among 10- to 14-year-old girls increased significantly over four decades; this might be explained by earlier pubertal timing and the high impact of social media on young adolescents. The existing data indicate that the overall incidence of anorexia nervosa among the total population appears to be rather stable over the last several decades, while the incidence of bulimia nervosa has declined. Binge-eating disorder is, worldwide, the most common eating disorder.

References

American Psychiatric Association (APA). (1987). *Diagnostic criteria from DSM-III-R.* American Psychiatric Association.

American Psychiatric Association (APA). (1994). *Diagnostic and statistical manual of mental disorders: DSM-IV.* American Psychiatric Association Publishing.

American Psychiatric Association (APA). (2013). *Diagnostic and statistical manual of mental disorders: DSM-5.* American Psychiatric Association Publishing.

Cuthbert, B. N., & Insel, T. R. (2013). Toward the future of psychiatric diagnosis: The seven pillars of RDoC. *BMC Medical Education, 11*, 126. https://doi.org/10.1186/1741-7015-11-126

Harrop, E. N., Mensinger, J. L., Moore, M., & Lindhorst, T. (2021). Restrictive eating disorders in higher weight persons: A systematic review of atypical anorexia nervosa prevalence and consecutive admission literature. *International Journal of Eating Disorders, 54*(8), 1328–1357. https://doi.org/10.1002/eat.23519

Hernandez, J. C., Perez, M., & Hoek, H. W. (2022). Update on the epidemiology and treatment of eating disorders among Hispanic/Latinx Americans in the United States. *Current Opinion in Psychiatry, 35*(6), 379–384. https://doi.org/10.1097/YCO.0000000000000819

Hoek, H. W. (2016). Review of the worldwide epidemiology of eating disorders. *Current Opinion in Psychiatry, 29*(6), 336–339. https://doi.org/10.1097/YCO.0000000000000282

Insel, T., Cuthbert, B., Garvey, M., Heinssen, R., Pine, D. S., Quinn, K., Sanislow, C., & Wang, P. (2010). Research domain criteria (RDoC): Toward a new classification framework for research on mental disorders. *American Journal of Psychiatry, 167*(7), 748–751. https://doi.org/10.1176/appi.ajp.2010.09091379

Keski-Rahkonen, A. (2021). Epidemiology of binge eating disorder: Prevalence, course, comorbidity, and risk factors. *Current Opinion in Psychiatry, 34*(6), 525–531. https://doi.org/10.1097/YCO.0000000000000750

Mangweth-Matzek, B., Kummer, K. K., & Hoek, H. W. (2023). Update on the epidemiology and treatment of eating disorders among older people. *Current Opinion Psychiatry, 36*(6), 405–411. https://doi.org/10.1097/YCO.0000000000000893

Quadflieg, N., Voderholzer, U., Meule, A., & Fichter, M. M. (2023). Comparing ICD-11 and DSM-5 eating disorder diagnoses with the Munich eating and feeding disorder questionnaire (ED-Quest). *International Journal of Eating Disorders, 56*(9), 1826–1831. https://doi.org/10.1002/eat.24010

Russell, G. (1979). Bulimia nervosa: An ominous variant of anorexia nervosa. *Psychological Medicine, 9*(3), 429–448. https://doi.org/10.1017/s0033291700031974

Schaefer, L. M., & Steinglass, J. E. (2021). Reward learning through the lens of RDoC: A review of theory, assessment, and empirical findings in the eating disorders. *Current Psychiatry Reports, 23*(1), 2. https://doi.org/10.1007/s11920-020-01213-9

Silen, Y., & Keski-Rahkonen, A. (2022). Worldwide prevalence of DSM-5 eating disorders among young people. *Current Opinions in Psychiatry, 35*(6), 362–371. https://doi.org/10.1097/YCO.0000000000000818

Silen, Y., Sipila, P. N., Raevuori, A., Mustelin, L., Marttunen, M., Kaprio, J., & Keski-Rahkonen, A. (2020). DSM-5 eating disorders among adolescents and young adults in Finland: A public health concern. *International Journal of Eating Disorders, 53*(5), 520–531. https://doi.org/10.1002/eat.23236

Smink, F. R., van Hoeken, D., Donker, G. A., Susser, E. S., Oldehinkel, A. J., & Hoek, H. W. (2016). Three decades of eating disorders in Dutch primary care: Decreasing incidence of bulimia nervosa but not of anorexia nervosa. *Psychological Medicine, 46*(6), 1189–1196. https://doi.org/10.1017/S003329171500272X

Stunkard, A. J. (1959). Eating patterns and obesity. *Psychiatric Quarterly, 33*, 284–295. https://doi.org/10.1007/BF01575455

Tsagkaris, C., Christopoulos, P., Papadakis, M., & Trompoukis, C. (2022). Anorexia and bulimia in late antiquity and early Byzantine period in the eastern Mediterranean region. *International Journal of Eating Disorders, 55*(5), 637–641. https://doi.org/10.1002/eat.23703

van Eeden, A. E., van Hoeken, D., Hendriksen, J. M. T., & Hoek, H. W. (2023). Increase in incidence of anorexia nervosa among 10- to 14-year-old girls: A nationwide study in the Netherlands over four decades. *International Journal of Eating Disorders, 56*(12), 2295–2303. https://doi.org/10.1002/eat.24064

van Eeden, A. E., van Hoeken, D., & Hoek, H. W. (2021). Incidence, prevalence and mortality of anorexia nervosa and bulimia nervosa. *Current Opinions in Psychiatry, 34*(6), 515–524. https://doi.org/10.1097/yco.0000000000000739

Walsh, B. T., Hagan, K. E., & Lockwood, C. (2023). A systematic review comparing atypical anorexia nervosa and anorexia nervosa. *International Journal of Eating Disorders, 56*(4), 798–820. https://doi.org/10.1002/eat.23856

World Health Organization (WHO) (2022). *International classification of diseases, 11th Revision (ICD-11).* WHO. https://icd.who.int/en

2

Neurobiology of Ingestive Behavior

William M. Howe and Alexandra G. DiFeliceantonio

Introduction

In our evolutionary past, decisions about what foods to consume were largely driven by availability and opportunity. However, in the modern food environment, enriched in readily accessible sources of calories, the decision-making process around what foods to eat is decidedly more complex. Many of these modern foods have been designed to be highly palatable (Demeke et al., 2023; Fazzino et al., 2019, 2024), and research has suggested that repeated exposure to them can allow reward-based ingestive behaviors to override signals of homeostatic need (Saper et al., 2002). These alterations can set the stage for pathological patterns of food choice that increase disease burden and underscore the critical need to more fully understand the neurobiological basis of reward-based ingestive behaviors. Here, we will discuss the interactions between peripheral and central mechanisms that can all modulate brain reward circuits and thereby ingestive behavior.

Biological Framework

Neurobiologists have historically placed emphasis on two major drivers of ingestive behavior. The first concerns satisfying physiological needs. Peripherally generated signals of metabolic, energetic, and nutritive demand determine the direction and voracity of appetitive behavior (Watts et al., 2022). Physiological needs are signaled by circulating hormones like the orexigenic ghrelin, anorexigenic cholecystokinin, insulin-stimulating glucagon-like-peptide 1, and the adipose hormone leptin (Jequier, 2002; Murphy and Bloom, 2006). These hormones act in the periphery, but also have action in the hypothalamus (Geary, 2004; Kanoski et al., 2016), a key brain region for the control of feeding behavior. Studies investigating the modulation of food intake from hypothalamic damage date back to the early 20th century (Brobeck et al., 1943; Tepperman et al., 1943). Recently, studies have further broken-down hypothalamic feeding circuits into molecularly distinct populations that appear to signal hunger and satiety. Those two primary groups are the Agouti-Related Peptide with neuropeptide-Y (AgRP/NPY) and proopiomelanocortin (POMC) expressing neurons, which are heavily expressed in the

William M. Howe and Alexandra G. DiFeliceantonio, *Neurobiology of Ingestive Behavior*. In: *The Handbook of the Neurobiology of Eating Disorders*. Edited by: Christina E. Wierenga and Joanna E. Steinglass, Oxford University Press.
 DOI: 10.1093/9780197675212.003.0003

arcuate nucleus (ARC) of the hypothalamus (Waterson & Horvath, 2015). In general terms, AgRP/NPY neurons facilitate feeding behavior, while POMC neurons inhibit feeding (Gropp et al., 2005). Leptin inhibits AgRP/NPY neurons, but depolarizes POMC neurons, increasing the activity of POMC neurons which decreases feeding behavior (Cowley et al., 2001; Gropp et al., 2005). Conversely, ghrelin activates AgRP/NPY neurons but inhibits POMC neurons and facilitates feeding (Cansell et al., 2012; Cowley et al., 2003; Van Den Top et al., 2004). ARC does not act alone, however, as both groups of neurons project to the lateral hypothalamus (LH) and paraventricular hypothalamus (PVN), and activation of either AgRP/NPY or POMC projections have the same effect as activating the cell types in the ARC (Betley et al., 2013). Importantly, POMC neurons project from ARC to the brainstem nucleus of the tractus solitarius (NTS; Zheng et al., 2010), and AgRP/NPY neurons in the ARC project to midbrain dopamine (DA) cells (Cansell et al., 2012), the parabrachial nucleus (Campos et al., 2016), and LH GABAergic neurons project to the ventral tegmental area (Nieh et al., 2015; Sheng et al., 2014). The interconnected AgRP/NPY and POMC neurons thus comprise a central push-pull control structure that regulates homeostatic feeding (Seely & Berridge, 2015).

It is also clear that the rewarding qualities of foods potently modulate ingestive behavior (Liu & Kanoski, 2018; Saper et al., 2002). Many models of such reward-based eating highlight the subjective value or hedonic "pleasure" associated with the orosensory qualities of a particular food. These values are stored in distributed brain circuits that can both bias future food choices, and, in particular contexts, supersede the role of homeostatic drives (Berridge et al., 2010; Rossi & Stuber, 2018). With respect to the central encoding of taste, there is a long and rich history of the study of individual differences in taste intensity perception. Perhaps the most well-known and well-studied are individual differences in sensitivity to phenylthiocarbamide (PTC) and the similar, 6-n-pro-pylthiouracil (PROP), discovered after a minor lab accident (Fox, 1931, 1932). Substantial individual variation in the capacity to perceive this bitter compound led to the identification of genetic factors that are key mediators (Blakeslee, 1932) of PTC and PROP sensitivity (for review, see Bartoshuk et al., 1994). Many biological explanations for individual differences in taste intensity perception have since focused on changes in peripheral signaling mechanisms, such as the density of fungiform papillae on the tongue (Bartoshuk et al., 1994; Duffy & Bartoshuk, 2000; Feeney & Hayes, 2014; Miller & Reedy, 1990), taste receptor coding, and function (Eny et al., 2010; Fushan et al., 2009; Kim et al., 2003, 2005). This emphasis is also true of diet-induced changes in taste perception, where studies have demonstrated reduced sensitivity of peripheral taste receptor cells (Ahart et al., 2020; Maliphol et al., 2013; May et al., 2019), and even their renewal (Kaufman et al., 2018), after high-fat, high-sugar diets.

Although individual variation in fungiform papillae, receptor distribution, and taste cell function certainly play an important role, they do not explain all the variance in taste perception (for review, see Hayes et al., 2013). Some evidence for the importance of central mechanisms comes from the existence of taste illusions.

Illusions are, by definition, perceptual phenomena and therefore centrally generated. The illusion of thermal taste, where individuals report sweet taste from temperature change alone, has been correlated with an individual's taste sensitivity (Cruz & Green, 2000; Green & George, 2004). Further, damage or anesthesia at the level of the chorda tympani, a branch of the facial nerve that relays information from the tongue, produces taste "phantoms," thought to be due to disinhibition of central circuits that govern taste (Bartoshuk et al., 2005; Yanagisawa et al., 1998).

For taste information to reach the brain from the periphery, it begins in the 7th (facial), 9th (glossopharyngeal), and 10th (vagus) cranial nerves, the afferents of which converge on the NTS of the hindbrain. In primates, afferents of NTS projection neurons go on to innervate the ventral posterior medial nucleus (VPM) of the thalamus. In rodents, this pathway bifurcates at the NTS with one pathway going to the pontine parabrachial nucleus (PBN), which in turn innervates the VPM and another targeting the amygdala and hypothalamus (Scott & Small, 2009). From the thalamus, taste information is relayed to primary gustatory cortex (insula and adjacent operculum), and then on to orbitofrontal cortex (OFC; often named secondary gustatory cortex) and amygdala, as well as back down to the thalamus, striatum, PBN (in rodents), and midbrain (Breslin, 2013; Carleton et al., 2010). Cortical processing of the relay of the sensory qualities of foods is key to taste perception. While there is substantial evidence for the role of the anterior insular cortex and operculum as primary gustatory cortex (Small, 2010; Yamamoto et al., 1980), some debate remains around the nature of the representation of taste. Studies in rodents using modern viral methods for functional circuit characterization have revealed evidence for a gustotopic map in the insula, similar to how other sensory systems, such as vision, are represented (Chen et al., 2011; Wang et al., 2018). In particular, sweet responsive neurons are clustered in the anterior gustatory cortex, whereas bitter responsive cells are concentrated in more posterior regions. Interestingly, these dissociable cortical ensembles have distinct efferent projections to the basolateral and central amygdala, respectively, forming dedicated channels for relaying taste information to limbic structures (Wang et al., 2018), although it should be noted not all studies in rodents find evidence for these topographic maps (Chen et al., 2021; Vincis et al., 2020). High-field (7T) functional magnetic resonance imaging (fMRI) studies have failed to find evidence for such a cleanly dissociable gustotopic map in the human insula, either finding sites of multi-taste representation (Chikazoe et al., 2019) or for population coding (Avery et al., 2020). This could represent species differences or reflect a lack of spatial resolution, as even at high-fields the spatial resolution of the blood oxygenation dependent level (BOLD) signal is orders of magnitude larger than that of calcium imaging. While the translatability of such clearly defined output channels from the insula to the amygdala controlling sweet versus bitter taste identity remains to be seen, it is clear that insula neurons indeed show physiological signatures of major components of taste, including intensity, texture, and temperatures (Rolls, 2020). Human insula is also responsive to breaches of taste expectation (Veldhuizen et al., 2011) and insula activity is blunted when participants expect a weaker bitter taste stimulus

(Nitschke et al., 2006). This indicates the insula must also encode or receive information about the expected taste. Working in concert, this mosaic of feedforward and feedback pathways sets the stage for the enormously variable and plastic nature of taste perception and influence on food intake and eating behavior.

Midbrain dopamine projections as the substrate of food reward

Once a taste perception is generated, how is it attributed with reward value? Midbrain DA neurons of the substantia nigra pars compacta (SNc) and ventral tegmental area (VTA) and their projections to the dorsal striatum and nucleus accumbens, respectively, have been the most heavily studied brain circuits within the neurobiology of reward. While still hotly debated, predominant theories propose that the circuits targeted by these cells support reward by broadcasting prediction-error signals (Mohebi et al., 2019; Montague et al., 1996; Schultz et al., 1997), signal stimulus salience (Kutlu et al., 2021; Robinson & Berridge, 1993; Saunders et al., 2018), or generally motivate reward seeking by representing internal states (Hamid et al., 2016; Howe et al., 2013; Mohebi et al., 2019) to brain areas like the striatum and amygdala. With regard to the domain of food reward specifically, it is known that intact DA function is essential for normal food intake (Palmiter, 2008; Szczypka et al., 2001), and in fact rodents become hypophagic when midbrain DA systems are depleted (Berridge et al., 1989). Diet and obesity also alter DA systems in rodent models (Geiger et al., 2009; Johnson & Kenny, 2010). In humans, it has been reported that expression of dopamine type 2 (D2) receptors is associated with body mass index (BMI) (Volkow et al., 2011). These findings have been inconsistent, however, with other studies finding no relationship between BMI and D2 receptor binding (Karlsson et al., 2015; Pak & Nummenmaa, 2023). Hypothesized reasons for these inconsistencies include a non-linear relationship (Horstmann et al., 2015; Janssen & Horstmann, 2022; van Galen et al., 2021) and differences in the binding properties of the radio-tracer used (Darcey et al., 2023). Despite these lingering inconsistencies, it is clear that midbrain DA systems are a key component of the brain machinery that instantiates and maintains a drive to consume food, but what about food specifically are fluctuations in DA encoding? It is clear that primary tastes evoke changes in striatal DA. Interestingly, sweet tastes increase, while aversive bitter tastes reduce, striatal DA release (McCutcheon et al., 2012; McCutcheon & Roitman, 2019). The latter observation could support the hypothesis that one role of DA in ingestive behavior is the encoding of the valence of the orosensory qualities of food.

Post-ingestive signals modifying food decisions

However, evidence suggests that taste is not the only determinant of food reward, nor is it the only component of ingestive behavior associated with changes in DA release. Studies dating back to the 1940s have also highlighted the importance of energetic density in determining food reward (Adolph, 1947). Major support for this idea comes from studies testing the reinforcing capacity of intra-gastric infusions of nutritive solutions, which bypass taste and olfactory inputs. Consistently, rats and mice will learn new behaviors to receive intragastric infusions of caloric solutions (Holman, 1969; Sclafani, 2006; Sclafani & Ackroff, 2006), and come to prefer flavors associated with intragastric infusions of calories over vehicle or caloric infusions adulterated with compounds to block their metabolism (de Araujo et al., 2020; Han, Tellez, Perkins, Perez, et al., 2018; Han, Tellez, Perkins, Shammah-Lagnado, et al., 2018; Tellez, Medina, et al., 2013). Furthermore, mice that lack the cellular mechanisms to transduce sweet taste (trmp5-/- mice) still show a robust preference for glucose-paired flavors (de Araujo et al., 2008). These findings demonstrate that these post-ingestive signals are important for the reinforcing properties of foods, and importantly, can both act independently and interact with perceptions of taste. Studies in humans also lend support for the idea that caloric density of foods can represent a major driver of food choice. Tang and colleagues (2014) conducted a study assessing the amount of money subjects were willing to pay for various food items and found that subjects' willingness to pay for foods was strongly correlated with the actual caloric density of the food items. Somewhat surprisingly, they found that subjects were not accurate in estimating the actual caloric density of the foods they bid on, and there was no relationship between their estimates of caloric density and their willingness to pay. Thus, the caloric density of food contributes to its subjective value, and this valuation appears to occur independently of explicit knowledge of caloric density. If true, post-ingestive signals of caloric density must somehow interact with brain circuits involved in the reward learning and value assignment.

Activity in the striatum is central to all theories of the neurobiological basis of reward and motivation, including for food. The striatum is the major target of midbrain DA systems and both human and animal studies have demonstrated that striatal "reward" systems are engaged by the intake of highly palatable foods (e.g., chocolate; Small, Zatorre, Dagher, et al., 2001), as well as the presentation of cues that have been associated with foods (Small et al., 2008). Accordingly, Tang and colleagues (2014) found that striatal activation to food cues also correlated with reported willingness to pay. Together, the available data support the possibility that post-ingestive signals of caloric density may modulate activity in striatal circuits to influence food reward. However, a recent study suggested that caloric density alone is not sufficient to explain the post-ingestive contribution to food reward (DiFeliceantonio et al., 2018). In this study, healthy participants were again presented with pictures of familiar foods and, similar to Tang and colleagues (2014), were asked to estimate caloric density and report their willingness to pay for each. However, whereas the food stimuli used in the Tang and colleagues' study varied in caloric content (low to high), in DiFeliceantonio and colleagues' study (2018) the food stimuli were grouped based on their macronutrient content (carbohydrates, fats, or combinations of the two), while caloric content was matched across macronutrient groups. Importantly, the foods in each macronutrient group were rated as equally pleasant, thereby controlling for potential differences in hedonic qualities. If caloric density determines food value, then subjects should have been willing to pay the same amount for foods regardless of their macronutrient makeup. However, subjects were consistently willing to pay more for foods made of fat and carbohydrate combinations than fats or carbs alone. Strikingly, this increased willingness to pay also correlated with neural activity in the caudate (dorsal striatum in rodents) but not the nucleus accumbens, as measured by fMRI. These data suggest that the macronutrient content of foods also exerts influence on food reward, and foods made of combinations of carbohydrates and fats, capable of recruiting both gut-to-midbrain pathways described above, are more reinforcing calorie for calorie than foods made of only one macronutrient.

Post-ingestive signals reach the midbrain and drive food reward

Although differential encoding in the caudate of the value of combination foods was demonstrated, fMRI can provide no information regarding the neurochemical source of that change in signal. Using modern recording techniques and viral methods, recent studies identified separable pathways that link signals generated in the gut by different macronutrients in food to midbrain dopamine cells, the source of dopamine in both the striatum as well as limbic structures like the amygdala (Small & DiFeliceantonio, 2019). Post-ingestive signals generated by intra-gastric delivery of fats recruit a pathway that is dependent on a proliferator-activated receptor α (PPAR-α) specific vagal activation, through right nodose ganglion, to hindbrain, to the midbrain (Han, Tellez, Perkins, Perez, et al., 2018). Activation of this pathway is sufficient to increase extracellular dopamine concentration in the striatum and support reward learning, supporting the notion of a generally excitatory effect of these signals on dopamine output neurons (Grove et al., 2022; Han, Tellez, Perkins, Perez, et al., 2018; Tellez, Medina, et al., 2013).

Information about carbohydrate availability appears to follow a different route from the periphery to the brain and is perhaps more complex. Generally, infusions directly into the stomach decrease AgRP neuronal activity in the hypothalamus, just as food does, as previously discussed (Goldstein et al., 2021). Vagotomy, severing the vagus, does not diminish the effect of intra-gastric nutrients to decrease AgRP neuron activity, indicating the vagus may not be a crucial pathway in signaling carbohydrates availability in the gut to the brain. Instead, a branch of the spinal nerve called the splanchnic nerve and its connections to the hepatic portal vein are necessary for hypothalamic and AgRP neuron response to intragastric glucose (Goldstein et al., 2021; Schmitt, 1973). In contrast to these findings, nutrient sensing studies that focus on brain dopamine as the central target of peripheral signaling have found conflicting results. The ability of intra-gastric sucrose to rapidly increase the firing of ventral tegmental area dopamine neurons appears to be vagally dependent (Fernandes et al., 2020). Accordingly, enteroendocrine cells ("neuropods") have been found to synapse onto the vagus and transduce nutrient information, including glucose (Kaelberer et al., 2018). The major central target of the vagus, the NTS, is responsive to intra-intestinal glucose infusions (but not non-nutritive sweeteners) (Tan et al., 2020). These findings seem to indicate the vagus is needed for peripheral nutrients to impact brain dopamine. In contrast, other studies have pointed to the hepatic portal vein as essential for mediating the rise in dorsal striatal dopamine, similar to what has been found to mediate AgRP neuron activity (Zhang et al., 2018). Identifying the exact signal for glucose reinforcement is further complicated by the fact that dopamine efflux in the striatum in response to intra-gastric glucose is dependent on glucose utilization and is therefore disrupted by infusion of 2-deoxy-D-glucose (2-DG) (Tellez, Ren, et al., 2013), adding another vagally independent signal with an unknown pathway to the brain.

The exact circuitry for relaying carbohydrate information to various brain sites remains unclear, but critically, these post-ingestive signals are able to change behavior. Experiments examining the role of post-ingestive signals on behavior often use a form of learning called flavor nutrient learning or conditioning (Sclafani, 1990). In this form of Pavlovian conditioning, instead of an external stimulus, such as a light or tone, acting as the conditional stimulus (CS) and food receipt acting as the unconditioned stimulus (US), the taste and olfactory sensation of a novel flavor is the CS and the post-ingestive consequences act as the US. This leads to an increase in consumption of the flavor, referred to as enhanced appetition, in contrast to satiating post-ingestive effects (Sclafani, 2013). Using these paradigms, infusions of carbohydrate or fat directly into the gut have been shown to change flavor preference (Lucas & Sclafani, 1989; Sclafani, 1988; Sclafani & Nissenbaum, 1988) and it has been hypothesized this process underlies a vast array of food and flavor preferences (Myers, 2018). These studies can also be used to help test potential mechanisms for carbohydrate reinforcement. For example, it is thought the sodium glucose co-transporter (SGLT-1) on the brush border membrane of the intestine is essential for the reinforcing properties of glucose. Evidence for this is alpha-methyl-D-glucopyranoside (MDG), which is transported by SGLT-1 but not metabolizable, is sufficient to condition a preference over non-nutritive sweeteners, such as saccharin (Zukerman et al., 2013) and acesulfame potassium (AceK) (Tan et al., 2020). However, activation of SGLT-1 is not sufficient as MDG does not condition a flavor preference over glucose, which both activates the SGLT-1 and is, of course, metabolized (Zhang et al., 2018). The uncertain involvement of the vagus in carbohydrate signaling is further complicated by studies demonstrating vagatomy (severing or damaging the vagus) leaves flavor nutrient learning to glucose intact (Qu et al., 2019; Sclafani & Lucas, 1996). Taken together, these studies indicate that nutrients in the gut can rapidly change brain activity and nutrient metabolism can influence both brain activity and food preference. However, there is still much work to be done to fully elucidate the mechanisms by which carbohydrate signals are conveyed to the brain to change behavior.

Using the flavor nutrient conditioning paradigm previously described, de Araujo and colleagues (de Araujo et al., 2013) reported increased rated liking to a novel flavor paired with a carbohydrate load in a sweetened beverage in humans. Further, they demonstrated that plasma glucose previously evoked by that flavor correlated with nucleus accumbens and hypothalamic activity in response to the flavor cue (this time containing no calories; i.e., tested in extinction). A later study replicated these findings and collected measures of metabolism using indirect calorimetry (Veldhuizen et al., 2017). This technique measures oxygen and carbon dioxide and applies the modified Weir's equation to calculate heat output (Weir, 1949) as a measure of metabolic rate. Specifically, they measured the increase in energy expenditure in response to a caloric load known as the thermic effect of food. Importantly, brain response in the nucleus accumbens to the carbohydrate-paired flavor was correlated with change in energy expenditure to that flavor. This provided evidence that glucose metabolism was important for brain response to food cues, confirming evidence from animals discussed previously. This demonstrates that in humans, these post-ingestive consequences are relayed to the brain, driving changes in neural activity, and changing food preference.

It is clear both homeostatic mechanisms and reward systems drive food intake. Given the nature of our modern food environment, with its abundance of calorically dense, extremely palatable foods, an understanding of the neurobiology of reward is essential for understanding human eating behavior. Much of our understanding of basic reward mechanisms is based on palatable food intake, normally sugar. As such we have a good understanding of how taste interacts with primary reward systems, including midbrain dopamine nuclei to encode reward and increase motivation. Emerging evidence points to additional post-ingestive mechanisms as being an important and understudied factor driving intake, especially in our modern food environment (see Figure 2.1). Next steps for the field in general are to integrate these two systems into a larger theoretical framework of food reward.

Alternative Perspectives

The role of the amygdala in taste perception and food reward

While substantial research has focused on the meso-striatal dopamine systems in mediating food reward, there is emerging and compelling evidence that the amygdala is supremely positioned to play a role in taste reward and food choice. Anatomical evidence is derived from its strong reciprocal connections with primary gustatory cortex, as previously noted (Wang et al., 2018). However, amygdala nuclei also receive direct input from the gustatory thalamus (Krettek & Price, 1977; Ottersen & Ben-Ari, 1979), and hindbrain gustatory relays (Norgren, 1976). There is also strong functional evidence, collected from patients with epilepsy

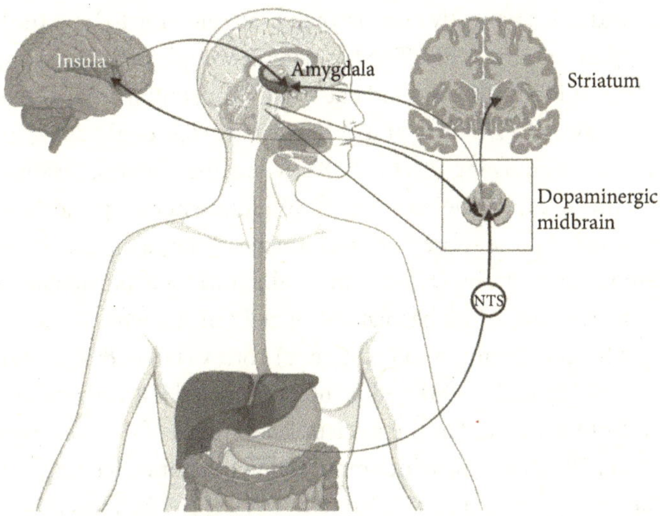

Figure 2.1 Taste and post-ingestive reward circuitries. Taste information travels from the tongue to the nucleus of the solitary track (NTS), to the ventral posterior nucleus of the thalamus, which in turns relays taste information to the gustatory cortex (insula). Gustatory cortex shares reciprocal connections with the amygdala, where tastes may be assigned with value in conjunction with ascending dopaminergic inputs. Post-ingestive signals are generated by nutrient sensors in the gut, which recruit an ascending pathway to the NTS via the vagus nerve. Vagal recipient NTS neurons in turn relay this nutrient information to midbrain dopamine cell bodies, enabling the modification of striatal DA release and associated reward computations. Created with BioRender.com

where structures within the temporal lobe are often targeted for surgical ablation. Specifically, in patients treated with surgical resections that included the amygdala, sour taste detection thresholds (increased sensitivity) were reduced (Small et al., 1997). These patients also reported stronger intensity of suprathreshold taste stimuli (Small, Zatorre, & Jones-Gotman, 2001a, 2001b). More recent studies have further supported a major role for the amygdala in taste perception, including that by Veldhuizen and colleagues (2020). Using fMRI of healthy participants concomitant with delivery of primary tastes whose intensity had been previously rated, this study revealed a strong association between taste intensity ratings of all tastes and amygdala activity as measured by the BOLD response. Further, the authors used effective connectivity to identify the VPM and mediodorsal (md) thalamus as key nodes modulated by the amygdala correlated with taste intensity perception.

While these studies provide evidence of the amygdala as a central modulator of taste perception, important questions remain unanswered. In the study by Veldhuizen and colleagues (2020), the authors present the peak BOLD response in the central nucleus of the amygdala (CEN); however, voxel size, normalization, and smoothing kernels can all distort the location of the functional signal.

The term "amygdala" is typically used as a catch-all referring to both the basolateral amygdala complex and the CEN. The basolateral complex has been implicated in neural encoding of food reward, food cue evaluation, and primary taste signaling (Holland et al., 2002; O'Doherty et al., 2002; Petrovich et al., 2002; Small et al., 2008; Sun et al., 2015; Wang et al., 2018). It includes lateral, basolateral, basomedial, and ventral sub nuclei composed of glutamatergic projection cells and interneurons. Each of these subregions is characterized by a unique pattern of efferent and afferent connections (Hintiryan et al., 2021). Of particular importance for gustatory processing is the basolateral nuclei (BLA), which is a major site of sensory inputs from thalamus and (gustatory) cortex (Janak & Tye, 2015; Krettek & Price, 1977; McDonald, 1998) and is interconnected with secondary gustatory cortex (orbitofrontal), as well as the nucleus accumbens of the mesolimbic system (Hintiryan et al., 2021), and provides input to hypothalamic feeding areas (lateral, ventromedial; Hintiryan et al., 2021; Krettek & Price, 1977). The CEN, in contrast, has been hypothesized to bind affective states with external stimuli (Balleine & Killcross, 2006), and is composed of a group of tightly packed GABAergic projection neurons. It is a major target of basal complex afferents, receives direct input from the gustatory thalamus, and in turn provides inhibitory input to a host of brain regions that might modulate taste perception including the basal forebrain, bed nucleus of the stria terminalis, lateral hypothalamus, midline thalamic nuclei, serotonin, dopamine, and norepinephine projection neurons of the midbrain and brainstem, as well as primary gustatory neurons of the NTS (Beckstead et al., 1980; Price & Amaral, 1981; Ricardo & Tongju Koh, 1978).

Straddling the border of the BLA and CEN is a band of intercalated GABAergic cells that provide inhibitory control over the interaction between the two major amygdala subdivisions (Ehrlich et al., 2009; Janak & Tye, 2015; Marowsky et al., 2005). Furthermore, BLA and CEN amygdala subregions have been shown to have dissociable roles in food reward behaviors (Balleine & Killcross, 2006; Corbit & Balleine, 2005; Janak & Tye, 2015; Wassum & Izquierdo, 2015). While research supports the hypothesis that the amygdala plays a major role in taste intensity perception, the unique information signaled by each subregion is unclear.

In discussing reward processes driving food intake, it is important to acknowledge the role ascending monoamine systems play in reward in general, as well as food reward. Dopamine is essential for learning and motivation (Berridge et al., 1989, 2009; Schultz et al., 1997). The role of serotonin in reward-guided appetitive behavior is much less clear, although emerging evidence suggests that serotonin and dopamine signals are opponent (Bang et al., 2020). Indeed, whereas dopamine is the canonical molecule signaling motivated pursuit of a primary food reward, serotonin may inhibit such appetitive drives (van Galen et al., 2021). The role of norepinephrine in food reward is even less clear. Noradrenergic tone does appear to modulate taste sensitivity (Heath et al., 2006), and recent studies indicated that ascending noradrenergic projections potently modulate the recall of learned taste aversions (Fukabori et al., 2020). Taken together, it seems reasonable to postulate a role for norepinephrine in central representations of food palatability although further work on this subject specifically is needed.

The amygdala receives dense projections from all ascending monoamine systems (Rainnie, 1999; Sengupta et al., 2017; Tang et al., 2020; Tully et al., 2007), positioning them to play a critical role in modulating amygdala physiology (Rainnie, 1999; Sengupta et al., 2017; Tang et al., 2020; Tully et al., 2007). Serotonergic fibers from the dorsal raphe innervate the BLA and CEN (Sadikot & Parent, 1990; Steinbusch, 1981), and serotonin release has been shown to inhibit sensory inputs into BLA via activation of local interneurons (Stutzmann et al., 1998; Stutzmann & LeDoux, 1999). Furthermore, there are relatively higher levels of inhibitory 5HT1A receptors in CEN compared to BLA, which itself appears to have a higher density of excitatory 5HT2 and 5HT3 receptors (Rainnie, 1999). Norepinephrine inputs from the locus coeruleus innervate both BLA and the CEN, although cross species data suggest that the densest input is directed to the CEN (Bowden et al., 1978; Swanson & Hartman, 1975). Norepinephrine effects on amygdala activity have been best characterized in the BLA, where it appears to have a net inhibitory effect (Buffalari & Grace, 2007). However more recent studies suggest that stimulation of locus coeruleus (norepinephrine source region) inputs to BLA can lead to a multitude of effects based on the presence of both excitatory beta adrenergic and inhibitory alpha2-adrenergic receptors expressed throughout the amygdala (Buffalari & Grace, 2007; McCall et al., 2017). There is dense dopaminergic input to CEN, BLA, and the intercalated cells ("transition zone"; Ehrlich et al., 2009; Marowsky et al., 2005; Sadikot & Parent, 1990). The impact of dopamine on amygdala activity is similarly complex, as it can act as both excitatory and inhibitory depending on the cell type (Rosenkranz & Grace, 1999, 2002). Cells in the BLA fire in a manner that is compatible with reinforcement learning models (a major hypothesized function of dopamine more globally in the brain); furthermore, these inputs are recruited in response to food rewards (Grove et al., 2022). Taken together with the general roles for ascending monoamine systems and the connectivity of the amygdala described above, it is clear that both the representation of the primary sensory qualities, as well as the learned values of foods and associated cues are relayed via the amygdala. Once there, these input signals are differentially modulated by local monoamine to shape output and can thereby potently affect multiple aspects of ingestive behavior.

Implications

Whereas neurobiologists interested in uncovering the circuitry supporting ingestive behavior historically focused on signals of homeostatic drive or reward, modern research has begun to paint a much more complex picture of the forces shaping food choice. Peripheral signals of nutrient need, food content, and taste perception and valuation are blended with learned associations of internal and external cues. These computations are distributed across expansive neural networks, including the insula, midbrain, striatum, and amygdala, containing feedforward and feedback loops modified by ever-shifting states of neurochemical modulation. Future research into the neurobiology of food intake will identify these key nodes and networks that integrate these signals. We suggest that the amygdala, which sits at the interface of canonical reward learning, gustatory, and post-ingestive input systems represents such a node. Furthermore, understanding the unique roles ascending systems like the monoamines, which possess the unique capacity to orchestrate activity across these circuits, will be key to uncovering the neurobiological basis of both adaptive and pathological eating behaviors.

References

Adolph, E. F. (1947). Urges to eat and drink in rats. *American Journal of Physiology, 151*(1), 110–125. https://doi.org/10.1152/ajplegacy.1947.151.1.110

Ahart, Z. C., Martin, L. E., Kemp, B. R., Dutta Banik, D., Roberts, S. G. E., Torregrossa, A.-M., & Medler, K. F. (2020). Differential effects of diet and weight on taste responses in diet-induced obese mice. *Obesity, 28*(2), 284–292. https://doi.org/10.1002/oby.22684

Avery, J. A., Liu, A. G., Ingeholm, J. E., Riddell, C. D., Gotts, S. J., & Martin, A. (2020). Taste quality representation in the human brain. *Journal of Neuroscience, 40*(5), 1042–1052. https://doi.org/10.1523/JNEUROSCI.1751-19.2019

Balleine, B. W., & Killcross, S. (2006). Parallel incentive processing: An integrated view of amygdala function. *Trends in Neurosciences, 29*(5), 272–279. https://doi.org/10.1016/j.tins.2006.03.002

Bang, D., Kishida, K. T., Lohrenz, T., White, J. P., Laxton, A. W., Tatter, S. B., Fleming, S. M., & Montague, P. R. (2020). Sub-second dopamine and serotonin signaling in human striatum during perceptual decision-making. *Neuron, 108*(5), 999–1010.e6. https://doi.org/10.1016/j.neuron.2020.09.015

Bartoshuk, L. M., Duffy, V. B., & Miller, I. J. (1994). PTC/PROP tasting: Anatomy, psychophysics, and sex effects. *Physiology & Behavior, 56*(6), 1165–1171. https://doi.org/10.1016/0031-9384(94)90361-1

Bartoshuk, L. M., Snyder, D. J., Grushka, M., Berger, A. M., Duffy, V. B., & Kveton, J. F. (2005). Taste damage: Previously unsuspected consequences. *Chemical Senses, 30*(suppl_1), i218–i219. https://doi.org/10.1093/chemse/bjh192

Beckstead, R. M., Morse, J. R., & Norgren, R. (1980). The nucleus of the solitary tract in the monkey: Projections to the thalamus and brain stem nuclei. *Journal of Comparative Neurology, 190*(2), 259–282. https://doi.org/10.1002/cne.901900205

Berridge, K. C., Ho, C.-Y., Richard, J. M., & Difeliceantonio, A. G. (2010). The tempted brain eats: Pleasure and desire circuits in obesity and eating disorders. *Brain Research, 1350*, 43–64. https://doi.org/10.1016/j.brainres.2010.04.003

Berridge, K. C., Robinson, T. E., & Aldridge, J. W. (2009). Dissecting components of reward: "Liking," "wanting," and learning. *Current Opinion in Pharmacology, 9*(1), 65–73. https://doi.org/10.1016/j.coph.2008.12.014

Berridge, K. C., Venier, I. L., & Robinson, T. E. (1989). Taste reactivity analysis of 6-hydroxydopamine-induced aphagia: Implications for arousal and anhedonia hypotheses of dopamine function. *Behavioral Neuroscience, 103*(1), 36–45. https://doi.org/10.1037//0735-7044.103.1.36

Betley, J. N., Cao, Z. F. H., Ritola, K. D., & Sternson, S. M. (2013). Parallel, redundant circuit organization for homeostatic control of feeding behavior. *Cell*, 155(6), 1337–1350. https://doi.org/10.1016/J.CELL.2013.11.002

Blakeslee, A. F. (1932). Genetics of sensory thresholds: Taste for phenyl thio carbamide. *Proceedings of the National Academy of Sciences of the United States of America, 18*(1), 120–130.

Bowden, D. M., German, D. C., & Douglas Poynter, W. (1978). An autoradiographic, semistereotaxic mapping of major projections from locus coeruleus and adjacent nuclei in Macaca mulatta. *Brain Research, 145*(2), 257–276. https://doi.org/10.1016/0006-8993(78)90861-2

Breslin, P. A. S. (2013). An evolutionary perspective on food and human taste. *Current Biology, 23*(9), R409–R418. https://doi.org/10.1016/j.cub.2013.04.010
Brobeck, J. R., Tepperman, J., & Long, C. N. H. (1943). Experimental hypothalamic hyperphagia in the albino rat. *Yale Journal of Biology and Medicine, 15*(6), 831.
Buffalari, D. M., & Grace, A. A. (2007). Noradrenergic modulation of basolateral amygdala neuronal activity: Opposing influences of alpha-2 and beta receptor activation. *Journal of Neuroscience, 27*(45), 12358–12366. https://doi.org/10.1523/JNEUROSCI.2007-07.2007
Campos, C. A., Bowen, A. J., Schwartz, M. W., & Palmiter, R. D. (2016). Parabrachial CGRP neurons control meal termination. *Cell Metabolism 23*(5), 811–820. https://doi.org/10.1016/J.CMET.2016.04.006
Cansell, C., Denis, R. G. P., Joly-Amado, A., Castel, J., & Luquet, S. (2012). Arcuate AgRP neurons and the regulation of energy balance. *Frontiers in Endocrinology (Lausanne), 3*(3), 169. https://doi.org/10.3389/FENDO.2012.00169/BIBTEX
Carleton, A., Accolla, R., & Simon, S. A. (2010). Coding in the mammalian gustatory system. *Trends in Neurosciences, 33*(7), 326–334. https://doi.org/10.1016/j.tins.2010.04.002
Chen, K., Kogan, J. F., & Fontanini, A. (2021). Spatially distributed representation of taste quality in the gustatory insular cortex of behaving mice. *Current Biology, 31*(2), 247–256.e4. https://doi.org/10.1016/j.cub.2020.10.014
Chen, X., Gabito, M., Peng, Y., Ryba, N. J. P., & Zuker, C. S. (2011). A gustotopic map of taste qualities in the mammalian brain. *Science, 333*(6047), 1262–1266. https://doi.org/10.1126/science.1204076
Chikazoe, J., Lee, D. H., Kriegeskorte, N., & Anderson, A. K. (2019). Distinct representations of basic taste qualities in human gustatory cortex. *Nature Communications, 10*(1), article 1. https://doi.org/10.1038/s41467-019-08857-z
Corbit, L. H., & Balleine, B. W. (2005). Double dissociation of basolateral and central amygdala lesions on the general and outcome-specific forms of Pavlovian-instrumental transfer. *Journal of Neuroscience, 25*(4), 962–970. https://doi.org/10.1523/JNEUROSCI.4507-04.2005
Cowley, M. A., Smart, J. L., Rubinstein, M., Cerdán, M. G., Diano, S., Horvath, T. L., Cone, R. D., & Low, M. J. (2001). Leptin activates anorexigenic POMC neurons through a neural network in the arcuate nucleus. *Nature, 411*(6836), 480–484. https://doi.org/10.1038/35078085
Cowley, M. A., Smith, R. G., Diano, S., Tschöp, M., Pronchuk, N., Grove, K. L., Strasburger, C. J., Bidlingmaier, M., Esterman, M., Heiman, M. L., Garcia-Segura, L. M., Nillni, E. A., Mendez, P., Low, M. J., Sotonyi, P., Friedman, J. M., Liu, H., Pinto, S., Colmers, W. F., Cone, R. D., . . . Horvath, T. L. (2003). The distribution and mechanism of action of ghrelin in the CNS demonstrates a novel hypothalamic circuit regulating energy homeostasis. *Neuron, 37*(4), 649–661. https://doi.org/10.1016/S0896-6273(03)00063-1
Cruz, A., & Green, B. G. (2000). Thermal stimulation of taste. *Nature, 403*(6772), 889–892. https://doi.org/10.1038/35002581
Darcey VL, Guo J, Chi M, Chung ST, Courville AB, Gallagher, I., Herscovitch, P., Howard, R., LaNoire, M., Milley, L., Schick, A., Stagliano, M., Turner, S., Urbanski, N., Yang, S., Yim, E., Zhai, N., Zhou, M. S., & Hall, K. D. (2023). Striatal dopamine tone is positively associated with body mass index in humans as determined by PET using dual dopamine type-2 receptor antagonist tracer. *medRxiv*. Preprint. https://doi.org/10.1101/2023.09.27.23296169
de Araujo, I. E., Lin, T., Veldhuizen, M. G., & Small, D. M. (2013). Metabolic regulation of brain response to food cues. *Current Biology, 23*(10), 878–883. https://doi.org/10.1016/j.cub.2013.04.001
de Araujo, I. E., Oliveira-Maia, A. J., Sotnikova, T. D., Gainetdinov, R. R., Caron, M. G., Nicolelis, M. A. L., & Simon, S. A. (2008). Food reward in the absence of taste receptor signaling. *Neuron, 57*(6), 930–941. https://doi.org/10.1016/j.neuron.2008.01.032
de Araujo, I. E., Schatzker, M., & Small, D. M. (2020). Rethinking food reward. *Annual Review of Psychology, 71*(1), 139–164. https://doi.org/10.1146/annurev-psych-122216-011643
Demeke, S., Rohde, K., Chollet-Hinton, L., Sutton, C., Kong, K. L., & Fazzino, T. L. (2023). Change in hyper-palatable food availability in the US food system over 30 years: 1988–2018. *Public Health Nutrition, 26*(1), 182–189. https://doi.org/10.1017/S1368980022001227
DiFeliceantonio, A. G., Coppin, G., Rigoux, L., Edwin Thanarajah, S., Dagher, A., Tittgemeyer, M., & Small, D. M. (2018). Supra-additive effects of combining fat and carbohydrate on food reward. *Cell Metabolism, 28*(1), 33–44.e3. https://doi.org/10.1016/j.cmet.2018.05.018
Duffy, V. B., & Bartoshuk, L. M. (2000). Food acceptance and genetic variation in taste. *Journal of the American Dietetic Association, 100*(6), 647–655. https://doi.org/10.1016/S0002-8223(00)00191-7
Ehrlich, I., Humeau, Y., Grenier, F., Ciocchi, S., Herry, C., & Lüthi, A. (2009). Amygdala inhibitory circuits and the control of fear memory. *Neuron, 62*(6), 757–771. https://doi.org/10.1016/j.neuron.2009.05.026

Eny, K. M., Wolever, T. M., Corey, P. N., & El-Sohemy, A. (2010). Genetic variation in TAS1R2 (Ile191Val) is associated with consumption of sugars in overweight and obese individuals in 2 distinct populations. *American Journal of Clinical Nutrition, 92*(6), 1501–1510. https://doi.org/10.3945/ajcn.2010.29836

Fazzino, T. L., Jun, D., Chollet-Hinton, L., & Bjorlie, K. (2024). US tobacco companies selectively disseminated hyper-palatable foods into the US food system: Empirical evidence and current implications. *Addiction (Abingdon, England), 119*(1), 62–71. https://doi.org/10.1111/add.16332

Fazzino, T. L., Rohde, K., & Sullivan, D. K. (2019). Hyper-palatable foods: development of a quantitative definition and application to the US food system database. *Obesity, 27*(11), 1761–1768. https://doi.org/10.1002/oby.22639

Feeney, E. L., & Hayes, J. E. (2014). Regional differences in suprathreshold intensity for bitter and umami stimuli. *Chemosensory Perception, 7*(3–4), 147–157. https://doi.org/10.1007/s12078-014-9166-3

Fernandes, A. B., Alves da Silva, J., Almeida, J., Cui, G., Gerfen, C. R., Costa, R. M., & Oliveira-Maia, A. J. (2020). Postingestive modulation of food seeking depends on vagus-mediated dopamine neuron activity. *Neuron, 106*(5), 778–788.e6. https://doi.org/10.1016/j.neuron.2020.03.009

Fox, A. L. (1931). Six in ten "tasteblind" to bitter chemical. *Science News-Letter, 9*, 249.

Fox, A. L. (1932). The relationship between chemical constitution and taste. *Proceedings of the National Academy of Sciences of the United States of America, 18*(1), 115–120.

Fukabori, R., Iguchi, Y., Kato, S., Takahashi, K., Eifuku, S., Tsuji, S., Hazama, A., Uchigashima, M., Watanabe, M., Mizuma, H., Cui, Y., Onoe, H., Hikishima, K., Yasoshima, Y., Osanai, M., Inagaki, R., Fukunaga, K., Nishijo, T., Momiyama, T., . . .Kobayashi, K. (2020). Enhanced retrieval of taste associative memory by chemogenetic activation of locus coeruleus norepinephrine neurons. *Journal of Neuroscience, 40*(43), 8367–8385. https://doi.org/10.1523/JNEUROSCI.1720-20.2020

Fushan, A. A., Simons, C. T., Slack, J. P., Manichaikul, A., & Drayna, D. (2009). Allelic polymorphism within the TAS1R3 promoter is associated with human taste sensitivity to sucrose. *Current Biology, 19*(15), 1288–1293. https://doi.org/10.1016/j.cub.2009.06.015

Geary N. (2004). Endocrine controls of eating: CCK, leptin, and ghrelin. *Physiology & Behavior, 81*(5), 719–733. https://doi.org/10.1016/J.PHYSBEH.2004.04.013

Geiger, B. M., Haburcak, M., Avena, N. M., Moyer, M. C., Hoebel, B. G., & Pothos, E. N. (2009). Deficits of mesolimbic dopamine neurotransmission in rat dietary obesity. *Neuroscience, 159*(4), 1193–1199. https://doi.org/10.1016/j.neuroscience.2009.02.007

Goldstein, N., McKnight, A. D., Carty, J. R. E., Arnold, M., Betley, J. N., & Alhadeff, A. L. (2021). Hypothalamic detection of macronutrients via multiple gut-brain pathways. *Cell Metabolism, 33*(3), 676–687.e5. https://doi.org/10.1016/j.cmet.2020.12.018

Green, B. G., & George, P. (2004). "Thermal taste" predicts higher responsiveness to chemical taste and flavor. *Chemical Senses, 29*(7), 617–628. https://doi.org/10.1093/chemse/bjh065

Gropp, E., Shanabrough, M., Borok, E., Xu, A. W., Janoschek, R., Buch, T., Plum, L., Balthasar, N., Hampel, B., Waisman, A., Barsh, G. S., Horvath, T. L., & Brüning, J. C. (2005). Agouti-related peptide–expressing neurons are mandatory for feeding. *Nature Neuroscience, 8*(10), 1289–1291. https://doi.org/10.1038/nn1548

Grove, J. C. R., Gray, L. A., La Santa Medina, N., Sivakumar, N., Ahn, J. S., Corpuz, T. V., Berke, J. D., Kreitzer, A. C., & Knight, Z. A. (2022). Dopamine subsystems that track internal states. *Nature, 608*(7922), article 7922. https://doi.org/10.1038/s41586-022-04954-0

Hamid, A. A., Pettibone, J. R., Mabrouk, O. S., Hetrick, V. L., Schmidt, R., Vander Weele, C. M., Kennedy, R. T., Aragona, B. J., & Berke, J. D. (2016). Mesolimbic dopamine signals the value of work. *Nature Neuroscience, 19*(1), 117–126. https://doi.org/10.1038/nn.4173

Han, W., Tellez, L. A., Perkins, M. H., Perez, I. O., Qu, T., Ferreira, J., Ferreira, T. L., Quinn, D., Liu, Z.-W., Gao, X.-B., Kaelberer, M. M., Bohórquez, D. V., Shammah-Lagnado, S. J., de Lartigue, G., & de Araujo, I. E. (2018). A neural circuit for gut-induced reward. *Cell, 175*(3), 665–678.e23. https://doi.org/10.1016/j.cell.2018.08.049

Hayes, J. E., Feeney, E. L., & Allen, A. L. (2013). Do polymorphisms in chemosensory genes matter for human ingestive behavior? *Food Quality and Preference, 30*(2), 202–216. https://doi.org/10.1016/j.foodqual.2013.05.013

Heath, T. P., Melichar, J. K., Nutt, D. J., & Donaldson, L. F. (2006). Human taste thresholds are modulated by serotonin and noradrenaline. *Journal of Neuroscience, 26*(49), 12664–12671. https://doi.org/10.1523/JNEUROSCI.3459-06.2006

Hintiryan, H., Bowman, I., Johnson, D. L., Korobkova, L., Zhu, M., Khanjani, N., Gou, L., Gao, L., Yamashita, S., Bienkowski, M. S., Garcia, L., Foster, N. N., Benavidez, N. L., Song, M. Y., Lo, D., Cotter, K. R., Becerra, M., Aquino, S., Cao, C., ... Dong, H.-W. (2021). Connectivity characterization of the mouse basolateral amygdalar complex. *Nature Communications, 12*(1), 2859. https://doi.org/10.1038/s41467-021-22915-5

Holland, P. C., Petrovich, G. D., & Gallagher, M. (2002). The effects of amygdala lesions on conditioned stimulus-potentiated eating in rats. *Physiology & Behavior, 76*(1), 117–129. https://doi.org/10.1016/S0031-9384(02)00688-1

Holman, G. L. (1969). Intragastric reinforcement effect. *Journal of Comparative and Physiological Psychology, 69*(3), 432–441. https://doi.org/10.1037/h0028233

Horstmann, A., Fenske, W. K., & Hankir, M. K. (2015). Argument for a non-linear relationship between severity of human obesity and dopaminergic tone: Relationship between obesity and dopaminergic tone. *Obesity Reviews 16*(10), 821–830. https://doi.org/10.1111/obr.12303

Howe, M.W., Tierney, P. L., Sandberg, S. G., Phillips, P. E., & Graybiel, A. M. (2013). Prolonged dopamine signalling in striatum signals proximity and value of distant rewards. *Nature, 500*(7464), 575–579. https://doi.org/10.1038/nature12475

Janak, P. H., & Tye, K. M. (2015). From circuits to behaviour in the amygdala. *Nature, 517*(7534), 284–292. https://doi.org/10.1038/nature14188

Janssen, L. K., & Horstmann, A. 2022. Molecular imaging of central dopamine in obesity: A qualitative review across substrates and radiotracers. *Brain Sciences 12*(4), 486 https://doi.org/10.3390/brainsci12040486

Jequier, E. (2002). Leptin signaling, adiposity, and energy balance. *Annals of the New York Academy of Sciences, 967*, 379–388. https://doi.org/10.1111/j.17496632.2002.tb04293.x

Johnson, P. M., & Kenny, P. J. (2010) Dopamine D2 receptors in addiction-like reward dysfunction and compulsive eating in obese rats. *Nature Neuroscience, 13*(5), 635–641. https://doi.org/10.1038/nn.2519

Kaelberer, M. M., Buchanan, K. L., Klein, M. E., Barth, B. B., Montoya, M. M., Shen, X., & Bohórquez, D. V. (2018). A gut-brain neural circuit for nutrient sensory transduction. *Science, 361*(6408), eaat5236–eaat5236. https://doi.org/10.1126/science.aat5236

Kanoski, S. E., Hayes, M. R., & Skibicka, K. P. (2016). GLP-1 and weight loss: Unraveling the diverse neural circuitry. *American Journal of Physiology. Regulatory, Integrative and Comparative Physiology, 310*(10), R885–R895. https://doi.org/101152/ajpregu005202015

Karlsson, H. K., Tuominen, L., Tuulari, J. J., Hirvonen, J., Parkkola, R., Helin, S., Salminen, P., Nuutila, P., & Nummenmaa, L. (2015). Obesity is associated with decreased μ-opioid but unaltered dopamine D2 receptor availability in the brain. *Journal of Neuroscience, 35*(9), 3959–3965. https://doi.org/10.1523/JNEUROSCI.4744-14.2015

Kaufman, A., Choo, E., Koh, A., & Dando, R. (2018). Inflammation arising from obesity reduces taste bud abundance and inhibits renewal. *PLOS Biology, 16*(3), e2001959. https://doi.org/10.1371/journal.pbio.2001959

Kim, U., Jorgenson, E., Coon, H., Leppert, M., Risch, N., & Drayna, D. (2003). Positional cloning of the human quantitative trait locus underlying taste sensitivity to phenylthiocarbamide. *Science, 299*(5610), 1221–1225. https://doi.org/10.1126/science.1080190

Kim, U., Wooding, S., Ricci, D., Jorde, L. B., & Drayna, D. (2005). Worldwide haplotype diversity and coding sequence variation at human bitter taste receptor loci. *Human Mutation, 26*(3), 199–204. https://doi.org/10.1002/humu.20203

Krettek, J. E., & Price, J. L. (1977). Projections from the amygdaloid complex to the cerebral cortex and thalamus in the rat and cat. *Journal of Comparative Neurology, 172*(4), 687–722. https://doi.org/10.1002/cne.901720408

Kutlu, M. G., Zachry, J. E., Melugin, P. R., Cajigas, S. A., Chevee, M. F., Kelly, S. J., Kutlu, B., Tian, L., Siciliano, C. A., & Calipari, E. S. (2021). Dopamine release in the nucleus accumbens core signals perceived saliency. *Current Biology, 31*(21), 4748–4761. https://doi.org/10.1016/j.cub.2021.08.052

Liu, C. M., & Kanoski, S. E. (2018). Homeostatic and non-homeostatic controls of feeding behavior: Distinct vs. common neural systems. *Physiology & Behavior, 193*(Pt B), 223–231. https://doi.org/10.1016/j.physbeh.2018.02.011

Lucas, F., & Sclafani, A. (1989). Flavor preferences conditioned by intragastric fat infusions in rats. *Physiology & Behavior, 46*(3), 403–412. https://doi.org/10.1016/0031-9384(89)90011-5

Maliphol, A. B., Garth, D. J., & Medler, K. F. (2013). Diet-induced obesity reduces the responsiveness of the peripheral taste receptor cells. *PLOS ONE, 8*(11), e79403. https://doi.org/10.1371/journal.pone.0079403

Marowsky, A., Yanagawa, Y., Obata, K., & Vogt, K. E. (2005). A specialized subclass of interneurons mediates dopaminergic facilitation of amygdala function. *Neuron, 48*(6), 1025–1037. https://doi.org/10.1016/j.neuron.2005.10.029

May, C. E., Vaziri, A., Lin, Y. Q., Grushko, O., Khabiri, M., Wang, Q.-P., Holme, K. J., Pletcher, S. D., Freddolino, P. L., Neely, G. G., & Dus, M. (2019). High dietary sugar reshapes sweet taste to promote feeding behavior in drosophila melanogaster. *Cell Reports*, *27*(6), 1675–1685.e7. https://doi.org/10.1016/j.celrep.2019.04.027

McCall, J. G., Siuda, E. R., Bhatti, D. L., Lawson, L. A., McElligott, Z. A., Stuber, G. D., & Bruchas, M. R. (2017). Locus coeruleus to basolateral amygdala noradrenergic projections promote anxiety-like behavior. *eLife*, *6*, e18247. https://doi.org/10.7554/eLife.18247

McCutcheon, J. E., Beeler, J. A., & Roitman, M. F. (2012). Sucrose-predictive cues evoke greater phasic dopamine release than saccharin-predictive cues. *Synapse*, 66(4), 346–351. https://doi.org/10.1002/syn.21519

McCutcheon, J. E., & Roitman, M. F. (2019). Mode of sucrose delivery alters reward-related phasic dopamine signals in nucleus accumbens. *ACS Chemical Neuroscience*, *10*(4), 1900–1907. https://doi.org/10.1021/acschemneuro.8b00262

McDonald, A. J. (1998). Cortical pathways to the mammalian amygdala. *Progress in Neurobiology*, *55*(3), 257–332. https://doi.org/10.1016/s0301-0082(98)00003-3

Miller, I. J., & Reedy, F. E. (1990). Variations in human taste bud density and taste intensity perception. *Physiology & Behavior*, *47*(6), 1213–1219. https://doi.org/10.1016/0031-9384(90)90374-d

Mohebi, A., Pettibone, J. R., Hamid, A. A., Wong, J. T., Vinson, L. T., Patriarchi, T., Tian, L., Kennedy, R. T., & Berke, J. D. (2019). Dissociable dopamine dynamics for learning and motivation. *Nature*, *570*(7759), 65–70. https://doi.org/10.1038/s41586-019-1235-y

Montague, P., Dayan, P., & Sejnowski, T. (1996). A framework for mesencephalic dopamine systems based on predictive Hebbian learning. *Journal of Neuroscience*, *16*(5), 1936–1947. https://doi.org/10.1523/JNEUROSCI.16-05-01936.1996

Murphy, K. G., & Bloom, S. R. (2006). Gut hormones and the regulation of energy homeostasis. *Nature*, *444*(7121), 854–859. https://doi.org/10.1038/nature05484

Myers, K. P. (2018). The convergence of psychology and neurobiology in flavor-nutrient learning. *Appetite*, *122*, 36–43. https://doi.org/10.1016/j.appet.2017.03.048

Nieh, E. H., Matthews, G. A., Allsop, S. A., Presbrey, K. N., Leppla, C. A., Wichmann, R., Neve, R., Wildes, C. P., & Tye, K. M. (2015). Decoding neural circuits that control compulsive sucrose seeking. *Cell*, *160*(3), 528–541. https://doi.org/10.1016/J.CELL.2015.01.003

Nitschke, J. B., Dixon, G. E., Sarinopoulos, I., Short, S. J., Cohen, J. D., Smith, E. E., Kosslyn, S. M., Rose, R. M., & Davidson, R. J. (2006). Altering expectancy dampens neural response to aversive taste in primary taste cortex. *Nature Neuroscience*, *9*(3), 435–442. https://doi.org/10.1038/nn1645

Norgren, R. (1976). Taste pathways to hypothalamus and amygdala. *Journal of Comparative Neurology*, *166*(1), 17–30. https://doi.org/10.1002/cne.901660103

O'Doherty, J. P., Deichmann, R., Critchley, H. D., & Dolan, R. J. (2002). Neural responses during anticipation of a primary taste reward. *Neuron*, *33*(5), 815–826. https://doi.org/10.1016/s0896-6273(02)00603-7

Ottersen, O. P., & Ben-Ari, Y. (1979). Afferent connections to the amygdaloid complex of the rat and cat. I. projections from the thalamus. *Journal of Comparative Neurology*, *187*(2), 401–424. https://doi.org/10.1002/cne.901870209

Pak, K., & Nummenmaa, L. (2023). Brain dopamine receptor system is not altered in obesity: Bayesian and frequentist meta-analyses. *Human Brain Mapping*, *44*(18), 6552–6560 https://doi.org/10.1002/hbm.26534

Palmiter, R. D. (2008). Dopamine signaling in the dorsal striatum is essential for motivated behaviors: Lessons from dopamine-deficient mice. *Annals of the New York Academy of Sciences*, (1129), 35–46. https://doi.org/10.1196/annals.1417.003.

Petrovich, G. D., Setlow, B., Holland, P. C., & Gallagher, M. (2002). Amygdalo-hypothalamic circuit allows learned cues to override satiety and promote eating. *Journal of Neuroscience*, *22*(19), 8748–8753.

Price, J. L., & Amaral, D. G. (1981). An autoradiographic study of the projections of the central nucleus of the monkey amygdala. *Journal of Neuroscience*, *1*(11), 1242–1259. https://doi.org/10.1523/JNEUROSCI.01-11-01242.1981

Qu, T., Han, W., Niu, J., Tong, J., & de Araujo, I. E. (2019). On the roles of the duodenum and the vagus nerve in learned nutrient preferences. *Appetite*, *139*, 145–151. https://doi.org/10.1016/j.appet.2019.04.014

Rainnie, D. G. (1999). Serotonergic modulation of neurotransmission in the rat basolateral amygdala. *Journal of Neurophysiology*, *82*(1), 69–85. https://doi.org/10.1152/jn.1999.82.1.69

Ricardo, J. A., & Tongju Koh, E. (1978). Anatomical evidence of direct projections from the nucleus of the solitary tract to the hypothalamus, amygdala, and other forebrain structures in the rat. *Brain Research*, *153*(1), 1–26. https://doi.org/10.1016/0006-8993(78)91125-3

Robinson, T. E., & Berridge, K. C. (1993). The neural basis of drug craving: An incentive-sensitization theory of addiction. *Brain Research. Brain Research Reviews, 18*(3), 247–291. https://doi.org/10.1016/0165-0173(93)90013-p

Rolls, E. T. (2020). The texture and taste of food in the brain. *Journal of Texture Studies, 51*(1), 23–44. https://doi.org/10.1111/JTXS.12488

Rosenkranz, J. A., & Grace, A. A. (1999). Modulation of basolateral amygdala neuronal firing and afferent drive by dopamine receptor activation in vivo. *Journal of Neuroscience, 19*(24), 11027–11039. https://doi.org/10.1523/JNEUROSCI.19-24-11027.1999

Rosenkranz, J. A., & Grace, A. A. (2002). Cellular mechanisms of infralimbic and prelimbic prefrontal cortical inhibition and dopaminergic modulation of basolateral amygdala neurons in vivo. *Journal of Neuroscience, 22*(1), 324–337. https://doi.org/10.1523/JNEUROSCI.22-01-00324.2002

Rossi, M. A., & Stuber, G. D. (2018). Overlapping brain circuits for homeostatic and hedonic feeding. *Cell Metabolism, 27*(1), 42–56. https://doi.org/10.1016/j.cmet.2017.09.021

Sadikot, A. F., & Parent, A. (1990). The monoaminergic innervation of the amygdala in the squirrel monkey: An immunohistochemical study. *Neuroscience, 36*(2), 431–447. https://doi.org/10.1016/0306-4522(90)90439-B

Saper, C. B., Chou, T. C., & Elmquist, J. K. (2002). The need to feed: Homeostatic and hedonic control of eating. *Neuron, 36*(2), 199–211. https://doi.org/10.1016/S0896-6273(02)00969-8

Saunders, B., Richard, J., Margolis, E., Janak, P. (2018). Dopamine neurons create Pavlovian conditioned stimuli with circuit-defined motivational properties. *Nature Neuroscience, 21*(8), 1072–1083. https://doi.org/10.1038/s41593-018-0191-4.

Schmitt, M. (1973). Influences of hepatic portal receptors on hypothalamic feeding and satiety centers. *American Journal of Physiology, 225*(5), 1089–1095. https://doi.org/10.1152/ajplegacy.1973.225.5.1089

Schultz, W., Dayan, P., & Montague, P. R. (1997). A neural substrate of prediction and reward. *Science, 275*(5306), 1593–1599. https://doi.org/10.1126/science.275.5306.1593

Sclafani, A. (1988). Carbohydrate appetite in rats: Taste and postingestive factors. *Appetite, 11*, 20–25. https://doi.org/10.1016/S0195-6663(88)80042-4

Sclafani, A. (1990). Nutritionally based learned flavor preferences in rats. In E. D. Capaldi & T. L. Powley(Eds.), *Taste, experience, and feeding* (pp. 139–156). American Psychological Association. https://doi.org/10.1037/10075-010

Sclafani, A. (2006). Sucrose motivation in sweet "sensitive" (C57BL/6J) and "subsensitive" (129P3/J) mice measured by progressive ratio licking. *Physiology & Behavior, 87*(4), 734–744. https://doi.org/10.1016/j.physbeh.2006.01.017

Sclafani, A. (2013). Gut-brain nutrient signaling. Appetition vs. satiation. *Appetite, 71*, 454–458. https://doi.org/10.1016/j.appet.2012.05.024

Sclafani, A., & Ackroff, K. (2006). Nutrient-conditioned flavor preference and incentive value measured by progressive ratio licking in rats. *Physiology & Behavior, 88*(1–2), 88–94. https://doi.org/10.1016/j.physbeh.2006.03.009

Sclafani, A., & Lucas, F. (1996). Abdominal vagotomy does not block carbohydrate-conditioned flavor preferences in rats. *Physiology & Behavior, 60*(2), 447–453. https://doi.org/10.1016/s0031-9384(96)80018-7

Sclafani, A., & Nissenbaum, J. W. (1988). Robust conditioned flavor preference produced by intragastric starch infusions in rats. *American Journal of Physiology, 255*(4 Pt 2), R672–675. https://doi.org/10.1152/ajpregu.1988.255.4.R672

Scott, T. R., & Small, D. M. (2009). The role of the parabrachial nucleus in taste processing and feeding. *Annals of the New York Academy of Sciences, 1170*(1), 372–377. https://doi.org/10.1111/j.1749-6632.2009.03906.x

Seeley, R. J., & Berridge, K. C. (2015). The hunger games. *Cell, 160*(5), 805–806. https://doi.org/10.1016/J.CELL.2015.02.028

Sengupta, A., Bocchio, M., Bannerman, D. M., Sharp, T., & Capogna, M. (2017). Control of amygdala circuits by 5-HT neurons via 5-HT and glutamate cotransmission. *Journal of Neuroscience, 37*(7), 1785–1796. https://doi.org/10.1523/JNEUROSCI.2238-16.2016

Sheng, Z., Santiago, A. M., Thomas, M. P., & Routh, V. H. (2014). Metabolic regulation of lateral hypothalamic glucose-inhibited orexin neurons may influence midbrain reward neurocircuitry. *Molecular and Cellular Neuroscience, 62*, 30–41. https://doi.org/10.1016/J.MCN.2014.08.001

Szczypka, M. S., Kwok, K., Brot, M., Matsumoto, A., Donahue, B., & Palmiter, R. (2001). Dopamine production in the caudate putamen restores feeding in dopamine-deficient mice. *Neuron, 30*(3), 819–828. https://doi.org/10.1016/s0896-6273(01)00319-1

Small, D. M. (2010). Taste representation in the human insula. *Brain Structure and Function, 214*(5), 551–561. https://doi.org/10.1007/s00429-010-0266-9

Small, D. M., & DiFeliceantonio, A. G. (2019). Processed foods and food reward. *Science, 363*(6425), 346–347. https://doi.org/10.1126/science.aav0556

Small, D. M., Jones-Gotman, M., Zatorre, R. J., Petrides, M., & Evans, A. C. (1997). A role for the right anterior temporal lobe in taste quality recognition. *Journal of Neuroscience, 17*(13), 5136–5142. https://doi.org/10.1523/JNEUROSCI.17-13-05136.1997

Small, D. M., Veldhuizen, M. G., Felsted, J., Mak, Y. E., & McGlone, F. (2008). Separable substrates for anticipatory and consummatory food chemosensation. *Neuron, 57*(5), 786–797. https://doi.org/10.1016/j.neuron.2008.01.021

Small, D. M., Zatorre, R. J., Dagher, A., Evans, A. C., & Jones-Gotman, M. (2001). Changes in brain activity related to eating chocolate: From pleasure to aversion. *Brain, 124*(9), 1720–1733.

Small, D. M., Zatorre, R. J., & Jones-Gotman, M. (2001a). Changes in taste intensity perception following anterior temporal lobe removal in humans. *Chemical Senses, 26*(4), 425–432. https://doi.org/10.1093/chemse/26.4.425

Small, D. M., Zatorre, R. J., & Jones-Gotman, M. (2001b). Increased intensity perception of aversive taste following right anteromedial temporal lobe removal in humans. *Brain, 124*(8), 1566–1575. https://doi.org/10.1093/brain/124.8.1566

Steinbusch, H. W. (1981). Distribution of serotonin-immunoreactivity in the central nervous system of the rat-cell bodies and terminals. *Neuroscience, 6*(4), 557–618. https://doi.org/10.1016/0306-4522(81)90146-9

Stutzmann, G. E., & LeDoux, J. E. (1999). GABAergic antagonists block the inhibitory effects of serotonin in the lateral amygdala: A mechanism for modulation of sensory inputs related to fear conditioning. *Journal of Neuroscience, 19*(11), RC8–RC8. https://doi.org/10.1523/JNEUROSCI.19-11-j0005.1999

Stutzmann, G. E., McEwen, B. S., & LeDoux, J. E. (1998). Serotonin modulation of sensory inputs to the lateral amygdala: Dependency on corticosterone. *Journal of Neuroscience, 18*(22), 9529–9538. https://doi.org/10.1523/JNEUROSCI.18-22-09529.1998

Sun, X., Kroemer, N. B., Veldhuizen, M. G., Babbs, A. E., de Araujo, I. E., Gitelman, D. R., Sherwin, R. S., Sinha, R., & Small, D. M. (2015). Basolateral amygdala response to food cues in the absence of hunger is associated with weight gain susceptibility. *Journal of Neuroscience, 35*(20), 7964–7976. https://doi.org/10.1523/JNEUROSCI.3884-14.2015

Swanson, L. W., & Hartman, B. K. (1975). The central adrenergic system. An immunofluorescence study of the location of cell bodies and their efferent connections in the rat utilizing dopamine-B-hydroxylase as a marker. *Journal of Comparative Neurology, 163*(4), 467–505. https://doi.org/10.1002/cne.901630406

Tan, H. E., Sisti, A. C., Jin, H., Vignovich, M., Villavicencio, M., Tsang, K. S., Goffer, Y., & Zuker, C. S. (2020). The gut–brain axis mediates sugar preference. *Nature, 580*(7804), 511–516. https://doi.org/10.1038/s41586-020-2199-7

Tang, D. W., Fellows, L. K., & Dagher, A. (2014). Behavioral and neural valuation of foods is driven by implicit knowledge of caloric content. *Psychological Science, 25*(12), 2168–2176. https://doi.org/10.1177/0956797614552081

Tang, W., Kochubey, O., Kintscher, M., & Schneggenburger, R. (2020). A VTA to basal amygdala dopamine projection contributes to signal salient somatosensory events during fear learning. *Journal of Neuroscience, 40*(20), 3969–3980. https://doi.org/10.1523/JNEUROSCI.1796-19.2020

Tellez, L. A., Medina, S., Han, W., Ferreira, J. G., Licona-Limón, P., Ren, X., Lam, T. K. T., Schwartz, G. J., & De Araujo, I. E. (2013). A gut lipid messenger links excess dietary fat to dopamine deficiency. *Science, 341*(6147), 800–802. https://doi.org/10.1126/science.1239275

Tellez, L. A., Ren, X., Han, W., Medina, S., Ferreira, J. G., Yeckel, C. W., & De Araujo, I. E. (2013). Glucose utilization rates regulate intake levels of artificial sweeteners. *Journal of Physiology, 591*(22), 5727–5744. https://doi.org/10.1113/jphysiol.2013.263103

Tepperman, J., Brobeck, J. R., & Long, C. N. H. (1943). The effects of hypothalamic hyperphagia and of alterations in feeding habits on the metabolism of the albino rat. *Yale Journal of Biology and Medicine 15*(6), 855.

Tully, K., Li, Y., Tsvetkov, E., & Bolshakov, V. Y. (2007). Norepinephrine enables the induction of associative long-term potentiation at thalamo-amygdala synapses. *Proceedings of the National Academy of Sciences, 104*(35), 14146–14150. https://doi.org/10.1073/pnas.0704621104

Van Den Top, M., Lee, K., Whyment, A. D., Blanks, A. M., & Spanswick, D. (2004). Orexigen-sensitive NPY/AgRP pacemaker neurons in the hypothalamic arcuate nucleus. *Nature Neuroscience*, *7*(5), 493–494. https://doi.org/10.1038/nn1226

van Galen, K. A., ter Horst, K. W., & Serlie, M. J. (2021). Serotonin, food intake, and obesity. *Obesity Reviews*, *22*(7), e13210. https://doi.org/10.1111/obr.13210

Veldhuizen, M. G., Babbs, R. K., Patel, B., Fobbs, W., Kroemer, N. B., Garcia, E., Yeomans, M. R., & Small, D. M. (2017). Integration of sweet taste and metabolism determines carbohydrate reward. *Current Biology*, *27*(16), 2476–2485.e6. https://doi.org/10.1016/j.cub.2017.07.018

Veldhuizen, M. G., Douglas, D., Aschenbrenner, K., Gitelman, D. R., & Small, D. M. (2011). The anterior insular cortex represents breaches of taste identity expectation. *Journal of Neuroscience*, *31*(41), 14735–14744. https://doi.org/10.1523/JNEUROSCI.1502-11.2011

Veldhuizen, M. G., Farruggia, M. C., Gao, X., Nakamura, Y., Green, B. G., & Small, D. M. (2020). Identification of an amygdala-thalamic circuit that acts as a central gain mechanism in taste perceptions. *Journal of Neuroscience*, *40*(26), 5051–5062. https://doi.org/10.1523/JNEUROSCI.2618-19.2020

Vincis, R., Chen, K., Czarnecki, L., Chen, J., & Fontanini, A. (2020). Dynamic representation of taste-related decisions in the gustatory insular cortex of mice. *Current Biology*, *30*(10), 1834–1844.e5. https://doi.org/10.1016/j.cub.2020.03.012

Volkow, N. D., Wang, G.-J., & Baler, R. D. 2011. Reward, dopamine and the control of food intake: implications for obesity. *Trends in Cognitive Sciences*, *15*(1), 37–46. https://doi.org/10.1016/j.tics.2010.11.001

Wang, L., Gillis-Smith, S., Peng, Y., Zhang, J., Chen, X., Salzman, C. D., Ryba, N. J. P., & Zuker, C. S. (2018). The coding of valence and identity in the mammalian taste system. *Nature*, *558*(7708), 127–131. https://doi.org/10.1038/s41586-018-0165-4

Wassum, K. M., & Izquierdo, A. (2015). The basolateral amygdala in reward learning and addiction. *Neuroscience & Biobehavioral Reviews*, *57*, 271–283. https://doi.org/10.1016/j.neubiorev.2015.08.017

Waterson, M. J., & Horvath, T. L. (2015). Neuronal regulation of energy homeostasis: Beyond the hypothalamus and feeding. *Cell Metabolism*, *22*(6), 962–970. https://doi.org/10.1016/J.CMET.2015.09.026

Watts, A. G., Kanoski, S. E., Sanchez-Watts, G., & Langhans, W. (2022). The physiological control of eating: Signals, neurons, and networks. *Physiological Reviews*, *102*(2), 689–813. https://doi.org/10.1152/physrev.00028.2020

Weir, J. B. de V. (1949). New methods for calculating metabolic rate with special reference to protein metabolism. *Journal of Physiology*, *109*(1–2), 1–9. https://doi.org/10.1113/jphysiol.1949.sp004363

Yamamoto, T., Matsuo, R., & Kawamura, Y. (1980). Localization of cortical gustatory area in rats and its role in taste discrimination. *Journal of Neurophysiology*, *44*(3), 440–455. https://doi.org/10.1152/jn.1980.44.3.440

Yanagisawa, K., Bartoshuk, L. M., Catalanotto, F. A., Karrer, T. A., & Kveton, J. F. (1998). Anesthesia of the chorda tympani nerve and taste phantoms. *Physiology & Behavior*, *63*(3), 329–335. https://doi.org/10.1016/s0031-9384(97)00423-x

Zhang, L., Han, W., Lin, C., Li, F., & de Araujo, I. E. (2018). Sugar metabolism regulates flavor preferences and portal glucose sensing. *Frontiers in Integrative Neuroscience*, *12*, 57. https://doi.org/10.3389/fnint.2018.00057

Zheng, H., Patterson, L. M., Rhodes, C. J., Louis, G. W., Skibicka, K. P., Grill, H. J., Myers, M. G., Jr, & Berthoud, H. R. (2010). A potential role for hypothalamomedullary POMC projections in leptin-induced suppression of food intake. *American Journal of Physiology. Regulatory, Integrative and Comparative Physiology*, *298*(3), R720–R728. https://doi.org/10.1152/AJPREGU.00619.2009

Zukerman, S., Ackroff, K., & Sclafani, A. (2013). Post-oral appetite stimulation by sugars and nonmetabolizable sugar analogs. *American Journal of Physiology. Regulatory, Integrative and Comparative Physiology*, *305*(7), R840–R853. https://doi.org/10.1152/ajpregu.00297.2013

3

Neuroendocrine Function and the Gut–Brain Axis in Eating Disorders

Diana L. Williams and Pamela K. Keel

Brief Definitional Overview

Satiation: Subjective state associated with termination of a meal due to achieving completion (or satisfaction) of the underlying drive state. Measured as the amount of food consumed in an ad lib meal.

Satiety: Subjective state associated with delay between the end of one meal (satiation) and the initiation of the next meal. Measured as the inter-meal interval.

Hunger: Subjective state associated with increased drive to consume food.

Binge eating: Consumption of a large amount of food in a limited period of time while experiencing a subjective feeling of loss of control over eating.

Gastrointestinal distress: Subjective feelings of nausea and stomachache following food intake.

Purging: Behaviors employed to forcefully evacuate matter from the body to influence weight or body shape.

Physiologic versus pharmacologic dose: Physiologic doses of a hormone are exogenously administered amounts that maintain the hormone within a normal endogenous range.

Pharmacologic doses elevate levels of the hormone above the normal endogenous range.

Biological Framework

Introduction to gut peptides

Many signals generated within the gut communicate to the brain about volume and nutrient content moving through the gastrointestinal (GI) tract (see Figure 3.1). The physiology and effects of gut peptides have been extensively reviewed elsewhere (e.g., Steinert et al., 2017) and a brief overview is provided here. The stomach contains a population of enteroendocrine cells that produce the hormone ghrelin, which is acylated in its active form. Ghrelin is unique among the peptides

Diana L. Williams and Pamela K. Keel, *Neuroendocrine Function and the Gut–Brain Axis in Eating Disorders*.
In: *The Handbook of the Neurobiology of Eating Disorders*. Edited by: Christina E. Wierenga and Joanna E. Steinglass, Oxford University Press. © Oxford University Press (2025). DOI: 10.1093/9780197675212.003.0004

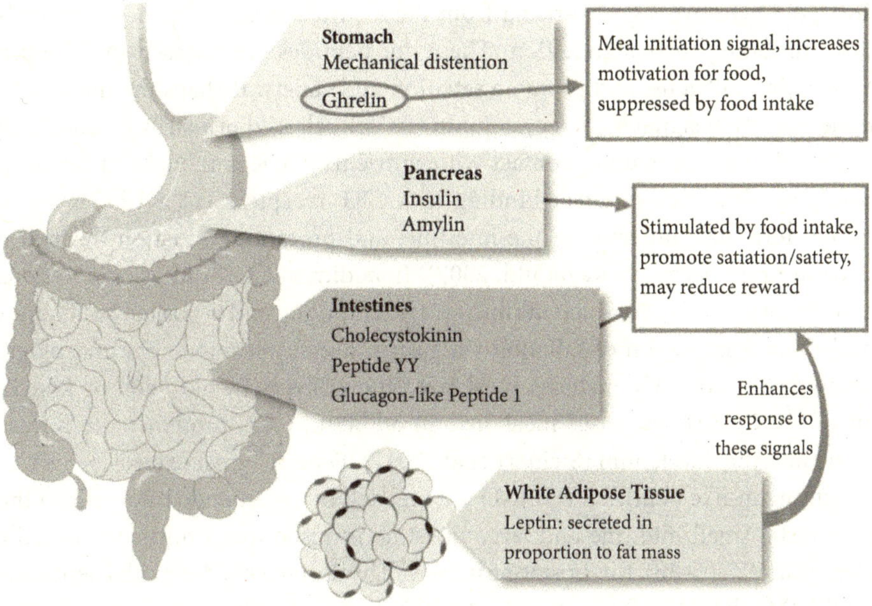

Figure 3.1 Illustration of the sources and eating-related functions of gut signals discussed in this chapter. Note that ghrelin is produced in the intestines as well as the stomach.

discussed here in that it promotes eating through its receptor, the growth hormone secretagogue receptor (GHSR), whereas other peptides limit food intake. Ghrelin-producing cells are also found in the small intestine, and ghrelin release from stomach and intestinal cells is suppressed by the presence of nutrients in the intestine. As such, circulating ghrelin levels are low immediately after a meal but gradually rise thereafter, peaking just before the next meal begins (Cummings et al., 2004), and ghrelin levels rise with fasting or food restriction (Hansen et al., 2002; Tschöp et al., 2000). Pharmacologic administration of ghrelin in rodents and humans promotes meal initiation (Overduin et al., 2012; Wren et al., 2001), and post-meal suppression of ghrelin may have a role in satiety. GHSRs are located on the afferent vagus nerve, and this may be a mechanism for some of ghrelin's effects on eating (Date et al., 2002; le Roux et al., 2005); however, ghrelin crosses the blood–brain barrier and GHSRs are located throughout the brain. In particular, ghrelin action at GHSRs expressed on neuropeptide Y (NPY) and agouti-related peptide (AgRP) neurons is considered a mechanism for its hyperphagic effects (Wang et al., 2014). Notably, the GHSR has an endogenous antagonist and inverse agonist liver expressed antimicrobial protein 2 (LEAP2), which blocks ghrelin action at these receptors. Therefore, a balance of ghrelin and LEAP2 levels may be an important consideration. In addition to promoting food intake, ghrelin has other physiological effects through the GHSR, including stimulation of growth hormone and increasing the rate of gastric emptying.

Most post-ingestive signals arising from the GI tract function as negative feedback, inhibiting further ingestion. These gut peptides are released in response to incoming nutrients and promote satiation and satiety. Perhaps the most well-studied satiation signal is cholecystokinin (CCK), released primarily by duodenal enteroendocrine cells upon contact with nutrients. CCK is thought to function mainly as a paracrine signal, binding to CCK1 receptors (CCK1R) on vagal afferent terminals innervating the intestine, and promoting satiation through a vagus-to-brain pathway (Raybould, 2007). In addition, CCK causes contractions of the pyloric sphincter, which inhibits gastric emptying and is posited to enhance mechanical stimulation of satiation via gastric stretch receptors. Pharmacologic administration of CCK reduces meal size, and conversely, blockade or knock-out of the CCK1R increases meal size. In addition, CCK promotes the release of bile into the duodenum (Steinert et al., 2017). Peptide tyrosine tyrosine (PYY) and glucagon-like peptide 1 (GLP-1) are secreted by enteroendocrine cells in the more distal small intestine and large intestine in response to nutrients. Initially released as PYY(1–36), this hormone is cleaved by the enzyme dipeptidyl peptidase 4 (DPP4) to the active form, PYY(3–36). PYY crosses the blood–brain barrier, and PYY(3–36) selectively activates the NPY2 receptor, through which it can suppress food intake. Data on the role of PYY(3–36) in physiological control of satiation or satiety are limited, and most studies in which PYY(3–36) impacts eating delivered pharmacologic doses (Steinert et al., 2017). To the extent that PYY(3–36) does suppress intake, it may act through the vagus nerve, as well as directly in the brain (Acuna-Goycolea & van den Pol, 2005; Koda et al., 2005; Stadlbauer et al., 2013). GLP-1 secreted by the intestine is also cleaved by DPP4; however, in this case, cleavage transforms it from active GLP-1(7–36) to the inactive form, GLP-1(9–36). Through action at GLP-1 receptors (GLP-1Rs), active GLP-1 appears to serve as a satiation signal (Krieger, 2020). GLP-1 is made by neurons in the hindbrain nucleus of the solitary tract (NTS) and reticular formation, as well, and in rodents, activation of neuronal GLP-1Rs potently suppresses food intake (Williams, 2022). Like CCK, the active form of GLP-1 does not appear to cross the blood–brain barrier due to rapid degradation. The peripheral and central GLP-1 systems are widely considered to be distinct, with intestine-derived GLP-1 exerting its effects primarily through nearby GLP-1Rs expressed on afferent vagal terminals (Brierley et al., 2021). Both PYY and GLP-1 slow gastric emptying rate, and GLP-1 is also well known as an incretin hormone, promoting insulin release.

While the pancreas is outside of the GI tract, the pancreatic peptides insulin and amylin are also meal-related signals that play important roles in energy balance. Pancreatic β cells co- release these peptides in response to elevated circulating glucose and incretin hormones. While insulin is best known for its role in glucose homeostasis, it can suppress feeding in rodents by acting at brain insulin receptors (Begg & Woods, 2012). Amylin receptors (AMYR) are expressed in a variety of brain areas, and secreted amylin crosses the blood–brain barrier to bind to these receptors. The area postrema, hypothalamus, and ventral tegmental area (VTA) are some of the key locations for amylin action to suppress feeding (Boccia et al., 2020; Geisler & Hayes, 2023). In addition to this hypophagic effect, amylin inhibits gastric emptying.

These gut signals are dynamic, changing rapidly in response to the status of the GI tract and incoming nutrients, making their disruption prime candidates to consider in dysregulated eating patterns, but their actions are modulated by longer-term signals of stored fuels. Leptin, perhaps the best known of these longer-term signals, is secreted by white adipose tissue in direct proportion to fat mass. Evidence from rodent models suggests that leptin has synergistic interactions with CCK and GLP-1, such that when leptin levels are elevated, individuals are more sensitive to the satiating effects of CCK and GLP-1, and conversely when leptin levels drop (as with fasting and weight loss), sensitivity to CCK and GLP-1 decreases (Wang et al., 2000; Williams et al., 2006). This is thought to be one reason why weight loss is difficult to maintain, because reduced sensitivity to satiation signals leads to increased food intake. Leptin resistance occurs when leptin is chronically elevated and fails to provoke the leptin receptor's normal intracellular signaling cascade (Myers et al., 2010), and this impairs responsiveness to satiation signals. Insulin is also considered an adiposity signal because basal insulin levels directly relate to white adipose tissue mass (Baskin et al., 1999), and rodent studies have shown that insulin synergistically interacts with CCK to reduce food intake (Riedy et al., 1995).

GI-meal related signals not only communicate to the brain about gut nutrient status, they also impact motivation and food reward through direct and indirect effects on brain reward-related circuitry (Geisler & Hayes, 2023). Vagal afferents stimulated by many of these gut signals synapse in the hindbrain NTS, and these neurons (including GLP-1-producing neurons) have ascending projections to many locations, including the VTA, where the dopaminergic cell bodies of the mesolimbic reward pathway reside, and the nucleus accumbens where many of those dopamine neurons project. Gut signals that cross the blood–brain barrier can act directly at these sites. For example, GHSRs are expressed in the VTA, and ghrelin stimulates feeding and motivation for food through these receptors (Skibicka et al., 2011), while VTA AMYR stimulation has the opposite effects (Mietlicki-Baase et al., 2017). In these ways, gut–brain communication is linked with brain mediation of reward, and dysfunction in gut–brain communication could lead to impairments in reward processing.

Laboratory animal models for eating disorders research

No rodent model can fully recapitulate a human eating disorder, but certain features of eating disorders can be modeled in lab animals (see Chapter 22). Use of non-human animal models allows a high degree of control over potential confounding variables, more invasive manipulations and measurements than would be possible in humans and strengthens the ability to make causal inferences. The most common approach to modeling features of anorexia nervosa (AN) is the activity-based anorexia (ABA) paradigm, which has been described in detail elsewhere (François & Zeltser, 2022; Spadini et al., 2021). Briefly, rodents are given time-limited access to food (e.g., a single 90-minute period per day), coupled with unlimited access to a running wheel. Subjects with limited food access but no running wheel adapt to consume more food during that time, and subjects with ad libitum food and wheel access maintain their body weight, but those receiving both the restricted feeding schedule and wheel consume less food and lose a substantial amount of weight. Rodents undergoing the ABA condition therefore share several features with humans who have AN: voluntary reduction of food intake, increased physical activity, and significant weight loss.

Rats and mice do not vomit or purge in other ways, so those features of some eating disorders cannot be addressed in these species; however, a number of different approaches to modeling binge eating have been used with rodents (Berger et al., 2023; Rehn et al., 2022). These commonly feature intermittent time-limited access to palatable high-fat (HF) and/or high-sugar (HS) food. During these palatable food access periods, rodents consume an amount that could be considered "excessive" relative to the amount consumed within that time when subjects receive standard chow only or have continuous access to the palatable food. Similar to patterns of binge eating in humans, rodents in the intermittent access paradigm consume a majority of food during the initial window of food access (e.g., the first 30 minutes of a 120-minute window of access) versus consuming food throughout the entire period of access. In some models, the limited access to palatable food is followed by voluntary reduction of chow intake, while others include experimenter-imposed cycles of food restriction.

State of the Science in Eating Disorders

Table 3.1 presents a summary of clinical findings reviewed below for altered endocrine factors in eating disorders.

Leptin

Clinical findings

Numerous studies document decreased plasma leptin in patients with AN compared with controls (Di Carlo et al., 2002; Föcker et al., 2011; Germain et al., 2007; Hebebrand et al., 1997; Lear et al., 1999; Mantzoros et al., 1997; Monteleone et al., 2000; Monteleone, Fabrazzo, et al., 2002; Tolle et al., 2003), likely representing a consequence of low fat mass. Supporting this, leptin levels improve after recovery from AN (de Alvaro et al., 2007; Manara et al., 2005; Oświecimska et al., 2005; van Elburg et al., 2007). During the course of weight gain, many patients

Table 3.1 Summary of altered endocrine factors in eating disorders

	Anorexia Nervosa	Bulimia Nervosa	Binge-Eating Disorder	Other Eating Disorders
Leptin	Reduced	Reduced	Elevated	Reduced in purging disorder
	Rapid increases with weight restoration may slow recovery		Mixed evidence that this remains true when controlling for adiposity	Mixed in night eating syndrome
Ghrelin	Elevated Predicts recovery	Mixed, with some evidence that postprandial levels remain high	Mixed, with some evidence of reduced fasting and postprandial ghrelin	Disrupted circadian pattern in night eating syndrome
				Higher in ARFID compared to AN but not controls
				Higher in purging disorder
CCK	Mixed	Reduced postprandial response	Mixed	Elevated fasting level in ARFID No difference in purging disorder
PYY	Mixed, with some evidence of Elevated postprandial response	Mixed, with some evidence of blunted postprandial response	Mixed	Elevated in purging disorder compared to BN and controls
GLP-1	Mixed	Reduced postprandial response	No difference	No difference in purging disorder
Insulin	Reduced levels, with evidence of higher insulin sensitivity	No differences in release, with evidence of reduced insulin	Elevated, with evidence of reduced insulin sensitivity	Higher in purging disorder compared to BN but not controls
Amylin	Limited evidence of reduced fasting amylin	No difference		No difference in purging disorder

with AN experience increases in leptin that exceed what would be expected from changes in fat mass (Hebebrand et al., 1997; Holtkamp et al., 2003; Mantzoros et al., 1997). Holtkamp and colleagues (2004) reported that leptin levels at discharge were higher than expected based on body mass index (BMI), and this discrepancy predicted risk for post-treatment weight loss and relapse (Holtkamp et al., 2004). In contrast, a meta-analysis of relapse predictors found that higher leptin levels predicted lower relapse in AN and noted that this effect emerged when leptin was measured at intake versus discharge (Sala et al., 2023). Relatedly, this meta-analysis also found that higher BMI at intake was associated with lower relapse risk in studies of AN.

Leptin findings in AN align with evidence of a significantly blunted developmental trajectory of premorbid BMI (measured over time as percentiles for age and biological sex), predicting onset of AN in adolescence (Stice et al., 2022; Yilmaz et al., 2019) and that genetic variants that impact metabolism are associated with AN (Watson et al., 2019). Collectively, findings suggest that individuals at risk for developing AN may maintain low weights, in part, because their bodies constitutionally fall at the lower end of the weight spectrum. Those with higher leptin concentrations (and BMIs) at intake are more likely to recover and maintain recovery; whereas those who experience a rebound of leptin at a lower discharge BMI may be fighting their own biology in attempting to maintain weight gain.

Leptin concentrations are lower in women with bulimia nervosa (BN) compared with healthy controls (Brewerton et al., 2000; Jimerson et al., 2000, 2010; Monteleone et al., 2000; Monteleone, Martiadis, et al., 2002). This may reflect the presence of weight suppression, defined as the difference between highest weight and current weight for adult height (Keel et al., 2019). Prior work has demonstrated greater weight suppression in BN compared to controls and that weight suppression is inversely correlated with leptin (Bodell & Keel, 2015; Keel et al., 2017). Greater weight suppression also predicts future onset of BN (Stice et al., 2020). This association is specifically linked to higher premorbid weight, consistent with evidence that future onset of BN is predicted by elevated developmental BMI trajectory (Yilmaz et al., 2019). Collectively, studies suggest that individuals with BN may present with reduced leptin as a consequence of efforts to maintain a weight below prior elevated weight. Importantly, reduced leptin may serve as a maintenance factor for binge eating in BN by modulating the strength of other signals that impact eating.

By contrast, elevated leptin levels have been found in individuals with binge-eating disorder (BED) (Adami et al., 2002; Monteleone et al., 2000; Monteleone, Fabrazzo, et al., 2002). In groups characterized by overweight and obesity, BED was associated with elevated leptin in some (Adami et al., 2002; Yagin et al., 2020) but not all studies (Brandao et al., 2010; Geliebter et al., 2005). Similar to BN, premorbid developmental BMI trajectories are elevated prior to BED onset (Yilmaz et al., 2019). However, unlike BN, weight suppression does not predict increased risk for BED (Stice et al., 2020). BED may be characterized by elevated drives toward food consumption, contributing to both increased weight which likely accounts for increased circulating leptin concentrations. The combination of elevated leptin with elevated food intake suggests disruption of leptin sensitivity in BED.

Mixed findings have been reported for leptin in night eating syndrome, with one report of elevated levels (Stunkard, 2000) and another report of no significant difference from controls (Allison et al., 2005). Studies in separate samples of women with purging disorder (Jimerson et al., 2010; Keel et al., 2017) supported lower leptin compared to controls, with lower leptin associated with greater weight suppression (Keel et al., 2017). Similar to findings for BN, elevated developmental BMI trajectory predicted increased risk of purging disorder onset (Yilmaz et al., 2019), and greater weight suppression predicted onset of purging disorder (Stice et al., 2020). Combined with findings for AN, BN, and BED, results suggest that lower leptin is neither required nor sufficient to produce binge eating.

Animal models

Leptin levels have been measured in the rodent ABA model, and unsurprisingly, are consistent with body fat mass such that rats and mice undergoing ABA have lower leptin levels than controls (Gelegen et al., 2007; Gilman et al., 2019; Pardo et al., 2010). Because leptin has been shown to suppress starvation-induced hyperactivity in rats (Exner et al., 2000), Hillebrand and colleagues (2005) examined whether pharmacological leptin treatment may reduce weight loss during ABA. While chronic brain leptin administration did reduce wheel running in ABA rats, it also increased energy expenditure and suppressed food intake further, so these subjects lost even more weight than ABA rats receiving vehicle treatment.

In models for binge eating in which rats are given intermittent access to HF and HS food, leptin levels appear to track body fat mass. In most studies, rats receiving less frequent access to palatable food gain less weight than those receiving ad libitum access over the duration of the feeding manipulation, and leptin levels in the intermittent groups fall between control chow-only and ad libitum palatable food groups (Bake et al., 2014; Davis et al., 2007; Kinzig et al., 2008).

Ghrelin

Clinical findings

Ghrelin appears to be a biomarker of low weight in AN. Studies of individuals with AN support higher fasting concentrations of ghrelin than controls (Kim et al., 2023; Mancuso et al., 2020; Prince et al., 2009; Rossi et al., 2021; Sedláčková et al., 2011; Tong & D'Alessio, 2011), and a meta-analysis supported these differences across both AN subtypes for total and acyl ghrelin (Seidel et al., 2021). Following a fixed test meal, ghrelin remained higher in AN compared to controls (Heruc et al., 2018; Mancuso et al., 2020). Elevated ghrelin predicted weight gain in adolescents with AN (Kim et al., 2023), and others reported that circulating ghrelin decreased after treatment and associated weight recovery (Otto et al., 2001; Wu et al., 2021).

Individuals with BN maintain higher levels of ghrelin after food intake than control participants (Keel et al., 2018; Kojima et al., 2005; Monteleone et al., 2003) despite no consistent differences in fasting ghrelin (Prince et al., 2009; Sedláčková et al., 2011). Others found no differences between BN and control participants

(Nakazato et al., 2004; Monteleone et al., 2008; Sedlackova et al., 2012), which may reflect challenges in accurate measurement of acyl ghrelin or different test meal sizes across studies, with less robust differences seen after smaller test meals (Devlin et al., 2012).

Studies of BED have also produced mixed results. One study found no differences in fasting ghrelin concentrations or in ghrelin response to food intake between control and BED participants (Munsch et al., 2009), while others suggested that BED patients have lower fasting concentrations of ghrelin and a less robust decrease in ghrelin after food intake (Geliebter et al., 2005, 2008). Monteleone, Fabrazzo, and colleagues (2005) reported reduced fasting ghrelin concentrations were associated with the presence of obesity, binge-eating disorder, or both. In a study of participants with body weight in the obese range, binge eating was associated with lower fasting acyl ghrelin and less robust postprandial reductions in acyl ghrelin (Hernandez et al., 2019). Carnell and colleagues (2018) found no differences in ghrelin response to a liquid test meal between BED and non-BED participants with body weights in the obese range; however, they reported differences in time-of-day effects. Specifically, those with BED demonstrated lower preprandial ghrelin in the morning compared to the afternoon whereas controls showed the opposite. Given expected patterns for ghrelin over the course of the day and the timing of binge- eating episodes, results suggest that disrupted meal patterns in BED may impact and be impacted by ghrelin. Specifically, ghrelin levels reach their apex in the morning after an overnight fast, reducing rapidly after the morning meal and slowly rising to reach a secondary peak near the midday meal. For those with BED, higher than expected ghrelin levels in the afternoon may predispose them to increased food intake later in the day, a time when binge-eating episodes are more likely to occur.

The disrupted circadian rhythm in night eating syndrome is associated with changes in circadian release of ghrelin (Allison et al., 2005; Birketvedt et al., 2012; Goel et al., 2009; Rosenhagen et al., 2005). Avoidant/restrictive food intake disorder (ARFID) is an eating disorder characterized by malnutrition in the absence of significant concerns about gaining weight or becoming fat. Despite not differing from AN on BMI percentile, ARFID was associated with lower fasting and postprandial ghrelin compared to AN and did not differ from controls (Becker et al., 2021). Like BN, purging disorder was associated with higher fasting and postprandial acyl ghrelin compared to non-eating disorder controls (Keel et al., 2018). Given evidence of elevated ghrelin in AN, regardless of subtype, and purging disorder, GI hunger signals cannot fully account for excessive food intake during binge eating.

Animal models

Ghrelin levels rise with fasting and weight loss, so perhaps not surprisingly, plasma ghrelin is high in male rats undergoing ABA with a one-hour food access schedule, significantly more so than subjects undergoing food restriction with no running wheel access (Pardo et al., 2010). A recent study using mice suggests that this increase could be due to an ABA-induced elevation in the number of ghrelin-producing cells in the stomach (François et al., 2015). Other data suggest that elevated ghrelin levels during ABA are one of the mechanisms for increased food- anticipatory activity, the hyperactivity observed shortly before scheduled food access (Tezenas du Montcel et al., 2023; Verhagen et al., 2011). If ghrelin promotes food intake and ghrelin levels are high in animals undergoing ABA, why do these subjects eat less? One study found that pharmacologic ghrelin treatment could prevent the development of ABA in male mice (Legrand et al., 2016). This raises the possibility that ABA reduces sensitivity to the orexigenic effects of ghrelin, and elevating ghrelin levels even further may overcome this.

Plasma ghrelin levels have also been examined in rodent models of binge eating, with mixed results. In one study, male rats maintained on standard rodent chow received intermittent chow restriction followed by access to sucrose-sweetened vegetable shortening for two hours twice weekly, while control groups experienced food restriction alone or had continuous access to the sweetened shortening (Bello et al., 2009). After eight weeks, ghrelin levels were elevated in the intermittent group compared with the continuous access group, although not significantly different from the restriction-only group. In another study in which male rats were given daily access to 60% fat diet for two-hour periods, with no food restriction, ghrelin levels were unaffected (Bake et al., 2014), and similar results have been reported for mice receiving daily two-hour access to high fat food (Cornejo et al., 2019). Food restriction or frequency of palatable food "binge" periods may determine whether ghrelin levels are altered in these paradigms.

Others have examined whether ghrelin may have a causal role in the elevated intake of palatable food in these models using loss-of-function approaches. King and colleagues (2016) found that in mice given access to high-fat diet for a two-hour period on three days per week, transgenic mice lacking the GHSR consumed less high-fat diet during those access periods than wild-type mice. However, there was no effect of genotype on intake in mice receiving two-hour access every day, a finding replicated in a later study (Bake et al., 2017). These findings suggest that different physiological mechanisms underlie elevated intake during more versus less frequent palatable food, offering some insights into potential differences observed between studies of BN and studies of BED. Relative to wild-type mice, GHSR knock-out mice have impaired high-fat diet-induced activation of NAc neurons (King et al., 2016), suggesting that GHSR-mediated activation in this brain area could play a role in elevated palatable food intake in the intermittent access model. Taking a different approach, Cornejo and colleagues (2019) showed that brain administration of LEAP2 or a synthetic GHSR antagonist reduced high-fat diet intake in male mice receiving daily two-hour access periods. Taken together, these data support the idea that endogenous GHSR signaling contributes to the elevated food intake observed in the limited- access model, at least under some circumstances.

Cholecystokinin

Clinical findings

Studies of CCK in AN have produced inconsistent results (Prince et al., 2009; Tong & D'Alessio, 2011). Harty and colleagues (1991) reported that patients with AN demonstrated an earlier and higher peak in postprandial CCK compared to controls. Others reported that CCK response did not differ between controls and patients acutely ill with AN or those recovered from AN post-treatment (Geracioti et al., 1992) or at four-year follow-up (Pirke et al., 1994). Finally, one study found no differences in fasting or postprandial CCK response between patients with AN and age-matched controls; however, during initial weight restoration, patients with AN had an elevated CCK response compared to controls, and this was normalized at the time of discharge (Cuntz et al., 2013). The authors posited that initial findings of "normal" CCK response represent an abnormal adaption to low nutritional intake.

Several studies have demonstrated reduced CCK response to food in women with BN compared with controls (Devlin et al., 1997; Geracioti et al., 1989; Geracioti & Liddle, 1988; Keel et al., 2007; Pirke et al., 1994). Others reported no differences between BN and controls on CCK response (Hannon-Engel et al., 2013; Phillipp et al., 1991), which may reflect differences in test meal size or composition (Devlin et al., 1997). Treatment with antidepressants was associated with symptom remission and with improved CCK response in two studies (Geracioti et al., 1989; Geracioti & Liddle, 1988). Efforts to increase postprandial CCK response with a prokinetic medication (erythromycin) had no impact on CCK response and was not associated with symptom improvement (Devlin et al., 2012). One study reported elevated fasting CCK in participants with ARFID compared to controls (Burton Murray et al., 2022). Studies of BED (Geliebter et al., 2004) and purging disorder (Keel et al., 2007) indicate normal CCK response to food intake, with the exception of one report of elevated CCK response to food in BED compared to controls (Munsch et al., 2009). Across studies, the more consistent patterns for suppressed CCK response in BN suggest a role for this GI signal in maintenance of binge eating among those who do not maintain elevated body weight.

Animal models

To our knowledge, there has been no investigation of CCK in the context of the rodent ABA model, and there are limited data for rodent models of binge eating. One study gave male mice, maintained continuously on HF and HS diet, access to 12.3% sucrose solution for a two-hour window on five randomly chosen days of the week, compared with controls that had water only (Gharibeh et al., 2022). After five weeks, they found that the satiating effect of CCK injection was impaired in the mice that had intermittent sucrose access relative to controls, suggesting that elevated intake in that setting could be mediated in part by reduced sensitivity to CCK.

Peptide tyrosine tyrosine

Clinical findings

Reports on PYY levels in eating disorders show very mixed results. One group reported that fasting PYY was elevated in AN at intake and normalized following two weeks of treatment (Heruc et al., 2018) while another study reported no differences in fasting PYY between individuals with AN and controls (Tam et al., 2020). A significantly decreased PYY response to food intake in patients with AN was found in one study (Stock et al., 2005), a significantly increased response seen in others (Mancuso et al., 2020; Nakahara et al., 2007; Sedlackova et al., 2012), and others found no significant difference (Becker et al., 2021; Otto et al., 2007). Collectively, findings reduce confidence that alterations in PYY contribute to or result from restrictions in food intake relative to energy needs in AN.

Two studies have supported blunted PYY responses to food intake in BN compared with controls (Kojima et al., 2005; Monteleone, Martiadis, et al., 2005), while another observed no difference (Devlin et al., 2012). For BED, no differences from controls in post-meal PYY release were reported by two studies (Carnell et al., 2018; Geliebter et al., 2008), while another study suggested an elevated PYY response (Munsch et al., 2009). One study supported elevated postprandial PYY response to a fixed meal in purging disorder compared to both BN and non- eating disorder controls, and PYY response predicted changes in gastrointestinal distress (Keel et al., 2018). ARFID demonstrated minimal differences in PYY response compared to both AN and controls in one study (Becker et al., 2021).

Animal models

To our knowledge, there are no laboratory animal studies addressing PYY in models for eating disorders.

Glucagon-like peptide 1

Clinical findings

Compared to controls, patients with AN have been reported to have both higher (Germain et al., 2007) and lower levels of GLP-1 (Tomasik et al., 2004). Research indicates lower levels of GLP-1 in women with BN than in controls (Dossat et al., 2015; Naessén et al., 2011). Women with BN also had significantly lower GLP-1 levels than women with purging disorder (Dossat et al., 2015), suggesting a unique association with the presence of binge eating in the absence of weight dysregulation. No differences have been reported in GLP-1 levels between controls and women with BED (Geliebter et al., 2008) or purging disorder (Dossat et al., 2015).

Animal models

GLP-1 levels in rodent models of intermittent palatable food access have been examined in two studies. Mukherjee and colleagues (2020) examined male rats receiving one-hour access to vegetable shortening either daily or on three days per week. After 8.5 weeks, plasma levels of GLP-1 were significantly higher in the rats that had shortening access three days/week, although this is difficult to interpret because it was not meal-evoked. The same study examined hindbrain expression of mRNA for the GLP-1 precursor preproglucagon (PPG) and found that it was substantially reduced in the three days/week group. Another study examining female rats used a different feeding schedule in which some rats received vegetable shortening only every fourth day for 24 hours, compared with groups maintained on chow only or ad libitum access to chow and shortening (Mukherjee et al., 2022). The intermittent group consumed more shortening on their access days than the ad libitum group, but this had no impact on PPG mRNA expression in brain or gut. Different feeding schedules or the sex of the rats may account for the differing results.

Because GLP-1R stimulation both promotes satiation and reduces motivation for palatable food, it has been suggested that GLP-1R agonists could reduce binge eating. One study examined this in mice on an intermittent access schedule. Ovariectomized females were maintained on standard chow but given HF diet access for one day/week (Cao et al., 2014), and in this setting, subcutaneous injection of GLP-1 suppressed HF diet intake. This could reflect GLP-1's ability to suppress food intake in general, because this experiment included no other feeding schedule comparison groups. While GLP-1 and long-acting GLP-1R agonists can effectively suppress palatable food intake, several studies have shown that maintenance on a HF diet impairs sensitivity to these treatments (Duca et al., 2013, 2015; Williams et al., 2011). It would therefore be valuable to determine whether there is a change in responsiveness in these intermittent access models, and if so, whether that can be explained by HF diet exposure alone.

Insulin

Clinical findings

Fasting insulin and insulin response to glucose and test meals was lower among patients with AN (Letiexhe et al., 1997; Tanaka et al., 2003). Delayed postprandial insulin peak to a glucose load as well as improved insulin response to intravenous versus oral glucose tolerance tests among some patients with AN likely reflects delays in gastric emptying associated with AN (Kinzig et al., 2007; Nozaki et al., 1994; Tanaka et al., 2003). Although insulin may be depressed in AN, sensitivity to its effects may be heightened and partially account for hypoglycemia commonly observed as a medical complication in patients. A recent meta-analysis supported heightened insulin sensitivity in AN compared to controls (Ilyas et al., 2019). In one study that subdivided patients with AN based on the pattern of insulin response to oral glucose, a subset of patients demonstrated blunted insulin response regardless of glucose administration route (Nozaki et al., 1994). Follow-up of patients with

AN following refeeding and weight restoration supported partial normalization of meal-induced insulin response (Kinzig et al., 2007; Nakahara et al., 2007). Supporting a potential etiological role for these physiological abnormalities, Adams and colleagues (2021) reported that genetic variants linked to elevated fasting insulin concentrations were associated with reduced risk for developing AN, with no associations for other psychiatric disorders.

Studies of insulin response in BN largely show no evidence of alterations compared to controls (Blouin et al., 1991; Casper et al., 1988; Dynesen et al., 2008; Raphael et al., 1995). Despite no difference in insulin response to food intake, a meta-analysis suggested lower insulin sensitivity in BN compared to controls (Ilyas et al., 2019). Maske, Williams, and colleagues (2020) found that women with purging disorder demonstrated significantly greater insulin response to a fixed test meal compared to women with BN; however, neither group differed significantly from controls.

Compared to individuals with BMI in the overweight or obese range without BED, those with BED and overweight or obesity exhibited higher fasting insulin concentrations and evidence of greater insulin resistance (Ilyas et al., 2019; Succurro et al., 2015) as well as higher insulin response to a fixed test meal at specific time points but not overall (Geliebter et al., 2004, 2005). Findings in BED support reduced sensitivity to the satiating effects of insulin in BED.

Animal models

Given the critical role of insulin in energy homeostasis, it is surprising that there is little data on insulin in rodent studies modeling eating disorders. One study examined insulin levels in male and female rats in the ABA paradigm where blood was collected post-prandially, and found no differences compared with control groups. Similarly, in rodent intermittent access studies in which insulin levels have been measured, there seems to be no effect of this pattern of food intake (Artiga et al., 2007; Bake et al., 2017; Mukherjee et al., 2020). However, these studies all examined insulin in blood collected when subjects were euthanized at the end of the experiment, with no relation to a meal. As a result, further assessment is warranted.

Amylin

Clinical findings

Limited findings are available for amylin in eating disorders. Several reviews of bone mineral density deficiency in AN refer to reduced amylin (Jada et al., 2021; Misra et al., 2016). However, evidence of associations with bone density come from a small study reporting reduced fasting amylin concentrations in AN (Wojcik et al., 2010), and reports of significant differences in meal-induced amylin response have not been cited. No differences in amylin responses to food intake were found among women with BN, purging disorder, or non-eating disorder controls (Maske, Williams, et al., 2020). Thus, excess food intake in BN occurs despite intact amylin responses.

Animal models

Circulating amylin levels have not been reported in rodent models of eating disorders; however, one study examined sensitivity to the hypophagic effects of amylin treatment after intermittent access to palatable food. There, female rats were maintained on standard chow only, chow and HF diet ad libitum, or chow ad libitum and the HF diet for twenty hours every fourth day (Maske, Coiduras, et al., 2020). After two weeks on this schedule, rats received amylin or vehicle injections, and the intermittent group was tested on a day with HF diet access as well as on a day with chow only. In this model, amylin significantly suppressed intake in the chow and ad libitum HF diet groups but was less effective in the intermittent rats tested on chow, and not at all effective in the intermittent rats tested on HF diet. This suggests that the pattern of eating resulting from intermittent HF diet access impairs rats' ability to respond to this satiation signal.

Limitations

A limitation of much of the clinical research in this area is that these studies cannot determine whether differences in plasma levels of gut hormones or responses to gut hormones precede the development of disordered eating or arise as consequence. In most cases, particularly when examining studies of AN, alterations appear to reflect biological defenses against reduced food intake and body weight. Similarly, in these studies, it is impossible to determine whether any observed differences in gut hormone responses have a causal role in the disordered eating or if they are merely a biomarker. Rodent models can be useful in this respect. In studies with laboratory animals, subjects are randomly assigned to their feeding conditions, so when groups differ, we can conclude that the feeding regimen produced changes. That said, proving that weight loss in the ABA model causes reduced leptin provides limited insight into factors that would produce initial weight loss in AN. Rodent models also allow experimental manipulation of hormones and their receptors in a way that would often be impossible or unethical in humans, such as genetic loss-of-function studies or delivery of experimental drugs. Although not all gut peptides have been examined in this way in rodent models, evidence discussed above suggests that dysfunction in these systems may have a causal role in at least some aspects of disordered eating and that interventions targeting these systems could enhance treatments for eating disorders.

There are also limitations to rodent studies. The best designs include multiple control groups to allow clearer conclusions; however, it can still be difficult to identify exactly what aspect of the manipulation is most relevant. For example, are the elevated ghrelin levels observed in intermittent access subjects in some studies caused by the temporal pattern of palatable food access, the reduced chow intake during times when the palatable food is not available, or the intermittent experience of extremely large meals? Further studies will be required to answer this question. Comparison across studies is complicated by the lack of standardization of these rodent models. Another limitation of the rodent literature is that the majority of published studies used only male subjects, which is inconsistent with the higher prevalence of eating disorders in women. Each of these may contribute to differences in findings across human subjects and rodent model research attempting to address the same questions.

Turning to the literature in humans, eating disorders comprise disparate symptoms, such as the combination of restriction, low weight, and binge eating in the binge-purge subtype of AN or the combination of restricting, binge eating, and purging in BN. Simple comparisons to control groups make it impossible to determine what feature of an eating disorder is linked to observed alterations in GI signals. Studies that include comparison groups that isolate specific aspects of dysregulated eating provide greater confidence that differences are linked to disordered eating behaviors. This approach has been used to isolate the effects of binge eating from elevated body weight in comparisons of BED to weight-matched controls. Similarly, comparisons of purging BN with purging disorder facilitate conclusions regarding correlates of binge eating. This approach is less viable in studies of AN because medically low weight is rare among individuals who are otherwise healthy; however, recent efforts to compare AN and ARFID have offered new insights. The greatest challenge remains lack of replication, largely due to the absence of a sufficient number of studies with adequate sample sizes.

Alternative Perspectives

Dysfunction in brain reward-related circuitry, especially the striatum and its major connections, has been a major focus of the literature on neurobiological underpinnings of eating disorders. Substantial evidence supports this hypothesis, with studies in human subjects as well as animal models finding that disordered eating is associated with structural and functional changes in corticostriatal pathways (Bello & Hajnal, 2010; Foldi et al., 2017; Frank, 2021; Leenaerts et al., 2022). This work highlights the central nervous system (CNS) as primary; however, this does not exclude gut–brain communication as an important factor. Rather, it is well established that nutrient detection in the GI tract is communicated to reward-related brain areas through poly-synaptic pathways. Under healthy conditions, vagally mediated nutrient-related signals can be not only satiating but also reinforcing, and these effects are thought to be mediated at least in part through mesocorticolimbic circuitry (de Araujo, Schatzker, et al., 2020). As discussed earlier in this chapter, ghrelin, leptin, insulin, and many gut satiation and satiety hormones impact neural activity in brain regions associated with reward. Therefore, altered release of these signals or processing at the level of the afferent vagus or subsequent CNS mediatory pathways could contribute to the differences between individuals with and without eating disorders observed in studies focused on brain reward circuitry. We hypothesize that this is an important mechanism, and ongoing work explores whether deficient GLP-1 function may serve as a maintenance factor for eating disorders characterized by recurrent binge eating via its influences on reward satiation and reward valuation (see Keel et al., 2019 for details).

In clinical research examining brain structure, connectivity, and activity, food reward has typically been addressed with tasks using visual food cues or taste, sometimes under fed versus fasted conditions, but with limited consideration of ongoing GI processes. Similarly, research using rodent models for eating disorders has focused on assessment of either gut hormones or brain reward circuitry. Future studies should directly examine potential relationships between the two. Basic research in rodents can further map the circuitry that connects the gut to more rostral subcortical and cortical structures, and also examine how this may be impacted in the ABA or intermittent palatable food access paradigms. In humans, it will be valuable to examine neural responses to food and food cues concurrently with gut nutrient load and measurement of gut hormone responses to determine how these may differ in people with eating disorders.

Implications

Although correlational studies cannot distinguish causes from consequences of dysregulated eating behavior, normalization of eating remains the goal of all eating disorder treatments. Thus, key issues are whether or not endocrine abnormalities produce resistance to change in treatment or contribute to medical morbidity. Each has important implications for clinical practice.

Starvation-induced endocrine changes, including reduced leptin, increased ghrelin, and reduced insulin release, largely promote food intake. In the treatment of AN, nutritional rehabilitation is critical to normalization of most endocrine factors. Reduced leptin and elevated ghrelin likely represent consequences of low weight that facilitate weight gain; however, evidence that patients with AN may experience greater insulin sensitivity and potentially greater postprandial PYY responses could serve as barriers. Metabolically, some alterations in AN may contribute to hypoglycemia and reduced bone mineral density, requiring multimodal care to address patients psychological and physical needs throughout treatment.

Although BN is not associated with medically low weight, many patients strive to maintain a weight that is below an elevated premorbid weight—a state referred to as weight suppression. This likely accounts for serum profiles that resemble those of AN in terms of reduced leptin and elevated ghrelin. However, unlike patterns in AN, BN is associated with reduced satiation signals in the form of blunted postprandial CCK release and GLP-1 levels compared to controls. Combined, these changes may produce both an increased drive toward food consumption that is related to elevated hunger and reward as well as reduced ability to achieve a state of satisfaction. In the context of treatment, behavioral interventions, including increased frequency of meals and snacks, may help to retrain physiological responses to food intake and gradually reinstate a greater sense of control over eating. Although there is no clear evidence of alterations in either insulin or amylin response in BN, presence of binge eating may be associated with insulin resistance across the weight spectrum. This may contribute to excess risk for Type 2 diabetes in patients with BN.

BED is associated with excess adiposity, and many alterations appear to be a consequence of elevated weight. However, some changes, such as elevated leptin and reduced ghrelin have been found in BED compared to weight-matched controls. This suggests that dysregulated eating likely accounts for metabolic complications. These patterns, in addition to insulin resistance, may explain excess morbidity with Type 2 diabetes in BED. However, unlike patterns in BN, BED does not show consistent alterations in endocrine factors linked to satiation or satiety. The continuation of binge eating despite endocrine signals to reduce food intake and intact satiation and satiety signals highlight the role of contextual factors in eating as well as insensitivity to interoceptive signals in BED. Rodent models provide some support for the idea that BED could involve reduced sensitivity to GI satiation signals (Gharibeh et al., 2022; Maske, Coiduras, et al., 2020), raising the possibility that greater stimulation of receptors for GI satiation signals could have a beneficial effect. Consistent with this, preliminary data from an open trial in people with Type 2 diabetes and BED suggest that the long-acting GLP1R agonist, dulaglutide (vs. gliclazide, a Type 2 diabetes treatment that increases insulin levels) reduced binge eating (Da Porto et al., 2020). However, a randomized controlled trial found no differences in binge-eating frequency following treatment with liraglutide, a different long-acting GLP-1R agonist versus a placebo for BED, despite finding significant differences in weight loss (Allison et al., 2023).

Finally, other eating disorders, such as ARFID and purging disorder, appear to present with some, but not all, of the physiological correlates of closely related eating disorders. At this early stage of investigation, findings for both conditions have yet to be independently replicated. That said, results largely point to physiological alterations that would contribute to patients' subjective reports. As such, clinicians should work with patients to devise strategies to cope with excess feelings of fullness that make it challenging to consume normal amounts of food in both ARFID and purging disorder. Use of staged exposure with response prevention along with techniques adapted to increase distress tolerance may be particularly useful to normalize eating in these patients.

Conclusion and Future Directions

The clinical and basic scientific evidence discussed in this chapter points to differences in gut–brain signaling and eating-related neuroendocrine factors in eating disorders. Some of these differences likely result from disordered eating patterns but may contribute to pathology maintenance. Identifying mechanisms of maintenance is critical to identifying targets for novel interventions. The most consistent findings that bridge clinical and rodent studies are for altered leptin and ghrelin levels in AN and the rodent ABA model. For many of the gut hormones we discussed, there has been limited investigation in laboratory animal models, so this is an area for further research. Studies in humans and rodents vary substantially in their methodological details (e.g., test meal size, time of testing relative to last meal, macronutrient composition of test meal, palatable food access for rodents, and biological sex [human studies focus mostly on females whereas rodent models focus mostly on males]), making it difficult to interpret whether findings differ across species or just across methods. Future research will benefit from collaboration between clinical and basic scientists to develop truly translational standard testing procedures that allow us to evaluate the same constructs in humans and rodents.

References

Acuna-Goycolea, C., & van den Pol, A. N. (2005). Peptide YY(3-36) inhibits both anorexigenic proopiomelanocortin and orexigenic neuropeptide Y neurons: Implications for hypothalamic regulation of energy homeostasis. *Journal of Neuroscience, 25*(45), 10510–10519. https://doi.org/10.1523/JNEUROSCI.2552-05.2005

Adami, G. F., Campostano, A., Cella, F., & Scopinaro, N. (2002). Serum leptin concentration in obese patients with binge eating disorder. *International Journal of Obesity and Related Metabolic Disorders, 26*(8), 1125–1128. https://doi.org/10.1038/sj.ijo.0802010

Adams, D. M., Reay, W. R., Geaghan, M. P., & Cairns, M. J. (2021). Investigation of glycaemic traits in psychiatric disorders using Mendelian randomisation revealed a causal relationship with anorexia nervosa. *Neuropsychopharmacology, 46*(6), 1093–1102. https://doi.org/10.1038/s41386-020-00847-w

Allison, K. C., Ahima, R. S., O'Reardon, J. P., Dinges, D. F., Sharma, V., Cummings, D. E., Heo, M., Martino, N. S., & Stunkard, A. J. (2005). Neuroendocrine profiles associated with energy intake, sleep, and stress in the night eating syndrome. *Journal of Clinical Endocrinology and Metabolism, 90*(11), 6214–6217. https://doi.org/10.1210/jc.2005-1018

Allison, K. C., Chao, A. M., Bruzas, M. B., McCuen-Wurst, C., Jones, E., McAllister, C., Gruber, K., Berkowitz, R. I., Wadden, T. A., & Tronieri, J. S. (2023). A pilot randomized controlled trial of liraglutide 3.0 mg for binge eating disorder. *Obesity Science & Practice, 9*(2), 127–136. https://doi.org/10.1002/osp4.619

Artiga, A. I., Viana, J. B., Maldonado, C. R., Chandler-Laney, P. C., Oswald, K. D., & Boggiano, M. M. (2007). Body composition and endocrine status of long-term stress-induced binge-eating rats. *Physiology & Behavior, 91*(4), 424–431. https://doi.org/10.1016/j.physbeh.2007.04.001

Bake, T., Hellgren, K. T., & Dickson, S. L. (2017). Acute ghrelin changes food preference from a high-fat diet to chow during binge-like eating in rodents. *Journal of Neuroendocrinology, 29*(4). https://doi.org/10.1111/jne.12463

Bake, T., Morgan, D. G. A., & Mercer, J. G. (2014). Feeding and metabolic consequences of scheduled consumption of large, binge-type meals of high fat diet in the Sprague-Dawley rat. *Physiology & Behavior, 128*(100), 70–79. https://doi.org/10.1016/j.physbeh.2014.01.018

Baskin, D. G., Figlewicz Lattemann, D., Seeley, R. J., Woods, S. C., Porte, D., & Schwartz, M. W. (1999). Insulin and leptin: Dual adiposity signals to the brain for the regulation of food intake and body weight. *Brain Research, 848*(1–2), 114–123. https://doi.org/10.1016/s0006-8993(99)01974-5

Becker, K. R., Mancuso, C., Dreier, M. J., Asanza, E., Breithaupt, L., Slattery, M., Plessow, F., Micali, N., Thomas, J. J., Eddy, K. T., Misra, M., & Lawson, E. A. (2021). Ghrelin and PYY in low-weight females with avoidant/restrictive food intake disorder compared to anorexia nervosa and healthy controls. *Psychoneuroendocrinology, 129*, 105243. https://doi.org/10.1016/j.psyneuen.2021.105243

Begg, D. P., & Woods, S. C. (2012). The central insulin system and energy balance. In M. C. Michel (Ed.), *Handbook of experimental pharmacology*, (pp. 111–129). Springer. https://doi.org/10.1007/978-3-642-24716-3_5

Bello, N. T., & Hajnal, A. (2010). Dopamine and binge eating behaviors. *Pharmacology, Biochemistry, and Behavior, 97*(1), 25–33. https://doi.org/10.1016/j.pbb.2010.04.016

Bello, N. T., Guarda, A. S., Terrillion, C. E., Redgrave, G. W., Coughlin, J. W., & Moran, T. H. (2009). Repeated binge access to a palatable food alters feeding behavior, hormone profile, and hindbrain c-Fos responses to a test meal in adult male rats. *American Journal of Physiology. Regulatory, Integrative and Comparative Physiology, 297*(3), R622–631. https://doi.org/10.1152/ajpregu.00087.2009

Berger, G., Corris, J. D., Fields, S. E., Hao, L., Scarpa, L. L., & Bello, N. T. (2023). Systematic review of binge eating rodent models for developing novel or repurposing existing pharmacotherapies. *Biomolecules, 13*(5), 742. https://doi.org/10.3390/biom13050742

Birketvedt, G. S., Geliebter, A., Kristiansen, I., Firgenschau, Y., Goll, R., & Florholmen, J. R. (2012). Diurnal secretion of ghrelin, growth hormone, insulin binding proteins, and prolactin in normal weight and overweight subjects with and without the night eating syndrome. *Appetite, 59*(3), 688–692. https://doi.org/10.1016/j.appet.2012.07.015

Blouin, A., Blouin, J., Braaten, J., Sarwar, G., Bushnik, T., & Walker, J. (1991). Physiological and psychological responses to a glucose challenge in bulimia. *International Journal of Eating Disorders, 10*(3), 285–296.

Boccia, L., Gamakharia, S., Coester, B., Whiting, L., Lutz, T. A., & Le Foll, C. (2020). Amylin brain circuitry. *Peptides, 132*, 170366. https://doi.org/10.1016/j.peptides.2020.170366

Bodell, L. P., & Keel, P. K. (2015). Weight suppression in bulimia nervosa: Associations with biology and behavior. *Journal of Abnormal Psychology, 124*(4), 994–1002. https://doi.org/10.1037/abn0000077

Brandao, P. P., Garcia-Souza, E. P., Neves, F. A., Pereira, M. J. dos S., Sichieri, R., Moura, E. G. de, Silva, P. C. L. da, & Moura, A. S. (2010). Leptin/adiponectin ratio in obese women with and without binge eating disorder. *Neuro Endocrinology Letters, 31*(3), 353–358.

Brewerton, T. D., Lesem, M. D., Kennedy, A., & Garvey, W. T. (2000). Reduced plasma leptin concentrations in bulimia nervosa. *Psychoneuroendocrinology, 25*(7), 649–658. https://doi.org/10.1016/s0306-4530(00)00016-0

Brierley, D. I., Holt, M. K., Singh, A., de Araujo, A., McDougle, M., Vergara, M., Afaghani, M. H., Lee, S. J., Scott, K., Maske, C., Langhans, W., Krause, E., de Kloet, A., Gribble, F. M., Reimann, F., Rinaman, L., de Lartigue, G., & Trapp, S. (2021). Central and peripheral GLP-1 systems independently suppress eating. *Nature Metabolism, 3*(2), 258–273. https://doi.org/10.1038/s42255-021-00344-4

Burton Murray, H., Becker, K. R., Harshman, S., Breithaupt, L., Kuhnle, M., Dreier, M. J., Hauser, K., Freizinger, M., Eddy, K. T., Misra, M., Kuo, B., Micali, N., Thomas, J. J., & Lawson, E. A. (2022). Elevated fasting satiety-promoting cholecystokinin (CCK) in avoidant/restrictive food intake disorder compared to healthy controls. *Journal of Clinical Psychiatry, 83*(5), 21m14111. https://doi.org/10.4088/JCP.21m14111

Cao, X., Xu, P., Oyola, M. G., Xia, Y., Yan, X., Saito, K., Zou, F., Wang, C., Yang, Y., Hinton, A., Yan, C., Ding, H., Zhu, L., Yu, L., Yang, B., Feng, Y., Clegg, D. J., Khan, S., DiMarchi, R., . . . Xu, Y. (2014). Estrogens stimulate serotonin neurons to inhibit binge-like eating in mice. *Journal of Clinical Investigation, 124*(10), 4351–4362. https://doi.org/10.1172/JCI74726

Carnell, S., Grillot, C., Ungredda, T., Ellis, S., Mehta, N., Holst, J., & Geliebter, A. (2018). Morning and afternoon appetite and gut hormone responses to meal and stress challenges in obese individuals with and without binge eating disorder. *International Journal of Obesity, 42*(4), 841–849. https://doi.org/10.1038/ijo.2017.307

Casper, R. C., Pandy, G. N., Jaspan, J. B., & Rubenstein, A. H. (1988). Hormone and metabolite plasma levels after oral glucose in bulimia and healthy controls. *Biological Psychiatry, 24*(6), 663–674. https://doi.org/10.1016/0006-3223(88)90140-0

Cornejo, M. P., Castrogiovanni, D., Schiöth, H. B., Reynaldo, M., Marie, J., Fehrentz, J.-A., & Perello, M. (2019). Growth hormone secretagogue receptor signalling affects high-fat intake independently of plasma levels of ghrelin and LEAP2, in a 4-day binge eating model. *Journal of Neuroendocrinology, 31*(10), e12785. https://doi.org/10.1111/jne.12785

Cummings, D. E., Frayo, R. S., Marmonier, C., Aubert, R., & Chapelot, D. (2004). Plasma ghrelin levels and hunger scores in humans initiating meals voluntarily without time- and food-related cues. *American Journal of Physiology. Endocrinology and Metabolism, 287*(2), E297–304. https://doi.org/10.1152/ajpendo.00582.2003

Cuntz, U., Enck, P., Frühauf, E., Lehnert, P., Riepl, R. L., Fichter, M. M., & Otto, B. (2013).Cholecystokinin revisited: CCK and the hunger trap in anorexia nervosa. *PLOS One, 8*(1), e54457. https://doi.org/10.1371/journal.pone.0054457

Da Porto, A., Casarsa, V., Colussi, G., Catena, C., Cavarape, A., & Sechi, L. (2020). Dulaglutide reduces binge episodes in type 2 diabetic patients with binge eating disorder: A pilot study. *Diabetes & Metabolic Syndrome, 14*(4), 289–292. https://doi.org/10.1016/j.dsx.2020.03.009

Date, Y., Murakami, N., Toshinai, K., Matsukura, S., Niijima, A., Matsuo, H., Kangawa, K., & Nakazato, M. (2002). The role of the gastric afferent vagal nerve in ghrelin-induced feeding and growth hormone secretion in rats. *Gastroenterology, 123*(4), 1120–1128. https://doi.org/10.1053/gast.2002.35954

Davis, J. F., Melhorn, S. J., Shurdak, J. D., Heiman, J. U., Tschöp, M. H., Clegg, D. J., & Benoit, S. C. (2007). Comparison of hydrogenated vegetable shortening and nutritionally complete high-fat diet on limited access-binge behavior in rats. *Physiology & Behavior, 92*(5), 924–930. https://doi.org/10.1016/j.physbeh.2007.06.024

de Alvaro, M. T. G., Muñoz-Calvo, M. T., Barrios, V., Martínez, G., Martos-Moreno, G. A., Hawkins, F., & Argente, J. (2007). Regional fat distribution in adolescents with anorexia nervosa: Effect of duration of malnutrition and weight recovery. *European Journal of Endocrinology, 157*(4), 473–479. https://doi.org/10.1530/EJE-07-0459

de Araujo, I. E., Schatzker, M., & Small, D. M. (2020). Rethinking food reward. *Annual Review of Psychology, 71*, 139–164. https://doi.org/10.1146/annurev-psych-122216-011643

Devlin, M. J., Kissileff, H. R., Zimmerli, E. J., Samuels, F., Chen, B. E., Brown, A. J., Geliebter, A., & Walsh, B. T. (2012). Gastric emptying and symptoms of bulimia nervosa: Effect of a prokinetic agent. *Physiology & Behavior, 106*(2), 238–242. https://doi.org/10.1016/j.physbeh.2012.02.009

Devlin, M. J., Walsh, B. T., Guss, J. L., Kissileff, H. R., Liddle, R. A., & Petkova, E. (1997). Postprandial cholecystokinin release and gastric emptying in patients with bulimia nervosa. *American Journal of Clinical Nutrition, 65*(1), 114–120. https://doi.org/10.1093/ajcn/65.1.114

Di Carlo, C., Tommaselli, G. A., De Filippo, E., Pisano, G., Nasti, A., Bifulco, G., Contaldo, F., & Nappi, C. (2002). Menstrual status and serum leptin levels in anorectic and in menstruating women with low body mass indexes. *Fertility and Sterility, 78*(2), 376–382. https://doi.org/10.1016/s0015-0282(02)03221-1

Dossat, A. M., Bodell, L. P., Williams, D. L., Eckel, L. A., & Keel, P. K. (2015). Preliminary examination of glucagon-like peptide-1 levels in women with purging disorder and bulimia nervosa. *International Journal of Eating Disorders, 48*(2), 199–205. https://doi.org/10.1002/eat.22264

Duca, F. A., Katebzadeh, S., & Covasa, M. (2015). Impaired GLP-1 signaling contributes to reduced sensitivity to duodenal nutrients in obesity-prone rats during high-fat feeding. *Obesity, 23*(11), 2260–2268. https://doi.org/10.1002/oby.21231

Duca, F. A., Sakar, Y., & Covasa, M. (2013). Combination of obesity and high-fat feeding diminishes sensitivity to GLP-1R agonist exendin-4. *Diabetes, 62*(7), 2410–2415. https://doi.org/10.2337/db12-1204

Dynesen, A. W., Bardow, A., Astrup, A., Petersson, B., Holst, J. J., & Nauntofte, B. (2008). Meal-induced compositional changes in blood and saliva in persons with bulimia nervosa. *American Journal of Clinical Nutrition, 87*(1), 12–22. https://doi.org/10.1093/ajcn/87.1.12

Exner, C., Hebebrand, J., Remschmidt, H., Wewetzer, C., Ziegler, A., Herpertz, S., Schweiger, U., Blum, W. F., Preibisch, G., Heldmaier, G., & Klingenspor, M. (2000). Leptin suppresses semi-starvation induced hyperactivity in rats: Implications for anorexia nervosa. *Molecular Psychiatry, 5*(5), 476–481. https://doi.org/10.1038/sj.mp.4000771

Föcker, M., Timmesfeld, N., Scherag, S., Bühren, K., Langkamp, M., Dempfle, A., Sheridan, E. M., de Zwaan, M., Fleischhaker, C., Herzog, W., Egberts, K., Zipfel, S., Herpertz- Dahlmann, B., & Hebebrand, J. (2011). Screening for anorexia nervosa via measurement of serum leptin levels. *Journal of Neural Transmission, 118*(4), 571–578. https://doi.org/10.1007/s00702-010-0551-z

Foldi, C. J., Milton, L. K., & Oldfield, B. J. (2017). A focus on reward in anorexia nervosa through the lens of the activity-based anorexia rodent model. *Journal of Neuroendocrinology, 29*(10). 10.1111/jne.12479. https://doi.org/10.1111/jne.12479

François, M., Barde, S., Achamrah, N., Breton, J., Do Rego, J.-C., Coëffier, M., Hökfelt, T., Déchelotte, P., & Fetissov, S. O. (2015). The number of preproghrelin mRNA expressing cells is increased in mice with activity-based anorexia. *Neuropeptides, 51*, 17–23. https://doi.org/10.1016/j.npep.2015.04.003

François, M., & Zeltser, L. M. (2022). Rethinking the approach to preclinical models of anorexia nervosa. *Current Psychiatry Reports, 24*(1), 71–76. https://doi.org/10.1007/s11920-022-01319-2

Frank G. K. W. (2021). From desire to dread—A neurocircuitry based model for food avoidance in anorexia nervosa. *Journal of Clinical Medicine, 10*(11), 2228. https://doi.org/10.3390/jcm10112228

Geisler, C. E., & Hayes, M. R. (2023). Metabolic hormone action in the VTA: Reward-directed behavior and mechanistic insights. *Physiology & Behavior, 268*, 114236. https://doi.org/10.1016/j.physbeh.2023.114236

Gelegen, C., Collier, D. A., Campbell, I. C., Oppelaar, H., van den Heuvel, J., Adan, R. A. H., & Kas, M. J. H. (2007). Difference in susceptibility to activity-based anorexia in two inbred strains of mice. *European Neuropsychopharmacology, 17*(3), 199–205. https://doi.org/10.1016/j.euroneuro.2006.04.007

Geliebter, A., Gluck, M. E., & Hashim, S. A. (2005). Plasma ghrelin concentrations are lower in binge-eating disorder. *Journal of Nutrition, 135*(5), 1326–1330. https://doi.org/10.1093/jn/135.5.1326

Geliebter, A., Hashim, S. A., & Gluck, M. E. (2008). Appetite-related gut peptides, ghrelin, PYY, and GLP-1 in obese women with and without binge eating disorder (BED). *Physiology & Behavior, 94*(5), 696–699. https://doi.org/10.1016/j.physbeh.2008.04.013

Geliebter, A., Yahav, E. K., Gluck, M. E., & Hashim, S. A. (2004). Gastric capacity, test meal intake, and appetitive hormones in binge eating disorder. *Physiology & Behavior, 81*(5), 735–740. https://doi.org/10.1016/j.physbeh.2004.04.014

Geracioti, T. D., Kling, M. A., Joseph-Vanderpool, J. R., Kanayama, S., Rosenthal, N. E., Gold, P. W., & Liddle, R. A. (1989). Meal-related cholecystokinin secretion in eating and affective disorders. *Psychopharmacology Bulletin, 25*(3), 444–449.

Geracioti, T. D., & Liddle, R. A. (1988). Impaired cholecystokinin secretion in bulimia nervosa. *New England Journal of Medicine, 319*(11), 683–688. https://doi.org/10.1056/NEJM198809153191105

Geracioti, T. D., Liddle, R. A., Altemus, M., Demitrack, M. A., & Gold, P. W. (1992). Regulation of appetite and cholecystokinin secretion in anorexia nervosa. *American Journal of Psychiatry, 149*(7), 958–961. https://doi.org/10.1176/ajp.149.7.958

Germain, N., Galusca, B., Le Roux, C. W., Bossu, C., Ghatei, M. A., Lang, F., Bloom, S. R., & Estour, B. (2007). Constitutional thinness and lean anorexia nervosa display opposite concentrations of peptide YY, glucagon-like peptide 1, ghrelin, and leptin. *American Journal of Clinical Nutrition, 85*(4), 967–971. https://doi.org/10.1093/ajcn/85.4.967

Gharibeh, N., Chaumontet, C., Darcel, N., Fromentin, G., Denis, I., & Zeeni, N. (2022). Intermittent sucrose solution intake and its schedule of access modulate energy intake and weight gain in response to chronic variable stress in mice. *Appetite, 176*, 106123. https://doi.org/10.1016/j.appet.2022.106123

Gilman, T. L., Owens, W. A., George, C. M., Metzel, L., Vitela, M., Ferreira, L., Bowman, M. A., Gould, G. G., Toney, G. M., & Daws, L. C. (2019). Age- and sex-specific plasticity in dopamine transporter function revealed by food restriction and exercise in a rat activity-based anorexia paradigm. *Journal of Pharmacology and Experimental Therapeutics, 371*(2), 268–277. https://doi.org/10.1124/jpet.119.260794

Goel, N., Stunkard, A. J., Rogers, N. L., Van Dongen, H. P. A., Allison, K. C., O'Reardon, J. P., Ahima, R. S., Cummings, D. E., Heo, M., & Dinges, D. F. (2009). Circadian rhythm profiles in women with night eating syndrome. *Journal of Biological Rhythms, 24*(1), 85–94. https://doi.org/10.1177/0748730408328914

Hannon-Engel, S. L., Filin, E. E., & Wolfe, B. E. (2013). CCK response in bulimia nervosa and following remission. *Physiology & Behavior, 122*, 56–61. https://doi.org/10.1016/j.physbeh.2013.08.014

Hansen, T. K., Dall, R., Hosoda, H., Kojima, M., Kangawa, K., Christiansen, J. S., & Jørgensen, J. O. L. (2002). Weight loss increases circulating levels of ghrelin in human obesity. *Clinical Endocrinology, 56*(2), 203–206. https://doi.org/10.1046/j.0300-0664.2001.01456.x

Harty, R. F., Pearson, P. H., Solomon, T. E., & McGuigan, J. E. (1991). Cholecystokinin, vasoactive intestinal peptide and peptide histidine methionine responses to feeding in anorexia nervosa. *Regulatory Peptides, 36*(1), 141–150. https://doi.org/10.1016/0167-0115(91)90202-r

Hebebrand, J., Blum, W. F., Barth, N., Coners, H., Englaro, P., Juul, A., Ziegler, A., Warnke, A., Rascher, W., & Remschmidt, H. (1997). Leptin levels in patients with anorexia nervosa are reduced in the acute stage and elevated upon short-term weight restoration. *Molecular Psychiatry, 2*(4), 330–334. https://doi.org/10.1038/sj.mp.4000282

Hernandez, D., Mehta, N., & Geliebter, A. (2019). Meal-related acyl and des-acyl ghrelin and other appetite-related hormones in people with obesity and binge eating. *Obesity, 27*(4), 629–635. https://doi.org/10.1002/oby.22431

Heruc, G. A., Little, T. J., Kohn, M., Madden, S., Clarke, S., Horowitz, M., & Feinle-Bisset, C. (2018). Appetite perceptions, gastrointestinal symptoms, ghrelin, peptide yy and state anxiety are disturbed in adolescent females with anorexia nervosa and only partially restored with short-term refeeding. *Nutrients, 11*(1), 59. https://doi.org/10.3390/nu11010059

Hillebrand, J. J. G., Koeners, M. P., de Rijke, C. E., Kas, M. J. H., & Adan, R. A. H. (2005). Leptin treatment in activity-based anorexia. *Biological Psychiatry, 58*(2), 165–171. https://doi.org/10.1016/j.biopsych.2005.03.011

Holtkamp, K., Hebebrand, J., Mika, C., Grzella, I., Heer, M., Heussen, N., & Herpertz-Dahlmann, B. (2003). The effect of therapeutically induced weight gain on plasma leptin levels in patients with anorexia nervosa. *Journal of Psychiatric Research, 37*(2), 165–169. https://doi.org/10.1016/s0022-3956(02)00100-0

Holtkamp, K., Hebebrand, J., Mika, C., Heer, M., Heussen, N., & Herpertz-Dahlmann, B. (2004). High serum leptin levels subsequent to weight gain predict renewed weight loss in patients with anorexia nervosa. *Psychoneuroendocrinology, 29*(6), 791–797. https://doi.org/10.1016/S0306-4530(03)00143-4

Ilyas, A., Hübel, C., Stahl, D., Stadler, M., Ismail, K., Breen, G., Treasure, J., & Kan, C. (2019). The metabolic underpinning of eating disorders: A systematic review and meta-analysis of insulin sensitivity. *Molecular and Cellular Endocrinology, 497*, 110307. https://doi.org/10.1016/j.mce.2018.10.005

Jada, K., Djossi, S. K., Khedr, A., Neupane, B., Proskuriakova, E., & Mostafa, J. A. (2021). The pathophysiology of anorexia nervosa in hypothalamic endocrine function and bone metabolism. *Cureus, 13*(12), e20548. https://doi.org/10.7759/cureus.20548

Jimerson, D. C., Mantzoros, C., Wolfe, B. E., & Metzger, E. D. (2000). Decreased serum leptin in bulimia nervosa. The Journal of Clinical Endocrinology and *Metabolism, 85*(12), 4511–4514. https://doi.org/10.1210/jcem.85.12.7051

Jimerson, D. C., Wolfe, B. E., Carroll, D. P., & Keel, P. K. (2010). Psychobiology of purging disorder: Reduction in circulating leptin levels in purging disorder in comparison with controls. *International Journal of Eating Disorders, 43*(7), 584–588. https://doi.org/10.1002/eat.20738

Keel, P. K., Bodell, L. P., Forney, K. J., Appelbaum, J., & Williams, D. (2019). Examining weight suppression as a transdiagnostic factor influencing illness trajectory in bulimic eating disorders. *Physiology & Behavior, 208*, 112565. https://doi.org/10.1016/j.physbeh.2019.112565

Keel, P. K., Bodell, L. P., Haedt-Matt, A. A., Williams, D. L., & Appelbaum, J. (2017). Weight suppression and bulimic syndrome maintenance: Preliminary findings for the mediating role of leptin. *International Journal of Eating Disorders, 50*(12), 1432–1436. https://doi.org/10.1002/eat.22788

Keel, P. K., Eckel, L. A., Hildebrandt, B. A., Haedt-Matt, A. A., Appelbaum, J., & Jimerson, D. C. (2018). Disturbance of gut satiety peptide in purging disorder. *International Journal of Eating Disorders, 51*(1), 53–61. https://doi.org/10.1002/eat.22806

Keel, P. K., Wolfe, B. E., Liddle, R. A., De Young, K. P., & Jimerson, D. C. (2007). Clinical features and physiological response to a test meal in purging disorder and bulimia nervosa. *Archives of General Psychiatry, 64*(9), 1058–1066. https://doi.org/10.1001/archpsyc.64.9.1058

Kim, Y. R., Lauze, M. S., Slattery, M., Perlis, R. H., Holsen, L. M., Breithaupt, L., Stern, C. M., Fava, M., Thomas, J. J., Lawson, E. A., Misra, M., & Eddy, K. T. (2023). Association between ghrelin and body weight trajectory in individuals with anorexia nervosa. *JAMA Network Open, 6*(3), e234625. https://doi.org/10.1001/jamanetworkopen.2023.4625

King, S. J., Rodrigues, T., Watts, A., Murray, E., Wilson, A., & Abizaid, A. (2016). Investigation of a role for ghrelin signaling in binge-like feeding in mice under limited access to high-fat diet. *Neuroscience, 319*, 233–245. https://doi.org/10.1016/j.neuroscience.2016.01.004

Kinzig, K. P., Coughlin, J. W., Redgrave, G. W., Moran, T. H., & Guarda, A. S. (2007). Insulin, glucose, and pancreatic polypeptide responses to a test meal in restricting type anorexia nervosa before and after weight restoration. *American Journal of Physiology. Endocrinology and Metabolism, 292*(5), E1441–1446. https://doi.org/10.1152/ajpendo.00347.2006

Kinzig, K. P., Hargrave, S. L., & Honors, M. A. (2008). Binge-type eating attenuates corticosterone and hypophagic responses to restraint stress. *Physiology & Behavior, 95*(1–2), 108–113. https://doi.org/10.1016/j.physbeh.2008.04.026

Koda, S., Date, Y., Murakami, N., Shimbara, T., Hanada, T., Toshinai, K., Niijima, A., Furuya, M., Inomata, N., Osuye, K., & Nakazato, M. (2005). The role of the vagal nerve in peripheral PYY3-36-induced feeding reduction in rats. *Endocrinology, 146*(5), 2369–2375. https://doi.org/10.1210/en.2004-1266

Kojima, S., Nakahara, T., Nagai, N., Muranaga, T., Tanaka, M., Yasuhara, D., Masuda, A., Date, Y., Ueno, H., Nakazato, M., & Naruo, T. (2005). Altered ghrelin and peptide YY responses to meals in bulimia nervosa. *Clinical Endocrinology, 62*(1), 74–78. https://doi.org/10.1111/j.1365-2265.2004.02176.x

Krieger, J.-P. (2020). Intestinal glucagon-like peptide-1 effects on food intake: Physiological relevance and emerging mechanisms. *Peptides, 131*, 170342. https://doi.org/10.1016/j.peptides.2020.170342

le Roux, C. W., Neary, N. M., Halsey, T. J., Small, C. J., Martinez-Isla, A. M., Ghatei, M. A., Theodorou, N. A., & Bloom, S. R. (2005). Ghrelin does not stimulate food intake in patients with surgical procedures involving vagotomy. *Journal of Clinical Endocrinology and Metabolism, 90*(8), 4521–4524. https://doi.org/10.1210/jc.2004-2537

Lear, S. A., Pauly, R. P., & Birmingham, C. L. (1999). Body fat, caloric intake, and plasma leptin levels in women with anorexia nervosa. *International Journal of Eating Disorders, 26*(3), 283–288. https://doi.org/10.1002/(sici)1098-108x(199911)26:3<283::aid-eat5>3.0.co;2-k

Leenaerts, N., Jongen, D., Ceccarini, J., Van Oudenhove, L., & Vrieze, E. (2022). The neurobiological reward system and binge eating: A critical systematic review of neuroimaging studies. *International Journal of Eating Disorders, 55*(11), 1421–1458. https://doi.org/10.1002/eat.23776

Legrand, R., Lucas, N., Breton, J., Azhar, S., Do Rego, J.-C., Déchelotte, P., Coëffier, M., & Fetissov, S. O. (2016). Ghrelin treatment prevents development of activity based anorexia in mice. *European Neuropsychopharmacology, 26*(6), 948–958. https://doi.org/10.1016/j.euroneuro.2016.03.010

Letiexhe, M. R., Scheen, A. J., & Lefèbvre, P. J. (1997). Plasma leptin levels, insulin secretion, clearance and action on glucose metabolism in anorexia nervosa. *Eating and Weight Disorders, 2*(2), 79–86. https://doi.org/10.1007/BF03339953

Manara, F., Manara, A., & Todisco, P. (2005). Correlation between psychometric and biological parameters in anorexic and bulimic patients during and after an intensive day hospital treatment. *Eating and Weight Disorders, 10*(4), 236–244. https://doi.org/10.1007/BF03327490

Mancuso, C., Izquierdo, A., Slattery, M., Becker, K. R., Plessow, F., Thomas, J. J., Eddy, K. T., Lawson, E. A., & Misra, M. (2020). Changes in appetite-regulating hormones following food intake are associated with changes in reported appetite and a measure of hedonic eating in girls and young women with anorexia nervosa. *Psychoneuroendocrinology, 113*, 104556. https://doi.org/10.1016/j.psyneuen.2019.104556

Mantzoros, C., Flier, J. S., Lesem, M. D., Brewerton, T. D., & Jimerson, D. C. (1997). Cerebrospinal fluid leptin in anorexia nervosa: Correlation with nutritional status and potential role in resistance to weight gain. *Journal of Clinical Endocrinology and Metabolism, 82*(6), 1845–1851. https://doi.org/10.1210/jcem.82.6.4006

Maske, C. B., Coiduras, I. I., Ondriezek, Z. E., Terrill, S. J., & Williams, D. L. (2020). Intermittent high-fat diet intake reduces sensitivity to intragastric nutrient infusion and exogenous amylin in female rats. *Obesity, 28*(5), 942–952. https://doi.org/10.1002/oby.22779

Maske, C. B., Williams, D. L., & Keel, P. K. (2020). Preliminary examination of insulin and amylin levels in women with purging disorder. *International Journal of Eating Disorders, 53*(6), 997–1001. https://doi.org/10.1002/eat.23230

Mietlicki-Baase, E. G., McGrath, L. E., Koch-Laskowski, K., Krawczyk, J., Reiner, D. J., Pham, T., Nguyen, C. T. N., Turner, C. A., Olivos, D. R., Wimmer, M. E., Schmidt, H. D., & Hayes, M. R. (2017). Amylin receptor activation in the ventral tegmental area reduces motivated ingestive behavior. *Neuropharmacology, 123*, 67–79. https://doi.org/10.1016/j.neuropharm.2017.05.024

Misra, M., Golden, N. H., & Katzman, D. K. (2016). State of the art systematic review of bone disease in anorexia nervosa. *International Journal of Eating Disorders, 49*(3), 276–292. https://doi.org/10.1002/eat.22451

Monteleone, P., Di Lieto, A., Tortorella, A., Longobardi, N., & Maj, M. (2000). Circulating leptin in patients with anorexia nervosa, bulimia nervosa or binge-eating disorder: Relationship to body weight, eating patterns, psychopathology and endocrine changes. *Psychiatry Research, 94*(2), 121–129. https://doi.org/10.1016/s0165-1781(00)00144-x

Monteleone, P., Fabrazzo, M., Tortorella, A., Fuschino, A., & Maj, M. (2002). Opposite modifications in circulating leptin and soluble leptin receptor across the eating disorder spectrum. *Molecular Psychiatry, 7*(6), 641–646. https://doi.org/10.1038/sj.mp.4001043

Monteleone, P., Fabrazzo, M., Tortorella, A., Martiadis, V., Serritella, C., & Maj, M. (2005). Circulating ghrelin is decreased in non-obese and obese women with binge eating disorder as well as in obese non-binge eating women, but not in patients with bulimia nervosa. *Psychoneuroendocrinology, 30*(3), 243–250. https://doi.org/10.1016/j.psyneuen.2004.07.004

Monteleone, P., Martiadis, V., Colurcio, B., & Maj, M. (2002). Leptin secretion is related to chronicity and severity of the illness in bulimia nervosa. *Psychosomatic Medicine, 64*(6), 874–879. https://doi.org/10.1097/01.psy.0000024239.11538.a5

Monteleone, P., Martiadis, V., Fabrazzo, M., Serritella, C., & Maj, M. (2003). Ghrelin and leptin responses to food ingestion in bulimia nervosa: Implications for binge-eating and compensatory behaviours. *Psychological Medicine, 33*(8), 1387–1394. https://doi.org/10.1017/s0033291703008316

Monteleone, P., Martiadis, V., Rigamonti, A. E., Fabrazzo, M., Giordani, C., Muller, E. E., & Maj, M. (2005). Investigation of peptide YY and ghrelin responses to a test meal in bulimia nervosa. *Biological Psychiatry, 57*(8), 926–931. https://doi.org/10.1016/j.biopsych.2005.01.004

Monteleone, P., Serritella, C., Martiadis, V., Scognamiglio, P., & Maj, M. (2008). Plasma obestatin, ghrelin, and ghrelin/obestatin ratio are increased in underweight patients with anorexia nervosa but not in symptomatic patients with bulimia nervosa. *Journal of Clinical Endocrinology and Metabolism, 93*(11), 4418–4421. https://doi.org/10.1210/jc.2008-1138

Mukherjee, A., DiBrog, A. M., & Mietlicki-Baase, E. G. (2022). The impact of binge-like palatable food intake on the endogenous glucagon-like peptide-1 system in female rats. *Behavioural Brain Research, 428*, 113869. https://doi.org/10.1016/j.bbr.2022.113869

Mukherjee, A., Hum, A., Gustafson, T. J., & Mietlicki-Baase, E. G. (2020). Binge-like palatable food intake in rats reduces preproglucagon in the nucleus tractus solitarius. *Physiology & Behavior, 219*, 112830. https://doi.org/10.1016/j.physbeh.2020.112830

Munsch, S., Biedert, E., Meyer, A. H., Herpertz, S., & Beglinger, C. (2009). CCK, ghrelin, and PYY responses in individuals with binge eating disorder before and after a cognitive behavioral treatment (CBT). *Physiology & Behavior, 97*(1), 14–20. https://doi.org/10.1016/j.physbeh.2009.01.015

Myers, M. G., Leibel, R. L., Seeley, R. J., & Schwartz, M. W. (2010). Obesity and leptin resistance: Distinguishing cause from effect. *Trends in Endocrinology and Metabolism, 21*(11), 643–651. https://doi.org/10.1016/j.tem.2010.08.002

Naessén, S., Carlström, K., Holst, J. J., Hellström, P. M., & Hirschberg, A. L. (2011). Women with bulimia nervosa exhibit attenuated secretion of glucagon-like peptide 1, pancreatic polypeptide, and insulin in response to a meal. *American Journal of Clinical Nutrition, 94*(4), 967–972. https://doi.org/10.3945/ajcn.111.014837

Nakahara, T., Kojima, S., Tanaka, M., Yasuhara, D., Harada, T., Sagiyama, K., Muranaga, T., Nagai, N., Nakazato, M., Nozoe, S., Naruo, T., & Inui, A. (2007). Incomplete restoration of the secretion of ghrelin and PYY compared to insulin after food ingestion following weight gain in anorexia nervosa. *Journal of Psychiatric Research, 41*(10), 814–820. https://doi.org/10.1016/j.jpsychires.2006.07.021

Nakazato, M., Hashimoto, K., Shiina, A., Koizumi, H., Mitsumoti, M., Imai, M., Shimizu, E., & Iyo, M. (2004). No changes in serum ghrelin levels in female patients with bulimia nervosa. *Progress in Neuro-Psychopharmacology & Biological Psychiatry, 28*(7), 1181–1184. https://doi.org/10.1016/j.pnpbp.2004.06.012

Nozaki, T., Tamai, H., Matsubayashi, S., Komaki, G., Kobayashi, N., & Nakagawa, T. (1994). Insulin response to intravenous glucose in patients with anorexia nervosa showing low insulin response to oral glucose. *Journal of Clinical Endocrinology and Metabolism, 79*(1), 217–222. https://doi.org/10.1210/jcem.79.1.8027230

Oświecimska, J., Ziora, K., Geisler, G., & Broll-Waśka, K. (2005). Prospective evaluation of leptin and neuropeptide Y (NPY) serum levels in girls with anorexia nervosa. *Neuro Endocrinology Letters, 26*(4), 301–304.

Otto, B., Cuntz, U., Fruehauf, E., Wawarta, R., Folwaczny, C., Riepl, R. L., Heiman, M. L., Lehnert, P., Fichter, M., & Tschöp, M. (2001). Weight gain decreases elevated plasma ghrelin concentrations of patients with anorexia nervosa. *European Journal of Endocrinology, 145*(5), 669–673.

Otto, B., Cuntz, U., Otto, C., Heldwein, W., Riepl, R. L., & Tschöp, M. H. (2007). Peptide YY release in anorectic patients after liquid meal. *Appetite, 48*(3), 301–304. https://doi.org/10.1016/j.appet.2006.06.008

Overduin, J., Figlewicz, D., Bennett-Jay, J., Kittleson, S., & Cummings, D. (2012). Ghrelin increases the motivation to eat, but does not alter food palatability. *American Journal of Physiology. Regulatory, Integrative and Comparative Physiology, 303*(3). https://doi.org/10.1152/ajpregu.00488.2011

Pardo, M., Roca-Rivada, A., Al-Massadi, O., Seoane, L. M., Camiña, J. P., & Casanueva, F. F. (2010). Peripheral leptin and ghrelin receptors are regulated in a tissue-specific manner in activity-based anorexia. *Peptides, 31*(10), 1912–1919. https://doi.org/10.1016/j.peptides.2010.06.022

Phillipp, E., Pirke, K. M., Kellner, M. B., & Krieg, J. C. (1991). Disturbed cholecystokinin secretion in patients with eating disorders. *Life Sciences, 48*(25), 2443–2450. https://doi.org/10.1016/0024-3205(91)90379-p

Pirke, K. M., Kellner, M. B., Friess, E., Krieg, J. C., & Fichter, M. M. (1994). Satiety and cholecystokinin. *International Journal of Eating Disorders, 15*(1), 63–69. https://doi.org/10.1002/1098-108x(199401)15:1<63::aid-eat2260150108>3.0.co;2-v

Prince, A. C., Brooks, S. J., Stahl, D., & Treasure, J. (2009). Systematic review and meta- analysis of the baseline concentrations and physiologic responses of gut hormones to food in eating disorders. *American Journal of Clinical Nutrition, 89*(3), 755–765. https://doi.org/10.3945/ajcn.2008.27056

Raphael, F. J., Rodin, D. A., Peattie, A., Bano, G., Kent, A., Nussey, S. S., & Lacey, J. H. (1995). Ovarian morphology and insulin sensitivity in women with bulimia nervosa. *Clinical Endocrinology, 43*(4), 451–455. https://doi.org/10.1111/j.1365-2265.1995.tb02617.x

Raybould, H. E. (2007). Mechanisms of CCK signaling from gut to brain. *Current Opinion in Pharmacology, 7*(6), 570–574. https://doi.org/10.1016/j.coph.2007.09.006

Rehn, S., Raymond, J. S., Boakes, R. A., & Leenaars, C. H. C. (2022). A systematic review and meta-analysis of animal models of binge eating—Part 1: Definitions and food/drink intake outcomes. *Neuroscience and Biobehavioral Reviews, 132*, 1137–1156. https://doi.org/10.1016/j.neubiorev.2021.10.036

Riedy, C. A., Chavez, M., Figlewicz, D. P., & Woods, S. C. (1995). Central insulin enhances sensitivity to cholecystokinin. *Physiology & Behavior, 58*(4), 755–760. https://doi.org/10.1016/0031-9384(95)00108-u

Rosenhagen, M. C., Uhr, M., Schüssler, P., & Steiger, A. (2005). Elevated plasma ghrelin levels in night-eating syndrome. *American Journal of Psychiatry, 162*(4), 813. https://doi.org/10.1176/appi.ajp.162.4.813

Rossi, E., Cassioli, E., Gironi, V., Idrizaj, E., Garella, R., Squecco, R., Baccari, M. C., Maggi, M., Vignozzi, L., Comeglio, P., Ricca, V., & Castellini, G. (2021). Ghrelin as a possible biomarker and maintaining factor in patients with eating disorders reporting childhood traumatic experiences. *European Eating Disorders Review, 29*(4), 588–599. https://doi.org/10.1002/erv.2831

Sala, M., Keshishian, A., Song, S., Moskowitz, R., Bulik, C. M., Roos, C. R., & Levinson, C. A. (2023). Predictors of relapse in eating disorders: A meta-analysis. *Journal of Psychiatric Research, 158*, 281–299. https://doi.org/10.1016/j.jpsychires.2023.01.002

Sedlackova, D., Kopeckova, J., Papezova, H., Hainer, V., Kvasnickova, H., Hill, M., & Nedvidkova, J. (2012). Comparison of a high-carbohydrate and high-protein breakfast effect on plasma ghrelin, obestatin, NPY and PYY levels in women with anorexia and bulimia nervosa. *Nutrition & Metabolism, 9*(1), 52. https://doi.org/10.1186/1743-7075-9-52

Sedláčková, D., Kopečková, J., Papežová, H., Vybíral, S., Kvasničková, H., Hill, M., & Nedvídková, J. (2011). Changes of plasma obestatin, ghrelin and NPY in anorexia and bulimia nervosa patients before and after a high-carbohydrate breakfast. *Physiological Research, 60*(1), 165–173. https://doi.org/10.33549/physiolres.931952

Seidel, M., Markmann Jensen, S., Healy, D., Dureja, A., Watson, H. J., Holst, B., Bulik, C. M., & Sjögren, J. M. (2021). A systematic review and meta-analysis finds increased blood levels of all forms of ghrelin in both restricting and binge-eating/purging subtypes of anorexia nervosa. *Nutrients, 13*(2), 709. https://doi.org/10.3390/nu13020709

Skibicka, K. P., Hansson, C., Alvarez-Crespo, M., Friberg, P. A., & Dickson, S. L. (2011). Ghrelin directly targets the ventral tegmental area to increase food motivation. *Neuroscience, 180*, 129–137. https://doi.org/10.1016/j.neuroscience.2011.02.016

Spadini, S., Ferro, M., Lamanna, J., & Malgaroli, A. (2021). Activity-based anorexia animal model: A review of the main neurobiological findings. *Journal of Eating Disorders, 9*(1), 123. https://doi.org/10.1186/s40337-021-00481-x

Stadlbauer, U., Arnold, M., Weber, E., & Langhans, W. (2013). Possible mechanisms of circulating PYY-induced satiation in male rats. *Endocrinology, 154*(1), 193–204. https://doi.org/10.1210/en.2012-1956

Steinert, R. E., Feinle-Bisset, C., Asarian, L., Horowitz, M., Beglinger, C., & Geary, N. (2017). Ghrelin, CCK, GLP-1, and PYY(3-36): Secretory controls and physiological roles in eating and glycemia in health, obesity, and after RYGB. *Physiological Reviews, 97*(1), 411–463. https://doi.org/10.1152/physrev.00031.2014

Stice, E., Desjardins, C. D., & Rohde, P. (2022). Young women who develop anorexia nervosa exhibit a persistently low premorbid body weight on average: A longitudinal investigation of an important etiologic clue. *Journal of Psychopathology and Clinical Science, 131*(5), 479–492. https://doi.org/10.1037/abn0000762

Stice, E., Rohde, P., Shaw, H., & Desjardins, C. (2020). Weight suppression increases odds for future onset of anorexia nervosa, bulimia nervosa, and purging disorder, but not binge eating disorder. *American Journal of Clinical Nutrition, 112*(4), 941–947. https://doi.org/10.1093/ajcn/nqaa146

Stock, S., Leichner, P., Wong, A. C. K., Ghatei, M. A., Kieffer, T. J., Bloom, S. R., & Chanoine, J.-P. (2005). Ghrelin, peptide YY, glucose-dependent insulinotropic polypeptide, and hunger responses to a mixed meal in anorexic, obese, and control female adolescents. *Journal of Clinical Endocrinology and Metabolism, 90*(4), 2161–2168. https://doi.org/10.1210/jc.2004-1251

Stunkard, A. (2000). Two eating disorders: Binge eating disorder and the night eating syndrome. *Appetite, 34*(3), 333–334. https://doi.org/10.1006/appe.1999.0337

Succurro, E., Segura-Garcia, C., Ruffo, M., Caroleo, M., Rania, M., Aloi, M., De Fazio, P., Sesti, G., & Arturi, F. (2015). Obese patients with a binge eating disorder have an unfavorable metabolic and inflammatory profile. *Medicine, 94*(52), e2098. https://doi.org/10.1097/MD.0000000000002098

Tam, F. I., Seidel, M., Boehm, I., Ritschel, F., Bahnsen, K., Biemann, R., Weidner, K., Roessner, V., & Ehrlich, S. (2020). Peptide YY3-36 concentration in acute- and long-term recovered anorexia nervosa. *European Journal of Nutrition, 59*(8), 3791–3799. https://doi.org/10.1007/s00394-020-02210-7

Tanaka, M., Tatebe, Y., Nakahara, T., Yasuhara, D., Sagiyama, K., Muranaga, T., Ueno, H., Nakazato, M., Nozoe, S., & Naruo, T. (2003). Eating pattern and the effect of oral glucose on ghrelin and insulin secretion in patients with anorexia nervosa. *Clinical Endocrinology, 59*(5), 574–579. https://doi.org/10.1046/j.1365-2265.2003.01886.x

Tezenas du Montcel, C., Cao, J., Mattioni, J., Hamelin, H., Lebrun, N., Ramoz, N., Gorwood, P., Tolle, V., & Viltart, O. (2023). Chronic food restriction in mice and increased systemic ghrelin induce preference for running wheel activity. *Psychoneuroendocrinology, 155*, 106311. https://doi.org/10.1016/j.psyneuen.2023.106311

Tolle, V., Kadem, M., Bluet-Pajot, M.-T., Frere, D., Foulon, C., Bossu, C., Dardennes, R., Mounier, C., Zizzari, P., Lang, F., Epelbaum, J., & Estour, B. (2003). Balance in ghrelin and leptin plasma levels in anorexia nervosa patients and constitutionally thin women. *Journal of Clinical Endocrinology and Metabolism, 88*(1), 109–116. https://doi.org/10.1210/jc.2002-020645

Tomasik, P. J., Sztefko, K., & Starzyk, J. (2004). Cholecystokinin, glucose dependent insulinotropic peptide and glucagon-like peptide 1 secretion in children with anorexia nervosa and simple obesity. *Journal of Pediatric Endocrinology & Metabolism, 17*(12), 1623–1631. https://doi.org/10.1515/jpem.2004.17.12.1623

Tong, J., & D'Alessio, D. (2011). Eating disorders and gastrointestinal peptides. *Current Opinion in Endocrinology, Diabetes, and Obesity, 18*(1), 42–49. https://doi.org/10.1097/MED.0b013e328341e12b

Tschöp, M., Smiley, D. L., & Heiman, M. L. (2000). Ghrelin induces adiposity in rodents. *Nature, 407*(6806), 908–913. https://doi.org/10.1038/35038090

van Elburg, A. A., Kas, M. J. H., Hillebrand, J. J. G., Eijkemans, R. J. C., & van Engeland, H. (2007). The impact of hyperactivity and leptin on recovery from anorexia nervosa. *Journal of Neural Transmission, 114*(9), 1233–1237. https://doi.org/10.1007/s00702-007-0740-6

Verhagen, L. A. W., Egecioglu, E., Luijendijk, M. C. M., Hillebrand, J. J. G., Adan, R. A. H., & Dickson, S. L. (2011). Acute and chronic suppression of the central ghrelin signaling system reveals a role in food anticipatory activity. *European Neuropsychopharmacology, 21*(5), 384–392. https://doi.org/10.1016/j.euroneuro.2010.06.005

Wang, L., Barachina, M. D., Martínez, V., Wei, J. Y., & Taché, Y. (2000). Synergistic interaction between CCK and leptin to regulate food intake. *Regulatory Peptides, 92*(1–3), 79–85. https://doi.org/10.1016/s0167-0115(00)00153-1

Wang, Q., Liu, C., Uchida, A., Chuang, J.-C., Walker, A., Liu, T., Osborne-Lawrence, S., Mason, B. L., Mosher, C., Berglund, E. D., Elmquist, J. K., & Zigman, J. M. (2014). Arcuate AgRP neurons mediate orexigenic and glucoregulatory actions of ghrelin. *Molecular Metabolism, 3*(1), 64–72. https://doi.org/10.1016/j.molmet.2013.10.001

Watson, H. J., Yilmaz, Z., Thornton, L. M., Hübel, C., Coleman, J. R. I., Gaspar, H. A., Bryois, J., Hinney, A., Leppä, V. M., Mattheisen, M., Medland, S. E., Ripke, S., Yao, S., Giusti- Rodríguez, P., Anorexia Nervosa Genetics Initiative, Hanscombe, K. B., Purves, K. L., Eating Disorders Working Group of the Psychiatric Genomics Consortium, Adan, R. A. H., . . . Bulik, C. M. (2019). Genome-wide association study identifies eight risk loci and implicates metabo-psychiatric origins for anorexia nervosa. *Nature Genetics, 51*(8), 1207–1214. https://doi.org/10.1038/s41588-019-0439-2

Williams, D. L. (2022). The diverse effects of brain glucagon-like peptide 1 receptors on ingestive behaviour. *British Journal of Pharmacology, 179*(4), 571–583. https://doi.org/10.1111/bph.15535

Williams, D. L., Baskin, D. G., & Schwartz, M. W. (2006). Leptin regulation of the anorexic response to glucagon-like peptide-1 receptor stimulation. *Diabetes, 55*(12), 3387–3393. https://doi.org/10.2337/db06-0558

Williams, D. L., Hyvarinen, N., Lilly, N., Kay, K., Dossat, A., Parise, E., & Torregrossa, A.-M. (2011). Maintenance on a high-fat diet impairs the anorexic response to glucagon-like- peptide-1 receptor activation. *Physiology & Behavior, 103*(5), 557–564. https://doi.org/10.1016/j.physbeh.2011.04.005

Wojcik, M. H., Meenaghan, E., Lawson, E. A., Misra, M., Klibanski, A., & Miller, K. K. (2010). Reduced amylin levels are associated with low bone mineral density in women with anorexia nervosa. *Bone, 46*(3), 796–800. https://doi.org/10.1016/j.bone.2009.11.014

Wren, A. M., Seal, L. J., Cohen, M. A., Brynes, A. E., Frost, G. S., Murphy, K. G., Dhillo, W. S., Ghatei, M. A., & Bloom, S. R. (2001). Ghrelin enhances appetite and increases food intake in humans. *Journal of Clinical Endocrinology and Metabolism, 86*(12), 5992. https://doi.org/10.1210/jcem.86.12.8111

Wu, Y.-K., Brownley, K. A., Bardone-Cone, A. M., Bulik, C. M., & Baker, J. H. (2021). Associations of stress and appetite hormones with binge eating in females with anorexia nervosa after weight restoration: A longitudinal study. *Journal of Personalized Medicine, 11*(10), 1020. https://doi.org/10.3390/jpm11101020

Yagin, N. L., Aliasgari, F., Alizadeh, M., Aliasgharzadeh, S., & Mahdavi, R. (2020). Comparison of endocannabinoids levels, FAAH gene polymorphisms, and appetite regulatory substances in women with and without binge eating disorder: A cross-sectional study. *Nutrition Research, 83*, 86–93. https://doi.org/10.1016/j.nutres.2020.09.001

Yilmaz, Z., Gottfredson, N. C., Zerwas, S. C., Bulik, C. M., & Micali, N. (2019). Developmental premorbid body mass index trajectories of adolescents with eating disorders in a longitudinal population cohort. *Journal of the American Academy of Child and Adolescent Psychiatry, 58*(2), 191–199. https://doi.org/10.1016/j.jaac.2018.11.008

4

Genetics of Eating Disorders

Jet D. Termorshuizen, Stefana Aicoboaie, Mohamed Abdulkadir, and Zeynep Yilmaz

Brief Definitional Overview

Psychiatric genetics: The scientific field that investigates the interplay between genetic factors and psychiatric disorders, aiming to unravel their complex etiology.

Genome-wide association study: A research approach that systematically examines genetic variants across the entire genome to identify variants statistically associated with a disease or a trait, requiring large sample sizes to ensure statistical power and robustness.

Common disease–common variant hypothesis: The hypothesis that the genetic contribution to common disorders is likely due to numerous disease-causing variants with small effect sizes, occurring frequently in the population.

Biological Framework

Eating disorder genetic research has advanced in tandem with the field of *psychiatric genetics*, which focuses on elucidating the genetics of psychopathology. *Family* and *twin studies* have shown that eating disorders are heritable: on a population level, genetic differences account for a substantial proportion of the variation in eating disorders. This led many researchers to search for the genes that are responsible for this heritable component, first through *linkage and candidate gene association studies*, and later by *genome-wide association studies* (GWASs) and *epigenetic studies*. There are several GWAS applications/methodologies, including *cross-disorder* approaches and research on *polygenic scores* (PGS). Whereas GWAS typically focuses on common genetic variation, there are also other forms of genetic variation to study, such as *copy number variation* (CNV); and while GWAS typically uses genotyping arrays—capturing scattered bits of the genome—*sequencing methods* (cover complete sections of the genome). A glossary of key terms and abbreviations are provided in Table 4.1, and an overview of the most significant results for each section is summarized in Table 4.2.

Jet D. Termorshuizen et al., *Genetics of Eating Disorders*. In: *The Handbook of the Neurobiology of Eating Disorders*. Edited by: Christina E. Wierenga and Joanna E. Steinglass, Oxford University Press.
DOI: 10.1093/9780197675212.003.0005

Table 4.1 Glossary providing the definitions of key terms and abbreviations

Term/Abbreviation	Definition
Base pair	A connection between nitrogenous bases (A, C, G, and T) that holds two nucleotides together in DNA
CNV	Copy number variant
De novo mutation	A spontaneously occurring mutation not inherited from a parent
DNA	Deoxyribonucleic acid
EWAS	Exome-wide association analysis
Exome	Protein coding DNA region
Genome	The complete genetic material in a cell
GWAS	Genome-wide association study
Locus (plural: loci)	Physical position of a gene or DNA sequence on a chromosome
LD	Linkage disequilibrium
PGC	Psychiatric Genomics Consortium
PGS	Polygenic score
SNP	Single nucleotide polymorphism; a single base pair difference at a specific location of the DNA sequence

Table 4.2 An overview of the most notable genetic findings in eating disorders.

Category	Summary of Findings
Family studies	**AN:** The relative risk for AN is four times higher in relatives of AN probands and female relatives are eleven times more likely to develop AN compared to individuals without AN relatives. **BN:** The relative risk for BN is 4.4–9.6 times higher in relatives of BN probands compared to individuals without BN relatives. **BED:** The relative risk for BED is 2.2 times higher in relatives of BED probands compared to individuals without BED relatives. **ARFID:** –
Twin studies	**AN:** Heritability estimate: 0.48–0.74 **BN:** Heritability estimate: 0.55–0.62 **BED:** Heritability estimate: 0.39–0.45 **ARFID:** Heritability estimate: 0.79
Linkage studies	**AN:** Suggestive evidence for linkage on chromosome 1 for AN and chromosome 4 for AN restricting subtype has been reported. **BN/BED/ARFID:** –
Candidate gene association studies	**AN/BN/BED:** Various genes hypothesized to play a role in eating, mood, sleep, appetite, hunger, neuroplasticity, and sex hormones have been studied (especially in AN and BN) in small samples, but results have failed to consistently replicate. **ARFID:** –

continued

Table 4.2 *continued*

Category	Summary of Findings
GWAS	**AN:** Eight genome-wide significant loci have been identified in 16,992 cases and 55,525 controls, providing strong evidence for the role of polygenicity in the genetic architecture of AN and encouraging the reconceptualization of AN as a metabo-psychiatric disorder. **BN/BED/ARFID:** —
Cross-disorder approaches	**AN:** Significant positive genetic correlations with psychiatric phenotypes, education, physical activity, and high-density lipoprotein have been reported. Additionally, significant negative genetic correlations with metabolic and anthropometric traits such as body mass index (which may be bidirectionally causal with AN) have been observed. Cross-disorder GWASs identified numerous shared loci across psychiatric disorders including AN. **BN/ BED/ARFID:** —
PGS	**AN PGS:** AN PGS is significantly associated with AN diagnosis; no differences in AN PGS have been found between male and female AN cases or AN subtypes. Higher AN PGS has also been associated with weight loss trajectory, slower growth during childhood, emotional eating, separation anxiety, and compulsive exercise during development in the general population. **BN/BED/ARFID PGS:** —
Copy number variation	**AN:** Deletions in chromosome 13q12, microduplications in chromosome 15q11.2, and copy number variants with at least 50% reciprocal overlap with regions associated with psychiatric and neurodevelopmental disorders have been observed in a small number of AN cases. **BN/BED/ARFID:** —
High-throughput sequencing	**AN/BN:** Rare variants in genes pertaining to estrogen, dopamine, reward pathways, neural differentiation, neuropeptide hormone signaling, inflammatory pathways, and cholinergic neurotransmission have been identified in a small number of eating disorder cases (predominantly AN) in pedigrees. **BED/ARFID:** —
Epigenetic studies	**AN:** Altered methylation levels observed in genes involved in a range of psychological, metabolic and physical functions (e.g., dopamine and glutamate signaling; cholesterol storage; lipid transport) in small studies. **BN:** No differences in global methylation levels have been reported compared to controls. **BED/ARFID:** —

Abbreviations: AN = anorexia nervosa; BN = bulimia nervosa; BED = binge-eating disorder; ARFID = avoidant/restrictive food intake disorder; GWAS = genome-wide association study; PGS = polygenic score.

The application of GWAS methodology has significantly advanced knowledge about psychiatric disorders, including eating disorders. The Psychiatric Genomics Consortium (PGC) has been crucial in this effort and focuses on elucidating fundamental biology, guiding clinical practice, and discovering therapeutic targets (O'Donovan, 2015). Since the first use of GWAS methodology in psychiatric research in 2008, it has become evident that common psychiatric disorders with a prevalence of 1% to 5% are considerably influenced by common genetic variation, supporting the *Common Disease-Common Variant Hypothesis* (Sullivan et al., 2018). All complex traits, including eating disorders, are likely substantially influenced by hundreds, or even thousands, of genetic variants, each with a small effect. The identification of these common genetic variants will likely improve understanding of eating disorder biology, advance the generation and potential clinical application of polygenic scores, and will enhance understanding of gene-environment interplay in the etiology of eating disorders.

State of the Science in Eating Disorders

Family and twin studies

Family studies assess whether individuals have a higher risk of developing a disorder if they have family members with the disorder (i.e., affected relatives) compared to individuals without affected relatives or the general population (Thornton et al., 2011). Family members of anorexia nervosa (AN) probands are at a fourfold increased risk for AN compared to individuals without relatives with AN (Steinhausen et al., 2015), with female relatives of AN probands being 11 times more likely to develop AN compared to individuals without relatives with AN (Strober et al., 2000). Relatives of bulimia nervosa (BN) probands are at a 4.4 (Strober et al., 2000) to 9.6 (Kassett et al., 1989) times greater risk of developing BN compared to individuals without BN probands, while early research showed a non-significant incidence increase in the prevalence of eating disorders in the families of BN probands (Hudson et al., 1987). Binge-eating disorder (BED) is also reported to aggregate within families (Fowler & Bulik, 1997) independent of obesity (Hudson et al., 2006).

Family studies can also evaluate cross-disorder eating disorder risk. For instance, relatives of AN or BN probands are at increased risk for either threshold or subthreshold AN and BN compared with relatives of controls (Strober et al., 2000), suggesting that AN and BN might share genetic risk (Lilenfeld et al., 1998) and that eating disorders may be expressed as a broad spectrum of eating-related pathology in families (Thornton et al., 2011). Of note, BN and AN restricting subtype might have significantly lower degree of genetic overlap compared to BN and AN binge eating/purging subtype (Grigoroiu-Serbanescu et al., 2003).

While family studies have made significant contributions to our understanding of the heritability of eating disorders, they cannot provide conclusive evidence that genetic factors play a role in the etiology of the disorder as the aggregation of the trait in a family could be explained by either genetic or environmental factors, and more likely, a combination of the two (Thornton et al., 2011). Twin studies can address this limitation or help us disentangle the effect of genetic factors from shared and unique environmental factors (Thornton et al., 2011) by comparing the similarities and differences between monozygotic and dizygotic twins (Slof-Op 't Landt et al., 2005). Studies have estimated the twin-based heritability of AN to be between 0.48 and 0.74 (Bulik et al., 2006; Bulik et al., 2010; Dellava et al., 2011; Kipman et al., 1999; Klump et al., 2001; Kortegaard et al., 2001; Wade et al., 2000), with the heritability of strictly defined AN (i.e., cases meeting all diagnostic criteria for AN) being higher than the heritability of broadly defined AN (i.e., subthreshold cases that do not meet all diagnostic criteria for AN) (Bulik et al., 2010; Dellava et al., 2011). BN also has a notable genetic component, with heritability estimates in the range of 0.55 and 0.62 (Bulik et al., 1998; Bulik et al., 2010; Kortegaard et al., 2001; Trace, Thornton, et al., 2013). As for BED, the heritability estimates range from 0.39 to 0.45 (Javaras et al., 2008; Mitchell et al., 2010), while the estimates for binge-eating behavior vary between 0.17 and 0.49 (Bulik et al., 2003; Munn et al., 2010; Reichborn-Kjennerud et al., 2004; Sullivan et al., 1998; Wade et al., 2008), with higher estimates for men compared to women (Root et al., 2010). While not as widely examined as the other eating disorders, a nationwide Swedish twin study showed the heritability of avoidant/restrictive food intake disorder (ARFID) to be 0.79 (Dinkler et al., 2023), although the heritability of ARFID-related phenotypes (e.g., nutrient intake, food fussiness, rejection of unfamiliar food, appetite) may be lower than for the ARFID diagnosis (Cooke et al., 2007; Fildes et al., 2016; Knaapila et al., 2007; Liu et al., 2013; Llewellyn et al., 2010; Smith et al., 2017). Finally, a large population-based twin study estimated the heritability of disordered eating behaviors and dysfunctional eating attitudes to be 0.43 to 0.49 (Munn et al., 2010).

Overall, family and twin studies provide us with crucial information toward understanding the heritability of eating disorders. This knowledge can in turn inform molecular genetic studies that have the power to identify specific genetic risk and thus elucidate the biological underpinning of eating disorder risk and maintenance (Thornton et al., 2011).

Linkage and candidate gene association studies

The classical approach to identifying genes for genetic disorders has historically involved family-based linkage analysis (Ott et al., 2015), which involves scanning the genome (using genetic markers) in a hypothesis-free manner to identify large segments of the genome that co-segregate with the trait of interest within a family. For AN, suggestive evidence for linkage on chromosomes 1 (AN) and 4 (AN restricting subtype) has been reported (Grice et al., 2002). While linkage analysis has been highly successful for single-gene disorders (Lipner & Greenberg, 2018), eating disorders—as will be reviewed in "Cross-disorder approaches"—have a complex genetic architecture involving many common genetic variants of small effect sizes (Bulik et al., 2022; Yilmaz et al., 2015), which are ill-suited for linkage analysis (Ott et al., 2015). Furthermore, recruiting multiple affected large families with an eating disorder is required for a well-powered linkage study (Chen & Abecasis, 2006), which has proven to be challenging.

In contrast to the whole-genome approach of family-based linkage studies, candidate gene association approach—carried out in unrelated individuals—focuses on genes with known biological functions hypothesized to be relevant to eating disorders or implicated in other psychiatric disorders (Helder & Collier, 2011; Trace, Baker, et al., 2013; Yilmaz et al., 2015). However, this method faces challenges due to the vast number of human genes, as the human genome is estimated to contain 19,969 protein-coding genes (Nurk et al., 2022) and the limited prior probability of association of a handful of genes that are being investigated. Despite these difficulties, candidate gene studies have been carried out extensively, particularly in AN (Yilmaz et al., 2015), often exploring neurotransmitter systems, hunger and appetite hormones, sex hormones, and neurotrophic factors (Watson et al., 2021; Yilmaz et al., 2015), yielding limited success. Notably, the largest candidate gene association replication study in AN examining 182 previously implicated genes found no associations after accounting for multiple testing (Pinheiro et al., 2010). The lack of consistent replication of candidate gene association studies, which has also been the case for other psychiatric disorders (Sullivan et al., 2018), may be attributed to factors such as small sample sizes, limited scope based on flawed hypotheses in gene or variant selection, methodological heterogeneity, and potential population stratification (Hübel et al., 2018).

Genome-wide association studies

GWASs have been, and continue to be, invaluable in facilitating gene discovery for complex traits such as eating disorders. GWAS leverages common variations in the form of single nucleotide polymorphisms (SNPs). SNPs are changes at specific spots in the genome that occur in a single base pair—A, C, G, or T—generally existing in more than 1% of the studied population. In other words, the less common (or *minor*) allele frequency is >1% for SNPs, but genetic variation can be rare (e.g., occurring in 0.01% of the population) or very common (e.g., occurring in as many as 50% of the population). GWAS comprises a hypothesis-free scan of the entire genome, tagging the genome strategically through hundreds of thousands of SNPs to provide a thorough coverage while taking advantage of the highly correlated structure of neighboring variants (a phenomenon referred to as linkage disequilibrium) and imputation methods. Most importantly, large sample sizes (i.e., ideally tens of thousands of unrelated individuals) are necessary to accurately detect and assess the effects of common variants, which are often present in controls as well as cases and therefore typically have small effect sizes. In addition, because over a million SNPs are tested, a stringent statistical correction is crucial to avoid false-positives, setting the genome-wide significance threshold to $p < 5 \times 10^{-8}$, determined by the number of independent common SNPs across the genome of European-ancestry individuals (Fadista et al., 2016).

To date, we know most about AN genomics, but global efforts are underway to expand GWAS efforts to other eating disorders. Early efforts suffered from significant limitations in sample size and methodological issues. An initial genome-wide microsatellite study of AN (Nakabayashi et al., 2009) reported associations with two loci, but results should be cautiously interpreted especially given the small sample size (320 AN cases and 341 controls), inadequate adjustment for multiple testing, and the use of DNA pooling which is susceptible to sequencing errors. Subsequent AN GWASs with larger sample sizes, comprising 1,033 cases and 3,733 controls (Wang et al., 2011)—and later, 2,907 cases and 14,860 controls (Boraska et al., 2014)— also did not yield genome-wide significant loci. A significant step forward in AN gene discovery was achieved by the two most recent AN GWASs under the umbrella of the Psychiatric Genomics Consortium Eating Disorders Working Group (PGC-ED). The Freeze 1 GWAS comprised 3,495 AN cases and 10,982 controls and identified one genome-wide significant SNP previously linked to type 1 diabetes and rheumatoid arthritis (Duncan et al., 2017). Furthermore, this was the first study to suggest that genetic factors influencing AN may also influence other psychiatric, anthropometric, and metabolic traits.

Building upon previous findings, the Freeze 2 PGC-ED AN GWAS—the largest AN GWAS published to date—expanded the sample size to 16,992 AN cases and 55,525 controls, leading to the discovery of eight genome-wide significant SNPs (Watson et al., 2019). This study further replicated previously reported genetic correlations (see the "Cross-disorder approaches" section of this chapter), showing genetic overlap between AN and psychiatric disorders. Importantly, the observation of the genetic overlap between AN and anthropometric and metabolic traits suggests a role for metabolic factors in the etiology of AN. Whereas PGC-ED Freeze 1 AN GWAS (Duncan et al., 2017) proposed shared genetics underlying extreme weight dysregulation, the newer findings suggest that metabolic factors may act on AN independently of body mass index (BMI) and potentially contribute to the pathophysiology of the disorder.

Two additional GWASs focused on studying eating disorder symptoms and related traits. The first study (Boraska et al., 2012) investigated the drive for thinness, body dissatisfaction, bulimia, weight fluctuation, breakfast skipping, and obsessive-compulsive personality disorder traits. The second study (Wade et al., 2013) aimed to identify genetic variants related to distinct eating disorder spectrums, including AN spectrum, BN spectrum, purging via substances, and disordered eating behaviors, established based on factor analyses. However, neither study identified genome-wide significant loci.

In sum, GWAS has proven to be a highly successful approach in complex traits genomics and significantly contributed to our understanding of the genetic architecture of AN. GWASs provide fundamental information through variant discovery and serve as an empirical starting point for follow-up studies to answer in-depth questions about genetic architecture, gene pathways and expression, functional annotation, tissue expression, and other inquiries geared toward dissecting the biological underpinnings of eating disorders.

Cross-disorder approaches

Recent developments in analytical tools have also made it possible to examine the genetic architecture of complex traits in relation to each other, allowing for the assessment of unique and shared genetic contributions. We will briefly summarize three methods: (1) genetic correlations; (2) cross-disorder GWAS; and (3) Mendelian randomization. PGS can also be used for cross-disorder examinations, which is covered in more detail in the "Polygenic Scoring" section of this chapter.

Genetic correlations

Genetic correlations allow for the pair-wise examination of the genetic overlap between complex traits for which GWAS results are available and do not require individual-level genetic data. A significant positive genetic correlation indicates that the genetic variants cumulatively increasing risk for one disorder also act in the same direction for the other disorder, whereas a significant negative genetic correlation means that the genetic variants cumulatively increasing risk for one disorder act in the opposite direction for the other disorder. The PGC-ED Freeze 2 AN GWAS examined 447 complex traits in relation to AN and revealed a range of intriguing significant genetic correlations (Watson et al., 2019). Specifically, positive genetic correlations were observed for AN with other psychiatric disorders such as schizophrenia, depression, anxiety, neuroticism, and obsessive-compulsive disorder (OCD)—yielding the most significant genetic overlap with AN—in line with the comorbidities reported in clinical and epidemiological studies. Additional significant positive genetic correlations were observed for AN with educational attainment, physical activity, and high-density lipoprotein. Intriguingly, the results also showed that AN may differ from other psychiatric disorders based on the negative genetic correlations with metabolic and anthropometric traits such as type 2 diabetes, insulin, leptin, fat mass, obesity, and BMI. These findings suggest that AN may be driven, at least in part, by metabolic mechanisms, leading some to consider the reconceptualization of AN as a metabo-psychiatric disorder (Bulik, Carroll, et al., 2021). Furthermore, the genetic correlation with body fat percentage appears to be stronger in female AN cases than male AN cases (Hübel, Gaspar, et al., 2019). A separate study reported a positive genetic correlation for AN and AN with binge eating with cannabis initiation, whereas smoking phenotypes had a negative genetic correlation with AN without binge eating (Munn-Chernoff et al., 2021).

Cross-disorder GWAS

Comorbidity among psychiatric disorders is common (Kessler et al., 2005; McGrath et al., 2020; Plana-Ripoll et al., 2019), and eating disorders are no exception (Momen et al., 2022). Many psychiatric diagnoses also have notable symptom overlap, and no biomarkers have been identified for psychiatric disorders, making accurate and differential diagnosis difficult. The high degree of genetic correlations among psychiatric disorders mirrors these clinical comorbidities (Anttila et al., 2018; Bulik-Sullivan et al., 2015; Cross-Disorder Group of the Psychiatric Genomics Consortium, 2019), providing additional challenges when it comes to the unique biological underpinnings of each disorder. Cross-disorder GWAS leverages the genetic overlap between two or more disorders to boost sample size for gene discovery. Three large-scale cross-disorder GWASs have been published to date (Cross-Disorder Group of the Psychiatric Genomics Consortium, 2013b, 2019; Cross-Disorder Phenotype Group of the Psychiatric et al., 2009), with the most recent one discovering more than 100 regions involved in more than one disorder and a region on chromosome 18 showing associations across all eight psychiatric disorders (AN, schizophrenia, bipolar disorder, major depressive disorder, attention-deficit/hyperactivity disorder, autism spectrum disorder, OCD, and Tourette syndrome) (Cross-Disorder Group of the Psychiatric Genomics Consortium, 2019). A more recent cross-disorder conditional GWAS analysis identified 58 novel AN loci; 38 unique loci shared between AN and schizophrenia, bipolar disorder, and major depressive disorder; and 45 loci shared between AN and traits such as mood instability and neuroticism (Bang et al., 2023). Considering the high degree of genetic overlap between AN and OCD and their notable comorbidity, two cross-disorder GWASs of AN and OCD have been published (Yilmaz et al., 2020; Yilmaz et al., 2023), with the most recent analysis of 19,680 AN or OCD cases and 62,556 controls reporting seven genome-wide significant loci, three of which were not previously identified in the AN and OCD disorder-specific GWASs (Yilmaz et al., 2023).

Mendelian randomization

Mendelian randomization employs genome-wide significant SNPs from GWAS as independent instrumental variables for a specific exposure to assess the extent to which the exposure is causally linked to the outcome (Smith & Ebrahim, 2003). To date, a causal bidirectional link between AN and BMI has been reported, suggesting that the genetic risk variants associated with AN are linked to lower BMI, whereby variants associated with lower BMI are associated with a higher risk of AN (Watson et al., 2019). For the time being, caution is advised in interpreting these and other Mendelian randomization results pertaining to AN and other eating disorder phenotypes because the strength of genetic instruments in Mendelian randomization is determined by well-powered GWAS and the presence of more than 30 genome-wide significant hits (Zhu et al., 2018).

Polygenic scoring

PGS is one of several applications of results obtained from GWAS and provides an individualized estimate of genetic risk for a certain trait, assessed using risk variants (see Figure 4.1 for a simplified illustration of the PGS concept). In practice, PGS is calculated by adding the risk-increasing genetic variants, weighted by their effect size estimates, from a discovery GWAS and can be used to predict a target phenotype same as or different from the discovery GWAS phenotype in an independent cohort without sample overlap (e.g., developing BMI PGS from BMI GWAS to predict AN risk). Importantly, PGS allows for the investigation of evidence for association from SNPs that do not necessarily reach the stringent threshold for genome-wide significance (Wray et al., 2007). Application of PGS is an emerging field that has seen a very sharp increase in the number of publications in the recent years, and considering the wide range of uses of PGS, this section will provide a very brief overview of the studies with large sample sizes and prioritize findings pertaining to AN PGS—the only eating disorder PGS available to date because no GWASs have been published in other eating disorders.

Individuals with AN have been shown to have a higher AN PGS than controls (Watson et al., 2019), providing evidence for the polygenic architecture of AN and the validity of AN PGS. AN PGS has also been used to study the

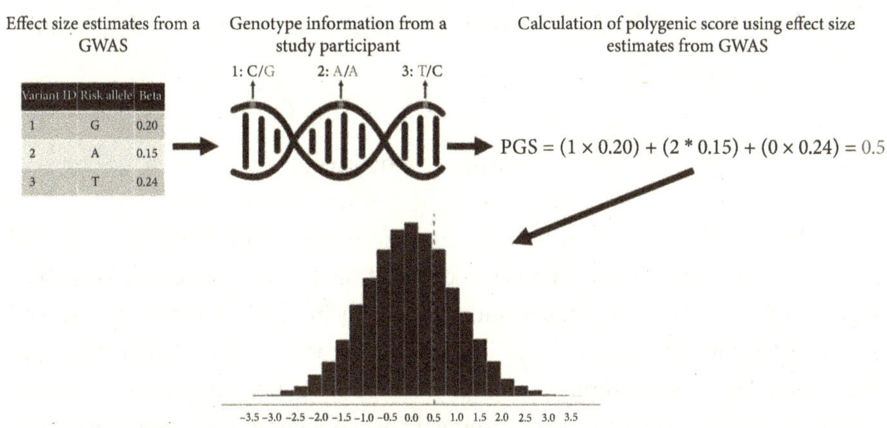

Figure 4.1 Simplified illustration of polygenic score (PGS) calculation for a phenotype using effect size estimates from three hypothetical genetic variants. In this example, the study participant has one copy of the risk allele of variant 1, two copies of the risk allele of variant 2, and no copies of the risk allele of variant 3, bringing the total of the PGS to 0.5 based on the effect size estimate associated with each risk variant. PGS is normally distributed after standardizing the scores and, through the visual examination of the distribution of PGSs across the study population, it is evident that this participant has a slightly higher PGS, and therefore a higher genetic load, for the phenotype of interest compared to the mean of the study population. *Abbreviations: GWAS = genome-wide association study.*

differences/similarities between eating disorder diagnoses, symptoms, and related traits. For instance, no differences have been found between AN cases with binge eating versus without binge eating in terms of their AN PGS (Watson et al., 2019). Our current sample size for AN PGS may be insufficient to predict disease course, whereas BMI PGS—which has much better statistical power—has been shown to be associated with severe and enduring eating disorders (Johansson et al., 2022). From a developmental perspective, higher AN PGS has been associated with slower growth during childhood (Abdulkadir et al., 2022) and weight loss trajectory among individuals without eating disorder diagnoses (Xu et al., 2022). Researchers also reported associations of AN PGS with emotional eating, separation anxiety, and compulsive exercise during development (Yilmaz et al., 2023). Interestingly, higher AN PGS is also associated with increased surface area of several brain regions in the prefrontal cortex including the lateral orbitofrontal cortex in participants with no eating disorder history (Leehr et al., 2019).

Additionally, there is particular interest in studying the genetic overlap between eating disorders and psychiatric, anthropometric, and metabolic traits, especially considering the genetic correlations discussed in the "Cross-disorder approaches" section of this chapter. One study using UK Biobank data calculated PGS for 269 traits and reported similar pattern of PGS associations for BN and BED regarding psychiatric and anthropometric traits (Hübel et al., 2021). Taken together, these genetic findings are in line with the clinical comorbidities of eating disorders and have the potential to serve as an important tool to uncover previously unknown correlates with other traits to further deepen our understanding of eating disorders.

Copy number variation

CNVs alter the number of copies of a genomic region in the form of additional copies of a sequence being present (i.e., duplications) or loss of genetic code (i.e., deletions). CNVs can be rare or common (especially in "CNV hotspots"), inherited or *de novo* (occurring spontaneously in the offspring and not found in the parents), affect a single gene or encompass multiple contiguous genes, and vary in size from a few base-pairs to an entire chromosome. Especially larger and rarer CNVs may alter DNA quantity, potentially impacting gene dosage, and are therefore more likely to have deleterious impact.

To date, two genome-wide CNV studies have been published in eating disorders, both of which focused on AN. The first study, comprising 1,033 AN cases and 3,773 controls, found no difference in CNV burden between AN cases and controls but reported a recurrent large deletion in chromosome 13q12 in two AN cases. The authors also identified CNVs disrupting the *CNTN6/CNTN4* region in multiple AN cases (Wang et al., 2011). The second study—the largest of its kind with 1,983 AN cases—similarly reported a large deletion in the 13q12 region in one AN case, as well as CNVs with at least 50% reciprocal overlap with regions associated with psychiatric and neurodevelopmental disorders in two AN cases (Yilmaz et al., 2017). More recently, another more targeted CNV analysis reported a significant association between AN and a microduplication in chromosome 15q11.2, previously linked to schizophrenia and autism (Chang et al., 2019). These results need to be replicated in larger independent samples, as there was significant case overlap among the three studies. Future efforts should also focus on structural variation in BN, BED, and ARFID, as our knowledge of the genetic architectures of these eating disorders is lagging.

High-throughput sequencing

GWAS primarily examines common genetic variations by genotyping up to millions of markers across the genome; however, it is not well-suited for studying rare variation. Rare variants are more likely to have a significant impact but may only relate to disease in a small subset of individuals due to their low frequency. High-throughput sequencing methods, such as exome sequencing and whole-genome sequencing, are the primary modern approaches for studying rare variations. Exome sequencing targets only gene exons, while whole-genome sequencing provides an individual's complete DNA sequence.

High-throughput sequencing of candidate genes has revealed associations involving the estrogen receptor 2 (*ESR2*) and the epoxide hydrolase 2 receptor (*EPHX2*) genes, shown to be associated with depression and anxiety in AN cases (Scott-Van Zeeland et al., 2014). Additionally, linkage analysis in combination with whole genome sequencing identified a missense mutation in the estrogen-related receptor alpha (*ESSRA*) in two families with multiple cases of eating disorders (Cui et al., 2013). Exome sequencing in the same two families also detected a potentially deleterious rare variant in the histone deacetylase 4 (*HDAC4*) gene, known to be involved in the estrogen system (Cui et al., 2013). A family whole-exome analysis of 144 females and eight males identified variants in the *NNAT* genes in two of the male AN cases—one nonsense variant and one rare variant in the 5'UTR (Lombardi et al., 2019). A more recent whole exome sequencing study detected ultra-rare deleterious variants of three reward-pathway related genes (*DRD4, NMS,* and *CCKAR)* in a family with three AN probands (Bienvenu et al., 2019). *De novo* missense mutations in genes involved in neuron differentiation and dopamine pathways have also been reported in nine AN probands (Bienvenu et al., 2020). One AN whole-exome sequencing study suggested grouping the mutated genes into three categories: neuropeptide hormone signaling, inflammatory pathways, and cholinergic neurotransmission (Lutter et al., 2017), which better fits with the complex AN etiology and its systemic impact.

Sequencing studies have the potential to elucidate the role of rare variants with deleterious effects, adding to our growing knowledge of the contribution of common variants on disease risk in the general population. Replication in independent samples of comparable sizes to GWAS is required to assess the validity of the findings outlined in this section for eating disorder pathophysiology (Munn-Chernoff et al., 2016).

Epigenetic studies

Epigenetics explores how cells regulate gene activity without altering the DNA sequence, leading to changes that influence gene expression while preserving the genetic code. Epigenetic change is an all-encompassing term that refers to DNA methylation, histone modification, and gene regulation at the transcriptional and post-transcriptional level by non-coding RNAs (Himmerich et al., 2019). Epigenetic factors are generally studied peripherally (blood, buccal cells, and saliva) through measures of global methylation, candidate gene approach or epigenome-wide association studies (EWAS).

Research is still inconclusive on the status of global methylation in patients with eating disorders, with some studies reporting global hypomethylation—which upregulates gene expression—in individuals with AN compared to controls (Frieling et al., 2007; Tremolizzo et al., 2014) with others reporting hypermethylation—which downregulates gene expression—(Booij et al., 2015) or no difference (Hübel, Marzi, et al., 2019). The limited literature on BN shows similar global DNA methylation levels compared with controls (Frieling et al., 2007), and others eating disorders have yet to be studied in terms of global methylation. Candidate gene methylation studies in AN to date, often conducted in small samples, tentatively suggest hypermethylation of genes for α-synuclein (Frieling et al., 2007), natriuretic peptide (Frieling et al., 2008), dopamine function (Frieling et al., 2010), and oxytocin (Kim et al., 2014). Preliminary methylation changes in BN and bulimia-spectrum patients resemble the variations observed in conditions often comorbid with BN, suggesting these changes may not be BN-specific (Groleau et al., 2012; Steiger et al., 2013). Just like candidate gene association studies, candidate gene methylation studies should also be interpreted with caution as they rely on limited prior hypotheses, small sample sizes, and heterogenous techniques (Himmerich et al., 2019; Hübel, Marzi, et al., 2019). The only EWAS published on AN reported altered methylation profiles in genes involved in dopamine and glutamate signaling, cholesterol storage and lipid transport (Booij et al., 2015), and duration of illness and age at onset were differentially associated with altered methylation profile in gene pathways involved in anxiety, bowel dysfunction, immunity, liver damage, brain development and morphology (Booij et al., 2015). However, these alterations observed in individuals with AN may normalize following remission (Steiger et al., 2019) and are likely secondary effects of the illness and not disease-specific vulnerabilities. To date, no EWASs have been conducted in other eating disorders.

Despite being in its infancy and having the same methodological challenges and limitations as other genetic methods during their earlier stages of research (e.g., small sample sizes and lack of multiple testing correction), epigenetic models of eating disorders have the potential to inform the design of personalized techniques that could improve screening and treatment of individual at high risk (Booij & Steiger, 2020).

Future Directions in Eating Disorders Genetic Research

We highlight several important future directions to advance the genetic research of eating disorders. These include: (1) increasing and diversifying samples and data; (2) studying developmental timing; (3) performing functional follow-up studies; (4) studying the contribution of genomic variants outside of common variation; and (5) adopting a patient-centered approach.

Increasing and diversifying samples and data

Based on the upward trajectories observed with the sample size boost in other psychiatric disorders (Sullivan et al., 2018), gene discovery for eating disorders will undoubtedly be advanced by increasing sample sizes and simultaneously collecting more diverse samples to increase generalizability. Major working groups of the PGC have demonstrated the necessity of increasing sample sizes for gene discovery and understanding trait genetic architecture (Sullivan et al., 2018). However, to be informative for larger populations, future studies should focus on collecting more diverse samples in terms of ancestry, sex, eating disorder diagnosis and symptomatology (Huckins et al., 2022).

Eating disorder genetic studies to date have predominantly included female participants of European ancestry with AN. While early replication efforts have shown promising preliminary signs that AN risk alleles identified in European-ancestry individuals act in the same direction in non-European samples (Boraska et al., 2014), studies point to the major limitations in generalizability of PGS across populations (Ding et al., 2023; Privé et al., 2022). Because eating disorders are most prevalent among young women (American Psychiatric Association, 2013; Solmi et al., 2022), genomic studies of AN to date have included a very limited number of male cases. However, research shows that AN in males can have a greater burden (Wu et al., 2020) and earlier age of onset (Kinasz et al., 2016; Yilmaz et al., 2023), although existing samples have not shown sex differences in risk prediction using AN PGS (Chatwin et al., 2023; Watson et al., 2019). Similarly, while AN was historically prioritized for GWAS due to its high mortality (Arcelus et al., 2011; Papadopoulos et al., 2009; Sullivan, 1995) and the lack of gold-standard treatments for adult patients (American Psychiatric Association, 2006; Watson & Bulik, 2013), GWASs for BN, BED, ARFID, as well as continuous measures of eating disorder symptoms, behaviors, and other related phenotypes are direly needed.

Global efforts are underway to significantly boost eating disorder genomic sample sizes, diversify populations, expand GWAS efforts to non-AN eating disorders, and incorporate detailed phenotype data through large studies such as the Anorexia Nervosa Genetics Initiative (ANGI) (Thornton et al., 2018), the Eating Disorders Genetics Initiative (EDGI) (Bulik, Thornton, et al., 2021), the Binge Eating Genetics Initiative (BEGIN) (Bulik et al., 2020), Genetic Links to Anxiety and Depression (GLAD; which comprises detailed eating disorder data collection) (Davies et al., 2019), and Avoidant Restrictive Food Intake Disorder Genes and Environment (ARFID-GEN) (Bulik et al., 2023). Inclusion of individuals with non-European or admixed ancestry, men (or more broadly, gender identities other than *cis* women), and have eating disorders other than AN will enhance our understanding of eating disorder genomics, improve the generalizability of findings, and help fight existing health disparities.

Developmental timing

Differences in the manifestation of genetic risk in the development of disordered eating have been demonstrated in previous twin studies, suggesting that genetic factors may contribute to risk in varying degrees depending on the developmental timepoint (Fairweather-Schmidt & Wade, 2015; O'Connor et al., 2020). It is important to also examine the contribution of specific genetic variants or PGS to eating disorder risk over time, which requires large population cohorts with longitudinal data collection and genotypes. This chapter highlights two such cohorts: the Avon Longitudinal Study of Parents and Children (ALSPAC); and the Norwegian Mother, Father and Child Study Cohort (MoBa). ALSPAC data have been widely used (with the findings highlighted in several sections of this chapter) to investigate the developmental impact of AN genetics, thanks to the detailed prospective data collection during childhood and adolescence (Fraser et al., 2013). MoBa is another large longitudinal cohort with rich developmental data (Magnus et al., 2016) and has made significant contributions to our understanding of eating disorder epidemiology (Perrin et al., 2015; Reba-Harrelson et al., 2010) and—more recently, with the addition of genotype data—genetics (Ayorech et al., 2021). As GWAS efforts for other eating disorders are underway and PGS for other eating disorders will become available, large developmental cohorts will continue to be useful resources in furthering our understanding on how genetic risk for an eating disorder is associated with developmental outcomes.

Functional follow-up

The goal of genetic studies is to reliably identify genes that increase risk for a disorder and elucidate the biological mechanisms associated with disease etiology. As reviewed, the PGC-ED Freeze 2 AN GWAS led to the discovery of eight risk loci (Watson et al., 2019), but linking these loci to specific genes is complicated due to linkage disequilibrium. Fine mapping these association signals to causal genetic variants (e.g., through re-sequencing) is crucial to advance our understanding of the biological relevance of the variants. Multiple approaches have been used to examine the function of the AN risk loci, resulting in the identification of four brain-expressed genes (*CADM1*, *MGMT*, *FOXP1*, and *PTBP2*) that have also been implicated in BMI (Locke et al., 2015), age at menarche (Pickrell et al., 2016), height (Yengo et al., 2022), body weight maintenance (Co et al., 2020), and axon development and regeneration (Dawicki-McKenna et al., 2023), mirroring aspects of the clinical presentation of AN and genetic correlations with other traits (Watson et al., 2019). However, these findings are very preliminary in nature, and as GWASs continue to uncover more risk loci, functional follow-up studies have the potential to aid the understanding of the biology of the risk variants, which in turn could facilitate drug discovery.

Moving beyond common variation

The GWAS approach has revolutionized our understanding of the genetic architecture of complex traits, including psychiatric disorders. However, it is important to be mindful of the fact that with current sample sizes, the effect sizes associated with individual GWAS risk variants are quite small, with relative risks ranging from 1.1 to 2.0 (Wray et al., 2007). Furthermore, SNP-based heritability estimates obtained through GWAS are notably lower that twin-based heritability estimates for AN (Watson et al., 2021) and other complex traits in general (Manolio et al., 2009; Zuk et al., 2012). While this may seem puzzling at first, GWAS is designed specifically to capture common variance and therefore is not the best tool to study other types of genetic contributions such as rare variation, structural variation, or epigenetic changes.

As discussed in the "High-throughput sequencing" section of this chapter, sequencing technology is the next step toward comprehensive molecular diagnostic testing that encompasses rare variation in unrelated cases and controls as well as in large densely affected pedigrees with a high incidence of eating disorders. Discovery of ultra-rare but deleterious mutations may not assist with risk prediction in the general population; however, once large sample sizes are reached, low-frequency rare variants could shed light on key biological pathways (Munn-Chernoff et al., 2016; Yilmaz et al., 2015). Carefully designed epigenetic studies can also advance our knowledge on the biological processes underlying eating disorders and help identify possible therapeutic targets (Hübel, Marzi, et al., 2019). Nevertheless, such work will require large-scale coordinated effort to increase sample sizes and standardizing measurement techniques, tissues tested, and diagnostic definitions (Booij & Steiger, 2020). Considering that they provide a snapshot at the time of sample collection as opposed to lifelong patterns, future epigenetic studies should look through a finer lens to characterize the epigenetic profile of different eating disorders by subtype, tissue and cell type, and also consider a large array of environmental factors such as diet, binge eating and purging behaviors, and medications (Horvath & Raj, 2018; Kubota et al., 2012; Moore et al., 2013).

Adopting a patient-centered approach

The concept of lived experience-focused clinical studies is gaining traction, leading to the development of protocols and guidelines for building collaborations with patients and advocacy groups (Giel et al., 2023). Because the ultimate goal of genomic research in eating disorders is to predict risk before the emergence of symptoms and improve clinical outcome for patients, adopting a patient-centered approach can empower patients and help dispel the stigma associated with eating disorders, lead to studies designed to better address patients' needs, reprioritize topics based on what is important for those with lived experience, and choose language in a manner that preserves the dignity of patients and respects their preferences.

Alternative Perspectives

In this section, we will consider three specific counter-perspectives to some of the existing assumptions and interpretation of current findings.

AN may not have a metabo-psychiatric nature

As explained in the "Cross-disorder approaches" section of this chapter, significant genetic correlations involving metabolic and anthropometric traits such as BMI (Watson et al., 2019) have provided the rationale for a potential reconceptualization of AN as a metabo-psychiatric disorder. However, because low body weight is the *sine qua non* of AN, low BMI could be the main factor driving these negative genetic correlations. Preliminary analyses suggest that there may be a mild but nonsignificant attenuation in the genetic correlations with AN when the BMI signal is covaried, suggesting that AN may share genetic variation with metabolic traits independent of BMI (Watson et al., 2019). Furthermore, the genetic architectures of AN and persistent thinness do not appear to significantly overlap (Hübel et al., 2024). Nonetheless, current sample sizes for AN and persistent thinness may not be sufficient to elucidate the relationship between the genetic architecture of AN and BMI. Notably, metabolic and anthropometric traits also show significant genetic correlations with other psychiatric disorders (Bahrami et al., 2020; Demontis et al., 2023; Hübel, Gaspar, et al., 2019; Wray et al., 2018)—albeit with different directionality—and therefore these associations are not necessarily unique to AN.

Genetics finding may not have sufficient specificity for any psychiatric disorder

Comorbidity among psychiatric disorders is common (Kessler et al., 2005; McGrath et al., 2020; Plana-Ripoll et al., 2019), and eating disorders are no exception (Momen et al., 2022). The high degree of genetic correlations among psychiatric disorders mirrors these clinical comorbidities (Anttila et al., 2018; Bulik-Sullivan et al., 2015; Cross-Disorder Group of the Psychiatric Genomics Consortium, 2019), providing additional challenges for unraveling the unique biological underpinnings of each disorder. However, genetic overlap is expected due to pleiotropy—the phenomenon where a single gene affects multiple seemingly unrelated traits—and there are also significant genetic differences among psychiatric disorders. Our view is that prioritizing cross-disorder genomic approaches alongside disorder-specific research could assist with finding loci unique to a specific disorder, examining the similarities and differences in genetic architectures, and assessing causality at a genetic level.

Genetic findings may not have clinical relevance

Despite the increase in the number of GWAS hits, these advancements have yet to lead to clinic-ready discoveries. As discussed in the "Future Directions" section of this chapter, functional follow-up is complex and advances slowly, thus it may be premature to expect immediate clinical applications. The clinical utility of PGS has also come into question despite the promising results (Koch et al., 2023). Some of the additional barriers for the use of PGS clinically include the cost of genotyping patients, the degree of training and willingness required by clinicians, managing expectations about the use of PGS, and privacy concerns about incorporating genomic data into medical records. Considering most genetic study participants are of European ancestry, the degree of transferability of genetic findings to other populations is unknown, which can lead to significant disparities in health care access (Martin et al., 2019). Collective efforts are underway to develop guidelines for the responsible use of PGS and build appropriate frameworks before PGS is ready for widespread clinical use (Adeyemo et al., 2021).

Implications

Genomic research in eating disorders shows promise in providing the field with a much-needed understanding of the biological underpinnings of these serious psychiatric disorders in the years to come. Two potential future applications of genomic research have particular clinical relevance: (1) informing and improving therapeutic approaches; and (2) development of multi-factorial prediction models for early identification and tailored treatment approaches.

The predominant eating disorder treatments with empirical support demonstrate limited effectiveness, typically achieve long-term success rates ranging from 25% to 65% (Berkman et al., 2007; Watson & Bulik, 2013). However, many individuals experience chronicity, partial recovery, or relapse, and there is currently no first-line established outpatient treatment with empirical support for adults with AN (Watson & Bulik, 2013). While there are a limited number of medications with evidence for efficacy in the treatment for BN and BED, no strong evidence base exists for any medication for the treatment of AN (Himmerich et al., 2023). Exploring the biological pathways associated with eating disorders and identifying potential drug target genes hold promise for developing advanced interventions. A relevant example is the case of schizophrenia, with GWAS results revealing connections to antipsychotic drugs as well as selective calcium channel blockers and antiepileptics, offering opportunities for repurposing existing therapeutics (Gaspar & Breen, 2017). Similarly, if the metabo-psychiatric findings for AN continue to replicate, pharmacological agents addressing metabolic processes could potentially emerge as potential targets for treating AN.

As GWAS sample sizes continue to increase, the explanatory power of PGS is also expected to significantly improve (Dudbridge, 2013). In fact, the predictive value of PGS has been demonstrated across multiple studies and psychiatric phenotypes (Cross-Disorder Group of the Psychiatric Genomics Consortium, 2013a; Demontis et al., 2023; Grove et al., 2019; Schizophrenia Working Group of the Psychiatric Genomics Consortium, 2014), and more recently, PGS have been shown to correlate with chronicity (Meier et al., 2016) and treatment resistance (Frank et al., 2015) in schizophrenia. PGS has the potential to become more powerful in predicting key clinical features associated with eating disorders, identifying distinct subtypes, and developing prediction models toward personalized precision medicine. However, PGS should be viewed as a valuable but not exhaustive tool in the realm of clinical decision-making and understanding the biology of eating disorders. Despite its limitations and concerns surrounding its effective use, it is our view that PGS may be used in the future in combination with known risk factors and clinical correlates such as family history, age of onset, comorbidities, medical history, other types of genetic information such as CNVs and rare pathogenic variants, as well as biomarker data to create integrated prediction models (Lewis & Vassos, 2022).

References

Abdulkadir, M., Hübel, C., Herle, M., Loos, R. J. F., Breen, G., Bulik, C. M., & Micali, N. (2022). The impact of anorexia nervosa and BMI polygenic risk on childhood growth: A 20-year longitudinal population-based study. *American Journal of Human Genetics, 109*(7), 1242–1254. https://doi.org/10.1016/j.ajhg.2022.05.005

Adeyemo, A., Balaconis, M. K., Darnes, D. R., Fatumo, S., Granados Moreno, P., Hodonsky, C. J., Inouye, M., Kanai, M., Kato, K., Knoppers, B. M., Lewis, A. C. F., Martin, A. R., McCarthy, M. I., Meyer, M. N., Okada, Y., Richards, J. B., Richter, L., Ripatti, S., Rotimi, C. N., . . . The Polygenic Risk Score Task Force of the International Common Disease. (2021). Responsible use of polygenic risk scores in the clinic: Potential benefits, risks and gaps. *Nature Medicine, 27*(11), 1876–1884. https://doi.org/10.1038/s41591-021-01549-6

American Psychiatric Association. (2006). Treatment of patients with eating disorders. *American Journal of Psychiatry, 163*(7 Suppl), 4–54.

American Psychiatric Association. (2013). *Diagnostic and statistical manual of mental disorders* (5th ed.). American Psychiatric Association.

Anttila, V., Bulik-Sullivan, B., Finucane, H. K., Walters, R. K., Bras, J., Duncan, L., Escott-Price, V., Falcone, G. J., Gormley, P., Malik, R., Patsopoulos, N. A., Ripke, S., Wei, Z., Yu, D., Lee, P. H., Turley, P., Grenier-Boley, B., Chouraki, V., Kamatani, Y., . . . Murray, R. (2018). Analysis of shared heritability in common disorders of the brain. *Science, 360*(6395). https://doi.org/10.1126/science.aap8757

Arcelus, J., Mitchell, A. J., Wales, J., & Nielsen, S. (2011). Mortality rates in patients with anorexia nervosa and other eating disorders: A meta-analysis of 36 studies. *Archives of General Psychiatry, 68*(7), 724. https://doi.org/10.1001/archgenpsychiatry.2011.74

Ayorech, Z., Davies, N. M., Watson, H., Yilmaz, Z., Tesli, M., J., H. L., Askeland, R. B., Øyen, A. S., Knudsen, G. P., Johansson, S., Helgeland, Ø., Magnus, P. M., Njølstad, P. R., Stoltenberg, C., Andreassen, O. A., Reichborn-Kjennerud, T., Smith, G. D., Bulik, C., Havdahl, A., & Ask, H. (2021). Childhood phenotypic manifestations of genetic risk for anorexia nervosa in the Norwegian Mother, Father and Child Cohort Study (MoBA). *PsyArXiv*. https://doi.org/10.31234/osf.io/w57h9.

Bahrami, S., Steen, N. E., Shadrin, A., O'Connell, K., Frei, O., Bettella, F., Wirgenes, K. V., Krull, F., Fan, C. C., Dale, A. M., Smeland, O. B., Djurovic, S., & Andreassen, O. A. (2020). Shared genetic loci between body mass index and major psychiatric disorders: A genome-wide association study. *JAMA Psychiatry, 77*(5), 503–512. https://doi.org/10.1001/jamapsychiatry.2019.4188

Bang, L., Bahrami, S., Hindley, G., Smeland, O. B., Rødevand, L., Jaholkowski, P. P., Shadrin, A., Connell, K. S. O., Frei, O., Lin, A., Rahman, Z., Cheng, W., Parker, N., Fan, C. C., Dale, A. M., Djurovic, S., Bulik, C. M., & Andreassen, O. A. (2023). Genome-wide analysis of anorexia nervosa and major psychiatric disorders and related traits reveals genetic overlap and identifies novel risk loci for anorexia nervosa. *Translational Psychiatry, 13*(1), 291. https://doi.org/10.1038/s41398-023-02585-1

Berkman, N. D., Lohr, K. N., & Bulik, C. M. (2007). Outcomes of eating disorders: A systematic review of the literature. *International Journal of Eating Disorders, 40*(4), 293–309. http://www.ncbi.nlm.nih.gov/entrez/query.fcgi?cmd=Retrieve&db=PubMed&dopt=Citation&list_uids=17370291

Bienvenu, T., Lebrun, N., Clarke, J., Duriez, P., Gorwood, P., & Ramoz, N. (2019). Exome sequencing in a familial form of anorexia nervosa supports multigenic etiology. *Journal of Neural Transmission, 126*(11), 1505–1511. https://doi.org/10.1007/s00702-019-02056-2

Bienvenu, T., Lebrun, N., Clarke, J., Duriez, P., Gorwood, P., & Ramoz, N. (2020). De novo deleterious variants that may alter the dopaminergic reward pathway are associated with anorexia nervosa. *Eating and Weight Disorders, 25*(6), 1643–1650. https://doi.org/10.1007/s40519-019-00802-9

Booij, L., Casey, K. F., Antunes, J. M., Szyf, M., Joober, R., Israel, M., & Steiger, H. (2015). DNA methylation in individuals with anorexia nervosa and in matched normal-eater controls: A genome-wide study. *International Journal of Eating Disorders, 48*(7), 874–882. https://doi.org/10.1002/eat.22374

Booij, L., & Steiger, H. (2020). Applying epigenetic science to the understanding of eating disorders: A promising paradigm for research and practice. *Current Opinion in Psychiatry, 33*(6), 515–520. https://doi.org/10.1097/yco.0000000000000632

Boraska, V., Davis, O. S., Cherkas, L. F., Helder, S. G., Harris, J., Krug, I., Pei-Chi Liao, T., Treasure, J., Ntalla, I., Karhunen, L., Keski-Rahkonen, A., Christakopoulou, D., Raevuori, A., Shin, S. Y., Dedoussis, G. V., Kaprio, J., Soranzo, N., Spector, T. D., Collier, D. A., & Zeggini, E. (2012). Genome-wide association analysis of eating disorder-related symptoms, behaviors, and personality traits. *American Journal of Medical Genetics. Part B, Neuropsychiatric Genetics, 159B*(7), 803. https://doi.org/10.1002/ajmg.b.32087

Boraska, V., Franklin, C. S., Floyd, J. A., Thornton, L. M., Huckins, L. M., Southam, L., Rayner, N. W., Tachmazidou, I., Klump, K. L., Treasure, J., Lewis, C. M., Schmidt, U., Tozzi, F., Kiezebrink, K., Hebebrand, J., Gorwood, P., Adan, R. A., Kas, M. J., Favaro, A., . . . Bulik, C. M. (2014). A genome-wide association study of anorexia nervosa. *Molecular Psychiatry, 19*(10), 1085–1094. https://doi.org/10.1038/mp.2013.187

Bulik-Sullivan, B., Finucane, H. K., Anttila, V., Gusev, A., Day, F. R., Loh, P. R., Duncan, L., Perry, J. R., Patterson, N., Robinson, E. B., Daly, M. J., Price, A. L., & Neale, B. M. (2015). An atlas of genetic correlations across human diseases and traits. *Nature Genetics, 47*(11), 1236–1241. https://doi.org/10.1038/ng.3406

Bulik, C., Thornton, L., Root, T., Pisetsky, E., Lichtenstein, P., & Pedersen, N. (2010). Understanding the relation between anorexia nervosa and bulimia nervosa in a Swedish national twin sample. *Biological Psychiatry, 67*, 71–77.

Bulik, C. M., Butner, J. E., Tregarthen, J., Thornton, L. M., Flatt, R. E., Smith, T., Carroll, I. M., Baucom, B. R. W., & Deboeck, P. R. (2020). The Binge Eating Genetics Initiative (BEGIN): Study protocol. *BMC Psychiatry, 20*(1), 307. https://doi.org/10.1186/s12888-020-02698-7

Bulik, C. M., Carroll, I. M., & Mehler, P. (2021). Reframing anorexia nervosa as a metabo-psychiatric disorder. *Trends in Endocrinology & Metabolism, 32*(10), 752–761. https://doi.org/10.1016/j.tem.2021.07.010

Bulik, C. M., Coleman, J. R. I., Hardaway, J. A., Breithaupt, L., Watson, H. J., Bryant, C. D., & Breen, G. (2022). Genetics and neurobiology of eating disorders. *Nature Neuroscience, 25*(5), 543–554. https://doi.org/10.1038/s41593-022-01071-z

Bulik, C. M., Micali, N., Ba, C. M. M., Qi, B., Munn-Chernoff, M. A., Thornton, L. M., White, J., Dinkler, L., Pisetsky, E. M., Johnson, J., Devine, K. R., Ortiz, S. N., Silverman, A. E., Berthold, N., Ba, A. D., Guintivano, J., Halvorsen, M., & J, J. (2023). ARFID Genes and Environment (ARFID-GEN): Study Protocol. Research Square. https://doi.org/10.21203/rs.3.rs-3186174/v1

Bulik, C. M., Sullivan, P. F., & Kendler, K. S. (1998). Heritability of binge-eating and broadly defined bulimia nervosa. *Biological Psychiatry, 44*(12), 1210.

Bulik, C. M., Sullivan, P. F., & Kendler, K. S. (2003). Genetic and environmental contributions to obesity and binge eating. *International Journal of Eating Disorders, 33*(3), 293–298. https://doi.org/10.1002/eat.10140

Bulik, C. M., Sullivan, P. F., Tozzi, F., Furberg, H., Lichtenstein, P., & Pedersen, N. L. (2006). Prevalence, heritability, and prospective risk factors for anorexia nervosa. *Archives of General Psychiatry, 63*(3), 305–312. https://doi.org/10.1001/archpsyc.63.3.305

Bulik, C. M., Thornton, L. M., Parker, R., Kennedy, H., Baker, J. H., MacDermod, C., Guintivano, J., Cleland, L., Miller, A. L., Harper, L., Larsen, J. T., Yilmaz, Z., Grove, J., Sullivan, P. F., Petersen, L. V., Jordan, J., Kennedy, M. A., & Martin, N. G. (2021). The Eating Disorders Genetics Initiative (EDGI): Study protocol. *BMC Psychiatry, 21*(1), 234. https://doi.org/10.1186/s12888-021-03212-3

Chang, X., Qu, H., Liu, Y., Glessner, J., Hou, C., Wang, F., Li, J., Sleiman, P., & Hakonarson, H. (2019). Microduplications at the 15q11.2 BP1-BP2 locus are enriched in patients with anorexia nervosa. *Journal of Psychiatric Research, 113*, 34–38. https://doi.org/10.1016/j.jpsychires.2019.01.021

Chatwin, H., Holde, K., Yilmaz, Z., Larsen, J. T., Albiñana, C., Vilhjálmsson, B. J., Mortensen, P. B., Thornton, L. M., Bulik, C. M., & Petersen, L. V. (2023). Risk factors for anorexia nervosa: A population-based investigation of sex differences in polygenic risk and early life exposures. *International Journal of Eating Disorders, 56*(9), 1703–1716. https://doi.org/10.1002/eat.23997

Chen, W. M., & Abecasis, G. R. (2006). Estimating the power of variance component linkage analysis in large pedigrees. *Genetic Epidemiology, 30*(6), 471–484. https://doi.org/10.1002/gepi.20160

Co, M., Anderson, A. G., & Konopka, G. (2020). FOXP transcription factors in vertebrate brain development, function, and disorders. *Wiley Interdisciplinay Reviews. Developmental Biology, 9*(5), e375. https://doi.org/10.1002/wdev.375

Cooke, L. J., Haworth, C. M., & Wardle, J. (2007). Genetic and environmental influences on children's food neophobia. *American Journal of Clinical Nutrition, 86*(2), 428–433. https://doi.org/10.1093/ajcn/86.2.428

Cross-Disorder Group of the Psychiatric Genomics Consortium. (2013a). Genetic relationship between five psychiatric disorders estimated from genome-wide SNPs. *Nature Genetics, 45*(9), 984–994. https://doi.org/10.1038/ng.2711

Cross-Disorder Group of the Psychiatric Genomics Consortium. (2013b). Identification of risk loci with shared effects on five major psychiatric disorders: A genome-wide analysis. *Lancet, 381*(9875), 1371–1379. https://doi.org/10.1016/s0140-6736(12)62129-1

Cross-Disorder Group of the Psychiatric Genomics Consortium. (2019). Genomic relationships, novel loci, and pleiotropic mechanisms across eight psychiatric disorders. *Cell, 179*(7), 1469–1482.e1411. https://doi.org/10.1016/j.cell.2019.11.020

Cross-Disorder Phenotype Group of the Psychiatric GWAS Consortium, Craddock, N., Kendler, K., Neale, M., Nurnberger, J., Purcell, S., Rietschel, M., Perlis, R., Santangelo, S. L., Schulze, T. G., Smoller, J. W., & Thapar, A. (2009). Dissecting the phenotype in genome-wide association studies of psychiatric illness. *British Journal of Psychiatry, 195*(2), 97–99. https://doi.org/10.1192/bjp.bp.108.063156

Cui, H., Moore, J., Ashimi, S. S., Mason, B. L., Drawbridge, J. N., Han, S., Hing, B., Matthews, A., McAdams, C. J., Darbro, B. W., Pieper, A. A., Waller, D. A., Xing, C., & Lutter, M. (2013). Eating disorder predisposition is associated with ESRRA and HDAC4 mutations. *Journal of Clinical Investigation, 123*(11), 4706–4713. https://doi.org/10.1172/jci71400

Davies, M. R., Kalsi, G., Armour, C., Jones, I. R., McIntosh, A. M., Smith, D. J., Walters, J. T. R., Bradley, J. R., Kingston, N., Ashford, S., Beange, I., Brailean, A., Cleare, A. J., Coleman, J. R. I., Curtis, C. J., Curzons, S. C. B., Davis, K. A. S., Dowey, L. R. C., Gault, V. A., . . . Breen, G. (2019). The Genetic Links to Anxiety and Depression (GLAD) Study: Online recruitment into the largest recontactable study of depression and anxiety. *Behaviour Research and Therapy, 123*, 103503. https://doi.org/10.1016/j.brat.2019.103503

Dawicki-McKenna, J. M., Felix, A. J., Waxman, E. A., Cheng, C., Amado, D. A., Ranum, P. T., Bogush, A., Dungan, L. V., Maguire, J. A., Gagne, A. L., Heller, E. A., French, D. L., Davidson, B. L., & Prosser, B. L. (2023). Mapping PTBP2 binding in human brain identifies SYNGAP1 as a target for therapeutic splice switching. *Nature Communications, 14*(1), 2628. https://doi.org/10.1038/s41467-023-38273-3

Dellava, J. E., Thornton, L. M., Lichtenstein, P., Pedersen, N. L., & Bulik, C. M. (2011). Impact of broadening definitions of anorexia nervosa on sample characteristics. *Journal of Psychiatric Research, 45*(5), 691. https://doi.org/10.1016/j.jpsychires.2010.10.003

Demontis, D., Walters, G. B., Athanasiadis, G., Walters, R., Therrien, K., Nielsen, T. T., Farajzadeh, L., Voloudakis, G., Bendl, J., Zeng, B., Zhang, W., Grove, J., Als, T. D., Duan, J., Satterstrom, F. K., Bybjerg-Grauholm, J., Bækved-Hansen, M., Gudmundsson, O. O., Magnusson, S. H., . . . Børglum, A. D. (2023). Genome-wide analyses of ADHD identify 27 risk loci, refine the genetic architecture and implicate several cognitive domains. *Nature Genetics, 55*(2), 198–208. https://doi.org/10.1038/s41588-022-01285-8

Ding, Y., Hou, K., Xu, Z., Pimplaskar, A., Petter, E., Boulier, K., Privé, F., Vilhjálmsson, B. J., Olde Loohuis, L. M., & Pasaniuc, B. (2023). Polygenic scoring accuracy varies across the genetic ancestry continuum. *Nature, 618*(7966), 774–781. https://doi.org/10.1038/s41586-023-06079-4

Dinkler, L., Wronski, M. L., Lichtenstein, P., Lundström, S., Larsson, H., Micali, N., Taylor, M. J., & Bulik, C. M. (2023). Etiology of the broad avoidant restrictive food intake disorder phenotype in Swedish twins aged 6 to 12 years. *JAMA Psychiatry, 80*(3), 260–269. https://doi.org/10.1001/jamapsychiatry.2022.4612

Dudbridge, F. (2013). Power and predictive accuracy of polygenic risk scores. *PLOS Genetics, 9*(3), e1003348. https://doi.org/10.1371/journal.pgen.1003348

Duncan, L., Yilmaz, Z., Gaspar, H., Walters, R., Goldstein, J., Anttila, V., Bulik-Sullivan, B., Ripke, S., Thornton, L., Hinney, A., Daly, M., Sullivan, P. F., Zeggini, E., Breen, G., & Bulik, C. M. (2017). Significant locus and metabolic genetic correlations revealed in genome-wide association study of anorexia nervosa. *American Journal of Psychiatry, 174*(9), 850–858. https://doi.org/10.1176/appi.ajp.2017.16121402

Fadista, J., Manning, A. K., Florez, J. C., & Groop, L. (2016). The (in)famous GWAS P-value threshold revisited and updated for low-frequency variants. *European Journal of Human Genetics, 24*(8), 1202–1205. https://doi.org/10.1038/ejhg.2015.269

Fairweather-Schmidt, A. K., & Wade, T. D. (2015). Changes in genetic and environmental influences on disordered eating between early and late adolescence: A longitudinal twin study. *Psychological Medicine, 45*(15), 3249–3258. https://doi.org/10.1017/s0033291715001257

Fildes, A., van Jaarsveld, C. H., Cooke, L., Wardle, J., & Llewellyn, C. H. (2016). Common genetic architecture underlying young children's food fussiness and liking for vegetables and fruit. *American Journal of Clinical Nutrition, 103*(4), 1099–1104. https://doi.org/10.3945/ajcn.115.122945

Fowler, S. J., & Bulik, C. M. (1997). Family environment and psychiatric history in women with binge-eating disorder and obese controls. *Behaviour Change, 14*(2), 106–112. https://doi.org/10.1017/S0813483900003569

Frank, J., Lang, M., Witt, S. H., Strohmaier, J., Rujescu, D., Cichon, S., Degenhardt, F., Nöthen, M. M., Collier, D. A., Ripke, S., Naber, D., & Rietschel, M. (2015). Identification of increased genetic risk scores for schizophrenia in treatment-resistant patients. *Molecular Psychiatry, 20*(2), 150–151. https://doi.org/10.1038/mp.2014.56

Fraser, A., Macdonald-Wallis, C., Tilling, K., Boyd, A., Golding, J., Davey Smith, G., Henderson, J., Macleod, J., Molloy, L., Ness, A., Ring, S., Nelson, S. M., & Lawlor, D. A. (2013). Cohort profile: The

Avon Longitudinal Study of Parents and Children: ALSPAC mothers cohort. *International Journal of Epidemiology*, *42*(1), 97–110. https://doi.org/10.1093/ije/dys066

Frieling, H., Bleich, S., Otten, J., Römer, K. D., Kornhuber, J., de Zwaan, M., Jacoby, G. E., Wilhelm, J., & Hillemacher, T. (2008). Epigenetic downregulation of atrial natriuretic peptide but not vasopressin mRNA expression in females with eating disorders is related to impulsivity. *Neuropsychopharmacology*, *33*(11), 2605–2609. https://doi.org/10.1038/sj.npp.1301662

Frieling, H., Gozner, A., Romer, K. D., Lenz, B., Bonsch, D., Wilhelm, J., Hillemacher, T., de Zwaan, M., Kornhuber, J., & Bleich, S. (2007). Global DNA hypomethylation and DNA hypermethylation of the alpha synuclein promoter in females with anorexia nervosa. *Molecular Psychiatry*, *12*(3), 229. https://doi.org/10.1038/sj.mp.4001931

Frieling, H., Romer, K. D., Scholz, S., Mittelbach, F., Wilhelm, J., De Zwaan, M., Jacoby, G. E., Kornhuber, J., Hillemacher, T., & Bleich, S. (2010). Epigenetic dysregulation of dopaminergic genes in eating disorders. *International Journal of Eating Disorders*, *43*(7), 577. https://doi.org/10.1002/eat.20745

Gaspar, H. A., & Breen, G. (2017). Drug enrichment and discovery from schizophrenia genome-wide association results: an analysis and visualisation approach. *Scientific Reports*, *7*(1), 12460. https://doi.org/10.1038/s41598-017-12325-3

Giel, K. E., Bremer, J., Rieß-Stumm, S., Gregg, B., Fritz, A., Klemm, I., Daugelat, M. C., & Schag, K. (2023). Enriching a randomized controlled treatment trial for anorexia nervosa by lived experience—Chances and effects of a lived experience council in the SUSTAIN study. *International Journal of Eating Disorders*, *57*(6): 1300–1310. https://doi.org/10.1002/eat.24050

Grice, D. E., Halmi, K. A., Fichter, M. M., Strober, M., Woodside, D. B., Treasure, J. T., Kaplan, A. S., Magistretti, P. J., Goldman, D., Bulik, C. M., Kaye, W. H., & Berrettini, W. H. (2002). Evidence for a susceptibility gene for anorexia nervosa on chromosome 1. *American Journal of Human Genetics*, *70*(3), 787. https://doi.org/10.1086/339250

Grigoroiu-Serbanescu, M., Magureanu, S., Milea, S., Dobrescu, I., & Marinescu, E. (2003). Modest familial aggregation of eating disorders in restrictive anorexia nervosa with adolescent onset in a Romanian sample. *European Child & Adolescent Psychiatry*, *12*(Suppl 1), i47–i53. https://doi.org/10.1007/s00787-003-1107-7

Groleau, P., Steiger, H., Joober, R., Bruce, K. R., Israel, M., Badawi, G., Zeramdini, N., & Sycz, L. (2012). Dopamine-system genes, childhood abuse, and clinical manifestations in women with bulimia-spectrum disorders. *Journal of Psychiatric Research*, *46*(9), 1139–1145. https://doi.org/10.1016/j.jpsychires.2012.05.018

Grove, J., Ripke, S., Als, T. D., Mattheisen, M., Walters, R. K., Won, H., Pallesen, J., Agerbo, E., Andreassen, O. A., Anney, R., Awashti, S., Belliveau, R., Bettella, F., Buxbaum, J. D., Bybjerg-Grauholm, J., Baekvad-Hansen, M., Cerrato, F., Chambert, K., Christensen, J. H., . . . Borglum, A. D. (2019). Identification of common genetic risk variants for autism spectrum disorder. *Nature Genetics*, *51*(3), 431–444. https://doi.org/10.1038/s41588-019-0344-8

Helder, S. G., & Collier, D. A. (2011). The genetics of eating disorders. *Current Topics in Behavioral Neurosciences*, *6*, 157. https://doi.org/10.1007/7854_2010_79

Himmerich, H., Bentley, J., Kan, C., & Treasure, J. (2019). Genetic risk factors for eating disorders: An update and insights into pathophysiology. *Therapeutic Advances in Psychopharmacology*, *9*, 2045125318814734. https://doi.org/10.1177/2045125318814734

Himmerich, H., Lewis, Y. D., Conti, C., Mutwalli, H., Karwautz, A., Sjögren, J. M., Uribe Isaza, M. M., Tyszkiewicz-Nwafor, M., Aigner, M., McElroy, S. L., Treasure, J., & Kasper, S. (2023). World Federation of Societies of Biological Psychiatry (WFSBP) guidelines update 2023 on the pharmacological treatment of eating disorders. *World Journal of Biological Psychiatry*, *24*(8), 643–706. https://doi.org/10.1080/15622975.2023.2179663

Horvath, S., & Raj, K. (2018). DNA methylation-based biomarkers and the epigenetic clock theory of ageing. *Nature Reviews Genetics*, *19*(6), 371–384. https://doi.org/10.1038/s41576-018-0004-3

Hübel, C., Abdulkadir, M., Herle, M., Loos, R. J. F., Breen, G., Bulik, C. M., & Micali, N. (2021). One size does not fit all: Genomics differentiates among anorexia nervosa, bulimia nervosa, and binge-eating disorder. *International Journal of Eating Disorders*, *54*(5), 785–793. https://doi.org/10.1002/eat.23481

Hübel, C., Abdulkadir, M., Herle, M., Palmos, A. B., Loos, R. J. F., Breen, G., Micali, N., & Bulik, C. M. (2024). Persistent thinness and anorexia nervosa differ on a genomic level. *European Journal of Human Genetics*, *32*(1), 117–124. https://doi.org/10.1038/s41431-023-01431-8

Hübel, C., Gaspar, H. A., Coleman, J. R. I., Hanscombe, K. B., Purves, K., Prokopenko, I., Graff, M., Ngwa, J. S., Workalemahu, T., O'Reilly, P. F., Bulik, C. M., & Breen, G. (2019). Genetic correlations of psychiatric traits with body composition and glycemic traits are sex- and age-dependent. *Nature Communications, 10*(1), 5765. https://doi.org/10.1038/s41467-019-13544-0

Hübel, C., Leppä, V., Breen, G., & Bulik, C. M. (2018). Rigor and reproducibility in genetic research on eating disorders. *International Journal of Eating Disorders, 51*(7), 593–607. https://doi.org/10.1002/eat.22896

Hübel, C., Marzi, S. J., Breen, G., & Bulik, C. M. (2019). Epigenetics in eating disorders: A systematic review. *Molecular Psychiatry, 24*(6), 901–915. https://doi.org/10.1038/s41380-018-0254-7

Huckins, L. M., Signer, R., Johnson, J., Wu, Y. K., Mitchell, K. S., & Bulik, C. M. (2022). What next for eating disorder genetics? Replacing myths with facts to sharpen our understanding. *Molecular Psychiatry, 27*(10), 3929–3938. https://doi.org/10.1038/s41380-022-01601-y

Hudson, J. I., Lalonde, J. K., Berry, J. M., Pindyck, L. J., Bulik, C. M., Crow, S. J., McElroy, S. L., Laird, N. M., Tsuang, M. T., Walsh, B. T., Rosenthal, N. R., & Pope, H. G., Jr. (2006). Binge-eating disorder as a distinct familial phenotype in obese individuals. *Archives of General Psychiatry, 63*(3), 313–319. https://doi.org/10.1001/archpsyc.63.3.313

Hudson, J. I., Pope, H. G., Jr., Jonas, J. M., Yurgelun-Todd, D., & Frankenburg, F. R. (1987). A controlled family history study of bulimia. *Psychological Medicine, 17*(4), 883–890. https://doi.org/10.1017/s0033291700000684

Javaras, K. N., Laird, N. M., Reichborn-Kjennerud, T., Bulik, C. M., Pope, H. G., Jr., & Hudson, J. I. (2008). Familiality and heritability of binge eating disorder: results of a case-control family study and a twin study. *International Journal of Eating Disorders, 41*(2), 174–179. http://www.ncbi.nlm.nih.gov/entrez/query.fcgi?cmd=Retrieve&db=PubMed&dopt=Citation&list_uids=18095307

Johansson, T., Birgegård, A., Zhang, R., Bergen, S. E., Landén, M., Petersen, L. V., Bulik, C. M., & Hübel, C. (2022). Polygenic association with severity and long-term outcome in eating disorder cases. *Translational Psychiatry, 12*(1), 61. https://doi.org/10.1038/s41398-022-01831-2

Kassett, J. A., Gershon, E. S., Maxwell, M. E., Guroff, J. J., Kazuba, D. M., Smith, A. L., Brandt, H. A., & Jimerson, D. C. (1989). Psychiatric disorders in the first-degree relatives of probands with bulimia nervosa. *American Journal of Psychiatry, 146*(11), 1468–1471. https://doi.org/10.1176/ajp.146.11.1468

Kessler, R. C., Chiu, W. T., Demler, O., Merikangas, K. R., & Walters, E. E. (2005). Prevalence, severity, and comorbidity of 12-month DSM-IV disorders in the National Comorbidity Survey Replication. *Archives of General Psychiatry, 62*(6), 617–627. https://doi.org/10.1001/archpsyc.62.6.617

Kim, Y. R., Kim, J. H., Kim, M. J., & Treasure, J. (2014). Differential methylation of the oxytocin receptor gene in patients with anorexia nervosa: a pilot study. *PLOS One, 9*(2), e88673. https://doi.org/10.1371/journal.pone.0088673

Kinasz, K., Accurso, E. C., Kass, A. E., & Le Grange, D. (2016). Does sex matter in the clinical presentation of eating disorders in youth? *Journal of Adolescent Health, 58*(4), 410–416. https://doi.org/10.1016/j.jadohealth.2015.11.005

Kipman, A., Gorwood, P., Mouren-Simeoni, M. C., & Ades, J. (1999). Genetic factors in anorexia nervosa. *European Psychiatry, 14*(4), 189.

Klump, K. L., Miller, K. B., Keel, P. K., McGue, M., & Iacono, W. G. (2001). Genetic and environmental influences on anorexia nervosa syndromes in a population-based twin sample. *Psychological Medicine, 31*(4), 737–740. https://doi.org/10.1017/s0033291701003725

Knaapila, A., Tuorila, H., Silventoinen, K., Keskitalo, K., Kallela, M., Wessman, M., Peltonen, L., Cherkas, L. F., Spector, T. D., & Perola, M. (2007). Food neophobia shows heritable variation in humans. *Physiology & Behavior, 91*(5), 573–578. https://doi.org/10.1016/j.physbeh.2007.03.019

Koch, S., Schmidtke, J., Krawczak, M., & Caliebe, A. (2023). Clinical utility of polygenic risk scores: a critical 2023 appraisal. *Journal of Community Genetics, 14*(5), 471–487. https://doi.org/10.1007/s12687-023-00645-z

Kortegaard, L. S., Hoerder, K., Joergensen, J., Gillberg, C., & Kyvik, K. O. (2001). A preliminary population-based twin study of self-reported eating disorder. *Psychological Medicine, 31*(2), 361–365.

Kubota, T., Miyake, K., & Hirasawa, T. (2012). Epigenetic understanding of gene-environment interactions in psychiatric disorders: a new concept of clinical genetics. *Clinical Epigenetics, 4*(1), 1. https://doi.org/10.1186/1868-7083-4-1

Leehr, E. J., Opel, N., Werner, J., Redlich, R., Repple, J., Grotegerd, D., Dohm, K., Goltermann, J., Böhnlein, J., Amare, A. T., Sindermann, L., Förster, K., Meinert, S., Enneking, V., Richter, M., Hahn, T., Baune, B. T., & Dannlowski, U. (2019). Evidence for a sex-specific contribution of polygenic load for anorexia nervosa to body weight and prefrontal brain structure in nonclinical individuals. *Neuropsychopharmacology, 44*(13), 2212–2219. https://doi.org/10.1038/s41386-019-0461-1

Lewis, C. M., & Vassos, E. (2022). Polygenic scores in psychiatry: On the road from discovery to implementation. *American Journal of Psychiatry, 179*(11), 800–806. https://doi.org/10.1176/appi.ajp.20220795

Lilenfeld, L. R., Kaye, W. H., Greeno, C. G., Merikangas, K. R., Plotnicov, K., Pollice, C., Rao, R., Strober, M., Bulik, C. M., & Nagy, L. (1998). A controlled family study of anorexia nervosa and bulimia nervosa: Psychiatric disorders in first-degree relatives and effects of proband comorbidity. *Archives of General Psychiatry, 55*(7), 603.

Lipner, E. M., & Greenberg, D. A. (2018). The rise and fall and rise of linkage analysis as a technique for finding and characterizing inherited influences on disease expression. *Methods in Molecular Biology, 1706*, 381–397. https://doi.org/10.1007/978-1-4939-7471-9_21

Liu, J., Tuvblad, C., Raine, A., & Baker, L. (2013). Genetic and environmental influences on nutrient intake. *Genes & Nutrition, 8*(2), 241–252. https://doi.org/10.1007/s12263-012-0320-8

Llewellyn, C. H., van Jaarsveld, C. H., Johnson, L., Carnell, S., & Wardle, J. (2010). Nature and nurture in infant appetite: Analysis of the Gemini twin birth cohort. *American Journal of Clinical Nutrition, 91*(5), 1172–1179. https://doi.org/10.3945/ajcn.2009.28868

Locke, A. E., Kahali, B., Berndt, S. I., Justice, A. E., Pers, T. H., Day, F. R., Powell, C., Vedantam, S., Buchkovich, M. L., Yang, J., Croteau-Chonka, D. C., Esko, T., Fall, T., Ferreira, T., Gustafsson, S., Kutalik, Z., Luan, J., Magi, R., Randall, J. C., . . . Speliotes, E. K. (2015). Genetic studies of body mass index yield new insights for obesity biology. *Nature, 518*(7538), 197–206. https://doi.org/10.1038/nature14177

Lombardi, L., Blanchet, C., Poirier, K., Lebrun, N., Ramoz, N., Rose Moro, M., Gorwood, P., & Bienvenu, T. (2019). Anorexia nervosa is associated with neuronatin variants. *Psychiatric Genetics, 29*(4), 103–110. https://doi.org/10.1097/ypg.0000000000000224

Lutter, M., Bahl, E., Hannah, C., Hofammann, D., Acevedo, S., Cui, H., McAdams, C. J., & Michaelson, J. J. (2017). Novel and ultra-rare damaging variants in neuropeptide signaling are associated with disordered eating behaviors. *PLOS One, 12*(8), e0181556. https://doi.org/10.1371/journal.pone.0181556

Magnus, P., Birke, C., Vejrup, K., Haugan, A., Alsaker, E., Daltveit, A. K., Handal, M., Haugen, M., Høiseth, G., Knudsen, G. P., Paltiel, L., Schreuder, P., Tambs, K., Vold, L., & Stoltenberg, C. (2016). Cohort profile update: The Norwegian Mother and Child Cohort Study (MoBa). *International Journal of Epidemiology, 45*(2), 382–388. https://doi.org/10.1093/ije/dyw029

Manolio, T. A., Collins, F. S., Cox, N. J., Goldstein, D. B., Hindorff, L. A., Hunter, D. J., McCarthy, M. I., Ramos, E. M., Cardon, L. R., Chakravarti, A., Cho, J. H., Guttmacher, A. E., Kong, A., Kruglyak, L., Mardis, E., Rotimi, C. N., Slatkin, M., Valle, D., Whittemore, A. S., . . . Visscher, P. M. (2009). Finding the missing heritability of complex diseases. *Nature, 461*(7265), 747. https://doi.org/10.1038/nature08494

Martin, A. R., Kanai, M., Kamatani, Y., Okada, Y., Neale, B. M., & Daly, M. J. (2019). Clinical use of current polygenic risk scores may exacerbate health disparities. *Nature Genetics, 51*(4), 584–591. https://doi.org/10.1038/s41588-019-0379-x

McGrath, J. J., Lim, C. C. W., Plana-Ripoll, O., Holtz, Y., Agerbo, E., Momen, N. C., Mortensen, P. B., Pedersen, C. B., Abdulmalik, J., Aguilar-Gaxiola, S., Al-Hamzawi, A., Alonso, J., Bromet, E. J., Bruffaerts, R., Bunting, B., de Almeida, J. M. C., de Girolamo, G., De Vries, Y. A., Florescu, S., . . . de Jonge, P. (2020). Comorbidity within mental disorders: A comprehensive analysis based on 145,990 survey respondents from 27 countries. *Epidemiology and Psychiatric Sciences, 29*, e153. https://doi.org/10.1017/s2045796020000633

Meier, S. M., Agerbo, E., Maier, R., Pedersen, C. B., Lang, M., Grove, J., Hollegaard, M. V., Demontis, D., Trabjerg, B. B., Hjorthoj, C., Ripke, S., Degenhardt, F., Nothen, M. M., Rujescu, D., Maier, W., Moo, D. S. S. C. Z. C., Werge, T., Mors, O., Hougaard, D. M., . . . Mattheisen, M. (2016). High loading of polygenic risk in cases with chronic schizophrenia. *Molecular Psychiatry, 21*(7), 969–974. https://doi.org/10.1038/mp.2015.130

Mitchell, K. S., Neale, M. C., Bulik, C. M., Aggen, S. H., Kendler, K. S., & Mazzeo, S. E. (2010). Binge eating disorder: A symptom-level investigation of genetic and environmental influences on liability. *Psychological Medicine, 40*(11), 1899. https://doi.org/10.1017/s0033291710000139;10.1017/s0033291710000139

Momen, N. C., Plana-Ripoll, O., Yilmaz, Z., Thornton, L. M., McGrath, J. J., Bulik, C. M., & Petersen, L. V. (2022). Comorbidity between eating disorders and psychiatric disorders. *International Journal of Eating Disorders, 55*(4), 505–517. https://doi.org/10.1002/eat.23687

Moore, L. D., Le, T., & Fan, G. (2013). DNA Methylation and Its Basic Function. *Neuropsychopharmacology, 38*(1), 23–38. https://doi.org/10.1038/npp.2012.112

Munn-Chernoff, M. A., Johnson, E. C., Chou, Y. L., Coleman, J. R. I., Thornton, L. M., Walters, R. K., Yilmaz, Z., Baker, J. H., Hübel, C., Gordon, S., Medland, S. E., Watson, H. J., Gaspar, H. A., Bryois, J., Hinney, A., Leppä, V. M., Mattheisen, M., Ripke, S., Yao, S., . . . Agrawal, A. (2021). Shared genetic risk between eating disorder- and substance-use-related phenotypes: Evidence from genome-wide association studies. *Addiction Biology, 26*(1), e12880. https://doi.org/10.1111/adb.12880

Munn-Chernoff, M. A., Yilmaz, Z., Lin, S., & Baker, J. H. (2016). Molecular genetics of eating disorders. In *Encyclopedia of Life Sciences* (pp. 1–9). John Wiley. https://doi.org/https://doi.org/10.1002/9780470015902.a0023609

Munn, M. A., Stallings, M. C., Rhee, S. H., Sobik, L. E., Corley, R. P., Rhea, S. A., & Hewitt, J. K. (2010). Bivariate analysis of disordered eating characteristics in adolescence and young adulthood. *International Journal of Eating Disorders, 43*(8), 751. https://doi.org/10.1002/eat.20854

Nakabayashi, K., Komaki, G., Tajima, A., Ando, T., Ishikawa, M., Nomoto, J., Hata, K., Oka, A., Inoko, H., Sasazuki, T., Japanese Genetic Research Group for Eating, & Shirasawa, S. (2009). Identification of novel candidate loci for anorexia nervosa at 1q41 and 11q22 in Japanese by a genome-wide association analysis with microsatellite markers. *Journal of Human Genetics, 54*(9), 531. https://doi.org/10.1038/jhg.2009.74

Nurk, S., Koren, S., Rhie, A., Rautiainen, M., Bzikadze, A. V., Mikheenko, A., Vollger, M. R., Altemose, N., Uralsky, L., Gershman, A., Aganezov, S., Hoyt, S. J., Diekhans, M., Logsdon, G. A., Alonge, M., Antonarakis, S. E., Borchers, M., Bouffard, G. G., Brooks, S. Y., . . . Phillippy, A. M. (2022). The complete sequence of a human genome. *Science, 376*(6588), 44–53. https://doi.org/10.1126/science.abj6987

O'Connor, S. M., Culbert, K. M., Mayhall, L. A., Burt, S. A., & Klump, K. L. (2020). Differences in genetic and environmental influences on body weight and shape concerns across pubertal development in females. *Journal of Psychiatric Research, 121*, 39–46. https://doi.org/10.1016/j.jpsychires.2019.11.001

O'Donovan, M. C. (2015). What have we learned from the Psychiatric Genomics Consortium. *World Psychiatry, 14*(3), 291–293. https://doi.org/10.1002/wps.20270

Ott, J., Wang, J., & Leal, S. M. (2015). Genetic linkage analysis in the age of whole-genome sequencing. *Nature Reviews Genetics, 16*(5), 275–284. https://doi.org/10.1038/nrg3908

Papadopoulos, F. C., Ekbom, A., Brandt, L., & Ekselius, L. (2009). Excess mortality, causes of death and prognostic factors in anorexia nervosa. *British Journal of Psychiatry, 194*(1), 10. https://doi.org/10.1192/bjp.bp.108.054742

Perrin, E. M., Von Holle, A., Zerwas, S., Skinner, A. C., Reba-Harrelson, L., Hamer, R. M., Stoltenberg, C., Torgersen, L., Reichborn-Kjennerud, T., & Bulik, C. M. (2015). Weight-for-length trajectories in the first year of life in children of mothers with eating disorders in a large Norwegian Cohort. *International Journal of Eating Disorders, 48*(4), 406–414. https://doi.org/10.1002/eat.22290

Pickrell, J. K., Berisa, T., Liu, J. Z., Ségurel, L., Tung, J. Y., & Hinds, D. A. (2016). Detection and interpretation of shared genetic influences on 42 human traits. *Nature Genetics, 48*(7), 709–717. https://doi.org/10.1038/ng.3570

Pinheiro, A. P., Bulik, C. M., Thornton, L. M., Sullivan, P. F., Root, T. L., Bloss, C. S., Berrettini, W. H., Schork, N. J., Kaye, W. H., Bergen, A. W., Magistretti, P., Brandt, H., Crawford, S., Crow, S., Fichter, M. M., Goldman, D., Halmi, K. A., Johnson, C., Kaplan, A. S., . . . Woodside, D. B. (2010). Association study of 182 candidate genes in anorexia nervosa. *American Journal of Medical Genetics. Part B, Neuropsychiatric Genetics, 153B*(5), 1070. https://doi.org/10.1002/ajmg.b.31082

Plana-Ripoll, O., Pedersen, C. B., Holtz, Y., Benros, M. E., Dalsgaard, S., de Jonge, P., Fan, C. C., Degenhardt, L., Ganna, A., Greve, A. N., Gunn, J., Iburg, K. M., Kessing, L. V., Lee, B. K., Lim, C. C. W., Mors, O., Nordentoft, M., Prior, A., Roest, A. M., . . . McGrath, J. J. (2019). Exploring Comorbidity Within Mental Disorders Among a Danish National Population. *JAMA Psychiatry, 76*(3), 259–270. https://doi.org/10.1001/jamapsychiatry.2018.3658

Privé, F., Aschard, H., Carmi, S., Folkersen, L., Hoggart, C., O'Reilly, P. F., & Vilhjálmsson, B. J. (2022). Portability of 245 polygenic scores when derived from the UK Biobank and applied to 9 ancestry groups from the same cohort. *American Journal of Human Genetics, 109*(1), 12–23. https://doi.org/10.1016/j.ajhg.2021.11.008

Reba-Harrelson, L., Von Holle, A., Hamer, R. M., Torgersen, L., Reichborn-Kjennerud, T., & Bulik, C. M. (2010). Patterns of maternal feeding and child eating associated with eating disorders in the Norwegian Mother and Child Cohort Study (MoBa). *Eating Behaviors, 11*(1), 54–61. https://doi.org/10.1016/j.eatbeh.2009.09.004

Reichborn-Kjennerud, T., Bulik, C. M., Tambs, K., & Harris, J. R. (2004). Genetic and environmental influences on binge eating in the absence of compensatory behaviors: A population-based twin study. *International Journal of Eating Disorders, 36*(3), 307–314. https://doi.org/10.1002/eat.20047

Root, T. L., Pisetsky, E. M., Thornton, L., Lichtenstein, P., Pedersen, N. L., & Bulik, C. M. (2010). Patterns of co-morbidity of eating disorders and substance use in Swedish females. *Psychological Medicine, 40*(1), 105. https://doi.org/10.1017/s0033291709005662;10.1017/s0033291709005662

Schizophrenia Working Group of the Psychiatric Genomics Consortium. (2014). Biological insights from 108 schizophrenia-associated genetic loci. *Nature, 511*(7510), 421–427. https://doi.org/10.1038/nature13595

Scott-Van Zeeland, A. A., Bloss, C. S., Tewhey, R., Bansal, V., Torkamani, A., Libiger, O., Duvvuri, V., Wineinger, N., Galvez, L., Darst, B. F., Smith, E. N., Carson, A., Pham, P., Phillips, T., Villarasa, N., Tisch, R., Zhang, G., Levy, S., Murray, S., . . . Schork, N. J. (2014). Evidence for the role of EPHX2 gene variants in anorexia nervosa. *Molecular Psychiatry, 19*(6), 724–732. https://doi.org/10.1038/mp.2013.91

Slof-Op 't Landt, M. C., van Furth, E. F., Meulenbelt, I., Slagboom, P. E., Bartels, M., Boomsma, D. I., & Bulik, C. M. (2005). Eating disorders: From twin studies to candidate genes and beyond. *Twin Research and Human Genetics, 8*(5), 467–482. https://doi.org/10.1375/183242705774310114

Smith, A. D., Herle, M., Fildes, A., Cooke, L., Steinsbekk, S., & Llewellyn, C. H. (2017). Food fussiness and food neophobia share a common etiology in early childhood. *Journal of Child Psychology and Psychiatry, 58*(2), 189–196. https://doi.org/10.1111/jcpp.12647

Smith, G. D., & Ebrahim, S. (2003). "Mendelian randomization": Can genetic epidemiology contribute to understanding environmental determinants of disease? *International Journal of Epidemiology, 32*(1), 1–22. https://doi.org/10.1093/ije/dyg070

Solmi, M., Radua, J., Olivola, M., Croce, E., Soardo, L., Salazar de Pablo, G., Il Shin, J., Kirkbride, J. B., Jones, P., Kim, J. H., Kim, J. Y., Carvalho, A. F., Seeman, M. V., Correll, C. U., & Fusar-Poli, P. (2022). Age at onset of mental disorders worldwide: Large-scale meta-analysis of 192 epidemiological studies. *Molecular Psychiatry, 27*(1), 281–295. https://doi.org/10.1038/s41380-021-01161-7

Steiger, H., Booij, L., Kahan, McGregor, K., Thaler, L., Fletcher, E., Labbe, A., Joober, R., Israël, M., Szyf, M., Agellon, L. B., Gauvin, L., St-Hilaire, A., & Rossi, E. (2019). A longitudinal, epigenome-wide study of DNA methylation in anorexia nervosa: Results in actively ill, partially weight-restored, long-term remitted and non-eating-disordered women. *Journal of Psychiatry and Neuroscience, 44*(3), 205–213. https://doi.org/10.1503/jpn.170242

Steiger, H., Labonte, B., Groleau, P., Turecki, G., & Israel, M. (2013). Methylation of the glucocorticoid receptor gene promoter in bulimic women: Associations with borderline personality disorder, suicidality, and exposure to childhood abuse. *International Journal of Eating Disorders, 46*(3), 246. https://doi.org/10.1002/eat.22113

Steinhausen, H. C., Jakobsen, H., Helenius, D., Munk-Jorgensen, P., & Strober, M. (2015). A nation-wide study of the family aggregation and risk factors in anorexia nervosa over three generations. *International Journal of Eating Disorders, 48*(1), 1–8. https://doi.org/10.1002/eat.22293

Strober, M., Freeman, R., Lampert, C., Diamond, J., & Kaye, W. (2000). Controlled family study of anorexia nervosa and bulimia nervosa: Evidence of shared liability and transmission of partial syndromes. *American Journal of Psychiatry, 157*(3), 393.

Sullivan, P. F. (1995). Mortality in anorexia nervosa. *American Journal of Psychiatry, 152*(7), 1073–1074. https://doi.org/10.1176/ajp.152.7.1073

Sullivan, P. F., Agrawal, A., Bulik, C. M., Andreassen, O. A., Borglum, A. D., Breen, G., Cichon, S., Edenberg, H. J., Faraone, S. V., Gelernter, J., Mathews, C. A., Nievergelt, C. M., Smoller, J. W., & O'Donovan, M. C. (2018). Psychiatric genomics: An update and an agenda. *American Journal of Psychiatry, 175*(1), 15–27. https://doi.org/10.1176/appi.ajp.2017.17030283

Sullivan, P. F., Bulik, C. M., & Kendler, K. S. (1998). Genetic epidemiology of binging and vomiting. *British Journal of Psychiatry, 173*, 75–79. https://doi.org/10.1192/bjp.173.1.75

Thornton, L. M., Mazzeo, S. E., & Bulik, C. M. (2011). The heritability of eating disorders: Methods and current findings. *Current Topics in Behavioral Neurosciences, 6*, 141. https://doi.org/10.1007/7854_2010_91

Thornton, L. M., Munn-Chernoff, M. A., Baker, J. H., Jureus, A., Parker, R., Henders, A. K., Larsen, J. T., Petersen, L., Watson, H. J., Yilmaz, Z., Kirk, K. M., Gordon, S., Leppa, V. M., Martin, F. C., Whiteman, D. C., Olsen, C. M., Werge, T. M., Pedersen, N. L., Kaye, W., . . . Bulik, C. M. (2018). The Anorexia Nervosa Genetics Initiative (ANGI): Overview and methods. *Contemporary Clinical Trials, 74*, 61–69. https://doi.org/10.1016/j.cct.2018.09.015

Trace, S. E., Baker, J. H., Penas-Lledo, E., & Bulik, C. M. (2013). The genetics of eating disorders. *Annual Review of Clinical Psychology, 9*, 589. https://doi.org/10.1146/annurev-clinpsy-050212-185546;10.1146/annurev-clinpsy-050212-185546

Trace, S. E., Thornton, L. M., Baker, J. H., Root, T. L., Janson, L. E., Lichtenstein, P., Pedersen, N. L., & Bulik, C. M. (2013). A behavioral-genetic investigation of bulimia nervosa and its relationship with alcohol use disorder. *Psychiatry Research, 208*(3), 232–237. https://doi.org/10.1016/j.psychres.2013.04.030

Tremolizzo, L., Conti, E., Bomba, M., Uccellini, O., Rossi, M. S., Marfone, M., Corbetta, F., Santarone, M. E., Raggi, M. E., Neri, F., Ferrarese, C., & Nacinovich, R. (2014). Decreased whole-blood global DNA methylation is related to serum hormones in anorexia nervosa adolescents. *World Journal of Biological Psychiatry, 15*(4), 327–333. https://doi.org/10.3109/15622975.2013.860467

Wade, T. D., Bulik, C. M., Neale, M., & Kendler, K. S. (2000). Anorexia nervosa and major depression: Shared genetic and environmental risk factors. *American Journal of Psychiatry, 157*(3), 469–471. https://doi.org/10.1176/appi.ajp.157.3.469

Wade, T. D., Gordon, S., Medland, S., Bulik, C. M., Heath, A. C., Montgomery, G. W., & Martin, N. G. (2013). Genetic variants associated with disordered eating. *International Journal of Eating Disorders, 46*(6), 594–608. https://doi.org/10.1002/eat.22133

Wade, T. D., Treloar, S., & Martin, N. G. (2008). Shared and unique risk factors between lifetime purging and objective binge eating: A twin study. *Psychological Medicine, 38*(10), 1455–1464. https://doi.org/10.1017/s0033291708002791

Wang, K., Zhang, H., Bloss, C. S., Duvvuri, V., Kaye, W., Schork, N. J., Berrettini, W., Hakonarson, H., & Price Foundation Collaborative Group. (2011). A genome-wide association study on common SNPs and rare CNVs in anorexia nervosa. *Molecular Psychiatry, 16*(9), 949–959. https://doi.org/10.1038/mp.2010.107

Watson, H. J., & Bulik, C. M. (2013). Update on the treatment of anorexia nervosa: Review of clinical trials, practice guidelines and emerging interventions. *Psychological Medicine, 43*(12), 2477–2500. https://doi.org/10.1017/s0033291712002620

Watson, H. J., Palmos, A. B., Hunjan, A., Baker, J. H., Yilmaz, Z., & Davies, H. L. (2021). Genetics of eating disorders in the genome-wide era. *Psychological Medicine, 51*(13), 2287–2297. https://doi.org/10.1017/s0033291720005474

Watson, H. J., Yilmaz, Z., Thornton, L. M., Hubel, C., Coleman, J. R. I., Gaspar, H. A., Bryois, J., Hinney, A., Leppa, V. M., Mattheisen, M., Medland, S. E., Ripke, S., Yao, S., Giusti-Rodriguez, P., Hanscombe, K. B., Purves, K. L., Adan, R. A. H., Alfredsson, L., Ando, T., . . . Bulik, C. M. (2019). Genome-wide association study identifies eight risk loci and implicates metabo-psychiatric origins for anorexia nervosa. *Nature Genetics, 51*(8), 1207–1214. https://doi.org/10.1038/s41588-019-0439-2

Wray, N. R., Goddard, M. E., & Visscher, P. M. (2007). Prediction of individual genetic risk to disease from genome-wide association studies. *Genome Research, 17*(10), 1520–1528. https://doi.org/10.1101/gr.6665407

Wray, N. R., Ripke, S., Mattheisen, M., Trzaskowski, M., Byrne, E. M., Abdellaoui, A., Adams, M. J., Agerbo, E., Air, T. M., Andlauer, T. M. F., Bacanu, S. A., Baekvad-Hansen, M., Beekman, A. F. T., Bigdeli, T. B., Binder, E. B., Blackwood, D. R. H., Bryois, J., Buttenschon, H. N., Bybjerg-Grauholm, J., . . . Sullivan, P. F. (2018). Genome-wide association analyses identify 44 risk variants and refine the genetic architecture of major depression. *Nature Genetics, 50*(5), 668–681. https://doi.org/10.1038/s41588-018-0090-3

Wu, J., Liu, J., Li, S., Ma, H., & Wang, Y. (2020). Trends in the prevalence and disability-adjusted life years of eating disorders from 1990 to 2017: Results from the Global Burden of Disease Study 2017. *Epidemiology and Psychiatric Sciences, 29*, e191. https://doi.org/10.1017/s2045796020001055

Xu, J., Johnson, J. S., Signer, R., Birgegård, A., Jordan, J., Kennedy, M. A., Landén, M., Maguire, S. L., Martin, N. G., Mortensen, P. B., Petersen, L. V., Thornton, L. M., Bulik, C. M., & Huckins, L. M. (2022). Exploring the clinical and genetic associations of adult weight trajectories using electronic health records in a racially diverse biobank: A phenome-wide and polygenic risk study. *Lancet Digital Health, 4*(8), e604–e614. https://doi.org/10.1016/s2589-7500(22)00099-1

Yengo, L., Vedantam, S., Marouli, E., Sidorenko, J., Bartell, E., Sakaue, S., Graff, M., Eliasen, A. U., Jiang, Y., Raghavan, S., Miao, J., Arias, J. D., Graham, S. E., Mukamel, R. E., Spracklen, C. N., Yin, X., Chen, S. H., Ferreira, T., Highland, H. H., . . . Hirschhorn, J. N. (2022). A saturated map of common genetic variants associated with human height. *Nature, 610*(7933), 704–712. https://doi.org/10.1038/s41586-022-05275-y

Yilmaz, Z., Halvorsen, M., Bryois, J., Yu, D., Thornton, L. M., Zerwas, S., Micali, N., Moessner, R., Burton, C. L., Zai, G., Erdman, L., Kas, M. J., Arnold, P. D., Davis, L. K., Knowles, J. A., Breen,

G., Scharf, J. M., Nestadt, G., Mathews, C. A., . . . Crowley, J. J. (2020). Examination of the shared genetic basis of anorexia nervosa and obsessive-compulsive disorder. *Molecular Psychiatry*, *25*(9), 2036–2046. https://doi.org/10.1038/s41380-018-0115-4

Yilmaz, Z., Hardaway, J. A., & Bulik, C. M. (2015). Genetics and epigenetics of eating disorders. *Advances in Genomics and Genetics*, *5*, 131–150.

Yilmaz, Z., Schaumberg, K., Halvorsen, M., Goodman, E. L., Brosof, L. C., Crowley, J. J., Mathews, C. A., Mattheisen, M., Breen, G., Bulik, C. M., Micali, N., & Zerwas, S. C. (2023). Predicting eating disorder and anxiety symptoms using disorder-specific and transdiagnostic polygenic scores for anorexia nervosa and obsessive-compulsive disorder. *Psychological Medicine*, *53*(7), 3021–3035. https://doi.org/10.1017/s0033291721005079

Yilmaz, Z., Szatkiewicz, J. P., Crowley, J. J., Ancalade, N., Brandys, M. K., van Elburg, A., de Kovel, C. G. F., Adan, R. A. H., Hinney, A., Hebebrand, J., Gratacos, M., Fernandez-Aranda, F., Escaramis, G., Gonzalez, J. R., Estivill, X., Zeggini, E., Sullivan, P. F., & Bulik, C. M. (2017). Exploration of large, rare copy number variants associated with psychiatric and neurodevelopmental disorders in individuals with anorexia nervosa. *Psychiatric Genetics*, *27*(4), 152–158. https://doi.org/10.1097/ypg.0000000000000172

Zhu, Z., Zheng, Z., Zhang, F., Wu, Y., Trzaskowski, M., Maier, R., Robinson, M. R., McGrath, J. J., Visscher, P. M., Wray, N. R., & Yang, J. (2018). Causal associations between risk factors and common diseases inferred from GWAS summary data. *Nature Communications*, *9*(1), 224. https://doi.org/10.1038/s41467-017-02317-2

Zuk, O., Hechter, E., Sunyaev, S. R., & Lander, E. S. (2012). The mystery of missing heritability: Genetic interactions create phantom heritability. *Proceedings of the National Academy of Science USA*, *109*(4), 1193–1198. https://doi.org/10.1073/pnas.1119675109

5

Computational Psychiatry and Eating Disorders

Pradyumna Sepúlveda, Ines Aitsahalia, Stella Dong, and Kiyohito Iigaya

Introduction

Computational psychiatry aims to gain a deeper understanding of neural and cognitive mechanisms underlying mental illnesses using mathematical models and computational tools developed in computer science, mathematics, neuroscience, and psychology (Adams et al., 2016; Huys et al., 2016; Maia, 2015; Maia & Frank, 2011; Montague et al., 2012). One of the goals is to capture individual variations of neural and behavioral alterations underlying various computational functions using computational modeling of empirical task measures (Palminteri et al., 2017; Wilson & Collins, 2019). This approach is inherently dimensional and transdiagnostic because mathematical models of neural and behavioral processes do not usually target specific diseases or symptoms. Instead, models describe various computational constructs of brain functions, such as reward learning or working memory, which can be impacted across many psychiatric conditions (Cuthbert & Insel, 2013; Insel et al., 2010). Consequently, in line with the National Institute of Mental Health's (NIMH) Research Domain Criteria (RDoc), this approach has the potential to shift the focus from symptom-based diagnosis (e.g., the *Diagnostic and Statistical Manual of Mental Disorders*, or DSM) to a mechanistic diagnosis that may inform effective therapeutic targets. If successful, computational psychiatry could serve as a crucial step toward developing precision psychiatry, offering objective, dimensional assessments of altered computational functions that underlie psychiatric conditions and are unique to individuals.

This chapter aims to provide a high-level overview of computational psychiatry, with a particular emphasis on the mechanistic modeling of neural and behavioral processes, especially as they relate to eating disorders.

Biological Framework

Although the final objective of computational psychiatry is to understand biological processes involved in the development of psychiatric conditions, its basis relies on a computational framework. Mechanistic modeling of neural and behavioral

Pradyumna Sepúlveda et al., *Computational Psychiatry and Eating Disorders*. In: *The Handbook of the Neurobiology of Eating Disorders*. Edited by: Christina E. Wierenga and Joanna E. Steinglass, Oxford University Press.
 DOI: 10.1093/9780197675212.003.0006

processes has been primarily developed in computational neuroscience. David Marr, one of the founders of computational neuroscience, argued that it is possible to understand the brain as an information processing system that can be analyzed from three distinct levels. The three levels of questions are: (1) What computational problem does the brain solve?, (2) What computational algorithms (or code) does the brain use?, and (3) How does the brain implement the algorithm? (Marr, 2010).

For example, a person goes to the cafeteria and tries to decide what to eat. In this case, the brain is trying to solve the problem of selecting the best food item for lunch (the first level). The brain may compare the calorie contents and tastes across different lunch options (the second level). The neurons in the prefrontal cortex may implement such an algorithm through the firing patterns of neurons (the third level).

While these three levels are complementary, most computational psychiatry research has focused on the second, algorithmic level. This may be because of the great success of reinforcement learning models (the most popular second-level model) in describing neural and behavioral data in humans (as described later) and probably because of outstanding challenges in testing neural, third-level models in human neuroimaging data due to the limited spatial-temporal resolutions.

Therefore, this chapter will describe models of the second-level (reinforcement learning [RL] and drift-diffusion model [DDM] paradigms) as examples of how the computational psychiatry approach can help understand neural and behavioral mechanisms underlying psychiatric conditions and how they may help potential therapeutic developments.

Reinforcement learning

Rescorla Wagner model and the value of stimulus

RL models describe the learning algorithms to obtain rewards and avoid punishments. RL models have provided enormous insights into adaptive (Botvinick et al., 2020; Dayan & Daw, 2008; Niv, 2019; Sutton & Barto, 2018) and maladaptive (Maia & Frank, 2011; Pike & Robinson, 2022) learning and decision-making behavior relevant to psychiatric conditions.

One of the most influential models of learning is the Rescorla-Wagner model (Rescorla, 1972) which describes learning about associations between (neutral) conditioned stimulus (CS) (e.g., a sound or a light) and (appetitive or aversive) unconditioned stimulus (US) (e.g., food or an electric shock). The Rescorla-Wagner model describes this Pavlovian conditioning using the value of conditioned stimulus, V, being updated as a result of events that violate expectations (Kamin, 1967):

$$V_{new} \leftarrow V_{old} + \alpha\,\delta \tag{1}$$

Where V_{new} is the updated value of CS, V_{old} is the previous value of the CS, α is the learning rate and δ is the prediction error, described as:

$$\delta = R_{US} - V_{i,\,old} \tag{2}$$

Here, R_{US} is the value of experienced US (e.g., 1 if reward, −1 if punishment). The prediction error δ represents the difference between the value of what the subject actually experienced (R_{US}) and the subject's expectation (V_{old}). Using this prediction error-based learning rule, the value of CS (V) will reach the actual experienced value of US. An important parameter of the model is the learning rate (α) which captures how fast subjects learn the value V. When the value of α is close to 0, the subject does not change the value V. On the other hand, when the learning rate is high, the new CS value V quickly reaches the experienced value R_{US}.

Q-learning model and the selection of valuable actions

While the Rescorla-Wagner model can generate predictions for stimulus value in passive conditioning, it does not predict actions (Niv, 2019). In realistic situations, actions are taken to receive more rewards. Thus, in more sophisticated RL models, agents need to identify states (*S*) in the environment and perform actions (*a*) (Figure 5.1a). For a rat moving in a maze, the states would correspond to specific locations of the maze and the actions would be right, left, forward, or backward movements.

The RL agent makes actions to maximize future rewards. In the algorithm called Q-learning (Watkins, 1989), the agent learns the value Q(S, *a*) of making the action *a* at state S:

$$Q(S_t, a_t)_{new} = Q(S_t, a_t)_{old} + \alpha\delta_t \tag{3}$$

Where S_t is the state at time t, a_t is the action taken at time t and the prediction error (δ_t) is expressed as:

$$\delta_t = r_t + max_a\, \gamma Q(S_{t+1}, a) - Q(S_t, a_t) \tag{4}$$

Where r_t is the reward at t and γ is the temporal discounting rate that reduces the effect of future rewards, in this case, the immediate next state. Here the reward is estimated as the aggregate of the reward obtained in the current state (r_t) and potential future rewards (captured by the expression $max_a\, \gamma Q(S_{t+1}, a)$). The max operator indicates that the temporal difference is calculated with respect to the (believed) best action at the next state, the action with the highest predictive value.

The agent can then select an action based on these Q values. The simplest way to choose an action is to always follow the highest Q(S, *a*) value. A more relaxed

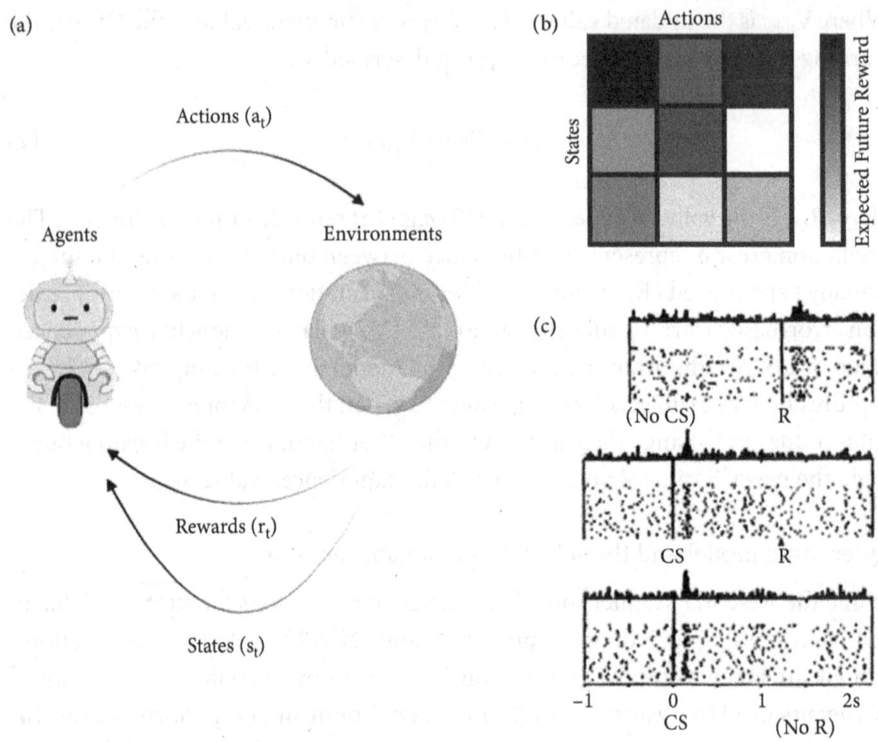

Figure 5.1 Reinforcement learning models. (a) The agent selects actions and transmits them to the environment, which sends back to the agent's observations and rewards. The agent selects the actions that will maximize long-term reward. (b) Tabular solution to a reinforcement learning problem. The agent computes the value of actions given several discrete states from their experience. (c) Temporal difference prediction errors that play key role in reinforcement learning have been shown to be encoded in midbrain dopaminergic neurons. Panel C reproduced with permission from Schultz et al. (1997). A neural substrate of prediction and reward. *Science, 275*(5306), 1593–1599. https://doi.org/10.1126/science.275.5306.1593

behavioral policy is to use a softmax function to generate a *probability* of choosing action a_i at state s:

$$p(a_i|s) = \frac{\exp(\beta Q(a_i|s))}{\sum_{a_j \in A} \exp(\beta Q(a_j|s))} \tag{5}$$

where β is the parameter that is often referred to as the inverse-temperature or the noise. At the limit of infinitely large β, or at an infinitely small temperature, this equation becomes the deterministic policy in which the agent always chooses the action with the highest Q value. In this regime, the agent strongly *exploits* the environment. On the other hand, at the limit of $\beta = 0$, or at an infinitely large temperature, the agent makes a completely random choice with no preference over actions. In this regime, the agent *explores* the environment with no bias. At a finite temperature, the agent makes a stochastic choice with the biases that are proportional to corresponding Q-values. This suggests that tuning the parameter

β enables the agent to address the known trade-off between exploitation and exploration. This trade-off between exploration/exploitation has been recognized as an important feature in human decisions, and the model could inform aspects of psychopathology (Addicott et al., 2017; Dubois & Hauser, 2022; Morris et al., 2016), including eating disorders (Hagan et al., 2024).

It is important to notice that the best action might not result in immediate reward but instead may lead to a new state where the reward can be available later. Simple representations of the environment, comprising a small number of states and actions that can be learned independently from each other, can be represented in tabular state representations (Figure 5.1b). This approach is usually insufficient in more complex environments. More sophisticated approaches, such as deep RL can be used to address this limitation (Botvinick et al., 2020; Mnih et al., 2015; Silver et al., 2016).

Sequential sampling model—Drift-diffusion model

While the RL models can predict the subject's choice, these models cannot predict how long it takes for the subjects to make each choice (response time, RT). In many experiments, the RT is an important behavioral measure that can provide insights into the decision processes impacted by psychiatric conditions. One of the most used models to capture RT distributions is the DDM.

Drift-diffusion model

The standard DDM (Ratcliff, 1978, 1981; Ratcliff & Rouder, 1998) assumes that decisions are made by accumulating stochastic information over time. In this model, the accumulation of information begins at a starting point and continues until the total amount of information reaches a predefined boundary (Figure 5.2a). In the DDM, the single accumulator is usually thought of as a particle that can move toward one of two boundaries (superior or inferior boundary in Figure 5.2a), one for each option (e.g., it could be a Yes/No, right /left options), which will trigger the choice. This type of model can be used in choices based on perceptual information (e.g., dot numerosity discrimination) or subjective value-based preferences (e.g., the snack to eat at lunch) (Gold & Shadlen, 2007). The response time in the model corresponds to the time required to reach the decision boundary. The model also can include a non-decision time parameter (t_0) to consider a constant time used for encoding and response-execution time, not for evidence accumulation. The rate at which the accumulation approaches the boundary (i.e., the average amount of information accumulated per unit of time) is captured by the drift rate parameter (v). The accumulation is not constant but varies depending on a noise term, usually obtained from a normal distribution with standard deviation σ, which is another parameter of the model. This captures the uncertainty in the decision, which makes the integration more unstable and delays reaching the final threshold. The model considers two boundaries, with the separation between them usually included as an additional parameter (a). The boundary separations

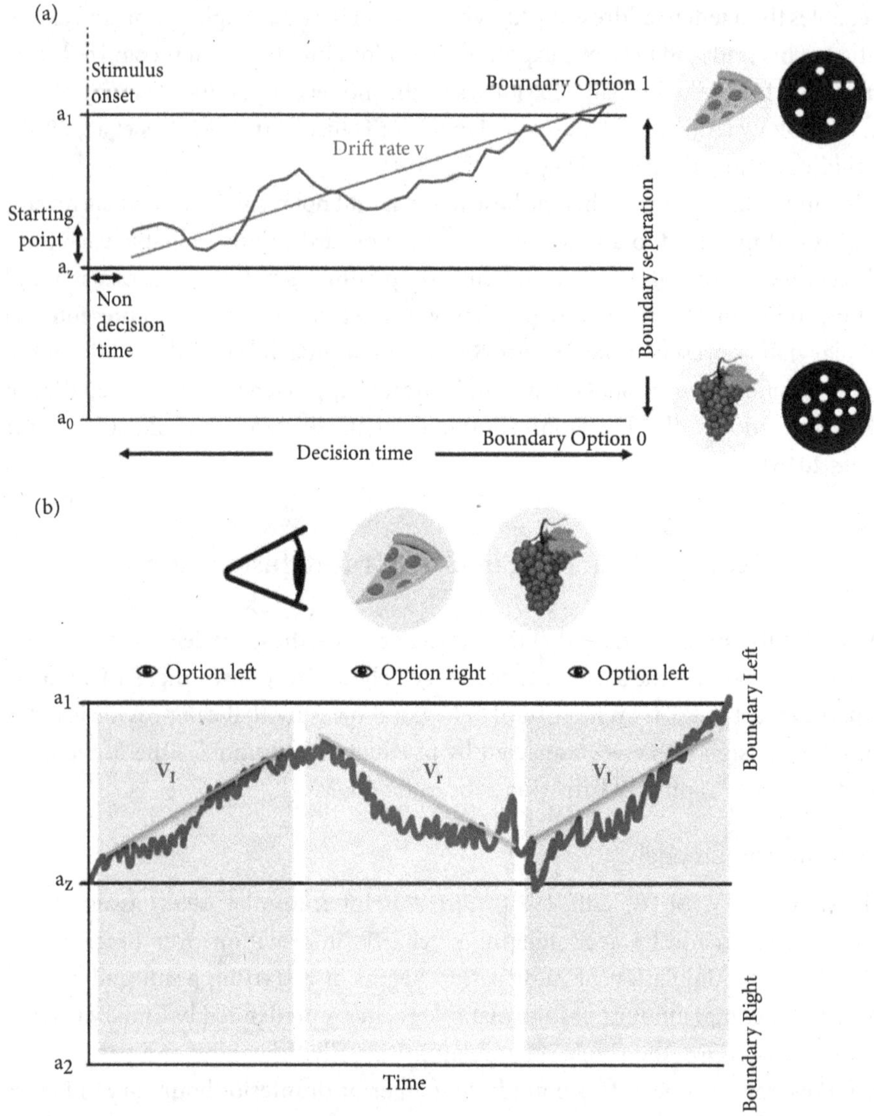

Figure 5.2 Drift diffusion models (DDM). The decision process is described as a sequential sampling with a diffusion signal, where the decision maker accumulates evidence until a stopping boundary is reached, choosing the alternative that corresponds to that boundary. (a) Visualization of the standard DDM parameters. The fixed drift rate, v, determines the speed at which the model moves to a boundary. (b) The attentional DDM. In this model, the drift rate is modulated by participant's attention, often approximated by eye-gaze.

can characterize specific decision-making styles. A high value of the parameter a is related to more conservative decisions, that require more evidence, with longer reaction times and fewer errors; a low boundary separation is associated with a riskier style, with faster response times and a higher error rate. The starting point of accumulation (z) is another parameter that can capture decisions biased toward one of the options. Further iterations of this model also consider choices driven by an "urgency signal," which translates into collapsing decision boundaries in time, to explain behavioral signatures such as incorrect responses being slower than correct choices (Milosavljevic et al., 2010; Thura et al., 2012).

An important feature of the DDM is that the evidence accumulation for the alternative option is anti-correlated; that is, an increase in evidence toward one option means a decrease in evidence toward the other. This is the main difference with race models, another type of sequential sampling model. In race models, each option is represented by an individual accumulator and a single boundary indicates when the decision is made (Forstmann et al., 2016; Sepulveda et al., 2020; Thomas et al., 2019).

Attentional drift diffusion model

DDM has been an important model for the characterization of the decision process, extendedly used in perceptual, memory (Ratcliff et al., 2004; Spaniol et al., 2006), and value-based (Milosavljevic et al., 2010) decision-making in healthy and clinical populations (Nejati et al., 2022; van Ravenzwaaij et al., 2012; White et al., 2010). However, the observation of everyday decisions suggests the deliberation process is likely to be more sophisticated. Consider an individual deciding whether to buy a bag of chips or popcorn at a supermarket. Instead of approaching the shelf and immediately choosing their preferred snack, the customer would likely stop for a second and gaze repeatedly between the two items, shifting their visual fixations between options. This observation inspired an extension to the DDM to include visual attention, the attentional DDM (aDDM) (Krajbich et al., 2010; Krajbich & Rangel, 2011). The standard DDM assumes fixations do not play a role in the accumulation process given that most of the decision experiments keep central fixation during the experiment. The aDDM assumes that attention can change the drift rate (Figure 5.2b), generating a choice bias toward the items that are fixated on more, which is in line with behavioral findings (Armel et al., 2008; Krajbich & Rangel, 2011).

The aDDM assumes that the brain computes a relative decision value that evolves over time as a Markov Gaussian process until one of the boundaries is reached, in a similar way to the DDM. The main difference is that the drift rate is modulated by fixated and non-fixated items. The accumulation process can be characterized by two expressions:

$$X_t = X_{t-1} + d\left(r_{left} - \theta r_{right}\right) + \varepsilon_t \tag{6}$$

$$X_t = X_{t-1} - d\left(r_{right} - \theta r_{left}\right) + \varepsilon_t \tag{7}$$

The first equation describes the accumulation when the item on the left side is fixated, and the second equation is when the right-side item is fixated. The variable X corresponds to the relative decision value (i.e., the accumulator variable) which is updated every timestep (t). The drift rate parameter defined in standard DDM is separated into two parts in the aDDM: (1) a constant parameter d that controls the speed of integration (units ms^{-1}) and (2) a term for the weighted difference between the evidence (r) of attended and unattended items. Because the original presentation of aDDM was developed for value-based decisions, r corresponds to the subjective preferences for each one of the items, which usually is quantified as how much participants like the item (e.g., the amount of money participants would be willing to pay for it) (Krajbich et al., 2010). This process can be adapted to quantify evidence in perceptual experiments (e.g., angles of lines relative to a target) (Tavares et al., 2017). Importantly, the second term includes the crucial attentional parameter (θ) which takes values between 0 and 1, multiplying the unattended item evidence. This means that the value of the unattended item is discounted favoring the accumulation of the attended item. A white Gaussian noise term (ε) with variance σ is randomly sampled every timestep.

Overall, the DDM and aDDM have been successful in integrating a dynamic dimension into the decision process in simple binary choice as previously described, but also in complex multi-alternative choice (Krajbich & Rangel, 2011). More recent models have complemented these findings, suggesting that attention could have a central role in controlling the reliability of the accumulated evidence and optimizing information gathering (Callaway et al., 2021; Jang et al., 2021).

Model fitting

While models on their own could be informative to understand how simulated (artificial) agents could behave (e.g., giving an idea of the relationship between the factors and outputs for simulated agents), a crucial step to understand actual human behavior is to identify a set of parameters that can predict empirical observations. The process of identifying model parameters that generate predictions resembling real-life data from a gigantic space of possible combinations of parameters is called model fitting (Palminteri et al., 2016). The free parameters in the model (e.g., the drift rate v in a DDM) are usually optimized to maximize the likelihood of the experimental data given the model. Methods to search for optimal parameters include standard maximum likelihood estimation applied to each participant's data, such as gradient descent or Newton–Raphson methods (Dedieu, 2015). More sophisticated ways can consider hierarchical relationships between parameters or participants and use Bayesian parameter inference and the Markov Chain Monte Carlo approach (Gershman et al., 2012; Piray et al., 2019; Salvatier et al., 2016). Additionally, multiple types of computational models can predict identical cognitive or behavioral manifestations; for example, there are unlimited ways to make a food choice, such as computing only the caloric content variable for the options or computing a full representation with multiple food-feature variables combined in internal option representations. To compare across models and identify the most parsimonious alternative, the likelihood of each fitted model can be used to calculate a relative quality-of-fit criterion (e.g., the Bayesian information criterion, BIC) which is used to compare between alternative models and identify the "winning" version (Wit et al., 2012). Further steps can include the simulation of behavior using the fitted model, which can be used to test the capacity of the model to predict data out-of-sample. This stage in conjunction with smart experimental design can help to distinguish between models, to keep the ones that capture the complexity of real animal behaviors. Overall, designing appropriate experimental tests, and contrasting actual human behavior with the models is fundamental to disentangling underlying computations and divergences in psychiatric disorders.

Neural evidence for the models

Experimental evidence supports that the brain may implement algorithms similar to RL models. One crucial finding is that midbrain dopaminergic neurons encode prediction error signals (Montague et al., 1996; Morris et al., 2006; Roesch et al., 2007; Schultz et al., 1993, 1997). In simple Pavlovian learning experiments, dopaminergic neurons in the ventral tegmental area (VTA) and substantia nigra (SN) initially respond to reward (Figure 5.1c, top). However, with the progress of learning, the neurons increase their response to the cues predicting reward, a key signature of the so-called temporal difference error (Figure 5.1c, center). Once the animals have learned the contingency between cues and rewards, if the animal experiences no reward following the cue a dip in dopaminergic firing has been observed, which has been interpreted as evidence of a negative prediction error (Figure 5.1c, bottom) (Schultz, 2002; Schultz et al., 1997). The connection between dopaminergic systems and RL has been further validated across species (Dayan, 2009; Ljungberg Paul; Schultz, Wolfram, 1992; Montague et al., 1996; Niv, 2019; Schultz, 1998). These circuits spark special interest given their importance in other conditions such as Parkinson's disease or addiction (Cheng et al., 2010; Obeso et al., 2009; Redish, 2004; Wise & Robble, 2020). Therefore, RL is a framework that is useful to understand how the brain learns values and makes decisions to interact in complex environments.

Neurons or brain areas that correlate with the decision variables in sequential sampling models must fulfill the requirement of not tracking a purely sensory or motor response. Perceptual experiments in monkeys found that neurons in the lateral intraparietal area (LIP) could be candidates to encode this variable (Roitman & Shadlen, 2002; Shadlen & Newsome, 1996). In a random dot motion task, subjects were presented with a display of randomly moving dots and were asked to determine the overall direction of motion. After the stimuli onset, the firing rate of LIP neurons was found proportional to the strength of evidence and choice. Even more, the rise in average neuronal firing (build-up rate) was also proportional to motion strength, which was interpreted as connected to the integration of evidence in time. These findings suggest that the integral of the sensory evidence signal (i.e., the accumulator) could be encoded by the neural activity, which has been shown to start after ~200 ms of the motion onset, a long time for a purely visual signal. The neuronal firing reaches a stereotyped level around ~85 ms before the response, which has been associated with the decision variable reaching an accumulation bound. It has been proposed that alternative populations may be encoding the different options involved in the decision, like in variations of a race architecture which allows extending the mechanism beyond binary choices (Usher & McClelland, 2001). Recent work has reported the relevance of the frontal eye field area in the human brain on the gaze bias, which means that gaze could indeed have a causal role in choice (Krajbich et al., 2021). Overall, the basis of decision is an area of active research with important open questions such as how the activity of this neuronal circuit is adjusted to process the evidence relevant to each one of the multiple tasks that animals need to perform in natural environments (Shadlen & Kiani, 2013).

State of the Science in Eating Disorders

Model-based versus model-free reinforcement learning

The RL models described in this chapter belong to the so-called model-free RL models. Another class of RL models, the so-called model-based RL models, have also been shown to be crucial to understand decision-making behavior (Adams et al., 2016; Collins & Cockburn, 2020; Daw et al., 2011; Doody et al., 2022; Hackel et al., 2019; Huys et al., 2016).

Model-based RL can be understood as a *deductive* approach for solving a problem (Sutton & Barto, 2018). In these types of models, an agent uses its general understanding of the system, or a cognitive map, to derive the best next action based on expected future reward (Dayan & Berridge, 2014). This is computationally costly because it means maintaining a representation of the transition probabilities between different states of the environment, but it is more flexible to unexpected changes. Because the agent has a complete mental map, changes in the environment can be easily incorporated into the model and "back-up plans" can be devised, without needing to rebuild the model from scratch (Drummond & Niv, 2020).

On the other hand, model-free RL is an *inductive* approach for solving a problem. An agent uses its past experiences as empirical evidence and uses frequency statistics to estimate the value of its actions directly. One example model-free algorithm is Q-learning, described above. Model-free methods are easier to use in terms of computational cost; however, much trial-and-error experience is required to make the computed values good estimates of future consequences, which could make them less flexible (Sutton & Barto, 2018).

The model-based versus model-free RL dichotomy is often seen as parallel to "goal-directed" versus "habitual" behavior (Dayan & Berridge, 2014). This has been the basis of much computational psychiatry research because people with psychiatric symptoms often present with disturbances in their habits and goals (American Psychiatric Association, 2013), and the two learning classes seem to be regulated by distinct (albeit overlapping) brain regions (Huang et al., 2020).

Studies have suggested impaired model-based reinforcement learning in clinical populations, such as in obsessive-compulsive disorder, binge-eating disorder, and substance use disorder, suggesting a potential link to compulsivity (Voon et al., 2015). However, one needs to be cautious about the interpretations of such results, as the models that participants use may not be the same as what experimentalists think (Collins & Cockburn, 2020), especially in individuals with psychiatric conditions. Also, many studies do not use naturalistic or behaviorally relevant stimuli, and the relationship of model-free learning to cognitive control is unclear. Patients with anorexia nervosa (AN) and bulimia nervosa (BN) present similarities in self-reported control or experimentally measured "self-control" (Tiggemann & Raven, 1998), contradicting some common hypotheses (Hay, 2020; Nunes et al., 2018).

Despite many researchers positing that restrictive disorders like AN are maintained by overreliance on goal-directed control (Haynos et al., 2022), reduced model-based reinforcement learning strategies have been found in patients with AN in lab experiments (Foerde et al., 2021; Wierenga et al., 2022). These mixed results depict the complexity of this process and the need for further work to clarify how goal-directed control toward food and additional factors interact to define decisions in eating disorders.

Anticipation and eating disorders

Many open questions about eating disorders remain in computational psychiatry. Recent research in our group has focused on the transition between AN and BN (Eddy et al., 2008; Serra et al., 2022), which could be explained by modeling and testing anticipation. Anticipatory value can be defined with a mathematical model from behavioral economics (Loewenstein, 1987). This value dynamically evolves over time, with its intensity exponentially increasing toward the delivery of reward or punishment (Loewenstein, 1987). People use this value throughout the duration of anticipation (anticipatory pleasure), affecting the enjoyable nature of the event beyond the mere consumption of the reward (consummatory pleasure). For example, in the case of a person who will dine in a fancy restaurant during the upcoming week, the value of their experience is not due only to the actual eating but is also derived from the entire week where they anticipate thinking about the possible dishes they can taste or the fancy atmosphere they will find. This intuition has been formalized in a model using the RL framework, with the exception that the total value of choice is computed from the sum of the value of anticipation and the reward the agent will obtain ($Total\ Value = \eta V^{anticipation} + V^{reward}$, with η a parameter modulating the relevance of anticipation). The value of anticipation can be represented as the total area under an anticipation signal exponentially increasing toward the delivery of the reward (Figure 5.3a, central panel; see Iigaya et al., 2016, 2020 for details on the modeling).

The importance of value anticipation in eating disorders is highlighted by patients scoring lower than healthy controls in anticipatory pleasure questionnaires (TEPS), without differences in consummatory pleasure (Dolan, Reilly, et al., 2022). Furthermore, patients with AN specifically display shallower discounting rates than healthy participants (Amlung et al., 2019; Decker et al., 2015; Steinglass et al., 2017). Among patients with eating disorders, reporting greater anticipatory pleasure was associated with lower overall restrictive symptom severity, but positively linked to the frequency of binge-eating episodes (Dolan, Brown, et al., 2022; Dolan, Khindri, et al., 2022; Dolan, Reilly, et al., 2022). Furthermore, neuroimaging studies of individuals with AN have found an emphasis on negative

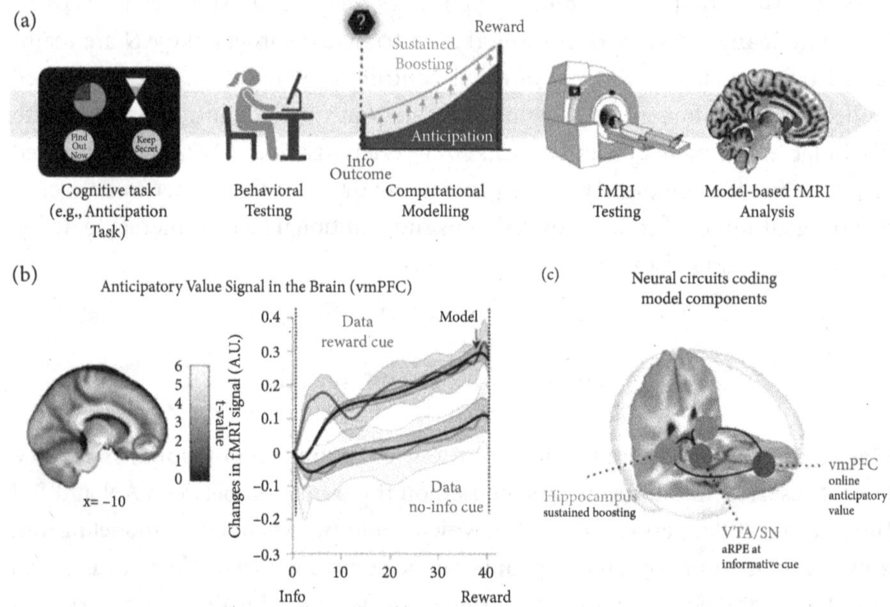

Figure 5.3 Model-Based fMRI, using a model of anticipatory value computation. (a) First a computational model is validated through behavioral testing (if it is a new model and/or tasks). Then participants perform the behavioral task in the fMRI scanner. The computational model capturing participants' behavior will make predictions about fMRI signals. (b) The temporal dynamics of the BOLD signal in the vmPFC matched the model's anticipatory value signal during the anticipation period. (c) The model-based fMRI uncovers the neural circuitry underlying anticipatory value computation. Adapted from K. Iigaya et al. (2020). The value of what's to come: Neural mechanisms coupling prediction error and the utility of anticipation. *Science Advances, 6*(25), eaba3828. Under a Creative Commons Attribution 4.0 International (CC BY 4.0).

emotions (associated with amygdala activation) during the expectation of a caloric taste stimulus (sucrose) but a normal response to the actual experience of the stimulus (Frank et al., 2023), suggesting that the primary difference may lie in the anticipation process.

Considering this evidence, it is possible that shifting from a positive anticipation of a rewarding future state—in patients with eating disorders, often a lower weight—to a negative anticipation of future punishment—a higher body weight and the psychological and social distress accompanying it—could relate to the well-documented transition from AN to BN (Eddy et al., 2008; Serra et al., 2022; Sepúlveda et al., 2025).

Anticipatory value computation allows for a systematic analysis of different factors in the anticipation process (Iigaya et al., 2020), which could be important to dissociate specific mechanisms for AN and BN. Consistent food deprivation in AN could further enhance dopamine (DA) activity, which may generate more intense dread in food anticipation in patients with BN. Patients who are primarily motivated by the dread of future punishment may be more at risk for self-hate and fear (Pearson et al., 2015, 2016), which are predictors of BN severity (Birgegård et al., 2009) compared to patients who focus more on the anticipation of future reward. Mesolimbic DA activity correlates with prediction errors that boost anticipatory utility (Iigaya et al., 2020), which presents a potential mechanism for the anticipation differences among eating disorder patients. Empirically delineating between anticipation and dread, could help predict the transition from AN to BN, aiding treatment. However, much future work is required to further develop computational models of eating disorders more broadly.

Model-based fMRI analysis

Combining the computational modeling approach with the so-called model-based fMRI (O'Doherty et al., 2007) enables uncovering how the computational model's signals are encoded in the brain (Figure 5.3a). For this, the computational model's parameters are fitted to participants' responses. The model adjusted to the participant's behavior can then generate predictions about the exact time course of fMRI signals encoding the model's variables. For example, in the case of an RL model developed to measure reward anticipation (Iigaya et al., 2016, 2020), the predicted signals include reward prediction error and value signals which change slowly over time till the delivery of the outcomes. The predicted signals are then convolved with hemodynamic response function (HRF) and compared directly with fMRI responses. The correlation between the convolved model's predictions and fMRI signals can be estimated using a standard GLM analysis using SPM, FSL, or performing a customized correlation analysis with cross-validation (Jenkinson et al., 2012; Penny et al., 2011). Thanks to this analysis in the anticipation model, it was possible to identify a precise time course of the anticipatory value signal in the vmPFC (Figure 5.3b). Model-based fMRI additionally found that the hippocampus, ventral tegmental area (VTA), and vmPFC orchestrate different aspects of the anticipatory value computation (Figure 5.3c) (for details, see Iigaya et al., 2020). Therefore, model-based fMRI can be an important avenue for understanding the decision-making mechanisms in eating disorders, such as the reward anticipation process (as previously mentioned) or the construction of food preferences (Suzuki et al., 2017; Xue et al., 2022).

Alternative Perspectives

Thus far, this chapter has focused on "theory-driven" computational psychiatry; that is, devising mathematical models and fitting behavioral and neural data to potentially explain the algorithmic mechanisms of mental illness. However, there are other avenues in computational psychiatry. The most-significant alternative perspective is the "data-driven" approach, which focuses on extracting patterns from high-dimensional datasets (Bennett et al., 2019; Huys et al., 2016; Rutledge et al., 2019). This "data-driven" perspective can be applied to many types of data: behavioral, self-report, clinical, or genetic (Cervin et al., 2021; Orrù et al., 2012; Wolfers et al., 2015).

These types of approaches can be used for a similar goal as theory-driven computational psychiatry: to lend explanatory power to brain processes, but they are also clinically useful for their predictive power. Machine learning tools have been used to help predict relapses as well as future risk of disorder development (Fardouly et al., 2022; Paulus & Thompson, 2021). Meta-analysis of questionnaires and behavioral data has already led to a shift in conceptions of mental illness, focusing on underlying commonalities that transcend specific diagnoses (Kotov et al., 2018). This has already been validated in longitudinal studies (Cervin et al., 2021), and could be useful to predict treatment response and improve treatment selection (Huys et al., 2016). These tools could also be used to help consolidate data from different human experiments, increasing the statistical power of neuroimaging analyses.

Implications

Therapeutic approaches: Neurofeedback

Computational modeling and neuroimaging could identify specific brain dynamics that may be associated with psychiatric symptoms. However, developing precise therapeutic methods leveraging these findings is challenging. A promising solution is fMRI-Neurofeedback (fMRI-NF), which uses machine learning methods to analyze real-time brain activity of a participant and provide online feedback (e.g., monetary reward) to the participant when detecting specific voxel activations. Research suggests that fMRI-NF enables participants to control their brain activity without conscious awareness of the target area (Cortese et al., 2016; Muñoz-Moldes & Cleeremans, 2020; Sepulveda et al., 2016; Shibata et al., 2011). These findings suggest fMRI-NF as a potential intervention for the treatment of phobias, post-traumatic stress disorder, and other psychiatric conditions (Cortese et al., 2016; Taschereau-Dumouchel et al., 2018). While NF studies in eating disorders are limited (Blume et al., 2022; Imperatori et al., 2018), machine-learning informed fMRI-NF approach could be a promising avenue to remediate the network imbalances in individuals with eating disorders (Ihssen et al., 2017; Spetter et al., 2017).

Conclusions

The standard use of the categorization system of the DSM, even when helpful to orient treatment in patients, can be insufficient to uncover the detailed causes and mechanisms underlying these disorders. Computational psychiatry, especially studies that consider the continuum of behaviors and traits from neurotypical to clinical diagnoses, could help to circumvent this problem. Computational psychiatry opens the possibility of transdiagnostic examination of psychiatric conditions and traits, fostering potential avenues for integral and individualized treatment.

References

Adams, R. A., Huys, Q. J. M., & Roiser, J. P. (2016). Computational psychiatry: Towards a mathematically informed understanding of mental illness. *Journal of Neurology, Neurosurgery & Psychiatry, 87*(1), article 1. https://doi.org/10.1136/jnnp-2015-310737

Addicott, M. A., Pearson, J. M., Sweitzer, M. M., Barack, D. L., & Platt, M. L. (2017). A primer on foraging and the explore/exploit trade-off for psychiatry research. *Neuropsychopharmacology, 42*(10), 1931–1939. https://doi.org/10.1038/npp.2017.108

American Psychiatric Association (Ed.). (2013). *Diagnostic and statistical manual of mental disorders: DSM-5* (5th ed). American Psychiatric Association.

Amlung, M., Marsden, E., Holshausen, K., Morris, V., Patel, H., Vedelago, L., Naish, K. R., Reed, D. D., & McCabe, R. E. (2019). Delay discounting as a transdiagnostic process in psychiatric disorders: A meta-analysis. *JAMA Psychiatry, 76*(11), article 11. https://doi.org/10.1001/jamapsychiatry.2019.2102

Armel, K. C., Beaumel, A., & Rangel, A. (2008). Biasing simple choices by manipulating relative visual attention. *Judgment and Decision Making, 3*(5), 396–403.

Bennett, D., Silverstein, S. M., & Niv, Y. (2019). The two cultures of computational psychiatry. *JAMA Psychiatry, 76*(6), 563. https://doi.org/10.1001/jamapsychiatry.2019.0231

Birgegård, A., Björck, C., Norring, C., Sohlberg, S., & Clinton, D. (2009). Anorexic self-control and bulimic self-hate: Differential outcome prediction from initial self-image. *International Journal of Eating Disorders, 42*(6), article 6. https://doi.org/10.1002/eat.20642

Blume, M., Schmidt, R., Schmidt, J., Martin, A., & Hilbert, A. (2022). EEG neurofeedback in the treatment of adults with binge-eating disorder: A randomized controlled pilot study. *Neurotherapeutics, 19*(1), 352–365. https://doi.org/10.1007/s13311-021-01149-9

Botvinick, M., Wang, J. X., Dabney, W., Miller, K. J., & Kurth-Nelson, Z. (2020). Deep reinforcement learning and its neuroscientific implications. *Neuron, 107*(4), 603–616. https://doi.org/10.1016/j.neuron.2020.06.014

Callaway, F., Rangel, A., & Griffiths, T. L. (2021). Fixation patterns in simple choice reflect optimal information sampling. *PLOS Computational Biology, 17*(3), 1–29. https://doi.org/10.1371/journal.pcbi.1008863

Cervin, M., Norris, L. A., Ginsburg, G., Gosch, E. A., Compton, S. N., Piacentini, J., Albano, A. M., Sakolsky, D., Birmaher, B., Keeton, C., Storch, E. A., & Kendall, P. C. (2021). The p factor consistently predicts long-term psychiatric and functional outcomes in anxiety-disordered youth. *Journal of the American Academy of Child and Adolescent Psychiatry, 60*(7), 902–912.e5. https://doi.org/10.1016/j.jaac.2020.08.440

Cheng, H.-C., Ulane, C. M., & Burke, R. E. (2010). Clinical progression in Parkinson disease and the neurobiology of axons. *Annals of Neurology, 67*(6), 715–725. https://doi.org/10.1002/ana.21995

Collins, A. G. E., & Cockburn, J. (2020). Beyond dichotomies in reinforcement learning. *Nature Reviews Neuroscience, 21*(10), 576–586. https://doi.org/10.1038/s41583-020-0355-6

Cortese, A., Amano, K., Koizumi, A., Kawato, M., & Lau, H. (2016). Multivoxel neurofeedback selectively modulates confidence without changing perceptual performance. *Nature Communications, 7*(1), 13669–13669. https://doi.org/10.1038/ncomms13669

Cuthbert, B. N., & Insel, T. R. (2013). Toward the future of psychiatric diagnosis: The seven pillars of RDoC. *BMC Medicine, 11*(1), 126. https://doi.org/10.1186/1741-7015-11-126

Daw, N. D., Gershman, S. J., Seymour, B., Dayan, P., & Dolan, R. J. (2011). Model-based influences on humans' choices and striatal prediction errors. *Neuron, 69*(6), 1204–1215. https://doi.org/10.1016/j.neuron.2011.02.027

Dayan, P. (2009). Dopamine, reinforcement learning, and addiction. *Pharmacopsychiatry, 42*(S 01), S56–S65. https://doi.org/10.1055/s-0028-1124107

Dayan, P., & Berridge, K. C. (2014). Model-based and model-free Pavlovian reward learning: Revaluation, revision, and revelation. *Cognitive, Affective & Behavioral Neuroscience, 14*(2), 473–492. https://doi.org/10.3758/s13415-014-0277-8

Dayan, P., & Daw, N. D. (2008). Decision theory, reinforcement learning, and the brain. *Cognitive, Affective & Behavioral Neuroscience, 8*(4), 429–453. https://doi.org/10.3758/CABN.8.4.429

Decker, J. H., Figner, B., & Steinglass, J. E. (2015). On weight and waiting: Delay discounting in anorexia nervosa pretreatment and posttreatment. *Biological Psychiatry, 78*(9), article 9. https://doi.org/10.1016/j.biopsych.2014.12.016

Dedieu, J.-P. (2015). Newton–Raphson method. In B. Engquist (Ed.), *Encyclopedia of applied and computational mathematics* (pp. 1023–1028). Springer. https://doi.org/10.1007/978-3-540-70529-1_374

Dolan, S. C., Brown, T. A., Wierenga, C. E., Kaye, W. H., & Reilly, E. E. (2022). Changes in anhedonia over the course of eating disorder treatment. *International Journal of Eating Disorders, 55*(3), article 3. https://doi.org/10.1002/eat.23673

Dolan, S. C., Khindri, R., Franko, D. L., Thomas, J. J., Reilly, E. E., & Eddy, K. T. (2022). Anhedonia in eating disorders: A meta-analysis and systematic review. *International Journal of Eating Disorders, 55*(2), article 2. https://doi.org/10.1002/eat.23645

Dolan, S. C., Reilly, E. E., Brown, T. A., Shott, M. E., & Frank, G. K. W. (2022). Anticipatory and consummatory pleasure in eating disorders. *Journal of Eating Disorders, 10*(1), article 1. https://doi.org/10.1186/s40337-022-00692-w

Doody, M., Van Swieten, M. M. H., & Manohar, S. G. (2022). Model-based learning retrospectively updates model-free values. *Scientific Reports, 12*(1), 2358. https://doi.org/10.1038/s41598-022-05567-3

Drummond, N., & Niv, Y. (2020). Model-based decision making and model-free learning. *Current Biology, 30*(15), R860–R865. https://doi.org/10.1016/j.cub.2020.06.051

Dubois, M., & Hauser, T. U. (2022). Value-free random exploration is linked to impulsivity. *Nature Communications, 13*(1), 4542. https://doi.org/10.1038/s41467-022-31918-9

Eddy, K. T., Dorer, D. J., Franko, D. L., Tahilani, K., Thompson-Brenner, H., & Herzog, D. B. (2008). Diagnostic crossover in anorexia nervosa and bulimia nervosa: Implications for DSM-V. *American Journal of Psychiatry, 165*(2), article 2. https://doi.org/10.1176/appi.ajp.2007.07060951

Fardouly, J., Crosby, R. D., & Sukunesan, S. (2022). Potential benefits and limitations of machine learning in the field of eating disorders: Current research and future directions. *Journal of Eating Disorders, 10*(1), 66. https://doi.org/10.1186/s40337-022-00581-2

Foerde, K., Daw, N. D., Rufin, T., Walsh, B. T., Shohamy, D., & Steinglass, J. E. (2021). Deficient goal-directed control in a population characterized by extreme goal pursuit. *Journal of Cognitive Neuroscience, 33*(3), article 3. https://doi.org/10.1162/jocn_a_01655

Forstmann, B. U., Ratcliff, R., & Wagenmakers, E.-J. (2016). Sequential sampling models in cognitive neuroscience: Advantages, applications, and extensions. *Annual Review of Psychology, 67*, 641.

Frank, G. K. W., Shott, M. E., Pryor, T., Swindle, S., Nguyen, T., & Stoddard, J. (2023). Trait anxiety is associated with amygdala expectation and caloric taste receipt response across eating disorders. *Neuropsychopharmacology, 48*(2), article 2. https://doi.org/10.1038/s41386-022-01440-z

Gershman, S., Hoffman, M., & Blei, D. (2012). Nonparametric variational inference. *arXiv.* https://doi.org/10.48550/ARXIV.1206.4665

Gold, J. I., & Shadlen, M. N. (2007). The neural basis of decision making. *Annual Review of Neuroscience, 30*(1), 535–574. https://doi.org/10.1146/annurev.neuro.29.051605.113038

Hackel, L. M., Berg, J. J., Lindström, B. R., & Amodio, D. M. (2019). Model-based and model-free social cognition: Investigating the role of habit in social attitude formation and choice. *Frontiers in Psychology, 10,* 2592. https://doi.org/10.3389/fpsyg.2019.02592

Hagan, K. E., Aimufua, I., Haynos, A. F., & Walsh, B. T. (2024). The explore/exploit trade-off: An ecologically valid and translational framework that can advance mechanistic understanding of eating disorders. *International Journal of Eating Disorders, 57*(5), 1102–1108. https://doi.org/10.1002/eat.24173

Hay, P. (2020). Current approach to eating disorders: A clinical update. *Internal Medicine Journal, 50*(1), article 1. https://doi.org/10.1111/imj.14691

Haynos, A. F., Widge, A. S., Anderson, L. M., & Redish, A. D. (2022). Beyond description and deficits: How computational psychiatry can enhance an understanding of decision-making in anorexia nervosa. *Current Psychiatry Reports, 24*(1), article 1. https://doi.org/10.1007/s11920-022-01320-9

Huang, Y., Yaple, Z. A., & Yu, R. (2020). Goal-oriented and habitual decisions: Neural signatures of model-based and model-free learning. *NeuroImage, 215,* 116834. https://doi.org/10.1016/j.neuroimage.2020.116834

Huys, Q. J. M., Maia, T. V., & Frank, M. J. (2016). Computational psychiatry as a bridge from neuroscience to clinical applications. *Nature Neuroscience, 19*(3), article 3. https://doi.org/10.1038/nn.4238

Ihssen, N., Sokunbi, M. O., Lawrence, A. D., Lawrence, N. S., & Linden, D. E. J. (2017). Neurofeedback of visual food cue reactivity: A potential avenue to alter incentive sensitization and craving. *Brain Imaging and Behavior, 11*(3), 915–924. https://doi.org/10.1007/s11682-016-9558-x

Iigaya, K., Hauser, T. U., Kurth-Nelson, Z., O'Doherty, J. P., Dayan, P., & Dolan, R. J. (2020). The value of what's to come: Neural mechanisms coupling prediction error and the utility of anticipation. *Science Advances, 6*(25), eaba3828.

Iigaya, K., Jolivald, A., Jitkrittum, W., Gilchrist, I. D., Dayan, P., Paul, E., & Mendl, M. (2016). Cognitive bias in ambiguity judgements: Using computational models to dissect the effects of mild mood manipulation in humans. *PLOS ONE, 11*(11), article 11. https://doi.org/10.1371/journal.pone.0165840

Imperatori, C., Mancini, M., Della Marca, G., Valenti, E., & Farina, B. (2018). Feedback-based treatments for eating disorders and related symptoms: A systematic review of the literature. *Nutrients, 10*(11), 1806. https://doi.org/10.3390/nu10111806

Insel, T., Cuthbert, B., Garvey, M., Heinssen, R., Pine, D. S., Quinn, K., Sanislow, C., & Wang, P. (2010). Research Domain Criteria (RDoC): Toward a new classification framework for research on mental disorders. *American Journal of Psychiatry, 167*(7), 748–751. https://doi.org/10.1176/appi.ajp.2010.09091379

Jang, A. I., Sharma, R., & Drugowitsch, J. (2021). Optimal policy for attention-modulated decisions explains human fixation behavior. *Elife, 10,* e63436.

Jenkinson, M., Beckmann, C. F., Behrens, T. E. J., Woolrich, M. W., & Smith, S. M. (2012). FSL. *NeuroImage, 62*(2), article 2. https://doi.org/10.1016/j.neuroimage.2011.09.015

Kamin, L. J. (1967). Predictability, surprise, attention, and conditioning. *Symposium on Punishment,* Report #*TR-13.* NASA.

Kotov, R., Krueger, R. F., & Watson, D. (2018). A paradigm shift in psychiatric classification: The Hierarchical Taxonomy Of Psychopathology (HiTOP). *World Psychiatry, 17*(1), 24–25. https://doi.org/10.1002/wps.20478

Krajbich, I., Armel, C., & Rangel, A. (2010). Visual fixations and the computation and comparison of value in simple choice. *Nature Neuroscience, 13*(10), 1292–1298.

Krajbich, I., Mitsumasu, A., Polania, R., Ruff, C. C., & Fehr, E. (2021). A causal role for the right frontal eye fields in value comparison. *Elife, 10,* e67477.

Krajbich, I., & Rangel, A. (2011). Multialternative drift-diffusion model predicts the relationship between visual fixations and choice in value-based decisions. *Proceedings of the National Academy of Sciences of the United States of America, 108*(33), 13852–13857. https://doi.org/10.1073/pnas.1101328108

Ljungberg, P., & Schultz, W. T. A. (1992). Responses of monkey dopamine neurons during learning of behavioral reactions. *Journal of Neurophysiology, 67*(1), 145–163. https://doi.org/10.1152/jn.1992.67.1.145

Loewenstein, G. (1987). Anticipation and the valuation of delayed consumption. *Economic Journal, 97*(387), 666. https://doi.org/10.2307/2232929

Maia, T. V. (2015). Introduction to the series on computational psychiatry. *Clinical Psychological Science, 3*(3), 374–377. https://doi.org/10.1177/2167702614567350

Maia, T. V., & Frank, M. J. (2011). From reinforcement learning models to psychiatric and neurological disorders. *Nature Neuroscience, 14*(2), 154–162. https://doi.org/10.1038/nn.2723

Marr, D. (2010). *Vision: A computational investigation into the human representation and processing of visual information.* MIT Press.

Milosavljevic, M., Malmaud, J., Huth, A., Koch, C., & Rangel, A. (2010). The Drift Diffusion Model can account for the accuracy and reaction time of value-based choices under high and low time pressure. *Judgment and Decision Making, 5*(6), 437–449. https://doi.org/10.1017/S1930297500001285

Mnih, V., Kavukcuoglu, K., Silver, D., Rusu, A. A., Veness, J., Bellemare, M. G., Graves, A., Riedmiller, M., Fidjeland, A. K., Ostrovski, G., Petersen, S., Beattie, C., Sadik, A., Antonoglou, I., King, H., Kumaran, D., Wierstra, D., Legg, S., & Hassabis, D. (2015). Human-level control through deep reinforcement learning. *Nature, 518*(7540), article 7540. https://doi.org/10.1038/nature14236

Montague, P., Dayan, P., & Sejnowski, T. (1996). A framework for mesencephalic dopamine systems based on predictive Hebbian learning. *Journal of Neuroscience, 16*(5), 1936–1947. https://doi.org/10.1523/JNEUROSCI.16-05-01936.1996

Montague, P. R., Dolan, R. J., Friston, K. J., & Dayan, P. (2012). Computational psychiatry. *Trends in Cognitive Sciences, 16*(1), 72–80. https://doi.org/10.1016/j.tics.2011.11.018

Morris, G., Nevet, A., Arkadir, D., Vaadia, E., & Bergman, H. (2006). Midbrain dopamine neurons encode decisions for future action. *Nature Neuroscience, 9*(8), 1057–1063. https://doi.org/10.1038/nn1743

Morris, L. S., Baek, K., Kundu, P., Harrison, N. A., Frank, M. J., & Voon, V. (2016). Biases in the explore–exploit tradeoff in addictions: The role of avoidance of uncertainty. *Neuropsychopharmacology, 41*(4), 940–948. https://doi.org/10.1038/npp.2015.208

Muñoz-Moldes, S., & Cleeremans, A. (2020). Delineating implicit and explicit processes in neurofeedback learning. *Neuroscience & Biobehavioral Reviews, 118*, 681–688. https://doi.org/10.1016/j.neubiorev.2020.09.003

Nejati, V., Rasanan, A. H. H., Rad, J. A., Alavi, M. M., Haghi, S., & Nitsche, M. A. (2022). Transcranial direct current stimulation (tDCS) alters the pattern of information processing in children with ADHD: Evidence from drift diffusion modeling. *Neurophysiologie Clinique, 52*(1), 17–27.

Niv, Y. (2019). Learning task-state representations. *Nature Neuroscience, 22*(10), 1544–1553. https://doi.org/10.1038/s41593-019-0470-8

Nunes, A., Helson, T. J., Dixon, L. M., Trappenberg, T. P., & Keshen, A. R. (2018). Characteristic impairments of goal-directed and habitual control in bulimia nervosa. *bioRxiv*, 348250. https://doi.org/10.1101/348250

Obeso, J. A., Marin, C., Rodriguez-Oroz, C., Blesa, J., Benitez-Temiño, B., Mena-Segovia, J., Rodríguez, M., & Olanow, C. W. (2009). The basal ganglia in Parkinson's disease: Current concepts and unexplained observations. *Annals of Neurology, 64*(S2), S30–S46. https://doi.org/10.1002/ana.21481

O'Doherty, J. P., Hampton, A., & Kim, H. (2007). Model-based fMRI and its application to reward learning and decision making. *Annals of the New York Academy of Sciences, 1104*, 35–53. https://doi.org/10.1196/annals.1390.022

Orrù, G., Pettersson-Yeo, W., Marquand, A. F., Sartori, G., & Mechelli, A. (2012). Using support vector machine to identify imaging biomarkers of neurological and psychiatric disease: A critical review. *Neuroscience & Biobehavioral Reviews, 36*(4), 1140–1152. https://doi.org/10.1016/j.neubiorev.2012.01.004

Palminteri, S., Kilford, E. J., Coricelli, G., & Blakemore, S.-J. (2016). The computational development of reinforcement learning during adolescence. *PLOS Computational Biology, 12*(6), e1004953. https://doi.org/10.1371/journal.pcbi.1004953

Palminteri, S., Wyart, V., & Koechlin, E. (2017). The importance of falsification in computational cognitive modeling. *Trends in Cognitive Sciences, 21*(6), 425–433. https://doi.org/10.1016/j.tics.2017.03.011

Paulus, M. P., & Thompson, W. K. (2021). Computational approaches and machine learning for individual-level treatment predictions. *Psychopharmacology, 238*(5), 1231–1239. https://doi.org/10.1007/s00213-019-05282-4

Pearson, C. M., Chester, D. S., Powell, D., Wonderlich, S. A., & Smith, G. T. (2016). Investigating the reinforcing value of binge anticipation. *International Journal of Eating Disorders, 49*(6), 539–541. https://doi.org/10.1002/eat.22547

Pearson, C. M., Wonderlich, S. A., & Smith, G. T. (2015). A risk and maintenance model for bulimia nervosa: From impulsive action to compulsive behavior. *Psychological Review, 122*(3), 516–535. https://doi.org/10.1037/a0039268

Penny, W. D., Friston, K. J., Ashburner, J. T., Kiebel, S. J., & Nichols, T. E. (2011). *Statistical parametric mapping: The analysis of functional brain images*. Elsevier.

Pike, A. C., & Robinson, O. J. (2022). Reinforcement learning in patients with mood and anxiety disorders vs control individuals: A systematic review and meta-analysis. *JAMA Psychiatry, 79*(4), 313–322. https://doi.org/10.1001/jamapsychiatry.2022.0051

Piray, P., Dezfouli, A., Heskes, T., Frank, M. J., & Daw, N. D. (2019). Hierarchical Bayesian inference for concurrent model fitting and comparison for group studies. *PLOS Computational Biology, 15*(6), e1007043. https://doi.org/10.1371/journal.pcbi.1007043

Ratcliff, R. (1978). A theory of memory retrieval. *Psychological Review, 85*(2), 59–108. https://doi.org/10.1037/0033-295X.85.2.59

Ratcliff, R. (1981). A theory of order relations in perceptual matching. *Psychological Review, 88*(6), 552–572. https://doi.org/10.1037/0033-295X.88.6.552

Ratcliff, R., & Rouder, J. N. (1998). Modeling response times for two-choice decisions. *Psychological Science, 9*(5), 347–356.

Ratcliff, R., Thapar, A., & McKoon, G. (2004). A diffusion model analysis of the effects of aging on recognition memory. *Journal of Memory and Language, 50*(4), 408–424. https://doi.org/10.1016/j.jml.2003.11.002

Redish, A. D. (2004). Addiction as a computational process gone awry. *Science, 306*(5703), article 5703. https://doi.org/10.1126/science.1102384

Rescorla, R. A. (1972). A theory of Pavlovian conditioning: Variations in the effectiveness of reinforcement and non-reinforcement. *Classical Conditioning, Current Research and Theory, 2*, 64–69.

Roesch, M. R., Calu, D. J., & Schoenbaum, G. (2007). Dopamine neurons encode the better option in rats deciding between differently delayed or sized rewards. *Nature Neuroscience, 10*(12), 1615–1624. https://doi.org/10.1038/nn2013

Roitman, J. D., & Shadlen, M. N. (2002). Response of neurons in the lateral intraparietal area during a combined visual discrimination reaction time task. *Journal of Neuroscience, 22*(21), 9475–9489.

Rutledge, R. B., Chekroud, A. M., & Huys, Q. J. (2019). Machine learning and big data in psychiatry: Toward clinical applications. *Current Opinion in Neurobiology, 55*, 152–159. https://doi.org/10.1016/j.conb.2019.02.006

Salvatier, J., Wiecki, T. V., & Fonnesbeck, C. (2016). Probabilistic programming in Python using PyMC3. *Computer Science, 2*, e55. https://doi.org/10.7717/peerj-cs.55

Schultz, W. (1998). Predictive reward signal of dopamine neurons. *Journal of Neurophysiology, 80*(1), 1–27. https://doi.org/10.1152/jn.1998.80.1.1

Schultz, W. (2002). Getting formal with dopamine and reward. *Neuron, 36*(2), 241–263.

Schultz, W., Apicella, P., & Ljungberg, T. (1993). Responses of monkey dopamine neurons to reward and conditioned stimuli during successive steps of learning a delayed response task. *Journal of Neuroscience, 13*(3), 900–913. https://doi.org/10.1523/JNEUROSCI.13-03-00900.1993

Schultz, W., Dayan, P., & Montague, P. R. (1997). A neural substrate of prediction and reward. *Science, 275*(5306), 1593–1599. https://doi.org/10.1126/science.275.5306.1593

Sepulveda, P., Sitaram, R., Rana, M., Montalba, C., Tejos, C., & Ruiz, S. (2016). How feedback, motor imagery, and reward influence brain self-regulation using real-time fMRI. *Human Brain Mapping, 37*(9), 3153–3171.

Sepulveda, P., Usher, M., Davies, N., Benson, A. A., Ortoleva, P., & De Martino, B. (2020). Visual attention modulates the integration of goal-relevant evidence and not value. *eLife, 9*, e60705. https://doi.org/10.7554/elife.60705

Sepúlveda, P., Aitsahalia, I., Kumar, K., Atkin, T., & Iigaya, K. (2025). Addressing altered anticipation as a transdiagnostic target through computational psychiatry. *Biological Psychiatry: Cognitive Neuroscience and Neuroimaging*. https://doi.org/10.1016/j.bpsc.2025.02.014

Serra, R., Di Nicolantonio, C., Di Febo, R., De Crescenzo, F., Vanderlinden, J., Vrieze, E., Bruffaerts, R., Loriedo, C., Pasquini, M., & Tarsitani, L. (2022). The transition from restrictive anorexia nervosa to binging and purging: A systematic review and meta-analysis. *Eating and Weight Disorders—Studies on Anorexia, Bulimia and Obesity*, *27*(3), article 3. https://doi.org/10.1007/s40519-021-01226-0

Shadlen, M. N., & Kiani, R. (2013). Decision making as a window on cognition. *Neuron*, *80*(3), 791–806. https://doi.org/10.1016/j.neuron.2013.10.047

Shadlen, M. N., & Newsome, W. T. (1996). Motion perception: Seeing and deciding. *Proceedings of the National Academy of Sciences*, *93*(2), 628–633.

Shibata, K., Watanabe, T., Sasaki, Y., & Kawato, M. (2011). Perceptual learning incepted by decoded fMRI neurofeedback without stimulus presentation. *Science*, *334*(6061), 1413–1415. https://doi.org/10.1126/science.1212003

Silver, D., Huang, A., Maddison, C. J., Guez, A., Sifre, L., Van Den Driessche, G., Schrittwieser, J., Antonoglou, I., Panneershelvam, V., Lanctot, M., Dieleman, S., Grewe, D., Nham, J., Kalchbrenner, N., Sutskever, I., Lillicrap, T., Leach, M., Kavukcuoglu, K., Graepel, T., & Hassabis, D. (2016). Mastering the game of Go with deep neural networks and tree search. *Nature*, *529*(7587), 484–489. https://doi.org/10.1038/nature16961

Spaniol, J., Madden, D. J., & Voss, A. (2006). A diffusion model analysis of adult age differences in episodic and semantic long-term memory retrieval. *Journal of Experimental Psychology: Learning, Memory, and Cognition*, *32*(1), 101.

Spetter, M. S., Malekshahi, R., Birbaumer, N., Lührs, M., Van Der Veer, A. H., Scheffler, K., Spuckti, S., Preissl, H., Veit, R., & Hallschmid, M. (2017). Volitional regulation of brain responses to food stimuli in overweight and obese subjects: A real-time fMRI feedback study. *Appetite*, *112*, 188–195. https://doi.org/10.1016/j.appet.2017.01.032

Steinglass, J. E., Lempert, K. M., Choo, T.-H., Kimeldorf, M. B., Wall, M., Walsh, B. T., Fyer, A. J., Schneier, F. R., & Simpson, H. B. (2017). Temporal discounting across three psychiatric disorders: Anorexia nervosa, obsessive compulsive disorder, and social anxiety disorder. *Depression and Anxiety*, *34*(5), article 5. https://doi.org/10.1002/da.22586

Sutton, R. S., & Barto, A. G. (2018). *Reinforcement learning: An introduction*. MIT Press.

Suzuki, S., Cross, L., & O'Doherty, J. P. (2017). Elucidating the underlying components of food valuation in the human orbitofrontal cortex. *Nature Neuroscience*, *20*(12), 1780–1786.

Taschereau-Dumouchel, V., Cortese, A., Chiba, T., Knotts, J. D., Kawato, M., & Lau, H. (2018). Towards an unconscious neural reinforcement intervention for common fears. *Proceedings of the National Academy of Sciences of the United States of America*, *115*(13), 3470–3475. https://doi.org/10.1073/pnas.1721572115

Tavares, G., Perona, P., & Rangel, A. (2017). The attentional drift diffusion model of simple perceptual decision-making. *Frontiers in Neuroscience*, *11*, 468. https://doi.org/10.3389/fnins.2017.00468

Thomas, A. W., Molter, F., Krajbich, I., Heekeren, H. R., & Mohr, P. N. (2019). Gaze bias differences capture individual choice behaviour. *Nature Human Behaviour*, *3*(6), 625–635.

Thura, D., Beauregard-Racine, J., Fradet, C.-W., & Cisek, P. (2012). Decision making by urgency gating: Theory and experimental support. *Journal of Neurophysiology*, *108*(11), 2912–2930. https://doi.org/10.1152/jn.01071.2011

Tiggemann, M., & Raven, M. (1998). Dimensions of control in bulimia and anorexia nervosa: Internal control, desire for control, or fear of losing self-control? *Eating Disorders*, *6*(1), article 1. https://doi.org/10.1080/10640269808249248

Usher, M., & McClelland, J. L. (2001). The time course of perceptual choice: The leaky, competing accumulator model. *Psychological Review*, *108*(3), 550–592. https://doi.org/10.1037/0033-295X.108.3.550

van Ravenzwaaij, D., Dutilh, G., & Wagenmakers, E.-J. (2012). A diffusion model decomposition of the effects of alcohol on perceptual decision making. *Psychopharmacology*, *219*(4), 1017–1025.

Voon, V., Derbyshire, K., Rück, C., Irvine, M. A., Worbe, Y., Enander, J., Schreiber, L. R. N., Gillan, C., Fineberg, N. A., Sahakian, B. J., Robbins, T. W., Harrison, N. A., Wood, J., Daw, N. D., Dayan, P., Grant, J. E., & Bullmore, E. T. (2015). Disorders of compulsivity: A common bias towards learning habits. *Molecular Psychiatry*, *20*(3), 345–352. https://doi.org/10.1038/mp.2014.44

Watkins, C. J. C. H. (1989). *Learning from delayed rewards* [Doctoral dissertation, Cambridge University].

White, C. N., Ratcliff, R., Vasey, M. W., & McKoon, G. (2010). Using diffusion models to understand clinical disorders. *Journal of Mathematical Psychology*, *54*(1), 39–52.

Wierenga, C. E., Reilly, E., Bischoff-Grethe, A., Kaye, W. H., & Brown, G. G. (2022). Altered reinforcement learning from reward and punishment in anorexia nervosa: Evidence from computational modeling. *Journal of the International Neuropsychological Society*, *28*(10), article 10. https://doi.org/10.1017/S1355617721001326

Wilson, R. C., & Collins, A. G. (2019). Ten simple rules for the computational modeling of behavioral data. *eLife*, *8*, e49547. https://doi.org/10.7554/eLife.49547

Wise, R. A., & Robble, M. A. (2020). Dopamine and addiction. *Annual Review of Psychology*, *71*(1), 79–106. https://doi.org/10.1146/annurev-psych-010418-103337

Wit, E., Heuvel, E. V. D., & Romeijn, J.-W. (2012). "All models are wrong . . . ": An introduction to model uncertainty. *Statistica Neerlandica*, *66*(3), 217–236. https://doi.org/10.1111/j.1467-9574.2012.00530.x

Wolfers, T., Buitelaar, J. K., Beckmann, C. F., Franke, B., & Marquand, A. F. (2015). From estimating activation locality to predicting disorder: A review of pattern recognition for neuroimaging-based psychiatric diagnostics. *Neuroscience & Biobehavioral Reviews*, *57*, 328–349. https://doi.org/10.1016/j.neubiorev.2015.08.001

Xue, A. M., Foerde, K., Walsh, B. T., Steinglass, J. E., Shohamy, D., & Bakkour, A. (2022). Neural representations of food-related attributes in the human orbitofrontal cortex during choice deliberation in anorexia nervosa. *Journal of Neuroscience*, *42*(1), 109–120.

PART II

BASIC NEUROSCIENCE DOMAINS IN EATING DISORDERS ("BOTTOM UP")

6

Appetite Regulation and Motivation to Eat in Eating Disorders

Susan Murray, Millie Kirchberg, and Walter H. Kaye

Brief Definitional Overview

Homeostatic feeding: Food intake that is regulated by physiological signals indicating current energy stores.
Hedonic feeding: Food intake that is influenced by the perceived and experienced rewarding properties of food.
Appetitive motivation: The drive to seek, obtain, and consume food which can be modulated by aspects of both homeostatic and hedonic feeding.

Biological Framework

Human feeding behavior is regulated by homeostatic and hedonic mechanisms within the peripheral and central nervous systems that signal the available amount of energy stores, process the reward value of food based on homeostatic need and sensory properties such taste, and promote or inhibit feeding accordingly. Homeostatic mechanisms include peripheral neuropeptides, such as ghrelin and leptin, which are produced by the stomach and adipose tissue, respectively, and have opposing actions on food intake, with ghrelin stimulating hunger and leptin suppressing appetite, via their effect on neurons within the hypothalamus, a homeostatic center within the brain (Arora & Anubhuti, 2006). There, ghrelin stimulates production of orexigenic (appetite-stimulating) neuropeptides such as neuropeptide Y (NPY) and agouti-related protein (AgRP) and inhibits the effects of leptin. Conversely, leptin signaling within the hypothalamus results in an inhibition of orexigenic peptides and the stimulation anorectic peptides such as proopiomelanocortin (POMC) neurons. Increasing evidence suggests that the hypothalamus, which regulates metabolic processes regarding hunger, interacts closely with motivation-reward systems associated with the hedonic drive to eat, to influence food intake (Ferrario et al., 2016).

Feeding and eating behavior is mediated by numerous factors and the underlying brain mechanisms are complex. One proposed brain circuit underlying appetitive motivation includes regions involved in motivation and reward

Susan Murray et al., *Appetite Regulation and Motivation to Eat in Eating Disorders. The Handbook of the Neurobiology of Eating Disorders*. Edited by: Christina E. Wierenga and Joanna E. Steinglass, Oxford University Press. © Oxford University Press (2025). DOI: 10.1093/9780197675212.003.0007 processing. In brief, signals regarding tastes of sucrose are transmitted from sweet taste receptors in the tongue through the brainstem and thalamus to the primary gustatory cortex in the insula. In humans, the anterior insula receives taste input from the mid-insula (Craig, 2002). Recent studies suggest that the insula taste cortex identifies sweetness and the amygdala, which is involved in processing emotions, codes the valence, specifies its hedonic value, and elicits execution of selective behaviors (Wang et al., 2018). The insula is a hub for interoception or the awareness and integration of internal body signals to regulate behavior (Craig, 2002). The human gustatory cortex maps to the anterior and mid-insula (Rolls, 2016). The mid-insula is a chemosensory region involved in relaying various somatosensory and viscerosensory signals to the anterior insula and striatum (Avery et al., 2017; Rolls, 2016). Specifically, the mid-dorsal insula integrates gustatory information with information about the body's homeostatic needs (hunger and satiety signaling) to modulate feeding behavior. The anterior insula projects along the ventromedial axis of the striatum, including the ventral and dorsal striatum (Fudge et al., 2005), which are engaged in goal-directed behavior, such as the consumption of palatable food (Rolls, 2016). This circuitry is integral to reward processing and the preparation for and control of actions triggered by external stimuli (Brass & Haggard, 2010). The ventral striatum consists of the nucleus accumbens, ventral rostral caudate, and ventral putamen and is implicated in reward valuation or value coding (Martinez et al., 2003). The dorsal striatum, in contrast, is made up of the dorsal caudate and putamen and has been implicated in reward learning that supports decision making (e.g., learning that certain cue or action is associated with reward [Balleine et al., 2007]). Animal studies suggest that dopamine signaling within the dorsal striatum plays a critical role in promoting feeding as dopamine-depleted mice do not initiate feeding behavior but will resume eating after selective restoration of dopamine in the dorsal striatum (Palmiter, 2008). Thus, it has been proposal that dopamine signaling within the dorsal striatum may serve as a permissive "action initiation" signal, promoting food retrieval and consumption in response to metabolic demand (Palmiter, 2008).

Taken together, taste information is integrated with reward value and homeostatic drive via projections from the anterior insula and amygdala to the striatum to guide motivated eating behavior, although it is important to note that brain regions (e.g., posterior cingulate cortex, medial orbitofrontal cortex [OFC]) that facilitate higher order cognitions (e.g., judgment and decision making) are also implicated in food choice (Xue et al., 2022). In healthy individuals, hunger increases brain response in reward, attention, and motivation regions (Haase et al., 2009; Rolls, 2016; Siep et al., 2009; Stice et al., 2013). Similarly, when hungry, there is a reduction in anorectic hormone secretion and an accompanying increase in orexigenic hormone secretion leading to increases in appetite and the reward value of food. The current chapter will review research designed to interrogate possible dysfunction within appetitive motivation circuits in anorexia nervosa (AN) and bulimia nervosa (BN) because these may be relevant to understanding the maintenance of symptoms.

State of the Science in Eating Disorders

Evidence of dysfunction within motivational circuitry in anorexia nervosa

While individuals with AN have been shown to have alterations in neural mechanisms coding motivation, salience, cognition, and valuation of food when ill and after weight restoration (Lloyd & Steinglass, 2018; Monteleone et al., 2018), few studies (Holsen et al., 2012; Wierenga et al., 2017) have systematically examined whether there is altered functioning in neurocircuitry in individuals with AN specifically when hungry that may contribute to restricted food intake. However, previous research does suggest that in those remitted from AN, reward valuation circuitry (e.g., ventral striatum) is less active during a monetary reward task compared to controls when fasted (Wierenga et al., 2015), suggesting decreased sensitivity to the typical motivational drive of hunger. Kaye and colleagues (2020) used a palatable taste task with functional MRI (fMRI) to compare response to tastants (i.e., sucrose and water) in the food reward-motivation circuit described above between AN and controls in both the hungry and fed state. To avoid the confounding effects of malnutrition on activation of this circuitry, women in remission from AN were studied as well as age- and weight-matched healthy control women. During the "hungry" condition, participants fasted for 16 hours prior to scanning. During the "fed" condition, participants consumed standardized meals the day before scanning as well as a weight-adjusted standardized breakfast before the scan. As expected, the circuitry that guides motivated behavior such as eating was activated by tastants in control women when hungry compared to when fed. However, women remitted from AN demonstrated reduced ventral caudal putamen and insular response to tastants when hungry. Moreover, the control group showed increased mid-insula-to-ventral caudal putamen functional connectivity to tastants when hungry compared with when fed, whereas the remitted AN group showed decreased functional connectivity between these regions when hungry compared to when fed and compared with control women when hungry. These findings suggest that neural response to tastants when hungry is altered in those with a history AN. Reduced recruitment of the striatal aspects of motivation circuitry in response to tastants when hungry may impair the translation of taste reward to motivated eating behavior in AN.

Interestingly, participants in the remitted AN group who were more harm avoidant showed less activation in response to tastants when hungry in regions of the rostral caudate known to receive input from orbitofrontal and medial prefrontal cortices as well as the dorsolateral prefrontal cortex. Harm avoidance is a construct based on anxiety, inhibition, and inflexibility (Cloninger et al., 1998). Cloninger describes harm avoidance as "a heritable tendency to respond intensely to signals of aversive stimuli, thereby learning to inhibit behavior to avoid punishment, novelty, and frustrative nonreward." Harm avoidance and anxiety have been associated with caudate dopamine availability in healthy human subjects (Kim et al., 2011) and dorsal striatum function has been linked to elevated anxiety, harm avoidance, and punishment sensitivity in AN (Bailer et al., 2017; DeGuzman et al., 2017; Frank et al., 2005). As mentioned, dopamine signaling within the dorsal striatum plays a role in feeding (Ferrario et al., 2016). It has been speculated that lower dorsal striatum response to taste when hungry among those with the most pronounced behavioral inhibition in the remitted AN group reflects a reduced eating action initiation signal.

These results are consistent with earlier reports showing hypoactive response within the insula, anterior cingulate, and striatum to the taste of sucrose and water in individuals recovered from AN compared to controls (Oberndorfer et al., 2013; Wagner et al., 2008). For example, when fasted, patients in remission from AN showed decreased cerebral blood flow in the right ventral striatum, right subgenual anterior cingulate cortex, and left posterior insula compared to when fed, opposite to the pattern seen in controls (Wierenga et al., 2017). These findings indicate aberrant resting neurovascular function within homeostatic and hedonic food motivation pathways during hunger in those remitted from AN, which is hypothesized to perpetuate food restriction. However, results remain mixed; in the only other study that assessed response to tastants when fasted and fed, individuals with AN showed greater activation in the right amygdala and left medial temporal gyrus when drinking chocolate milk compared to healthy controls when fasted for approximately eight hours (Vocks et al., 2011). Another study found that those recovered from AN exhibited heightened neural response in the ventral striatum to the taste of chocolate though participants were not fasting (Cowdrey et al., 2011). Mixed results across studies are likely due to differences in sample demographics (e.g., ill versus remitted, illness duration, AN subtype) and methodology (e.g., study design, including the types of food cues used, length of fasting, etc., and analytic approaches).

Studies investigating the effect of homeostatic state on neural response to images of food provide further evidence of reduced neural response to food cues in AN. For example, one study found that after a 12-hour fast, patients with AN showed reduced activation to images of food in the visual occipital cortex compared to healthy controls, and when satiated, patients with AN exhibited decreased activation in inferior parietal cortex relative to controls (Santel et al., 2006). In a separate study, neural response to images of high- and low-calorie foods was investigated after a 12-hour fast and again after a standardized meal. Compared to controls, those currently ill with AN showed hypoactivation in the hypothalamus, amygdala, hippocampus, OFC, and insula to high calorie foods when fasted. Effects were similar among weight-restored individuals with a history of AN; compared to controls, these women showed hypoactivation to images of high calorie foods in the hypothalamus, amygdala, and insula when fasted (Holsen et al., 2012). After the meal, decreased activation was observed in the insula of ill AN only. These findings point to both state and trait related deficits that may perpetuate starvation.

In contrast, other studies have reported increased activation of the amygdala and posterior cingulate cortex in response to images of high calorie foods in patients with AN compared to controls as well as increased activation of the left insula during satiation in AN under shorter fasting conditions (e.g., three- to six-hour; Gizewski et al., 2010; Joos et al., 2011).

To bypass the cephalic phase of food intake and directly examine gut/brain signaling, peripheral hormone response and neural function was examined in AN and control participants following intragastric infusions of glucose and water with subjects blind to the type of liquid administered (Simon et al., 2020). Participants with AN showed typical hormonal responses; glucose infusion led to an increase in blood glucose and insulin levels along with decreased active ghrelin levels. On the neural level, however, individuals with AN showed less de-activation within the hypothalamus, ventral striatum, and amygdala in response to glucose infusion compared to controls, implicating hypothalamic dysfunction in the pathophysiology of AN. Moreover, individuals with AN had reduced functional connectivity between the hypothalamus and reward-related brain regions (e.g., the ventral striatum) in response to intragastric glucose, suggesting a possible disruption of hypothalamic regulation of food intake via blunted hypothalamic reactivity and reduced engagement of circuits coding of hedonic and motivational aspects of food.

In addition to evidence from research suggesting dysfunction in neurocircuitry underling taste and motivation in AN, studies show that individuals with AN have alterations in circulating hormones that influence appetite. For example, individuals with AN show elevated levels of peptide YY (PYY), an anorexigenic hormone that typically reduces appetite (Misra et al., 2006). Thus, greater PYY has been proposed as one factor that might maintain food restriction in AN despite low body weight. Interestingly, patients with AN do not report significantly different hunger ratings than controls; however, they do report a significantly lower desire to eat their favorite food (Mancuso et al., 2020). These data provide additional support for the possibility that despite reporting similar levels of hunger, patients with AN may be less motivated by hunger to eat.

AN is also frequently associated with higher circulating levels of ghrelin (Heruc et al., 2018; Misra et al., 2005), consistent with what would be expected in a starvation-state. However, patients with AN do not show the positive relationship between ghrelin levels and self-reported hunger that healthy controls show (Holsen et al., 2014), suggesting that individuals with AN may be resistant to the effects of this appetite signal. Consistent with this, ghrelin infusion fails to increase hunger in those with AN (Miljic et al., 2006). Moreover, unlike healthy controls, both ill and weight-restored individuals with AN fail to show positive relationships between ghrelin levels and activation of the amygdala, hippocampus, insula, and orbitofrontal cortex in response to high-calorie foods (Holsen et al., 2014). Interestingly, one study found that twice daily ghrelin infusions did result in increased hunger and energy intake in women with AN (Hotta et al., 2009), suggesting that individuals with AN may require more ghrelin to stimulate hunger. Finally, one study examined the effect of eating a favorite or neutral food on ghrelin response in underweight AN, weight restored AN, and healthy controls (Monteleone et al., 2016). While the weight restored and healthy control group had higher ghrelin levels when consuming their favorite food and decreased ghrelin during the neutral food condition, underweight AN participants showed decreased ghrelin levels regardless of the food's palatability. This finding could contribute to the ability of those with AN to resist eating and remain dangerously underweight.

In summary, studies in individuals with AN demonstrate abnormal hypothalamic, insula, and striatal response to hunger compared to controls suggesting impaired function of neurocircuitry regulating goal-directed behavior such as food consumption. Simply put, those with AN appear to have a failure of signals regarding energy deficits that normally drive a motivation to eat. Dysfunction in these signaling pathways likely contribute to their ability to severely restrict eating despite emaciation. While a desire to lose weight may initially drive food restriction (i.e., dieting), individuals who fail to respond to homeostatic and reward signals that stimulate eating when hungry may be able to maintain food avoidance. This new understanding offers an opportunity to consider new treatment targets.

Evidence of dysfunction within motivational circuitry in bulimia nervosa

As mentioned, hunger enhances the motivational salience of food whereas food reward is attenuated by satiety, promoting the termination of food intake. Satiety signaling and its impact on food reward circuitry might have particular relevance for disorders characterized by binge eating, which reflect behavioral difficulties in stopping eating despite replete energy stores. However, there are very few studies that have examined the influence of homeostatic state on food reward circuit function in binge-type disorders. Initial evidence showed that self-report ratings of hunger and fullness in individuals with BN did not vary significantly between a fasted and fed state (Halmi et al., 1989). Moreover, it has been shown that those with BN exhibit an attenuated decrease in ghrelin after eating compared to control subjects (Monteleone et al., 2003). Together, these data suggest individuals with BN may be less responsive to changes in metabolic status and this may help explain patterns of continued eating despite fullness.

To test the theory of insensitivity to satiety in BN, one study compared taste processing in women with remitted BN and women without an eating disorder during two neuroimaging scans, one after 16 hours of fasting and another after a standardized meal (Ely et al., 2017). Consistent with the expected pattern of reduced responding to food stimuli when sated, control women showed a significant reduction in neural activation when tasting sucrose and water in the amygdala and putamen when fed compared to when fasted whereas women in remission from BN failed to show differential activation in these regions between fasting and fed conditions. Moreover, women remitted from BN showed elevated amygdala activation to taste compared to controls when fed. Although the amygdala is often known for its role in fear processing, more recently this region has been implicated in taste processing and feeding behavior; it is proposed that amygdala activation under conditions of satiety may promote eating behavior via projections to the hypothalamus (Sun et al., 2015). Previous neuroimaging studies have also found that, unlike healthy controls, women remitted from BN showed no difference in ventral striatal activation to monetary rewards when hungry versus sated. Moreover, while control women showed greater dorsal caudate activation to monetary reward when hungry, women remitted from BN showed greater activation of this region when fed than controls (Bischoff-Grethe et al., 2021). Thus, change in metabolic state may not alter the salience of food among individuals with BN as expected which may perpetuate eating beyond satiety.

Alternative Perspectives

It is important to consider alternative interpretations of these data to assess if and how the theories presented here may be incomplete and to develop them with greater nuance. For example, despite reporting a lower desire to eat (Mancuso et al., 2020), individuals with AN often engage in behaviors (e.g., reading recipes and preparing food for others) that suggest that the reinforcing value of food is increased while in a state of negative energy balance (Murray & Strigo, 2018). Indeed, individuals with AN will sometimes report a fear that if they start eating they may not be able to stop, which may increase fear of eating. On its face, this may suggest an intact motivational drive to eat. However, this may also be understood as a reflection of knowing that if one were to eat, one would find it particularly satisfying given one's degree of hunger which is distinct from experiencing motivation to initiate eating. It may be helpful to look to the ways in which the concept of reward is dissociated into related but separate sub-constructs (e.g., wanting, liking, reward learning, motivational effort; Berridge & Robinson, 2003) to see how the processes involved in feeding behavior can be deconstructed to identify precisely where dysfunction may occur in the case of eating disorders. Many previous examinations of appetitive dysfunction in eating disorders have focused on aberrations in either the experience of hunger (e.g., do individuals with eating disorders experience hunger differently?) or consumption (e.g., do individuals with eating disorders experience food as more or less enjoyable?) with less focus on the motivational circuitry that bridges the gap between hunger and consumption.

Importantly, motivated behavior is not solely determined by homeostatic and hedonic signaling; food intake, like most decisions, is influenced by several considerations. For example, it has been argued that subjective reward value should be considered when interpreting neurobiological response patterns (Haynos et al., 2020). Reduced striatal response to tastants during hunger in AN might, for example, be due to an altered relationship with food that develops over the course of the disorder. As mentioned, individuals with AN with the highest harm avoidance scores showed the lowest response to tastants when hungry in the caudate (Kaye et al., 2020). If food is coded as a threat for those with AN due to its perceived effect on weight, it is possible that a greater tendency to avoid aversive consequences leads to enhanced recruitment of cognitive control circuitry in response to food reward. During both anticipation and receipt of monetary reward, individuals remitted from AN exhibited greater activation of the dorsolateral prefrontal cortex, a region implicated in executive control, compared to controls (Ehrlich et al., 2015), suggesting that greater "top-down" cognitive control circuitry modulates responding to rewarding stimuli in this population. Additionally, anxiety associated with eating may disrupt or inhibit the typical response to food reward during hunger in AN. A recent study investigating neural response to reward during persistent threat found decreased insula and putamen activation in response to reward during threatening versus safe conditions (Penner et al., 2022), providing initial support for the notion that encountering feared stimuli may result in a downregulation of this neural circuitry. Along similar lines, a recent pilot study found that individuals with social anxiety disorder showed reduced activation in the putamen when receiving negative feedback about social performance compared to controls (Lin et al., 2023). It is worth mentioning, however, that one study found decreased activation patterns in response to both sucrose and water in those with a history of AN (Kaye et al., 2020); thus, fear of weight gain associated with caloric intake may not sufficiently explain decreased activation of motivation circuitry in this study. It has also been suggested that reduced striatal response to reward in AN may be confounded by symptoms of depression as AN is highly comorbid with major depressive disorder (Holsen & Goldstein, 2015), a hypothesis worthy of further exploration. Finally, the dorsal striatum has been implicated in habitual or automatic behavior (Lipton et al., 2019). Because individuals with AN tend to exhibit highly routinized eating patterns, it is possible that altered activity within the dorsal striatum during hunger may reflect habit-based responding to food cues (Steinglass & Walsh, 2006). However, it is worth noting that research suggests that it is the putamen, not the caudate, within the dorsal striatum that is associated with habit-based responding (Grahn et al., 2008).

The hypothesis that individuals with AN may not translate normal hunger cues into motivation to eat is not incompatible with the above theories. Instead, these factors may interact to perpetuate food restriction. To illustrate this, consider that each person may have a certain threshold at which hunger will lead to taking action to procure and consume food. Imagine that for someone with no risk of an eating disorder (person A), their threshold is a six out of a possible 10, whereas for someone predisposed to an eating disorder (person B), this threshold is eight. Both may experience hunger, but the point at which hunger initiates action may naturally vary. Now, imagine that person B develops an eating disorder and, over time, an accompanying fear of weight gain and sustained habits of eating; in addition to adaptations to hunger signaling that occur with prolonged food restriction, there may develop a conscious motivation to avoid eating that compounds an unconscious natural lower motivation to eat. This conceptualization may help shift the debate about whether there is impaired motivation to eat in eating disorders from one that argues its absence versus presence to one of relative thresholds. Moreover, it acknowledges the potential for both physiological alterations in bottom-up motivation to eat and higher-order cognitions which may influence motivation and decision making around food choice. Indeed, the combination of these factors may lend additional insight into why achieving and maintaining recovery from AN is so challenging.

Just as inhibitory control may interact with reward sensitivity to guide motivational bias and behavior in AN, it is increasingly recognized that along with a failure to devalue reward when sated, individuals with BN show deficits in cognitive control circuitry (Berner, Winter, et al., 2023). Using a task designed to measure one's predictions that inhibition is required, women in remission from BN showed reduced dorsal caudate activation specifically when fed (Berner, Harlé, et al., 2023). Importantly, this was associated with a history of more frequent binge eating and self-induced vomiting and was opposite to the pattern shown by control subjects who exhibited increased dorsal caudate activation when fed. Taken together, it is hypothesized that when sated those prone to BN may both fail to devalue food and be less able to engage inhibitory control circuitry.

Finally, it is worth considering the phenomenon of diagnostic migration within eating disorders and how this might pose a challenge to the theories proposed. For example, one longitudinal study found that one-third of those diagnosed with AN later met diagnostic criteria for BN and approximately half crossed between restrictive and binge/purge subtypes of AN over time (Eddy et al., 2008). How can this be explained if these disorders are marked by distinct neuropathophysiology? On the one hand, it is possible that despite lower motivation to eat in AN, over time, natural adaptions to starvation (e.g., increased bottom-up motivation to eat or decreased top-down inhibition) occur to support survival resulting in binge eating episodes. Given continued motivation for weight control, these individuals may begin engaging in compensatory behaviors. It is worth noting that relatively few individuals with the restricting subtype of AN crossed over to BN; it is mostly individuals with the binge/purge subtype of AN that go on to develop BN. Moreover, it is rare for those with a diagnosis of BN to develop AN, providing support for the notion that BN is characterized by distinct underlying neural mechanisms from AN.

Implications

Treatments for eating disorders are limited in efficacy because we lack a clear understanding of the underlying neural mechanisms of these disorders. The eating disorder field needs to consider new insights into maladaptive eating behavior to develop more effective methods for promoting regular food intake and reducing binge eating in AN and BN.

Recruitment of the neural circuitry implicated in translating appetitive reward signals into motivated behaviors when hungry may interfere with food approach and eating initiation in AN. Particularly among individuals with high anxiety, new pharmacological and psychotherapeutic strategies that directly target these processes may be beneficial. Preliminary findings from open and controlled trials of medications that act on dopaminergic and serotonergic systems, such as olanzapine and aripiprazole, support investigating strategies for enhancing initiation to eat or compensating for altered appetitive motivation (Kaye et al., 2015). These trials, most of which are not controlled, have suggested that olanzapine and aripiprazole may be associated with reduced distress around eating, fewer obsessional thoughts about food, weight and body image, significant lessening of eating-disordered behaviors, and improvement in body weight in AN (Attia et al., 2019; Frank et al., 2017; Marzola et al., 2015; Trunko et al., 2011). Patients with eating disorders may not be able to rely on natural motivation to normalize food intake and instead will likely have to engage in what is termed "mechanical eating" or eating despite low motivation to eat or strong hunger cues. Strategies to reduce the effort needed to initiate eating may also be helpful (e.g., having meals plated for patients during treatment, planning and procuring food before mealtimes so it is readily available, and relying on pre-prepared or packaged foods can reduce barriers to consumption).

In the case of BN, pharmacological agents targeting the reward system may be useful in addressing reduced devaluation of food reward when sated. Additionally, medications or interventions (e.g., cognitive training using neurofeedback) that enhance inhibitory control may be useful in shifting decision making around food when sated. Moreover, behavioral strategies including stimulus control techniques (e.g., portioning and plating food before eating, leaving the kitchen or dining area after meal completion, and engaging in distracting activities after eating) can be helpful in reducing the opportunity to continue to eat despite satiation.

As a relatively new avenue within the eating disorder field, greater research is needed to further refine the theories and associated neurocircuitry discussed. In particular, because maladaptive food choices are known to perpetuate eating disorders, it will be important to link neuroimaging with behavioral decision making (e.g., choosing food versus viewing food cues; Murray & Strigo, 2018) and to translate these findings into targeted treatments. Additionally, though prospective studies of disorders with low prevalence are challenging, evidence of altered motivational drive prior to the onset of eating disorders would assist in determining whether the findings discussed in this chapter reflect neurobiological vulnerabilities that increase risk for eating disorder development or patterns of responding secondary to having an eating disorder.

References

Arora, S., & Anubhuti. (2006). Role of neuropeptides in appetite regulation and obesity—A review. *Neuropeptides, 40*(6), 375–401. https://doi.org/10.1016/j.npep.2006.07.001

Attia, E., Steinglass, J. E., Walsh, B. T., Wang, Y., Wu, P., Schreyer, C., Wildes, J., Yilmaz, Z., Guarda, A. S., Kaplan, A. S., & Marcus, M. D. (2019). Olanzapine versus placebo in adult outpatients with anorexia nervosa: A randomized clinical trial. *American Journal of Psychiatry, 176*(6), 449–456. https://doi.org/10.1176/appi.ajp.2018.18101125

Avery, J. A., Gotts, S. J., Kerr, K. L., Burrows, K., Ingeholm, J. E., Bodurka, J., Martin, A., & Kyle Simmons, W. (2017). Convergent gustatory and viscerosensory processing in the human dorsal mid-insula. *Human Brain Mapping, 38*(4), 2150–2164. https://doi.org/10.1002/hbm.23510

Bailer, U. F., Price, J. C., Meltzer, C. C., Wagner, A., Mathis, C. A., Gamst, A., & Kaye, W. H. (2017). Dopaminergic activity and altered reward modulation in anorexia nervosa-insight from multimodal imaging. *International Journal of Eating Disorders, 50*(5), 593–596. https://doi.org/10.1002/eat.22638

Balleine, B. W., Delgado, M. R., & Hikosaka, O. (2007). The role of the dorsal striatum in reward and decision-making. *Journal of Neuroscience, 27*(31), 8161–8165. https://doi.org/10.1523/jneurosci.1554-07.2007

Berner, L. A., Harlé, K. M., Simmons, A. N., Yu, A., Paulus, M. P., Bischoff-Grethe, A., Wierenga, C. E., Bailer, U. F., & Kaye, W. H. (2023). State-specific alterations in the neural computations underlying inhibitory control in women remitted from bulimia nervosa. *Molecular Psychiatry, 28*(7), 3055–3062. https://doi.org/10.1038/s41380-023-02063-6

Berner, L. A., Winter, S. R., Ayaz, H., Shewokis, P. A., Izzetoglu, M., Marsh, R., Nasser, J. A., Matteucci, A. J., & Lowe, M. R. (2023). Altered prefrontal activation during the inhibition of eating responses in women with bulimia nervosa. *Psychological Medicine, 53*(8), 3580–3590. https://doi.org/10.1017/s0033291722000198

Berridge, K. C., & Robinson, T. E. (2003). Parsing reward. *Trends in Neurosciences, 26*(9), 507–513. 10.1016/s0166-2236(03)00233-9

Bischoff-Grethe, A., Wierenga, C. E., Bailer, U. F., McClure, S. M., & Kaye, W. H. (2021). Satiety does not alter the ventral striatum's response to immediate reward in bulimia nervosa. *Journal of abnormal psychology, 130*(8), 862–874. https://doi.org/10.1037/abn0000712

Brass, M., & Haggard, P. (2010). The hidden side of intentional action: The role of the anterior insular cortex. *Brain Structure and Function, 214*(5), 603–610. https://doi.org/10.1007/s00429-010-0269-6

Cloninger, C. R., Van Eerdewegh, P., Goate, A., Edenberg, H. J., Blangero, J., Hesselbrock, V., Reich, T., Nurnberger, J., Jr., Schuckit, M., Porjesz, B., Crowe, R., Rice, J. P., Foroud, T., Przybeck, T. R., Almasy, L., Bucholz, K., Wu, W., Shears, S., Carr, K., Crose, C., . . . Conneally, P. M. (1998). Anxiety proneness linked to epistatic loci in genome scan of human personality traits. *American Journal of Medical Genetics, 81*(4), 313–317. https://doi.org/10.1002/(sici)1096-8628(19980710)81:4<313::aid-ajmg7>3.0.co;2-u

Cowdrey, F. A., Park, R. J., Harmer, C. J., & McCabe, C. (2011). Increased neural processing of rewarding and aversive food stimuli in recovered anorexia nervosa. *Biological Psychiatry, 70*(8), 736–743. https://doi.org/10.1016/j.biopsych.2011.05.028

Craig, A. D. (2002). How do you feel? Interoception: The sense of the physiological condition of the body. *Nature Reviews Neuroscience, 3*(8), 655–666. https://doi.org/10.1038/nrn894

DeGuzman, M., Shott, M. E., Yang, T. T., Riederer, J., & Frank, G. K. W. (2017). Association of elevated reward prediction error response with weight gain in adolescent anorexia nervosa. *American Journal of Psychiatry, 174*(6), 557–565. https://doi.org/10.1176/appi.ajp.2016.16060671

Eddy, K. T., Dorer, D. J., Franko, D. L., Tahilani, K., Thompson-Brenner, H., & Herzog, D. B. (2008). Diagnostic crossover in anorexia nervosa and bulimia nervosa: Implications for DSM-V. *American Journal of Psychiatry, 165*(2), 245–250. 10.1176/appi.ajp.2007.07060951

Ehrlich, S., Geisler, D., Ritschel, F., King, J. A., Seidel, M., Boehm, I., Breier, M., Clas, S., Weiss, J., Marxen, M., Smolka, M. N., Roessner, V., & Kroemer, N. B. (2015). Elevated cognitive control over reward processing in recovered female patients with anorexia nervosa. *Journal of Psychiatry and Neuroscience, 40*(5), 307–315. https://doi.org/10.1503/jpn.140249

Ely, A. V., Wierenga, C. E., Bischoff-Grethe, A., Bailer, U. F., Berner, L. A., Fudge, J. L., Paulus, M. P., & Kaye, W. H. (2017). Response in taste circuitry is not modulated by hunger and satiety in women remitted from bulimia nervosa. *Journal of Abnormal Psychology, 126*(5), 519–530. https://doi.org/10.1037/abn0000218

Ferrario, C. R., Labouèbe, G., Liu, S., Nieh, E. H., Routh, V. H., Xu, S., & O'Connor, E. C. (2016). Homeostasis meets motivation in the battle to control food intake. *Journal of Neuroscience, 36*(45), 11469–11481. https://doi.org/10.1523/jneurosci.2338-16.2016

Frank, G. K., Bailer, U. F., Henry, S. E., Drevets, W., Meltzer, C. C., Price, J. C., Mathis, C. A., Wagner, A., Hoge, J., Ziolko, S., Barbarich-Marsteller, N., Weissfeld, L., & Kaye, W. H. (2005). Increased dopamine D2/D3 receptor binding after recovery from anorexia nervosa measured by positron emission tomography and [11c]raclopride. *Biological Psychiatry, 58*(11), 908–912. https://doi.org/10.1016/j.biopsych.2005.05.003

Frank, G. K. W., Shott, M. E., Hagman, J. O., Schiel, M. A., DeGuzman, M. C., & Rossi, B. (2017). The partial dopamine D2 receptor agonist aripiprazole is associated with weight gain in adolescent anorexia nervosa. *International Journal of Eating Disorders, 50*(4), 447–450. https://doi.org/10.1002/eat.22704

Fudge, J. L., Breitbart, M. A., Danish, M., & Pannoni, V. (2005). Insular and gustatory inputs to the caudal ventral striatum in primates. *Journal of Comparative Neurology, 490*(2), 101–118. https://doi.org/10.1002/cne.20660

Gizewski, E. R., Rosenberger, C., de Greiff, A., Moll, A., Senf, W., Wanke, I., Forsting, M., & Herpertz, S. (2010). Influence of satiety and subjective valence rating on cerebral activation patterns in response to visual stimulation with high-calorie stimuli among restrictive anorectic and control women. *Neuropsychobiology, 62*(3), 182–192. https://doi.org/10.1159/000319360

Grahn, J. A., Parkinson, J. A., & Owen, A. M. (2008). The cognitive functions of the caudate nucleus. *Progress in Neurobiology, 86*(3), 141–155. https://doi.org/10.1016/j.pneurobio.2008.09.004

Haase, L., Cerf-Ducastel, B., & Murphy, C. (2009). Cortical activation in response to pure taste stimuli during the physiological states of hunger and satiety. *NeuroImage, 44*(3), 1008–1021. https://doi.org/10.1016/j.neuroimage.2008.09.044

Halmi, K. A., Sunday, S., Puglisi, A., & Marchi, P. (1989). Hunger and satiety in anorexia and bulimia nervosa. *Annals of the New York Academy of Sciences, 575*, 431–445. https://doi.org/10.1111/j.1749-6632.1989.tb53264.x

Haynos, A. F., Lavender, J. M., Nelson, J., Crow, S. J., & Peterson, C. B. (2020). Moving towards specificity: A systematic review of cue features associated with reward and punishment in anorexia nervosa. *Clinical Psychology Review, 79*, 101872. https://doi.org/10.1016/j.cpr.2020.101872

Heruc, G. A., Little, T. J., Kohn, M., Madden, S., Clarke, S., Horowitz, M., & Feinle-Bisset, C. (2018). Appetite perceptions, gastrointestinal symptoms, ghrelin, peptide YY and state anxiety are disturbed in adolescent females with anorexia nervosa and only partially restored with short-term refeeding. *Nutrients, 11*(1). https://doi.org/10.3390/nu11010059

Holsen, L. M., & Goldstein, J. M. (2015). Valuation and cognitive circuitry in anorexia nervosa: disentangling appetite from the effort to obtain a reward. *Biological Psychiatry, 77*(7), 604–606. https://doi.org/10.1016/j.biopsych.2015.02.011

Holsen, L. M., Lawson, E. A., Blum, J., Ko, E., Makris, N., Fazeli, P. K., Klibanski, A., & Goldstein, J. M. (2012). Food motivation circuitry hypoactivation related to hedonic and nonhedonic aspects of hunger and satiety in women with active anorexia nervosa and weight-restored women with anorexia nervosa. *Journal of Psychiatry and Neuroscience, 37*(5), 322–332. https://doi.org/10.1503/jpn.110156

Holsen, L. M., Lawson, E. A., Christensen, K., Klibanski, A., & Goldstein, J. M. (2014). Abnormal relationships between the neural response to high- and low-calorie foods and endogenous acylated ghrelin in women with active and weight-recovered anorexia nervosa. *Psychiatry Research, 223*(2), 94–103. https://doi.org/10.1016/j.pscychresns.2014.04.015

Hotta, M., Ohwada, R., Akamizu, T., Shibasaki, T., Takano, K., & Kangawa, K. (2009). Ghrelin increases hunger and food intake in patients with restricting-type anorexia nervosa: A pilot study. *Endocrine Journal, 56*(9), 1119–1128. https://doi.org/10.1507/endocrj.k09e-168

Joos, A. A., Saum, B., van Elst, L. T., Perlov, E., Glauche, V., Hartmann, A., Freyer, T., Tüscher, O., & Zeeck, A. (2011). Amygdala hyperreactivity in restrictive anorexia nervosa. *Psychiatry Research, 191*(3), 189–195. https://doi.org/10.1016/j.pscychresns.2010.11.008

Kaye, W. H., Wierenga, C. E., Bischoff-Grethe, A., Berner, L. A., Ely, A. V., Bailer, U. F., Paulus, M. P., & Fudge, J. L. (2020). Neural insensitivity to the effects of hunger in women remitted from anorexia nervosa. *American Journal of Psychiatry, 177*(7), 601–610. https://doi.org/10.1176/appi.ajp.2019.19030261

Kaye, W. H., Wierenga, C. E., Knatz, S., Liang, J., Boutelle, K., Hill, L., & Eisler, I. (2015). Temperament-based treatment for anorexia nervosa. *European Eating Disorders Review, 23*(1), 12–18. https://doi.org/10.1002/erv.2330

Kim, J. H., Son, Y. D., Kim, H. K., Lee, S. Y., Cho, S. E., Kim, Y. B., & Cho, Z. H. (2011). Association of harm avoidance with dopamine D2/3 receptor availability in striatal subdivisions: A high resolution PET study. *Biological Psychology, 87*(1), 164–167. https://doi.org/10.1016/j.biopsycho.2011.02.011

Lin, H., Bruchmann, M., & Straube, T. (2023). Altered putamen activation for social comparison-related feedback in social anxiety disorder: A pilot study. *Neuropsychobiology, 82*(6), 359–372. https://doi.org/10.1159/000531762

Lipton, D. M., Gonzales, B. J., & Citri, A. (2019). Dorsal striatal circuits for habits, compulsions and addictions. *Frontiers in Systems Neuroscience, 13*, 28. https://doi.org/10.3389/fnsys.2019.00028

Lloyd, E. C., & Steinglass, J. E. (2018). What can food-image tasks teach us about anorexia nervosa? A systematic review. *Journal of Eating Disorders, 6*, 31. https://doi.org/10.1186/s40337-018-0217-z

Mancuso, C., Izquierdo, A., Slattery, M., Becker, K. R., Plessow, F., Thomas, J. J., Eddy, K. T., Lawson, E. A., & Misra, M. (2020). Changes in appetite-regulating hormones following food intake are associated with changes in reported appetite and a measure of hedonic eating in girls and young women with anorexia nervosa. *Psychoneuroendocrinology, 113*, 104556. https://doi.org/10.1016/j.psyneuen.2019.104556

Martinez, D., Slifstein, M., Broft, A., Mawlawi, O., Hwang, D.-R., Huang, Y., Cooper, T., Kegeles, L., Zarahn, E., Abi-Dargham, A., Haber, S. N., & Laruelle, M. (2003). Imaging human mesolimbic dopamine transmission with positron emission tomography. Part II: Amphetamine-induced dopamine release in the functional subdivisions of the striatum. *Journal of Cerebral Blood Flow & Metabolism, 23*(3), 285–300. https://doi.org/10.1097/01.WCB.0000048520.34839.1A

Marzola, E., Desedime, N., Giovannone, C., Amianto, F., Fassino, S., & Abbate-Daga, G. (2015). Atypical antipsychotics as augmentation therapy in anorexia nervosa. *PLOS ONE, 10*(4), e0125569. https://doi.org/10.1371/journal.pone.0125569

Miljic, D., Pekic, S., Djurovic, M., Doknic, M., Milic, N., Casanueva, F. F., Ghatei, M., & Popovic, V. (2006). Ghrelin has partial or no effect on appetite, growth hormone, prolactin, and cortisol release in patients with anorexia nervosa. *Journal of Clinical Endocrinology & Metabolism, 91*(4), 1491–1495. https://doi.org/10.1210/jc.2005-2304

Misra, M., Miller, K. K., Kuo, K., Griffin, K., Stewart, V., Hunter, E., Herzog, D. B., & Klibanski, A. (2005). Secretory dynamics of ghrelin in adolescent girls with anorexia nervosa and healthy adolescents. *American Journal of Physiology-Endocrinology Metabolism, 289*(2), E347–356. https://doi.org/10.1152/ajpendo.00615.2004

Misra, M., Miller, K. K., Tsai, P., Gallagher, K., Lin, A., Lee, N., Herzog, D. B., & Klibanski, A. (2006). Elevated peptide YY levels in adolescent girls with anorexia nervosa. *Journal of Clinical Endocrinology & Metabolism, 91*(3), 1027–1033. https://doi.org/10.1210/jc.2005-1878

Monteleone, A. M., Castellini, G., Volpe, U., Ricca, V., Lelli, L., Monteleone, P., & Maj, M. (2018). Neuroendocrinology and brain imaging of reward in eating disorders: A possible key to the treatment of anorexia nervosa and bulimia nervosa. *Progress in Neuro-Psychopharmacology and Biological Psychiatry, 80*, 132–142. https://doi.org/10.1016/j.pnpbp.2017.02.020

Monteleone, A. M., Monteleone, P., Dalle Grave, R., Nigro, M., El Ghoch, M., Calugi, S., Cimino, M., & Maj, M. (2016). Ghrelin response to hedonic eating in underweight and short-term weight restored patients with anorexia nervosa. *Psychiatry Research, 235*, 55–60. https://doi.org/10.1016/j.psychres.2015.12.001

Monteleone, P., Martiadis, V., Fabrazzo, M., Serritella, C., & Maj, M. (2003). Ghrelin and leptin responses to food ingestion in bulimia nervosa: implications for binge-eating and compensatory behaviours. *Psychological medicine, 33*(8), 1387–1394. https://doi.org/10.1017/s0033291703008316

Murray, S. B., & Strigo, I. A. (2018). Anorexia nervosa, neuroimaging research, and the contextual salience of food cues: The food approach–avoidance conundrum. *International Journal of Eating Disorders, 51*(8), 822–825. https://doi.org/10.1002/eat.22883

Oberndorfer, T. A., Frank, G. K., Simmons, A. N., Wagner, A., McCurdy, D., Fudge, J. L., Yang, T. T., Paulus, M. P., & Kaye, W. H. (2013). Altered insula response to sweet taste processing after recovery from anorexia and bulimia nervosa. *American Journal of Psychiatry, 170*(10), 1143–1151. https://doi.org/10.1176/appi.ajp.2013.11111745

Palmiter, R. D. (2008). Dopamine signaling in the dorsal striatum is essential for motivated behaviors. *Annals of the New York Academy of Sciences, 1129*(1), 35–46. https://doi.org/10.1196/annals.1417.003

Penner, A. E., White, E., Stoddard, J., & Gowin, J. L. (2022). The neural circuitry of reward during sustained threat. *Cognitive, Affective, & Behavioral Neuroscience, 22*(1), 134–144. https://doi.org/10.3758/s13415-021-00938-1

Rolls, E. T. (2016). Motivation explained: Ultimate and proximate accounts of hunger and appetite. In A. J. Elliot (Ed.), *Advances in Motivation Science* (Vol. 3, pp. 187–249). Elsevier. https://doi.org/10.1016/bs.adms.2015.12.004

Santel, S., Baving, L., Krauel, K., Münte, T. F., & Rotte, M. (2006). Hunger and satiety in anorexia nervosa: fMRI during cognitive processing of food pictures. *Brain Research, 1114*(1), 138–148. https://doi.org/10.1016/j.brainres.2006.07.045

Siep, N., Roefs, A., Roebroeck, A., Havermans, R., Bonte, M. L., & Jansen, A. (2009). Hunger is the best spice: An fMRI study of the effects of attention, hunger and calorie content on food reward processing in the amygdala and orbitofrontal cortex. *Behavioural Brain Research, 198*(1), 149–158. https://doi.org/10.1016/j.bbr.2008.10.035

Simon, J. J., Stopyra, M. A., Mönning, E., Sailer, S., Lavandier, N., Kihm, L. P., Bendszus, M., Preissl, H., Herzog, W., & Friederich, H. C. (2020). Neuroimaging of hypothalamic mechanisms related to glucose metabolism in anorexia nervosa and obesity. *Journal of Clinical Investigation, 130*(8), 4094–4103. https://doi.org/10.1172/jci136782

Steinglass, J., & Walsh, B. T. (2006). Habit learning and anorexia nervosa: A cognitive neuroscience hypothesis. *International Journal of Eating Disorders, 39*(4), 267–275. https://doi.org/10.1002/eat.20244

Stice, E., Burger, K., & Yokum, S. (2013). Caloric deprivation increases responsivity of attention and reward brain regions to intake, anticipated intake, and images of palatable foods. *NeuroImage, 67*, 322–330. https://doi.org/10.1016/j.neuroimage.2012.11.028

Sun, X., Kroemer, N. B., Veldhuizen, M. G., Babbs, A. E., Araujo, I. E. D., Gitelman, D. R., Sherwin, R. S., Sinha, R., & Small, D. M. (2015). Basolateral amygdala response to food cues in the absence of hunger is associated with weight gain susceptibility. *Journal of Neuroscience, 35*(20), 7964–7976. https://doi.org/10.1523/jneurosci.3884-14.2015

Trunko, M. E., Schwartz, T. A., Duvvuri, V., & Kaye, W. H. (2011). Aripiprazole in anorexia nervosa and low-weight bulimia nervosa: Case reports. *International Journal of Eating Disorders, 44*(3), 269–275. https://doi.org/10.1002/eat.20807

Vocks, S., Herpertz, S., Rosenberger, C., Senf, W., & Gizewski, E. R. (2011). Effects of gustatory stimulation on brain activity during hunger and satiety in females with restricting-type anorexia nervosa: An fMRI study. *Journal of Psychiatric Research, 45*(3), 395–403. https://doi.org/10.1016/j.jpsychires.2010.07.012

Wagner, A., Aizenstein, H., Mazurkewicz, L., Fudge, J., Frank, G. K., Putnam, K., Bailer, U. F., Fischer, L., & Kaye, W. H. (2008). Altered insula response to taste stimuli in individuals recovered from restricting-type anorexia nervosa. *Neuropsychopharmacology, 33*(3), 513–523. https://doi.org/10.1038/sj.npp.1301443

Wang, L., Gillis-Smith, S., Peng, Y., Zhang, J., Chen, X., Salzman, C. D., Ryba, N. J. P., & Zuker, C. S. (2018). The coding of valence and identity in the mammalian taste system. *Nature, 558*(7708), 127–131. https://doi.org/10.1038/s41586-018-0165-4

Wierenga, C. E., Bischoff-Grethe, A., Melrose, A. J., Irvine, Z., Torres, L., Bailer, U. F., Simmons, A., Fudge, J. L., McClure, S. M., Ely, A., & Kaye, W. H. (2015). Hunger does not motivate reward in women remitted from anorexia nervosa. *Biological Psychiatry, 77*(7), 642–652. https://doi.org/10.1016/j.biopsych.2014.09.024

Wierenga, C. E., Bischoff-Grethe, A., Rasmusson, G., Bailer, U. F., Berner, L. A., Liu, T. T., & Kaye, W. H. (2017). Aberrant cerebral blood flow in response to hunger and satiety in women remitted from anorexia nervosa [original research]. *Frontiers in Nutrition, 4.* 10.3389/fnut.2017.00032

Xue, A. M., Foerde, K., Walsh, B. T., Steinglass, J. E., Shohamy, D., & Bakkour, A. (2022). Neural representations of food-related attributes in the human orbitofrontal cortex during choice deliberation in anorexia nervosa. *The Journal of Neuroscience: The Official Journal of the Society for Neuroscience, 42*(1), 109–120. https://doi.org/10.1523/JNEUROSCI.0958-21.2021

7

Reward Processing and Reinforcement Learning in Eating Disorders

Adanya D. Johnson, Kira G. Venables, and Ann F. Haynos

Brief Definitional Overview

Reward processing: Operations initiated at the experiential level of reward responding, including the identification of rewarding stimuli, the production of emotional responses to these stimuli, and the motivation of approach toward rewarding experiences (Monteleone et al., 2018).

Reward/reinforcement learning: A subdomain of reward processing that refers to the activities through which an organism learns from the rewards in their environment. Behaviorally, reinforcement learning occurs when an organism acquires a tendency to repeat an action that has previously been rewarded (Skinner, 1976). Reinforcement learning also refers to a set of computational modeling algorithms that seek to mathematically capture the process through which an agent learns to pursue a reward through trial and error (Sutton & Barto, 1998).

Introduction

This chapter details the bottom-up processes involved in attending and responding to, as well as learning from, rewards that may initiate or perpetuate eating disorders. Rewards are salient stimuli that are pleasant or desired and that individuals feel motivated to pursue. Reward abnormalities may be particularly relevant to eating disorders because these disorders present with extreme drives for approach (i.e., binge eating) and avoidance (i.e., restrictive eating) behavior related to food, which is generally considered a primary reward. Additionally, individuals with eating disorders have been noted to demonstrate affective and temperamental features indicative of reward deficiencies (e.g., anhedonia; Keating et al., 2012) or surpluses (e.g., impulsivity; Waxman, 2009), depending on the eating disorder diagnosis and symptom profile. For this reason, a substantial body of research has aimed to understand reward functioning across the eating disorder spectrum and how such reward processes may impact the development and maintenance of these disorders. This chapter will specifically review reward processing (i.e., attending

Adanya D. Johnson, Kira G. Venables, and Ann F. Haynos, *Reward Processing and Reinforcement Learning in Eating Disorders*. In: *The Handbook of the Neurobiology of Eating Disorders*. Edited by: Christina E. Wierenga and Joanna E. Steinglass, Oxford University Press. © Oxford University Press (2025). DOI: 10.1093/9780197675212.003.0008 and responding to rewards) and reinforcement (i.e., learning from rewards) in eating disorders.

Biological Framework

The neural circuits associated with reward processing are complex, interconnected, and are incompletely understood in eating disorders, but rapid advances in neuroscientific methodology over recent decades (e.g., structural and functional neuroimaging, neurocognitive reward tasks) have allowed for the generation of novel insights into the relationship between aberrations in these areas and disordered eating pathology (Frank, 2015). The most canonical reward circuits include the mesolimbic and mesocortical reward circuits (see Figure 7.1), which are interconnected networks that are implicated in reward salience, reinforcement learning, and initial and sustained motivation to engage in reward-seeking behaviors (Morales & Berridge, 2020; Salamone et al., 2016). Both circuits involve the neurotransmitter dopamine, which has been implicated in food and other reward motivation (Kontis & Theochari, 2012). Dopamine signaling has also been highlighted as crucial to reward learning, as the spiking of dopamine neurons to environmental stimuli has been linked to subsequent decision-making regarding reward pursuit (Schultz, 2016).

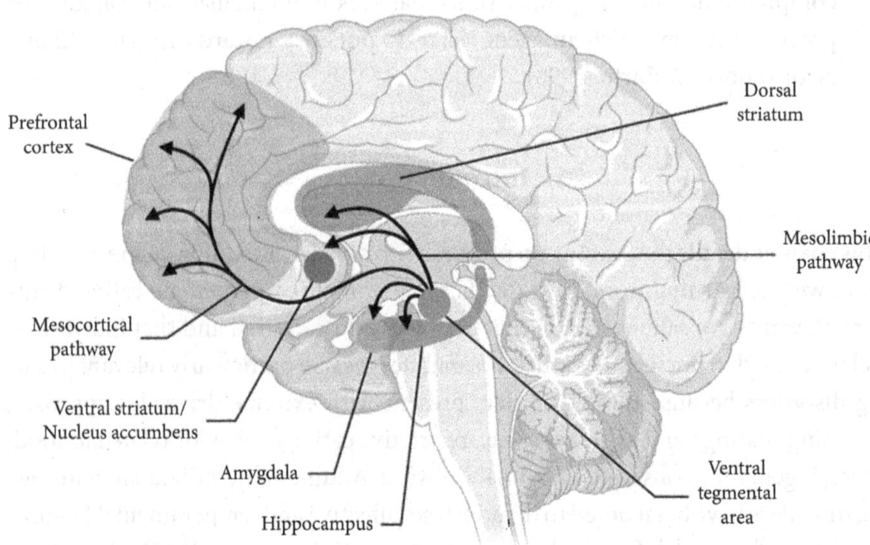

Figure 7.1 Visual representation of mesocortical and mesolimbic pathways involved in reward processing. Note: The ventral tegmental area serves as a major site of dopamine production. Outward arrows represent dopamine projections from the ventral tegmental area that signal along the mesolimbic pathway to limbic regions of the brain (e.g., ventral and dorsal striatum, hippocampus) and along the mesocortical pathway to the prefrontal cortex.

The ventral tegmental area (VTA) in the midbrain is the primary production site of dopamine, which is subsequently transmitted to limbic regions of the brain, including the ventral striatum, hippocampus, and ventral pallidum and to cortical regions, such as the prefrontal cortex (PFC) (Morales & Margolis, 2017). The primary site of dopaminergic inputs from the VTA is the ventral striatum, including the nucleus accumbens, which is often considered a central hub of the mesolimbic reward circuit. Activity within the ventral striatum is associated with tracking reward anticipation and receipt, as well as invigorating approach behavior (Daniel & Pollmann, 2014). Projections from the VTA to other limbic structures (e.g., amygdala, hippocampus) assist in tracking the reward salience and emotional responding that encourage associative learning and long-term memory formation from reward stimuli (Bromberg-Martin et al., 2010). Within the mesocortical circuit, the VTA and other limbic structures interface via structural and functional connections to cortical structures, including the orbitofrontal cortex (OFC) and other regions in the PFC. The OFC has been implicated in the monitoring of reward valuation and various other regions of the PFC support the higher-level cognitive functions (e.g., planning and decision-making) that allow individuals to moderate reward pursuit through balancing short- and long-term goals (Wallis, 2007; Rolls & Grabenhorst, 2008).

In addition to neurobiological responses, other physiological functions have been identified as correlates of reward processing among individuals with eating disorders. For instance, several psychophysiological measures have shown links to reward processing, including facial electromyography measures (e.g., zygomatic muscle that controls smiling) (Soussignan et al., 2010, 2011), the post-auricular muscle (which pulls the ear back) (Benning et al., 2004; Racine et al., 2021), startle eye blink (Frank et al., 2020), and heart rate variability (Peyser et al., 2021). Additionally, specific hormones or neuropeptides, such as oxytocin, have been associated with reward responding across healthy and psychiatric samples (Giel et al., 2018). Although the specific ways in which different psychophysiological, neurobiological, and emotional and cognitive processes interact in response to rewards requires further investigation, research indicates correspondence between these indices during reward processing (Wilson et al., 2020). Further, the relative non-invasiveness of such peripheral biological measures situates them as potentially useful indicators of reward processing and approach motivation.

State of the Science in Eating Disorders

Reward processing and learning are operations that can be measured in different ways. This section reviews evidence for alterations in reward processing and learning in individuals with eating disorders across multiple measures, including temperamental, behavioral, and biological metrics. Overall findings are summarized in Table 7.1.

Table 7.1 Summary of findings related to reward processing and reinforcement learning in anorexia nervosa (AN), bulimia nervosa (BN), and binge-eating disorder (BED)

Data Type	Summary of Method		Main Findings in Anorexia Nervosa	Main Findings in Bulimia Nervosa	Main Findings in Binge-Eating Disorder
Temperament	Measures personality traits via self-report questionnaires.		Sensation- and novelty-seeking lower in AN-R and higher in AN-BP.	Heightened sensation- and novelty-seeking.	Some evidence of heightened novelty-seeking, but overall mixed results.
Behavioral responses	Presents stimuli or conditions to measure cognitive or behavioral processes related to reward, learning, and decision making.	Delay Discounting	Reduced delay discounting (i.e., preference for larger-later vs. smaller-sooner rewards).	Elevated delay discounting (i.e., preference for smaller-sooner rewards).	Elevated delay discounting (i.e., preference for smaller-sooner rewards).
		Progressive Ratio	Significant effort exerted to engage in ED behaviors (e.g., calorie restriction, exercise).	Significant effort exerted to obtain palatable food.	Limited research.
		Reward Learning	Impaired model-based reinforcement learning. Potential deficits in reward learning deficits.	Impaired model-based reinforcement learning. Reduced reinforcement learning under dopamine deficiency.	Impaired model-based reinforcement learning.
Psychophysiology	Measures physiological reactions (e.g., heart rate, skin conductance, electromyography) that correspond with psychological states		Greater post-auricular response to low-calorie food linked to restrictive eating. Several psychophysiological indices reflect reward reactivity to thin images.	Greater post-auricular response to high-calorie food linked to binge eating.	Greater post-auricular response to high-calorie food linked to binge eating.
Neurotransmitter research	Measures metabolic or physiological function typically via the injection of radioactive tracers and the detection of radioactivity.		Reduced dopamine concentrations in cerebrospinal fluid and striatum. Dopamine release associated with anxiety.	Reduced dopamine concentrations across brain regions (e.g., putamen, insula, and amygdala). Dopamine activity has a negative association with binge/purge episodes.	Abnormal dopamine concentrations in the basal ganglia, caudate, and putamen. Directionality is inconsistent.

Structural MRI	Captures brain structure (e.g., grey and white matter) via magnetic field, excitation of photons that emit a radio signal, and measurement of hydrogen atoms.		Reduced grey and white matter across brain regions (e.g., striatum, OFC) in acute AN; mostly normalizes with weight restoration.	Enlarged volume of the ventral striatum and OFC, which is associated with severity of eating disorder symptoms.	Abnormal volume in ventral striatum, OFC, and caudate. Reduced vs. enlarged volume is inconsistent.
Resting state functional MRI	Correlation of blood oxygenation level-dependent contrast signals between brain regions.		Altered connectivity of mesocortical reward circuitry. Directionality is inconsistent.	Lower connectivity in cortical reward networks and between the striatum and prefrontal cortex.	Lower connectivity between limbic and prefrontal regions.
Task-based functional MRI	Correlation of blood oxygenation level-dependent contrast signals within and between brain regions in response to specific cues or actions.	In response to disorder-specific cues:	Abnormal activation in reward circuitry (e.g., OFC, striatum, VTA) to palatable food. Directionality is inconsistent. Increased activation in striatum and OFC to low-density food. Increased activation in reward-related brain regions to thin images.	Enhanced activation in regions related to reward and motivation (e.g., dorsal striatum, OFC, and vmPFC) to palatable foods. Reward responsivity may be dependent on hunger and satiety. No change in reward-related brain regions to images of thin bodies.	Enhanced activation in regions related to reward and motivation (e.g., dorsal striatum, OFC, and vmPFC) to palatable foods.
		In response to disorder-neutral cues:	Some evidence of lower activation in ACC and striatum during monetary reward tasks. Some evidence of decreased activation in the medial PFC and to social cues.	Limited research. Reward responsivity may be dependent on hunger and satiety states. Some evidence of increased caudate activation in anticipation of social touch.	Limited research. Some evidence of decreased activation in ventral striatum during anticipation of monetary reward and decreased activation in the medial PFC during receipt of monetary reward.

Temperament and personality traits

Temperament reflects a set of consistent traits within an individual that influence activity, reactivity, emotionality, and sociability (Goldsmith et al., 1987). A significant body of research has found differences in temperamental traits related to reward processing across eating disorder presentations. Responsivity to novel and high-intensity rewards can be measured through reward sensitivity, sensation-seeking, and novelty-seeking measures. Individuals with anorexia nervosa (AN), especially the restricting subtype (AN-R), typically score lower on measures of reward sensitivity, sensation-seeking, and novelty-seeking relative to healthy controls and those with other eating disorders (Atiye et al., 2015; Farstad et al., 2016; Harrison et al., 2010). However, elevated reward sensitivity and novelty-seeking has been reported in the binge eating/purging subtype of AN (AN-BP) compared to healthy controls and some other eating disorders, such as binge-eating disorder (BED) (Atiye et al., 2015; Harrison et al., 2010). Similarly, individuals with bulimia nervosa (BN) have also demonstrated elevated reward sensitive and sensation- and novelty-seeking (Atiye et al., 2015; Farstad et al., 2016; Harrison et al., 2010). The literature on temperament in BED is smaller, and existing results are mixed; some studies identified elevated novelty-seeking (Haynos, Wang, et al., 2021) and other studies found no differences from controls (Atiye et al., 2015; Farstad et al., 2016).

Responses to behavioral tasks

A number of neurocognitive tasks have been used to assess different aspects of how individuals with eating disorders respond to and learn from rewards. Findings emerging from several of the most commonly used reward-based neurocognitive paradigms that appraise the value-based decision-making and effort expenditure necessary to obtain rewards are described in this section.

Delay discounting

Delay discounting provides a complex assessment of reward processing that captures the degree to which a reward loses its value over time (Amlung et al., 2019). Delay discounting tasks capture a person's propensity to select immediate rewards rather than to delay gratification and has been related to numerous neural and behavioral outcomes across psychiatry and behavioral economics (Amlung et al., 2019; Odum, 2011). In these tasks, individuals are asked to choose between a smaller amount of money more immediately available (smaller-sooner reward) or a larger amount of money available on a later timescale (larger-later reward) (Odum, 2011). In the context of eating disorders, individuals with greater reward impulsivity are expected to prefer smaller-sooner rewards over the larger-later rewards on these tasks (see Chapter 12). Several studies have found that individuals with AN select more larger-later rewards on delay discounting tasks, which may reflect less reward sensitivity and/or greater self-control (Lempert et al., 2018; Steinglass et al., 2012). However, this effect may be less pronounced during adolescence or young adulthood (Doose et al., 2020; King et al., 2016) and appears to resolve with weight restoration (Decker et al., 2015; King et al., 2020; Wierenga et al., 2015). In contrast, individuals with BN and BED have generally demonstrated elevated discounting of monetary rewards (i.e., preference for smaller-sooner rewards) and self-reported a reduced ability to delay gratification relative to healthy controls (Amlung et al., 2019; Bartholdy et al., 2017; Kekic et al., 2016), although some studies report the opposite pattern of findings (Hagan et al., 2021). In general, these findings suggest differences in reward processing among individuals with eating disorders.

Progressive ratio

In these tasks, participants are asked to work (e.g., through button presses) to obtain a specific reward (e.g., money, food) and the amount of effort they are willing to expend is considered to correspond with the motivational value of the reward for the participant. On these tasks, individuals with restrictive eating pathology have been shown to expend significant amounts of effort to earn exercise (Gianini et al., 2016; Klein et al., 2010; O'Hara, Keyes, Renwick, Leyton, et al., 2016; Schebendach et al., 2007), caloric restriction (Haynos et al., 2016), and non-nutritive artificial sweetener (Schebendach et al., 2017). Similarly, individuals with BN have been shown to engage in greater effort than healthy controls to obtain palatable food (Bodell & Keel, 2015; Schebendach et al., 2013). These studies highlight heightened reward motivation in the context of illness-relevant rewards in these groups.

Reward learning

Reward or reinforcement learning tasks have been used to examine how individuals with eating disorders learn and execute strategies to maximize reward. In these tasks, participants are directed to detect information about the cues and/or environment within the task that signal the potential for reward and to use this information to select subsequent actions (Schaefer & Steinglass, 2021). In some paradigms, the reward contingencies or rules change over the course of the task, requiring participants to update their internal model of how to effectively obtain rewarding outcomes. Some studies using these tasks have revealed deficits in reward learning in AN (Foerde & Steinglass, 2017; Wierenga et al., 2022) and others have not (Bernardoni et al., 2018; Geisler et al., 2017). Similarly, two studies have not found group differences in general reward learning disturbances between individuals with BN and controls (Grob et al., 2012; Hagan & Forbush, 2021).

One set of reinforcement learning tasks (i.e., Two-Stage or Drifting Double-Bandit Tasks) require participants to understand how a sequence of actions and their outcomes leads to rewarding consequences (Schaefer & Steinglass, 2021).

In these tasks, there are two dominant decision strategies that emerge from computational modeling of the participants' responses: model-free learning and model-based learning (Sutton & Barto, 1998). In model-based learning, the individual uses an internal cognitive working model of the potential changes and outcomes in the environment to choose the behavior most likely to yield reward (Decker et al., 2016). In contrast, in model-free reinforcement learning, the individual uses simplistic trial-and-error strategies to obtain a reward. Across several investigations, individuals with eating disorders, including AN and BED, have demonstrated deficits in model-based learning for reward (Foerde et al., 2021; Reiter et al., 2017; Voon et al., 2015). Such deficits in model-based learning for reward may relate to the persistence of behavior, even after it becomes harmful or no longer reinforced (Schaefer & Steinglass, 2021).

Physiological response

A small literature has examined reward processing through psychophysiological assessments. In response to high-calorie food images, individuals with AN have displayed marked lower zygomatic activity, indicating less positive facial expression, compared to healthy controls (Soussignan et al., 2011). Further, greater restrictive eating has been associated with greater post-auricular reflex engagement to low-calorie foods, indicating greater reward response to cues for restriction (Racine et al., 2021). On the other hand, binge eating has been associated with greater post-auricular muscle engagement to high-calorie foods, reflecting heightened responsivity to cues for consumption (Racine et al., 2018). Studies have also detected elevated skin conductance, decreased eyeblink startle, and altered brain wave patterns on EEG to underweight stimuli among individuals with AN, which may reflect heightened response to illness-compatible reward cues (Clarke et al., 2016; Horndasch et al., 2012, 2018; O'Hara, Keyes, Renwick, Giel, et al., 2016).

Neurotransmitter activity

Dopamine is the primary neurotransmitter that has been linked with reward pathways. As such, several studies have investigated dopaminergic functioning in eating disorders. Across several studies, individuals with acute AN and those recovered from AN have been shown to have decreased cerebrospinal fluid concentrations of homovanillic acid, the primary metabolite of dopamine, relative to healthy individuals (Kontis & Theochari, 2012). Further, one study using positron emission tomography (PET), found that individuals recovered from AN had higher dopamine D2/D3 receptor binding potential in the antero-ventral striatum relative to healthy controls, indicating lower endogenous dopamine (Frank et al., 2005). In contrast, other PET studies have found no difference in striatal dopamine

D2 receptor binding potential between individuals with AN and healthy controls (Bailer et al., 2012; Broft et al., 2015). However, in one of the aforementioned studies, individuals with AN reported more anxiety than healthy controls in response to dopamine release in the dorsal caudate following an amphetamine challenge (Bailer et al., 2017). Given that food consumption yields dopamine release, this finding could provide insight on why individuals with AN might find food consumption unenjoyable and use restriction to suppress dopamine production.

There is also a growing focus on the relationship between dopamine and binge eating given the role of this neurotransmitter in food craving, impulsivity, and decision-making (Yu et al., 2022). Most research has identified a link between dopamine availability and binge eating; however, the direction of this relationship is not fully clear. Several studies using PET have identified reduced dopamine activity in putamen, insula, and amygdala, and a relationship between lesser dopamine activity and greater binge/purge episodes in BN (Broft et al., 2012; Frank et al., 2011). Similarly, one PET study found individuals with BED had lower D2 binding potential in the striatum and other subcortical regions relative to healthy controls (Majuri et al., 2017). However, a different PET study found individuals with BED had greater striatal dopamine release than higher-weight non-BED controls in response to food stimuli paired with methylphenidate, a drug that blocks dopamine reuptake transporters (Wang et al., 2011). Thus, more research is needed to clarify the specific pattern of dopamine production associated with binge eating.

Structural neuroimaging

Structural neuroimaging studies have revealed abnormalities in brain volume, as well as grey and white matter distributions, in regions associated with reward processing among individuals with eating disorders. Individuals with acute AN have been found to exhibit reduced global grey and white matter, regional reductions in the striatum, and regional grey matter increases in the OFC (Frank et al., 2013; Phillipou et al., 2018; Titova et al., 2013). Findings following weight restoration have been more mixed. Some studies have identified increased grey matter in the medial OFC relative to controls among weight-restored and recovered individuals with AN (Frank et al., 2013; Frank, 2015). However, several other studies have shown that grey matter volume is normalized by weight gain and clinical recovery in AN (Bernardoni et al., 2016; Castro-Fornieles et al., 2021; Joos et al., 2010). Structural alterations in white matter connectivity between reward regions (e.g., striatum and OFC) also have been reported in AN across various illness stages (Cha et al., 2016; Lloyd et al., 2023; Via et al., 2014).

In contrast to the pattern of structural findings in AN, individuals with BN have been found to have increased volume of the ventral striatum and OFC, which has been linked to severity of clinical symptoms (Abdo et al., 2020; Schäfer et al., 2010). For instance, in a study by Abdo and colleagues (2020), the left nucleus accumbens within the ventral striatum was enlarged in individuals with binge eating. Similarly, Schäfer and colleagues (2010) found greater ventral striatal volumes in individuals with BN were correlated with increased purging and lower body mass index (BMI). In BED, findings are inconsistent. Whereas some research has identified higher brain volume in the ventral striatum and OFC among individuals with BED that parallels the findings from BN (Abdo et al., 2020; Schäfer et al., 2010), other research has reported lower bilateral medial and lateral OFC volumes, along with lower left ventral striatal and bilateral caudate volumes, which were related to reward learning differences, in BED (Voon et al., 2015).

Functional neuroimaging

Resting state functional connectivity

Task-free functional imaging has revealed abnormalities in resting-state functional architecture of reward-related networks among individuals with eating disorders. The research in AN is mixed, with some studies finding hyperconnectivity in mesocortical reward networks in acute and weight-restored AN (Cha et al., 2016; Uniacke et al., 2019) and other studies finding hypoconnectivity of this same reward circuitry in AN (Haynos et al., 2019; Kullmann et al., 2014). Findings are more consistent among disorders characterized by binge eating, which have generally identified lower resting state functional connectivity between the striatum and prefrontal cortex (Leenaerts et al., 2022), as well as within cortical regions implicated in reward processing (Canna et al., 2017; Stopyra et al., 2019). Similarly, individuals with BED have shown lower connectivity between the striatum and prefrontal regions, such as the OFC and dorsomedial and dorsolateral PFC, compared to controls (Haynos, Camchong, et al., 2021; Murray et al., 2022; Stopyra et al., 2019); this pattern of findings has been linked to problems related to reward learning in BED (Haynos, Camchong, et al., 2021). Therefore, there is significant evidence of abnormal neural patterns in reward circuitry at rest, though the direction of the findings for AN remains unclear.

Task-based neural responses to disorder-relevant stimuli

Much of the task-based fMRI literature on reward responsivity in eating disorders has focused on neural responses to food stimuli (e.g., pictures, smells, or tastes of food, points to obtain food). In AN, the existing pattern of findings on brain responses to food cues is inconclusive. Several studies have found individuals with or recovered from AN to have diminished activation in reward-related regions (e.g., VTA, striatum, OFC) in response to palatable food images, scents, and taste compared to individuals with BN or healthy controls (Brooks et al., 2011; Holsen et al., 2012; Jiang et al., 2019; Kaye et al., 2020; Oberndorfer et al., 2013; Wagner et al., 2007). In contrast, other research has identified enhanced activation in reward circuitry (e.g., ventral and dorsal striatum, OFC) to the sight and taste of palatable food among individuals with AN in different illness stages compared to healthy controls (Cowdrey et al., 2011, 2013; Frank et al., 2012; Monteleone et al., 2017; Rothemund et al., 2011; Sanders et al., 2015). Additionally, one study revealed individuals with AN demonstrated a heightened response in the dorsal striatum and OFC to low-calorie and low-fat food images (Foerde et al., 2015), potentially indicating heightened reward processing related to low-density foods.

The literature is more consistent in demonstrating heightened reward responsivity to food among individuals with BN and BED (Bronleigh et al., 2022). Individuals with BN and BED have demonstrated increased activation in the dorsal striatum, ACC, insula, OFC, and ventromedial PFC in response to images of palatable foods (Fleck et al., 2019; Geliebter et al., 2016; Lee et al., 2017; Neveu et al., 2018; Schienle et al., 2009; Simon et al., 2016). In addition, increased activity in reward-related regions, such as the dorsal striatum or the medial OFC in response to food images or anticipated food receipt has correlated with greater food craving and external eating in binge-eating populations (Simon et al., 2016; Wonderlich et al., 2017). However, it should be noted that not all evidence has provided support for heightened reward activation to food in these populations (Bohon & Stice, 2011; Ely et al., 2017).

Other disorder-relevant stimuli have been investigated among patients with eating disorders. In several studies, images of thin or underweight bodies have evoked greater activation relative to healthy controls in reward-related brain regions (e.g., ventral striatum) among individuals with AN (Fladung et al., 2010, 2013; Vocks et al., 2010), but not in BN (Vocks et al., 2010). Further, Kullman and colleagues (2014) found increased PFC activation to exercise-related images in individuals with AN relative to athlete and non-athlete healthy controls, which the authors hypothesized was related to greater inhibitory control to moderate appetitive responses to these cues. Together, these studies suggest that weight-loss-related stimuli engage neural circuitry frequently associated with reward functions in AN. More research is needed to understand reactivity to such cues in other eating disorders.

Task-based neural responses to disorder-neutral stimuli

Monetary rewards have often been used as disorder-neutral stimuli to examine global reward processing. Relative to healthy controls, individuals with current and remitted AN have demonstrated less activation in the striatum during delay discounting paradigms (Decker et al., 2015; Wierenga et al., 2015), as well as poorer differentiation between monetary wins and losses in the ventral striatum (Wagner et al., 2007). However, some studies indicate that reward circuit activation to the anticipation or receipt of monetary gains is no different (Bernardoni et al., 2018; Bischoff-Grethe et al., 2013; Murao et al., 2017; Piccolo et al., 2019) in acute and recovered AN participants compared to healthy control participants. Further, other studies found elevated activation in reward circuitry in individuals with AN compared to healthy controls (Decker et al., 2015; DeGuzman et al., 2017; Wagner et al., 2007).

Fewer studies have examined neural response to monetary rewards in BN and BED. One study demonstrated individuals with BED had diminished activity in ventral striatum during the monetary reward anticipation, and decreased activity in the medial PFC during monetary reward receipt (Balodis et al., 2013, 2014). In contrast, Simon and colleagues (2016) found no differences in brain activity during the anticipation or receipt of monetary rewards in individuals with BN and BED. There is also some evidence that individuals with binge-eating pathology may adapt reward responsivity less in response to physiological state, such as hunger and satiety (Bischoff-Grethe et al., 2021; Mueller et al., 2018) and show diminished neural activation in the PFC, OFC, striatum, and caudate when learning to respond flexibly to rewards in their environment (Hartogsveld et al., 2022; Reiter et al., 2017; Voon et al., 2015).

Some studies have also examined reward circuitry responses to social cues among eating disorder samples. In AN, several studies have identified reduced activation in reward-related regions (e.g., caudate, medial PFC) to positive social cues, potentially highlighting social reward deficits in this population (Davidovic et al., 2018; Sala et al., 2018; Via et al., 2015). Other research has found no differences in reward circuit responsivity from controls (Boehm et al., 2018; Sweitzer et al., 2018) or even heightened responding in reward-related regions (e.g., medial PFC) (Mendoza et al., 2022) in response to social stimuli in AN. There is a much smaller body of research on social reward processing in BN. In one study, individuals recovered from BN demonstrated elevated caudate activation in response to the anticipation of positive social touch (Wierenga et al., 2020). In another study, individuals with BN demonstrated no differences from controls in neural responding to positive social interactions (Luo et al., 2022). Thus, more research is needed to understand responding to social reward across eating disorders (see Chapter 9 in this handbook).

Alternative Perspectives

Several major theories hypothesize a role of reward dysfunction in the pathogenesis of eating disorders. One influential set of theories situate eating disorders on a continuum of reward responding and inhibition, wherein individuals with primary restrictive eating pathology (e.g., AN-R) are conceptualized as being low on reward responsiveness and high in reward inhibition and individuals with primarily binge-eating pathology (e.g., BN, BED) as being high in reward responsiveness and low in reward inhibition (Kaye et al., 2013; Wierenga et al., 2014). This balance of reward responsiveness versus inhibition is thought to underlie the differences in food approach versus avoidance seen in different eating disorder diagnoses. Much of the evidence reviewed in this chapter supports this perspective. Individuals with primarily restrictive eating pathology self-report less reward responsiveness on temperament measures compared to those with binge-eating/purging pathology (Atiye et al., 2015; Farstad et al., 2016). Similarly, on delay discounting paradigms, individuals with AN have lower motivation and those with BN and BED have higher motivation to pursue immediately available rewards (Amlung et al., 2019; Lempert et al., 2018). Individuals with AN generally demonstrate lower structural brain volume, and individuals with BN show higher structural brain volume in reward regions (Donnelly et al., 2018; Walton et al., 2022). Further, a number of studies highlight under-responding in AN and over-responding in BN and BED on reward-related psychophysiological and neural markers in response to food cues and potentially other rewards (Haynos et al., 2020). These findings could reflect differing predispositions to bottom-up reward processing that increase risk of certain types of eating pathology.

However, a significant body of research does not correspond with this narrative. In some domains, individuals with eating disorders exhibit similar patterns of reward dysfunction, independent of the specific diagnosis or symptom profile. For instance, all eating disorder diagnoses studied appear to demonstrate deficiencies in dopamine production, although the mechanism of action could be different for AN versus BN and BED (Frank, 2015; Yu et al., 2022). Similarly, resting state functional connectivity patterns appear to be altered across eating pathology, with multiple studies suggesting shared cross-diagnostic tendencies toward mesocortical hypoconnectivity (Haynos, Camchong, et al., 2021; Haynos et al., 2019; Kullmann et al., 2014; Murray et al., 2022). Reward learning paradigms additionally suggest that an over-reliance on computationally simplistic reward-based decision strategies may be shared across eating pathology (Foerde et al., 2021; Voon et al., 2015). Finally, myriad results run counter to this model, finding enhanced reward responding to food and other rewards in AN and diminished reward responsivity in BN and BED (Donnelly et al., 2018; Haynos et al., 2020). Other research has identified subsets of individuals within a single eating disorder diagnosis that demonstrate differing patterns of reward responding, suggesting these distinctions do not vary neatly with diagnostic category (Haynos, Wang, et al., 2021; Steding et al., 2019). Finally, it is difficult to reconcile this theoretical framework with the robust literature showing substantial diagnostic crossover between eating disorder diagnoses, including AN and BN (Eddy et al., 2008).

Other theories conceptualize eating disorders as similar to addictive disorders in that they are at least initially perpetuated by a reward drive; in AN, the reward drive is presumed to be oriented toward thinness and weight loss and, in BN and BED, it is presumed to focus on food (Godier & Park, 2015; Smith & Robbins, 2013). There is also a notable body of research supporting this model of eating disorders. Progressive ratio tasks demonstrate that individuals with eating disorders will exert significant effort to access eating disorder-relevant experiences (i.e., restriction, exercise, binge eating) (Bodell & Keel, 2015; Gianini et al., 2016; Haynos et al., 2016; Schebendach et al., 2013). As previously noted, individuals with BN and

BED frequently demonstrate heightened psychophysiological and neural reward responding to food and those with restrictive eating disorders exhibit similar reward responses to weight-loss cues (Fladung et al., 2010, 2013; Racine et al., 2021; Vocks et al., 2010). Similar to addictive disorders, eating disorder behaviors tend to escalate over time and become increasingly compulsive (Godier & Park, 2015). However, one major issue with the addictive narrative is that this perspective cannot as clearly explain the generalization of reward processing anomalies beyond eating disorder contexts (Haynos et al., 2023).

To reconcile these perspectives, our group has suggested that individuals with varied eating disorder presentations may not differ in global reward processing, but rather on specific reward preferences based on discrete qualities of certain reward classes (Haynos et al., 2020). For instance, instead of having an overall reward deficiency, individuals with AN may be more drawn to rewards that are predictable, controllable, delayed, and effortful, rather than the immediate, high-intensity, and unpredictable rewards often used in reward paradigms. Accordingly, studies have found individuals with AN to show greater deficits in reward responsivity within uncertain contexts (Piccolo et al., 2019). Individuals with AN also exhibit greater delay (Lempert et al., 2018) and effort (Haynos et al., 2023; Patzelt et al., 2019) tolerance in pursuing rewards than those without an eating disorder. From this perspective, gravitation towards restrictive eating in AN may result from such behavior sharing reward properties (e.g., controllability, effortfulness) that correspond with their preferences. This perspective is newly formed, and more research is needed to determine its veracity.

Notably, limitations in the literature pose a major barrier to evaluating any theory of reward processing (Haynos et al., 2020). There has been considerable variability in the methods used to capture reward making it difficult to synthesize findings across studies. For example, food cues deviate widely between studies in terms of palatability, caloric and fat content, mode of presentation (i.e., visual, taste), and the conditions under which they are presented (e.g., fasting, fed). The conclusions derived from reward investigations are similarly discrepant across studies. For instance, the same patterns of neural activity are often interpreted as reflecting appetitive responding in one study and aversive responding in another. This problem is compounded through the examination of biological indices divorced from behavioral or self-report phenomena. The reward literature, like most eating disorder research, is plagued by small and non-representative samples, potentially rendering many studies under-powered and non-generalizable. Certain diagnoses, such as atypical anorexia nervosa and avoidant/restrictive food intake disorder, have been largely uninvestigated within this literature. Given these limitations, it is no surprise that mixed evidence can be found for several theories of reward processing in eating disorders. To more definitively determine the influence of reward processing on eating pathology, greater rigor and standardization is needed in the research in this area.

Implications

Despite the growing body of evidence implicating reward processing aberrations in the perpetuation of eating disorders, few clinical approaches have explicitly targeted these constructs (Haynos, Anderson, et al., 2021). Considering the limited efficacy of existing treatments (Bulik, 2021), incorporation of emerging neurobiological insights into practice may yield improved outcomes. Notably, the efficacy of such treatments relies heavily upon improving theoretical models of reward responding. Thus, reward-targeting treatment research can both investigate novel avenues for intervention and serve as a probe for testing theories of reward processing.

Pharmacological treatments

Despite increasing knowledge regarding the neurobiology of eating disorders, there remains insufficient evidence to support use of most pharmacological agents for these conditions. The only FDA-approved medications to treat eating disorders are lisdexamfetamine dimesylate for BED and fluoxetine for BN (Muratore & Attia, 2022). No medications have FDA-approval for the treatment of AN, although evidence increasingly supports the use of olanzapine to support weight restoration (Çöpür & Çöpür, 2020). There is some evidence that the effects of lisdexamfetamine dimesylate on BED may occur through reward alterations (Schneider et al., 2021). This drug increases dopamine transmission, which may rebalance the deficits in dopamine production linked to binge eating. Preclinical and non-clinical samples have found that lisdexamfetamine dimesylate reduces reward drive and responsivity of reward circuitry (e.g., ventromedial PFC) to food (Fleck et al., 2019; Vickers et al., 2015). Research is needed to determine whether this mechanism extends to binge-eating populations (Schneider et al., 2021). Some research provides additional support for dopamine reuptake inhibitors for binge-eating populations, but evidence is mixed (McElroy et al., 2020; Wang et al., 2011).

Alternately, olanzapine is a dopamine antagonist that blocks the action potential of this neurotransmitter. Although limited data suggest that individuals with AN may have lower circulating dopamine, they also have exhibited increased anxiety to dopamine release (Bailer et al., 2012), raising the potential of dopamine hypersensitivity in perpetuating restrictive eating. Thus, olanzapine may impact clinical change in AN by reducing the anxiogenic impact of the increases in dopamine that occur when normalizing food intake. However, the impacts of atypical antipsychotics upon reward responsivity in AN have not been examined. There may be a role for other psychopharmacology acting upon reward circuitry, such as anti-craving medications (Stancil et al., 2019), in eating disorder treatment. However, this research is in its infancy.

Psychosocial treatments

Standard, empirically supported treatments for eating disorders, such as cognitive behavioral therapy, primarily focus on encouraging more adaptive patterns of eating, weight-control, and body-focused behaviors (Fairburn, 2008) and do not directly address reward responsivity. For this reason, behavioral treatments aimed at targeting aspects of reward processing and learning implicated in eating pathology have been developed over recent years.

One example of this approach from the prevention literature is the Body Project, a dissonance-based prevention program aimed at decreasing reward responses to the thin body image ideal in young women (Stice & Presnell, 2007). This prevention program has garnered significant support (Stice, Onipede, et al., 2021) and recent research suggests that one mechanism of action may be through alterations of reward circuitry. Specifically, in one study, participants who participated in the Body Project displayed reductions in reward circuit activation in response to images of thin models (Stice, Yokum, et al., 2021). However, notably, this program only targets reward explicitly related to eating disorder content.

Other novel treatments targeting reward processing have been developed for individuals with existing eating pathology. Reward Re-Training is a recently developed treatment that aims to offset disorder-specific reward responsivity in binge-eating populations through increasing rewarding experiences outside of palatable food (Juarascio et al., 2022). In transdiagnostic samples with binge-eating symptomatology, Reward Re-Training has been shown to reduce palatable food reward responsiveness and eating pathology (Juarascio et al., 2022, 2023). Another emerging behavioral treatment, Temperament Based Therapy with Support, encourages tailoring interventions to correspond with individual differences in temperamental reward responsiveness (Kaye et al., 2015) (see Chapter 19). Preliminary results of this treatment suggest that it may improve eating disorder symptoms and increase BMI among individuals with AN (Wierenga et al., 2018). Finally, initial research is being conducted to examine the impact of an adaptation of a treatment called Positive Affect Treatment (PAT) on AN (Haynos, Anderson, et al., 2021). PAT was originally designed to treat anhedonia in depression and anxiety by increasing reward anticipation, experiencing, and learning (Craske et al., 2016). Research on PAT in AN is ongoing; however, the results in mood and anxiety disorders have been positive, suggesting that PAT improves mood and rectifies reward abnormalities (Craske et al., 2019, 2023). Initial research on reward processing interventions is promising, but the literature is small, highlighting the need for further research that integrates neurobiological findings into efficacious treatments.

Conclusions

Bottom-up reward processing and reinforcement learning have been investigated extensively among individuals with eating disorders, especially AN and BN. Extant findings suggest aberrations in reward processing may influence the development and maintenance of eating pathology. However, the literature is highly mixed and impacted by methodological limitations. As a result, it has been difficult to comprehend the precise pathways through which reward processing affects eating disorder symptoms, or to evaluate the theories emerging from this literature. Few clinical approaches have been developed to target identified reward processing disturbances; however, new studies suggest such approaches may be beneficial. Continued research on reward processing, and its interactions with other bottom-up and top-down systems, is needed to better understand and treat serious eating pathology.

References

Abdo, N., Boyd, E., Baboumian, S., Pantazatos, S. P., & Geliebter, A. (2020). Relationship between binge eating and associated eating behaviors with subcortical brain volumes and cortical thickness. *Journal of Affective Disorders, 274*, 1201–1205.

Amlung, M., Marsden, E., Holshausen, K., Morris, V., Patel, H., Vedelago, L., Naish, K. R., Reed, D. D., & McCabe, R. E. (2019). Delay discounting as a transdiagnostic process in psychiatric disorders: A meta-analysis. *JAMA Psychiatry, 76*(11), 1176–1186.

Atiye, M., Miettunen, J., & Raevuori-Helkamaa, A. (2015). A meta-analysis of temperament in eating disorders. *European Eating Disorders Review, 23*(2), 89–99.

Bailer, U. F., Narendran, R., Frankle, W. G., Himes, M. L., Duvvuri, V., Mathis, C. A., & Kaye, W. H. (2012). Amphetamine induced dopamine release increases anxiety in individuals recovered from anorexia nervosa. *International Journal of Eating Disorders, 45*, 263–271.

Bailer, U. F., Price, J. C., Meltzer, C. C., Wagner, A., Mathis, C. A., Gamst, A., & Kaye, W. H. (2017). Dopaminergic activity and altered reward modulation in anorexia nervosa—Insight from multimodal imaging. *International Journal of Eating Disorders, 50*(5), 593–596.

Balodis, I. M., Grilo, C. M., Kober, H., Worhunsky, P. D., White, M. A., Stevens, M. C., Pearlson, G. D., & Potenza, M. N. (2014). A pilot study linking reduced fronto-striatal recruitment during reward processing to persistent bingeing following treatment for binge-eating disorder. *International Journal of Eating Disorders, 47*(4), 376–384.

Balodis, I. M., Kober, H., Worhunsky, P. D., White, M. A., Stevens, M. C., Pearlson, G. D., Sinha, R., Grilo, C. M., & Potenza, M. N. (2013). Monetary reward processing in obese individuals with and without binge eating disorder. *Biological Psychiatry, 73*(9), 877–886.

Bartholdy, S., Rennalls, S., Danby, H., Jacques, C., Campbell, I. C., Schmidt, U., & O'Daly, O. G. (2017). Temporal discounting and the tendency to delay gratification across the eating disorder spectrum. *European Eating Disorders Review, 25*(5), 344–350.

Benning, S. D., Patrick, C. J., & Lang, A. R. (2004). Emotional modulation of the post-auricular reflex. *Psychophysiology, 41*(3), 426–432.

Bernardoni, F., Geisler, D., King, J. A., Javadi, A.-H., Ritschel, F., Murr, J., Reiter, A. M. F., Rössner, V., Smolka, M. N., Kiebel, S., & Ehrlich, S. (2018). Altered medial frontal feedback learning signals in anorexia nervosa. *Biological Psychiatry, 83*(3), 235–243.

Bernardoni, F., King, J. A., Geisler, D., Stein, E., Jaite, C., Nätsch, D., Tam, F. I., Boehm, I., Seidel, M., Roessner, V., & Ehrlich, S. (2016). Weight restoration therapy rapidly reverses cortical thinning in anorexia nervosa: A longitudinal study. *NeuroImage, 130*, 214–222.

Bischoff-Grethe, A., McCurdy, D., Grenesko-Stevens, E., Irvine, L. E. Z., Wagner, A., Yau, W., Fennema-Notestine, C., Wierenga, C. E., Fudge, J. L., Delgado, M. R., & Kaye, W. H. (2013). Altered brain response to reward and punishment in adolescents with anorexia nervosa. *Psychiatry Research, 214*(3), 331–340.

Bischoff-Grethe, A., Wierenga, C. E., Bailer, U. F., McClure, S. M., & Kaye, W. H. (2021). Satiety does not alter the ventral striatum's response to immediate reward in bulimia nervosa. *Journal of Abnormal Psychology, 130*(8), 862–874.

Bodell, L. P., & Keel, P. K. (2015). Weight suppression in bulimia nervosa: Associations with biology and behavior. *Journal of Abnormal Psychology, 124*(4), 994–1002.

Boehm, I., King, J. A., Bernardoni, F., Geisler, D., Seidel, M., Ritschel, F., Goschke, T., Haynes, J. D., Roessner, V., & Ehrlich, S. (2018). Subliminal and supraliminal processing of reward-related stimuli in anorexia nervosa. *Psychological Medicine, 48*(5), 790–800.

Bohon, C., & Stice, E. (2011). Reward abnormalities among women with full and subthreshold bulimia nervosa: A functional magnetic resonance imaging study. *International Journal of Eating Disorders, 44*(7), 585–595.

Broft, A., Shingleton, R., Kaufman, J., Liu, F., Kumar, D., Slifstein, M., Abi-Dargham, A., Schebendach, J., Van Heertum, R., Attia, E., Martinez, D., & Walsh, B. T. (2012). Striatal dopamine in bulimia nervosa: A PET imaging study. *International Journal of Eating Disorders, 45*(5), 648–656.

Broft, A., Slifstein, M., Osborne, J., Kothari, P., Morim, S., Shingleton, R., Kenney, L., Vallabhajosula, S., Attia, E., Martinez, D., & Walsh, B. T. (2015). Striatal dopamine type 2 receptor availability in anorexia nervosa. *Psychiatry Research, 233*(3), 380–387.

Bromberg-Martin, E. S., Matsumoto, M., & Hikosaka, O. (2010). Dopamine in motivational control: Rewarding, aversive, and alerting. *Neuron, 68*(5), 815–834.

Bronleigh, M., Baumann, O., & Stapleton, P. (2022). Neural correlates associated with processing food stimuli in anorexia nervosa and bulimia nervosa: An activation likelihood estimation meta-analysis of fMRI studies. *Eating and Weight Disorders*, 27(7), 2309–2320. https://doi.org/10.1007/s40519-022-01390-x

Brooks, S. J., O'Daly, O. G., Uher, R., Friederich, H.-C., Giampietro, V., Brammer, M., Williams, S. C., Schiöth, H. B., Treasure, J., & Campbell, I. C. (2011). Differential neural responses to food images in women with bulimia versus anorexia nervosa. *PLOS ONE, 6*(7), e22259.

Bulik, C. M. (2021). From awareness to action: An urgent call to address the inadequacy of treatment for anorexia nervosa. *American Journal of Psychiatry, 178*(9), 786–788.

Canna, A., Prinster, A., Monteleone, A. M., Cantone, E., Monteleone, P., Volpe, U., Maj, M., Di Salle, F., & Esposito, F. (2017). Interhemispheric functional connectivity in anorexia and bulimia nervosa. *European Journal of Neuroscience, 45*(9), 1129–1140.

Castro-Fornieles, J., de la Serna, E., Calvo, A., Pariente, J., Andrés-Perpiña, S., Plana, M. T., Romero, S., Flamarique, I., Gárriz, M., & Bargalló, N. (2021). Cortical thickness 20 years after diagnosis of anorexia nervosa during adolescence. *European Archives of Psychiatry and Clinical Neuroscience, 271*(6), 1133–1139.

Cha, J., Ide, J. S., Bowman, F. D., Simpson, H. B., Posner, J., & Steinglass, J. E. (2016). Abnormal reward circuitry in anorexia nervosa: A longitudinal, multimodal MRI study. *Human Brain Mapping, 37*(11), 3835–3846.

Clarke, J., Ramoz, N., Fladung, A.-K., & Gorwood, P. (2016). Higher reward value of starvation imagery in anorexia nervosa and association with the Val66Met BDNF polymorphism. *Translational Psychiatry, 6*(6), e829.

Çöpür, S., & Çöpür, M. (2020). Olanzapine in the treatment of anorexia nervosa: A systematic review. *Egyptian Journal of Neurology, Psychiatry and Neurosurgery, 56*(1), 60.

Cowdrey, F. A., Finlayson, G., & Park, R. J. (2013). Liking compared with wanting for high- and low-calorie foods in anorexia nervosa: Aberrant food reward even after weight restoration. *American Journal of Clinical Nutrition, 97*(3), 463–470.

Cowdrey, F. A., Park, R. J., Harmer, C. J., & McCabe, C. (2011). Increased neural processing of rewarding and aversive food stimuli in recovered anorexia nervosa. *Biological Psychiatry, 70*(8), 736–743.

Craske, M. G., Meuret, A. E., Echiverri-Cohen, A., Rosenfield, D., & Ritz, T. (2023). Positive affect treatment targets reward sensitivity: A randomized controlled trial. *Journal of Consulting and Clinical Psychology*, 91(6), 350–366.

Craske, M. G., Meuret, A. E., Ritz, T., Treanor, M., & Dour, H. J. (2016). Treatment for anhedonia: A neuroscience driven approach. *Depression and Anxiety, 33*(10), 927–938.

Craske, M. G., Meuret, A. E., Ritz, T., Treanor, M., Dour, H., & Rosenfield, D. (2019). Positive affect treatment for depression and anxiety: A randomized clinical trial for a core feature of anhedonia. *Journal of Consulting and Clinical Psychology, 87*(5), 457–471.

Daniel, R., & Pollmann, S. (2014). A universal role of the ventral striatum in reward-based learning: Evidence from human studies. *Neurobiology of Learning and Memory, 114*, 90–100.

Davidovic, M., Karjalainen, L., Starck, G., Wentz, E., Björnsdotter, M., & Olausson, H. (2018). Abnormal brain processing of gentle touch in anorexia nervosa. *Psychiatry Research: Neuroimaging, 281*, 53–60.

Decker, J. H., Figner, B., & Steinglass, J. E. (2015). On weight and waiting: Delay discounting in anorexia nervosa pretreatment and posttreatment. *Biological Psychiatry, 78*(9), 606–614.

Decker, J. H., Otto, A. R., Daw, N. D., & Hartley, C. A. (2016). From creatures of habit to goal-directed learners: Tracking the developmental emergence of model-based reinforcement learning. *Psychological Science, 27*(6), 848–858.

DeGuzman, M., Shott, M. E., Yang, T. T., Riederer, J., & Frank, G. K. W. (2017). Association of elevated reward prediction error response with weight gain in adolescent anorexia nervosa. *American Journal of Psychiatry, 174*(6), 557–565.

Donnelly, B., Touyz, S., Hay, P., Burton, A., Russell, J., & Caterson, I. (2018). Neuroimaging in bulimia nervosa and binge eating disorder: A systematic review. *Journal of Eating Disorders, 6*, 3.

Doose, A., King, J. A., Bernardoni, F., Geisler, D., Hellerhoff, I., Weinert, T., Roessner, V., Smolka, M. N., & Ehrlich, S. (2020). Strengthened default mode network activation during delay discounting in adolescents with anorexia nervosa after partial weight restoration: A longitudinal fMRI study. *Journal of Clinical Medicine, 9*(4), E900.

Eddy, K. T., Dorer, D. J., Franko, D. L., Tahilani, K., Thompson-Brenner, H., & Herzog, D. B. (2008). Diagnostic crossover in anorexia nervosa and bulimia nervosa: Implications for DSM-V. *American Journal of Psychiatry, 165*(2), 245–250. https://doi.org/10.1176/appi.ajp.2007.07060951

Ely, A. V., Wierenga, C. E., Bischoff-Grethe, A., Bailer, U. F., Berner, L. A., Fudge, J. L., Paulus, M. P., & Kaye, W. H. (2017). Response in taste circuitry is not modulated by hunger and satiety in women remitted from bulimia nervosa. *Journal of Abnormal Psychology, 126*(5), 519–530.

Fairburn, C. G. (2008). *Cognitive Behavior Therapy and Eating Disorders* (1st ed.). Guilford Press.

Farstad, S. M., McGeown, L. M., & von Ranson, K. M. (2016). Eating disorders and personality, 2004–2016: A systematic review and meta-analysis. *Clinical Psychology Review, 46*, 91–105.

Fladung, A.-K., Grön, G., Grammer, K., Herrnberger, B., Schilly, E., Grasteit, S., Wolf, R. C., Walter, H., & von Wietersheim, J. (2010). A neural signature of anorexia nervosa in the ventral striatal reward system. *American Journal of Psychiatry, 167*(2), 206–212.

Fladung, A.-K., Schulze, U. M. E., Schöll, F., Bauer, K., & Grön, G. (2013). Role of the ventral striatum in developing anorexia nervosa. *Translational Psychiatry, 3*, e315.

Fleck, D. E., Eliassen, J. C., Guerdjikova, A. I., Mori, N., Williams, S., Blom, T. J., Beckwith, T., Tallman, M. J., Adler, C. M., DelBello, M. P., Strakowski, S. M., & McElroy, S. L. (2019). Effect of lisdexamfetamine on emotional network brain dysfunction in binge eating disorder. *Psychiatry Research. Neuroimaging, 286*, 53–59.

Foerde, K., Daw, N. D., Rufin, T., Walsh, B. T., Shohamy, D., & Steinglass, J. E. (2021). Deficient goal-directed control in a population characterized by extreme goal pursuit. *Journal of Cognitive Neuroscience, 33*(3), 463–481.

Foerde, K., & Steinglass, J. E. (2017). Decreased feedback learning in anorexia nervosa persists after weight restoration. *International Journal of Eating Disorders, 50*(4), 415–423.

Foerde, K., Steinglass, J. E., Shohamy, D., & Walsh, B. T. (2015). Neural mechanisms supporting maladaptive food choices in anorexia nervosa. *Nature Neuroscience, 18*(11), 1571–1573.

Frank, G. K., Bailer, U. F., Henry, S. E., Drevets, W., Meltzer, C. C., Price, J. C., Mathis, C. A., Wagner, A., Hoge, J., Ziolko, S., Barbarich-Marsteller, N., Weissfeld, L., & Kaye, W. H. (2005). Increased dopamine D2/D3 receptor binding after recovery from anorexia nervosa measured by positron emission tomography and [11c]raclopride. *Biological Psychiatry, 58*(11), 908–912.

Frank, G. K., Shott, M. E., Hagman, J. O., & Mittal, V. A. (2013). Alterations in brain structures related to taste reward circuitry in ill and recovered anorexia nervosa and in bulimia nervosa. *American Journal of Psychiatry, 170*(10), 1152–1160.

Frank, G. K. W. (2015). Recent advances in neuroimaging to model eating disorder neurobiology. *Current Psychiatry Reports, 17*(4), 22.

Frank, G. K. W., Kalina, C., DeGuzman, M. C., & Shott, M. E. (2020). Eye blink and reward prediction error response in anorexia nervosa. *International Journal of Eating Disorders, 53*(9), 1544–1549.

Frank, G. K. W., Reynolds, J. R., Shott, M. E., Jappe, L., Yang, T. T., Tregellas, J. R., & O'Reilly, R. C. (2012). Anorexia nervosa and obesity are associated with opposite brain reward response. *Neuropsychopharmacology, 37*(9), 2031–2046.

Frank, G. K. W., Reynolds, J. R., Shott, M. E., & O'Reilly, R. C. (2011). Altered temporal difference learning in bulimia nervosa. *Biological Psychiatry, 70*(8), 728–735.

Geisler, D., Ritschel, F., King, J. A., Bernardoni, F., Seidel, M., Boehm, I., Runge, F., Goschke, T., Roessner, V., Smolka, M. N., & Ehrlich, S. (2017). Increased anterior cingulate cortex response precedes behavioural adaptation in anorexia nervosa. *Scientific Reports, 7*, 42066.

Geliebter, A., Benson, L., Pantazatos, S. P., Hirsch, J., & Carnell, S. (2016). Greater anterior cingulate activation and connectivity in response to visual and auditory high-calorie food cues in binge eating: Preliminary findings. *Appetite, 96*, 195–202.

Gianini, L. M., Klein, D. A., Call, C., Mayer, L., Foltin, R. W., Walsh, B. T., Wang, Y., Wu, P., & Attia, E. (2016). The reinforcing effect of exercise in anorexia nervosa: Clinical correlates and relationship to outcome. *Eating Disorders, 24*(5), 412–423.

Giel, K., Zipfel, S., & Hallschmid, M. (2018). Oxytocin and eating disorders: A narrative review on emerging findings and perspectives. *Current Neuropharmacology, 16*(8), 1111–1121.

Godier, L. R., & Park, R. J. (2015). Does compulsive behavior in anorexia nervosa resemble an addiction? A qualitative investigation. *Frontiers in Psychology, 6*, 1608.

Goldsmith, H. H., Buss, A. H., Plomin, R., Rothbart, M. K., Thomas, A., Chess, S., Hinde, R. A., & McCall, R. B. (1987). Roundtable: What is temperament? Four approaches. *Child Development, 58*(2), 505–529.

Grob, S., Pizzagalli, D. A., Dutra, S. J., Stern, J., Mörgeli, H., Milos, G., Schnyder, U., Hasler, G. (2012). Dopamine-related deficit in reward learning after catecholamine depletion in unmedicated, remitted subjects with bulimia nervosa. *Neuropsychopharmacology, 37*(8), 1945–1952.

Hagan, K. E., & Forbush, K. T. (2021). Reward learning in unmedicated women with bulimia nervosa: A pilot investigation. *Journal of Psychiatric Research, 136*, 63–70.

Hagan, K. E., Jarmolowicz, D. P., & Forbush, K. T. (2021). Reconsidering delay discounting in bulimia nervosa. *Eating Behaviors, 41*, 101506.

Harrison, A., O'Brien, N., Lopez, C., & Treasure, J. (2010). Sensitivity to reward and punishment in eating disorders. *Psychiatry Research, 177*(1–2), 1–11.

Hartogsveld, B., Quaedflieg, C. W. E. M., van Ruitenbeek, P., & Smeets, T. (2022). Volume and connectivity differences in brain networks associated with cognitive constructs of binge eating. *eNeuro, 9*(1), ENEURO.0080–21.2021.

Haynos, A. F., Anderson, L. M., Askew, A. J., Craske, M. G., & Peterson, C. B. (2021). Adapting a neuroscience-informed intervention to alter reward mechanisms of anorexia nervosa: A novel direction for future research. *Journal of Eating Disorders, 9*(1), 63.

Haynos, A. F., Camchong, J., Pearson, C. M., Lavender, J. M., Mueller, B. A., Peterson, C. B., Specker, S., Raymond, N., & Lim, K. O. (2021). Resting state hypoconnectivity of reward networks in binge eating disorder. *Cerebral Cortex, 31*(5), 2494–2504.

Haynos, A. F., Hall, L. M. J., Lavender, J. M., Peterson, C. B., Crow, S. J., Klimes-Dougan, B., Cullen, K. R., Lim, K. O., & Camchong, J. (2019). Resting state functional connectivity of networks associated with reward and habit in anorexia nervosa. *Human Brain Mapping, 40*(2), 652–662.

Haynos, A. F., Hill, B., & Fruzzetti, A. E. (2016). Emotion regulation training to reduce problematic dietary restriction: An experimental analysis. *Appetite, 103*, 265–274.

Haynos, A. F., Koithan, E., & Hagan, K. E. (2023). Learned industriousness as a translational mechanism in anorexia nervosa. *Nature Reviews Psychology, 2*, 112–126.

Haynos, A. F., Lavender, J. M., Nelson, J., Crow, S. J., & Peterson, C. B. (2020). Moving towards specificity: A systematic review of cue features associated with reward and punishment in anorexia nervosa. *Clinical Psychology Review, 79*, 101872.

Haynos, A. F., Wang, S. B., LeMay-Russell, S., Lavender, J. M., Pearson, C. M., Mathis, K. J., Peterson, C. B., & Crow, S. J. (2021). An empirical taxonomy of reward response patterns in a transdiagnostic eating disorder sample. *Eating Behaviors, 42*, 101531.

Holsen, L., Lawson, E., Blum, J., Ko, E., Makris, N., Fazeli, P., Klibanski, A., & Goldstein, J. (2012). Food motivation circuitry hypoactivation related to hedonic and nonhedonic aspects of hunger and satiety in women with active anorexia nervosa and weight-restored women with anorexia nervosa. *Journal of Psychiatry & Neuroscience, 37*(5), 322–332.

Horndasch, S., Kratz, O., Holczinger, A., Heinrich, H., Hönig, F., Nöth, E., & Moll, G. H. (2012). "Looks do matter"—Visual attentional biases in adolescent girls with eating disorders viewing body images. *Psychiatry Research, 198*(2), 321–323.

Horndasch, S., Roesch, J., Forster, C., Dörfler, A., Lindsiepe, S., Heinrich, H., Graap, H., Moll, G. H., & Kratz, O. (2018). Neural processing of food and emotional stimuli in adolescent and adult anorexia nervosa patients. *PLOS ONE, 13*(3), e0191059.

Jiang, T., Soussignan, R., Carrier, E., & Royet, J.-P. (2019). Dysfunction of the mesolimbic circuit to food odors in women with anorexia and bulimia nervosa: A fMRI study. *Frontiers in Human Neuroscience, 13*, 117.

Joos, A., Klöppel, S., Hartmann, A., Glauche, V., Tüscher, O., Perlov, E., Saum, B., Freyer, T., Zeeck, A., & van Elst, L. T. (2010). Voxel-based morphometry in eating disorders: Correlation of psychopathology with grey matter volume. *Psychiatry Research: Neuroimaging, 182*(2), 146–151.

Juarascio, A. S., Presseller, E. K., Wilkinson, M. L., Kelkar, A., Srivastava, P., Chen, J. Y., Dengler, J., Manasse, S. M., & Medaglia, J. (2022). Correcting the reward imbalance in binge eating: A pilot randomized trial of reward re-training treatment. *Appetite, 176*, 106103.

Juarascio, A. S., Srivastava, P., Manasse, S. M., Wilkinson, M. L., Felonis, C. R., & Drexler, S. A. (2023). Reward retraining: A pilot randomized controlled trial of a novel treatment approach for transdiagnostic binge eating. *International Journal of Eating Disorders, 56*(3), 662–670.

Kaye, W. H., Wierenga, C. E., Bailer, U. F., Simmons, A. N., & Bischoff-Grethe, A. (2013). Nothing tastes as good as skinny feels: The neurobiology of anorexia nervosa. *Trends in Neurosciences, 36*(2), 110–120.

Kaye, W. H., Wierenga, C. E., Bischoff-Grethe, A., Berner, L. A., Ely, A. V., Bailer, U. F., Paulus, M. P., & Fudge, J. L. (2020). Neural insensitivity to the effects of hunger in women remitted from anorexia nervosa. *American Journal of Psychiatry, 177*(7), 601–610.

Kaye, W. H., Wierenga, C. E., Knatz, S., Liang, J., Boutelle, K., Hill, L., & Eisler, I. (2015). Temperament-based treatment for anorexia nervosa. *European Eating Disorders Review, 23*(1), 12–18.

Keating, C., Tilbrook, A. J., Rossell, S. L., Enticott, P. G., & Fitzgerald, P. B. (2012). Reward processing in anorexia nervosa. *Neuropsychologia, 50*(5), 567–575.

Kekic, M., Bartholdy, S., Cheng, J., McClelland, J., Boysen, E., Musiat, P., O'Daly, O. G., Campbell, I. C., & Schmidt, U. (2016). Increased temporal discounting in bulimia nervosa. *International Journal of Eating Disorders, 49*(12), 1077–1081.

King, J. A., Bernardoni, F., Geisler, D., Ritschel, F., Doose, A., Pauligk, S., Pásztor, K., Weidner, K., Roessner, V., Smolka, M. N., & Ehrlich, S. (2020). Intact value-based decision-making during intertemporal choice in women with remitted anorexia nervosa? An fMRI study. *Journal of Psychiatry & Neuroscience, 45*(2), 108–116.

King, J. A., Geisler, D., Bernardoni, F., Ritschel, F., Böhm, I., Seidel, M., Mennigen, E., Ripke, S., Smolka, M. N., Roessner, V., & Ehrlich, S. (2016). Altered neural efficiency of decision making during temporal reward discounting in anorexia nervosa. *Journal of the American Academy of Child and Adolescent Psychiatry, 55*(11), 972–979.

Klein, D. A., Schebendach, J. E., Gershkovich, M., Bodell, L. P., Foltinb, R. W., & Walsh, B. T. (2010). Behavioral assessment of the reinforcing effect of exercise in women with anorexia nervosa: Further paradigm development and data. *International Journal of Eating Disorders, 43*(7), 611–618.

Kontis, D., & Theochari, E. (2012). Dopamine in anorexia nervosa: A systematic review. *Behavioural Pharmacology, 23*(5 and 6), 496.

Kullmann, S., Giel, K. E., Teufel, M., Thiel, A., Zipfel, S., & Preissl, H. (2014). Aberrant network integrity of the inferior frontal cortex in women with anorexia nervosa. *NeuroImage: Clinical, 4*, 615–622.

Lee, J. E., Namkoong, K., & Jung, Y.-C. (2017). Impaired prefrontal cognitive control over interference by food images in binge-eating disorder and bulimia nervosa. *Neuroscience Letters, 651*, 95–101.

Leenaerts, N., Jongen, D., Ceccarini, J., Van Oudenhove, L., & Vrieze, E. (2022). The neurobiological reward system and binge eating: A critical systematic review of neuroimaging studies. *International Journal of Eating Disorders, 55*(11), 1421–1458.

Lempert, K. M., Steinglass, J. E., Pinto, A., Kable, J. W., & Simpson, H. B. (2018). Can delay discounting deliver on the promise of RDoC? *Psychological Medicine, 49*(2), 190–199.

Lloyd, E. C., Foerde, K. E., Muratore, A. F., Aw, N., Semanek, D., Steinglass, J. E., & Posner, J. (2023). Large-scale exploration of whole-brain structural connectivity in anorexia nervosa: Alterations in the connectivity of frontal and subcortical networks. *Biological Psychiatry. Cognitive Neuroscience and Neuroimaging, 8*(8), 864–873.

Luo, Y., Mendoza, C., Pelfrey, S., Lohrenz, T., Gu, X., Montague, P. R., & McAdams, C. J. (2022). Elevated neurobehavioral responses to negative social interactions in women with bulimia nervosa. *Biological Psychiatry. Cognitive Neuroscience and Neuroimaging, 7*(7), 696–705.

Majuri, J., Joutsa, J., Johansson, J., Voon, V., Alakurtti, K., Parkkola, R., Lahti, T., Alho, H., Hirvonen, J., Arponen, E., Forsback, S., & Kaasinen, V. (2017). Dopamine and opioid neurotransmission in behavioral addictions: a comparative pet study in pathological gambling and binge eating. *Neuropsychopharmacology, 42*(5), 1169–1177.

McElroy, S. L., Hudson, J. I., Grilo, C. M., Guerdjikova, A. I., Deng, L., Koblan, K. S., Goldman, R., Navia, B., Hopkins, S., & Loebel, A. (2020). Efficacy and safety of dasotraline in adults with binge-eating disorder: A randomized, placebo-controlled, flexible-dose clinical trial. *Journal of Clinical Psychiatry, 81*(5), 5957.

Mendoza, C. J., Palka, J. M., Pelfrey, S. E., Hunt, B. J., Krawczyk, D. C., & McAdams, C. J. (2022). Neural processes related to negative self-concept in adult and adolescent anorexia nervosa. *European Eating Disorders Review, 30*(1), 23–35.

Monteleone, A. M., Castellini, G., Volpe, U., Ricca, V., Lelli, L., Monteleone, P., & Maj, M. (2018). Neuroendocrinology and brain imaging of reward in eating disorders: A possible key to the treatment of anorexia nervosa and bulimia nervosa. *Progress in Neuro-Psychopharmacology and Biological Psychiatry, 80,* 132–142.

Monteleone, A. M., Monteleone, P., Esposito, F., Prinster, A., Volpe, U., Cantone, E., Pellegrino, F., Canna, A., Milano, W., Aiello, M., Di Salle, F., & Maj, M. (2017). Altered processing of rewarding and aversive basic taste stimuli in symptomatic women with anorexia nervosa and bulimia nervosa: An fMRI study. *Journal of Psychiatric Research, 90,* 94–101.

Morales, I., & Berridge, K. C. (2020). "Liking" and "wanting" in eating and food reward: Brain mechanisms and clinical implications. *Physiology & Behavior, 227,* 113152.

Morales, M., & Margolis, E. B. (2017). Ventral tegmental area: Cellular heterogeneity, connectivity and behaviour. *Nature Reviews Neuroscience, 18*(2), 73–85.

Mueller, S. V., Morishima, Y., Schwab, S., Wiest, R., Federspiel, A., & Hasler, G. (2018). Neural correlates of impaired reward-effort integration in remitted bulimia nervosa. *Neuropsychopharmacology, 43*(4), 868–876. https://doi.org/10.1038/npp.2017.277

Murao, E., Sugihara, G., Isobe, M., Noda, T., Kawabata, M., Matsukawa, N., Takahashi, H., Murai, T., & Noma, S. (2017). Differences in neural responses to reward and punishment processing between anorexia nervosa subtypes: An fMRI study. *Psychiatry and Clinical Neurosciences, 71*(9), 647–658.

Muratore, A. F., & Attia, E. (2022). Psychopharmacologic management of eating disorders. *Current Psychiatry Reports, 24*(7), 345–351.

Murray, S. B., Alba, C., Duval, C. J., Nagata, J. M., Cabeen, R. P., Lee, D. J., Toga, A. W., Siegel, S. J., & Jann, K. (2022). Aberrant functional connectivity between reward and inhibitory control networks in pre-adolescent binge eating disorder. *Psychological Medicine,* 53(9), 3869–3878.

Neveu, R., Neveu, D., Carrier, E., Gay, A., Nicolas, A., & Coricelli, G. (2018). Goal directed and self-control systems in bulimia nervosa: An fMRI Study. *EBioMedicine, 34,* 214–222.

Oberndorfer, T. A., Frank, G. K. W., Simmons, A. N., Wagner, A., McCurdy, D., Fudge, J. L., Yang, T. T., Paulus, M. P., & Kaye, W. H. (2013). Altered insula response to sweet taste processing after recovery from anorexia and bulimia nervosa. *American Journal of Psychiatry, 170*(10), 1143–1151.

Odum, A. L. (2011). Delay discounting: I'm a k, you're a k. *Journal of the Experimental Analysis of Behavior, 96*(3), 427–439.

O'Hara, C. B., Keyes, A., Renwick, B., Giel, K. E., Campbell, I. C., & Schmidt, U. (2016). Evidence that illness-compatible cues are rewarding in women recovered from anorexia nervosa: A study of the effects of dopamine depletion on eye-blink startle responses. *PLOS ONE, 11*(10), e0165104.

O'Hara, C. B., Keyes, A., Renwick, B., Leyton, M., Campbell, I. C., & Schmidt, U. (2016). The effects of acute dopamine precursor depletion on the reinforcing value of exercise in anorexia nervosa. *PLOS ONE, 11*(1), e0145894.

Patzelt, E. H., Kool, W., Millner, A. J., & Gershman, S. J. (2019). The transdiagnostic structure of mental effort avoidance. *Scientific Reports, 9*(1), 1689.

Peyser, D., Scolnick, B., Hildebrandt, T., & Taylor, J. A. (2021). Heart rate variability as a biomarker for anorexia nervosa: A review. *European Eating Disorders Review, 29*(1), 20–31.

Phillipou, A., Carruthers, S. P., Di Biase, M. A., Zalesky, A., Abel, L. A., Castle, D. J., Gurvich, C., & Rossell, S. L. (2018). White matter microstructure in anorexia nervosa. *Human Brain Mapping, 39*(11), 4385–4392.

Piccolo, M., Milos, G., Bluemel, S., Schumacher, S., Müller-Pfeiffer, C., Fried, M., Ernst, M., & Martin-Soelch, C. (2019). Food vs money? Effects of hunger on mood and behavioral reactivity to reward in anorexia nervosa. *Appetite, 134,* 26–33.

Racine, S. E., Hebert, K. R., & Benning, S. D. (2018). Emotional reactivity and appraisal of food in relation to eating disorder cognitions and behaviours: Evidence to support the motivational conflict hypothesis. *European Eating Disorders Review, 26*(1), 3–10.

Racine, S. E., Suissa-Rocheleau, L., Martin, S. J., & Benning, S. D. (2021). Implicit and explicit motivational responses to high- and low-calorie food in women with disordered eating. *International Journal of Psychophysiology, 159,* 37–46.

Reiter, A. M. F., Heinze, H.-J., Schlagenhauf, F., & Deserno, L. (2017). Impaired flexible reward-based decision-making in binge eating disorder: Evidence from computational modeling and functional neuroimaging. *Neuropsychopharmacology, 42*(3), 628–637.

Rolls, E. T., & Grabenhorst, F. (2008). The orbitofrontal cortex and beyond: From affect to decision-making. *Progress in Neurobiology, 86*(3), 216–244. https://doi.org/10.1016/j.pneurobio.2008.09.001

Rothemund, Y., Buchwald, C., Georgiewa, P., Bohner, G., Bauknecht, H.-C., Ballmaier, M., Klapp, B. F., & Klingebiel, R. (2011). Compulsivity predicts fronto striatal activation in severely anorectic individuals. *Neuroscience, 197,* 242–250.

Sala, M., Han, K., Acevedo, S., Krawczyk, D. C., & McAdams, C. J. (2018). Oxytocin receptor polymorphism decreases midline neural activations to social stimuli in anorexia nervosa. *Frontiers in Psychology*, *9*, 2183.

Salamone, J. D., Pardo, M., Yohn, S. E., López-Cruz, L., SanMiguel, N., & Correa, M. (2016). Mesolimbic dopamine and the regulation of motivated behavior. *Current Topics in Behavioral Neurosciences*, *27*, 231–257.

Sanders, N., Smeets, P. A. M., van Elburg, A. A., Danner, U. N., van Meer, F., Hoek, H. W., & Adan, R. A. H. (2015). Altered food-cue processing in chronically ill and recovered women with anorexia nervosa. *Frontiers in Behavioral Neuroscience*, *9*, 46.

Schaefer, L. M., & Steinglass, J. E. (2021). Reward learning through the lens of RDoC: A review of theory, assessment, and empirical findings in the eating disorders. *Current Psychiatry Reports*, *23*(1), 2.

Schäfer, A., Vaitl, D., & Schienle, A. (2010). Regional grey matter volume abnormalities in bulimia nervosa and binge-eating disorder. *NeuroImage*, *50*(2), 639–643.

Schebendach, J., Broft, A., Foltin, R. W., & Walsh, B. T. (2013). Can the reinforcing value of food be measured in bulimia nervosa? *Appetite*, *62*, 70–75.

Schebendach, J. E., Klein, D. A., Foltin, R. W., Devlin, M. J., & Walsh, B. T. (2007). Relative reinforcing value of exercise in inpatients with anorexia nervosa: Model development and pilot data. *International Journal of Eating Disorders*, *40*(5), 446–453.

Schebendach, J., Klein, D. A., Mayer, L. E. S., Attia, E., Devlin, M. J., Foltin, R. W., & Walsh, B. T. (2017). Assessment of the motivation to use artificial sweetener among individuals with an eating disorder. *Appetite*, *109*, 131–136.

Schienle, A., Schäfer, A., Hermann, A., & Vaitl, D. (2009). Binge-eating disorder: Reward sensitivity and brain activation to images of food. *Biological Psychiatry*, *65*(8), 654–661.

Schneider, E., Higgs, S., & Dourish, C. T. (2021). Lisdexamfetamine and binge-eating disorder: A systematic review and meta-analysis of the preclinical and clinical data with a focus on mechanism of drug action in treating the disorder. *European Neuropsychopharmacology*, *53*, 49–78.

Schultz, W. (2016). Dopamine reward prediction error coding. Dialogues in Clinical Neuroscience, *18*(1), 23–32.

Simon, J. J., Skunde, M., Walther, S., Bendszus, M., Herzog, W., & Friederich, H.-C. (2016). Neural signature of food reward processing in bulimic-type eating disorders. *Social Cognitive and Affective Neuroscience*, *11*(9), 1393–1401.

Skinner, B. F. (1976). *About behaviorism* (1st ed.). Vintage.

Smith, D. G., & Robbins, T. W. (2013). The neurobiological underpinnings of obesity and binge eating: A rationale for adopting the food addiction model. *Biological Psychiatry*, *73*(9), 804–810.

Soussignan, R., Jiang, T., Rigaud, D., Royet, J. P., & Schaal, B. (2010). Subliminal fear priming potentiates negative facial reactions to food pictures in women with anorexia nervosa. *Psychological Medicine*, *40*(3), 503–514.

Soussignan, R., Schaal, B., Rigaud, D., Royet, J.-P., & Jiang, T. (2011). Hedonic reactivity to visual and olfactory cues: Rapid facial electromyographic reactions are altered in anorexia nervosa. *Biological Psychology*, *86*(3), 265–272.

Stancil, S. L., Adelman, W., Dietz, A., & Abdel-Rahman, S. (2019). Naltrexone reduces binge eating and purging in adolescents in an eating disorder program. *Journal of Child and Adolescent Psychopharmacology*, *29*(9), 721–724.

Steding, J., Boehm, I., King, J. A., Geisler, D., Ritschel, F., Seidel, M., Doose, A., Jaite, C., Roessner, V., Smolka, M. N., & Ehrlich, S. (2019). Goal-directed vs. habitual instrumental behavior during reward processing in anorexia nervosa: An fMRI study. *Scientific Reports*, *9*(1), 13529.

Steinglass, J. E., Figner, B., Berkowitz, S., Simpson, H. B., Weber, E. U., & Walsh, B. T. (2012). Increased capacity to delay reward in anorexia nervosa. *Journal of the International Neuropsychological Society*, *18*(4), 773–780.

Stice, E., Onipede, Z. A., & Marti, C. N. (2021). A meta-analytic review of trials that tested whether eating disorder prevention programs prevent eating disorder onset. *Clinical Psychology Review*, *87*, 102046.

Stice, E., & Presnell, K. (2007). *The body project: Promoting body acceptance and preventing eating disorders: Facilitator guide* (pp. vi, 140). Oxford University Press.

Stice, E., Yokum, S., Rohde, P., Gau, J., & Shaw, H. (2021). Evidence that a novel transdiagnostic eating disorder treatment reduces reward region response to the thin beauty ideal and high-calorie binge foods. *Psychological Medicine*, 53(6), 2252–2262.

Stopyra, M. A., Simon, J. J., Skunde, M., Walther, S., Bendszus, M., Herzog, W., & Friederich, H.-C. (2019). Altered functional connectivity in binge eating disorder and bulimia nervosa: A resting-state fMRI study. *Brain and Behavior, 9*(2), e01207.

Sutton, R. S., & Barto, A. G. (1998). *Reinforcement learning: An introduction*. MIT Press.

Sweitzer, M. M., Watson, K. K., Erwin, S. R., Winecoff, A. A., Datta, N., Huettel, S., Platt, M. L., & Zucker, N. L. (2018). Neurobiology of social reward valuation in adults with a history of anorexia nervosa. *PLOS ONE, 13*(12), e0205085.

Titova, O. E., Hjorth, O. C., Schiöth, H. B., & Brooks, S. J. (2013). Anorexia nervosa is linked to reduced brain structure in reward and somatosensory regions: A meta-analysis of VBM studies. *BMC Psychiatry, 13*, 110.

Uniacke, B., Wang, Y., Biezonski, D., Sussman, T., Lee, S., Posner, J., & Steinglass, J. (2019). Resting-state connectivity within and across neural circuits in anorexia nervosa. *Brain and Behavior, 9*(1), e01205.

Via, E., Soriano-Mas, C., Sánchez, I., Forcano, L., Harrison, B. J., Davey, C. G., Pujol, J., Martínez-Zalacaín, I., Menchón, J. M., Fernández-Aranda, F., & Cardoner, N. (2015). Abnormal social reward responses in anorexia nervosa: An fMRI Study. *PLOS ONE, 10*(7), e0133539.

Via, E., Zalesky, A., Sánchez, I., Forcano, L., Harrison, B. J., Pujol, J., Fernández-Aranda, F., Menchón, J. M., Soriano-Mas, C., Cardoner, N., & Fornito, A. (2014). Disruption of brain white matter microstructure in women with anorexia nervosa. *Journal of Psychiatry & Neuroscience, 39*(6), 367–375.

Vickers, S. P., Hackett, D., Murray, F., Hutson, P. H., & Heal, D. J. (2015). Effects of lisdexamfetamine in a rat model of binge-eating. *Journal of Psychopharmacology, 29*(12), 1290–1307.

Vocks, S., Busch, M., Grönemeyer, D., Schulte, D., Herpertz, S., & Suchan, B. (2010). Neural correlates of viewing photographs of one's own body and another woman's body in anorexia and bulimia nervosa: An fMRI study. *Journal of Psychiatry & Neuroscience, 35*(3), 163–176.

Voon, V., Derbyshire, K., Rück, C., Irvine, M. A., Worbe, Y., Enander, J., Schreiber, L. R., Gillan, C., Fineberg, N. A., Sahakian, B. J., Robbins, T. W., Harrison, N. A., Wood, J., Daw, N. D., Dayan, P., Grant, J. E., & Bullmore, E. T. (2015). Disorders of compulsivity: A common bias towards learning habits. *Molecular Psychiatry, 20*(3), 345–352.

Wagner, A., Aizenstein, H., Venkatraman, V. K., Fudge, J., May, J. C., Mazurkewicz, L., Frank, G. K., Bailer, U. F., Fischer, L., Nguyen, V., Carter, C., Putnam, K., & Kaye, W. H. (2007). Altered reward processing in women recovered from anorexia nervosa. *American Journal of Psychiatry, 164*(12), 1842–1849.

Wallis, J. D. (2007). Neuronal mechanisms in prefrontal cortex underlying adaptive choice behavior. *Annals of the New York Academy of Sciences, 1121*, 447–460. https://doi.org/10.1196/annals.1401.009

Walton, E., Bernardoni, F., Batury, V.-L., Bahnsen, K., Larivière, S., Abbate-Daga, G., Andres-Perpiña, S., Bang, L., Bischoff-Grethe, A., Brooks, S. J., Campbell, I. C., Cascino, G., Castro-Fornieles, J., Collantoni, E., D'Agata, F., Dahmen, B., Danner, U. N., Favaro, A., Feusner, J. D., Frank, G. K. W., . . . Ehrlich, S. (2022). Brain structure in acutely underweight and partially weight-restored individuals with anorexia nervosa—A coordinated analysis by the ENIGMA eating disorders working group. *Biological Psychiatry*, 92(9), 730–738.

Wang, G.-J., Geliebter, A., Volkow, N. D., Telang, F. W., Logan, J., Jayne, M. C., Galanti, K., Selig, P. A., Han, H., Zhu, W., Wong, C. T., & Fowler, J. S. (2011). Enhanced striatal dopamine release during food stimulation in binge eating disorder. *Obesity (Silver Spring, Md.), 19*(8), 1601–1608.

Waxman, S. E. (2009). A systematic review of impulsivity in eating disorders. *European Eating Disorders Review, 17*(6), 408–425.

Wierenga, C. E., Bischoff-Grethe, A., Berner, L. A., Simmons, A. N., Bailer, U., Paulus, M. P., & Kaye, W. H. (2020). Increased anticipatory brain response to pleasant touch in women remitted from bulimia nervosa. *Translational Psychiatry, 10*(1), 236.

Wierenga, C. E., Bischoff-Grethe, A., Melrose, A. J., Irvine, Z., Torres, L., Bailer, U. F., Simmons, A., Fudge, J. L., McClure, S. M., Ely, A., & Kaye, W. H. (2015). Hunger does not motivate reward in women remitted from anorexia nervosa. *Biological Psychiatry, 77*(7), 642–652.

Wierenga, C. E., Ely, A., Bischoff-Grethe, A., Bailer, U. F., Simmons, A. N., & Kaye, W. H. (2014). Are extremes of consumption in eating disorders related to an altered balance between reward and inhibition? *Frontiers in Behavioral Neuroscience, 8*, 410.

Wierenga, C. E., Hill, L., Knatz Peck, S., McCray, J., Greathouse, L., Peterson, D., Scott, A., Eisler, I., & Kaye, W. H. (2018). The acceptability, feasibility, and possible benefits of a neurobiologically-informed 5-day multifamily treatment for adults with anorexia nervosa. *International Journal of Eating Disorders, 51*(8), 863–869.

Wierenga, C. E., Reilly, E., Bischoff-Grethe, A., Kaye, W. H., & Brown, G. G. (2022). Altered reinforcement learning from reward and punishment in anorexia nervosa: Evidence from computational modeling. *Journal of the International Neuropsychological Society, 28*(10), 1003–1015.

Wilson, K. A., James, G. A., Kilts, C. D., & Bush, K. A. (2020). Combining physiological and neuroimaging measures to predict affect processing induced by affectively valent image stimuli. *Scientific Reports, 10*(1), 9298.

Wonderlich, J. A., Breithaupt, L. E., Crosby, R. D., Thompson, J. C., Engel, S. G., & Fischer, S. (2017). The relation between craving and binge eating: Integrating neuroimaging and ecological momentary assessment. *Appetite, 117*, 294–302.

Yu, Y., Miller, R., & Groth, S. W. (2022). A literature review of dopamine in binge eating. *Journal of Eating Disorders, 10*(1), article 1.

8

Interoception in Eating Disorders

Emily M. Choquette and Sahib S. Khalsa

Brief Definitional Overview

Interoception: The process by which the nervous systems senses, interprets, and integrates signals originating from inside the body, providing a moment-by-moment mapping of the body's internal landscape across conscious and unconscious levels. Most interoceptive processing is unconscious.

Interoceptive awareness: The conscious sensation and interpretation of signals originating from inside the body. Interoceptive awareness is a multifaceted construct with numerous dimensions including attention, detection, accuracy, perceived intensity, discrimination, sensibility, and insight. Interoceptive awareness facets can be targeted individually or in combination during conditions of physiological rest or interoceptive perturbation.

Homeostasis: The reactive regulatory process by which a living organism achieves physiological states within a range conducive to survival in the face of environmental perturbations. Homeostasis usually operates across rapid timescales.

Allostasis: The predictive regulatory process of maintaining stability, or homeostasis, by dynamically adjusting homeostatic setpoints through neural, physiological, or behavioral changes. Allostasis can operate across rapid or prolonged timescales, such as making adjustments prior to an anticipated homeostatic perturbation to avoid dyshomeostatic future states.

Central autonomic network (CAN): The CAN is a network of brain regions playing a key role in the regulation of visceromotor, neuroendocrine, nociceptive, and behavioral responses that are critical for ensuring the maintenance of homeostasis within the body.

Introduction

Interoception is a biological process broadly spanning the nervous system's sensation, interpretation, and integration of internal bodily signals (Khalsa et al., 2018). It involves all major organ systems involved in maintaining body homeostasis including the cardiovascular, pulmonary, gastrointestinal, genitourinary,

Emily M. Choquette and Sahib S. Khalsa, *Interoception in Eating Disorders*. In: *The Handbook of the Neurobiology of Eating Disorders*. Edited by: Christina E. Wierenga and Joanna E. Steinglass, Oxford University Press.
 DOI: 10.1093/9780197675212.003.0009

nociceptive (pain), chemosensory, osmotic, thermoregulatory, visceral, immune, and autonomic systems. It is a critical ingredient in the generation of reflexes, urges, motivational drives, emotions, and regulatory responses. Interoception thus entails a bidirectional (i.e., "top-down" and "bottom-up") process between the brain and body comprised of feedback and feedforward loops that continuously update the internal model and setpoints of homeostasis and develop anticipatory regulatory (reactive) or allostatic (anticipatory) strategies for potential future bodily threats.

Biological Framework

As a process fundamental to the maintenance of body homeostasis, most interoceptive signaling between the brain and body occurs unconsciously. Conscious perceptions usually arise when a disruption of homeostasis triggers the noticing of physiologic sensations (such as hunger, thirst, or heart palpitations), or when attention is purposefully shifted to the body (such as when choosing to focus one's attention on breathing sensations, or on the heartbeat sensation). Interoceptive awareness is currently defined as the conscious sensation and interpretation of bodily signals (Khalsa et al., 2018). The term was originally introduced during the development of the Eating Disorder Inventory (EDI; Garner et al., 1983), a self-report measure used to assess eating disorder symptom severity, with the relevant subscale items developed using clinicians' experience and previous empirical work on "gastric perceptivity" in eating disorders (Coddington & Bruch, 1970). Since then, interoceptive awareness has become a broad and multifaceted term embodying all aspects of the conscious experience of interoception. This includes facets such as interoceptive attention, detection, perceived intensity, discrimination, accuracy, insight, and sensibility (Grafinkel et al., 2015; Khalsa et al., 2018). These features work collectively to constitute patterns of thoughts and behaviors in response to an individual's environment, both internal and external, in service of promoting homeostasis and ultimately survival.

Interoceptive signals are detected via a range of molecular sensors located in the peripheral, enteric (intestinal), and central nervous systems (Berntson & Khalsa, 2021). These signals are then relayed to discrete sites within the central nervous system (CNS) (i.e., spinal cord and brain) for further processing (Figure 8.1). The vagus nerve (10th cranial nerve) is a major peripheral afferent neural pathway conveying interoceptive information from internal organs such as the heart, lungs, liver, and stomach/gastrointestinal tract and from the immune system to the brain (Browning et al., 2017; Karemaker, 2022; Rajendran et al., 2023; Taylor et al., 2022). However, afferent interoceptive signals are also relayed via other cranial nerves such as the trigeminal (5th cranial nerve), glossopharyngeal (9th cranial nerve), as well as via dedicated spinal nerves (e.g., the dorsal roots of sacral, lumbar, and thoracic nerves). Finally, there are thinly myelinated and

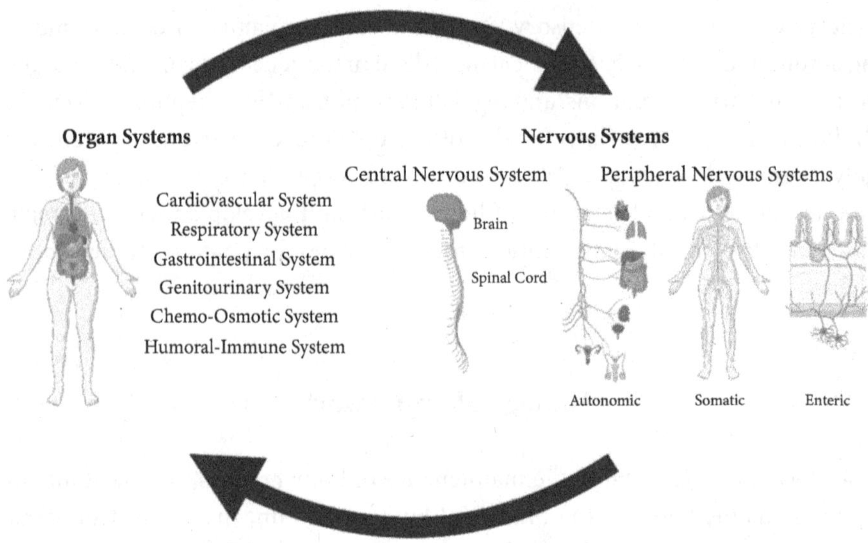

Figure 8.1 Biological systems of the brain–body feedback loop that constitutes interoception.

unmyelinated nerve fibers distributed widely throughout the skin and peripheral tissues that send information via the lamina I spinothalamic pathway to the brainstem and thalamus (Craig, 2022). Collectively, this allows for the neural sensing of extremely diverse inputs including mechanical signals associated with pressure, movement, exertion, pain, thermal (heat or cold) signals, inflammation, or tissue injury, and even biochemical signals related to chemo-osmosis, which is the process of chemical sensing whereby the movement of ions across cell membranes from high to low concentrations (or vice versa) leads to changes in cellular signaling.

Interoceptors—The molecular and cellular sensors of interoception

As the previous paragraph indicates, interoception depends on the nervous system's sensing of input that is transduced by various cells containing chemoreceptors, humoral receptors, specialized mechanoreceptors, and free nerve endings distributed across many organ systems throughout the body (Wang & Chang, 2024). Each of these receptors will be briefly considered. The breadth of this process has even evoked the concept of an "*interoceptive nervous system*," (Carvalho & Damasio, 2021) although such a system will not be found in modern textbooks. However, it is worth noting that the notion of an interoceptive nervous system encompasses vast subsets of the nervous system, such as the autonomic nervous system, the enteric nervous system, and aspects of the peripheral nervous system (Figure 8.1).

Chemoreceptors

Chemoreceptors are specialized molecules that are sensitive to certain types of chemicals. They may be peripheral (e.g., located in tongue or nose) or central (e.g., located in the heart or brain). Once they detect a specific chemical signal, they transmit this information to the CNS. Chemoreceptors are crucial to a range of vital bodily functions including, but not limited to, respiration and cardiovascular reflexes (Marshall, 1994), body temperature regulation (Nattie & Li, 2012), glucose regulation, and taste (Liu & Bohórquez, 2022). The circumventricular organs include the subfornical organ, which is especially sensitive on a rapid timescale to thirst and fluid intake (Zimmerman & Knight, 2020), the area postrema, and the organum vasculosum of the lamina terminalis. An important aspect of mammalian chemoreception is the fact that the circumventricular organs are a focal point of blood–brain barrier permeability, which allows these neural structures to have direct access to circulating chemicals.

Humoral receptors

Humoral receptors are characterized as receptors which detect specific hormones, enzymes, or other molecules regulating body functions as they circulate throughout the bloodstream and lymphatic system. Particularly relevant to eating disorders are the hormones which stimulate appetite, satiety, and food intake such as ghrelin, leptin, and cholecystokinin (Andermann & Lowell, 2017; Kaelberer & Bohórquez, 2018). Leptin and ghrelin work on hunger in an opposing fashion (i.e., stimulating satiety vs. stimulating appetite, respectively) typically by binding to specific receptors in the hypothalamus and triggering the release of other hormones (e.g., growth hormone, corticotrophin-releasing hormone, adrenocorticotropic hormone) through the hypothalamic–pituitary–adrenal (HPA) axis. Leptin and ghrelin also participate in information exchange with other brain regions (such as the insular cortex) which helps individuals to detect changes in energy balance in one's body and to sense changes in appetite (Zanchi et al., 2017).

Mechanoreceptors

Mechanoreceptors are molecular receptors that respond to mechanical forces, such as pressure or stretch. Baroreceptors are specialized mechanoreceptors that detect changes in blood pressure. These stretch-triggered receptors innervate discrete portions of arteries (e.g., the aortic arch and carotid sinus), and they are mechanically activated when changes in blood pressure associated with cardiac systole distend arteries. This initiates afferent signaling to the brainstem nucleus tractus solitarius (NTS), which in turn begins a process of complex compensatory reflexes and can involve additional brainstem nuclei (e.g., the dorsal motor nucleus [DMN] of the vagus), and result in momentary increases or decreases in heart rate, blood pressure, and digestive enzyme secretion and gut peristalsis (Pilowsky

& Goodchild, 2002; Travagli & Anselmi, 2016). PIEZOs are an important form of mechanoreceptor that were only recently discovered (Coste et al., 2010). These receptors are expressed in neurons innervating nearly every major internal organ system (Alcaino et al., 2017; Dalghi et al., 2021; Kaelberer et al., 2018; Min et al., 2021; Szczot et al., 2017; Williams et al., 2016), and as a result, they play key roles in the sensory processing of numerous interoceptive signals.

Brain networks of interoception

A detailed review of the brain networks of interoception would be voluminous, so a brief summary is listed with several pertinent references. Afferent interoceptive signals are relayed to the NTS, the classical visceral receiving area of the brain stem, and then via additional brainstem structures (such as the DMN and parabrachial nucleus [PB]) to higher level brain structures including the insular cortex, somatosensory cortices, anterior cingulate cortex, and the orbitofrontal and medial prefrontal cortices (Figure 8.2) (Berntson & Khalsa, 2021; Critchley & Harrison, 2013). Human and animal studies have firmly established the insular cortex as an interoceptive hub that plays many roles in behavior, processing, and integration of internal sensory information (Craig, 2002; Gogolla, 2017; Hassanpour et al., 2018; Schulz, 2016). Several other important functions relevant to eating disorders are the insula's role in appetite and energy balance (Al-Zubaidi et al., 2020; Kaye et al., 2020; Livneh et al., 2017; Simmons, Rapuano, et al., 2013), as well as its role in the mapping of gustatory signals from the tongue (Small, 2010; Veldhuizen et al., 2011). The constructivist perspective suggests that interoceptive perceptions are unconsciously influenced by (or may even directly reflect) the brain's predictions about the state of the body (Barrett & Simmons, 2015; Seth & Friston, 2016). Accordingly, discrepancies between predicted and actual bodily states, or so-called interoceptive prediction errors, prompt compensatory adjustments to restore balance (Paulus & Stein, 2010; Seth et al., 2011). Animal and human studies have shown that the insular cortex plays an integral role in estimating this difference between anticipated and experienced interoceptive stimulation, with specific roles hypothesized for insular subregions. For example, an emphasis on prediction error processing in the mid to posterior insula and emphasis on prediction generation in the anterior insula (for more details, see Adolfi et al., 2017; Barrett & Simmons, 2015; Critchley et al., 2004; Livneh & Andermann, 2021; Livneh et al., 2020; Nord et al., 2021; Paulus & Stein, 2010). The amygdala (Feinstein et al., 2022) and striatum are also involved in representing the valence and intensity of interoceptive signals. Further there is evidence that projections from the anterior and mid-cingulate and lateral prefrontal cortex to the anterior insula likely regulate cognitive reactions during interoceptive experiences (Critchley et al., 2004; Paulus & Khalsa, 2021; Simmons, Avery, et al., 2013).

While afferent cortical systems receive most of the attention when it comes to studying interoceptive neurocircuitry, there are important efferent or descending pathways that work to regulate the body's internal environment to maintain or return to homeostasis. These descending regulatory pathways appear to span all of the same systems as the afferent pathways, thus comprising a complete "brain–body feedback loop" for each system (Figure 8.2) (Berntson & Khalsa, 2021). Feedback loops are functionally engaged in the production of sympathetic (i.e., fight, flight, freeze behaviors) and parasympathetic (i.e., rest, digest, and recuperate) nervous system responses which produce opposing effects on body physiology, and are thus intimately connected with the autonomic nervous system in the periphery.

The central autonomic network (CAN) is established as an internal regulator through which the brain controls or influences essential visceromotor, neuroendocrine, nociceptive, and behavioral responses (Benarroch, 1993; Saper, 2002). Although the CAN's major neural components include the bilateral mid cingulate cortex, insular cortex, inferior parietal lobule, amygdala, hypothalamus, periaqueductal gray matter, parabrachial complex, NTS, locus coeruleus, and ventrolateral

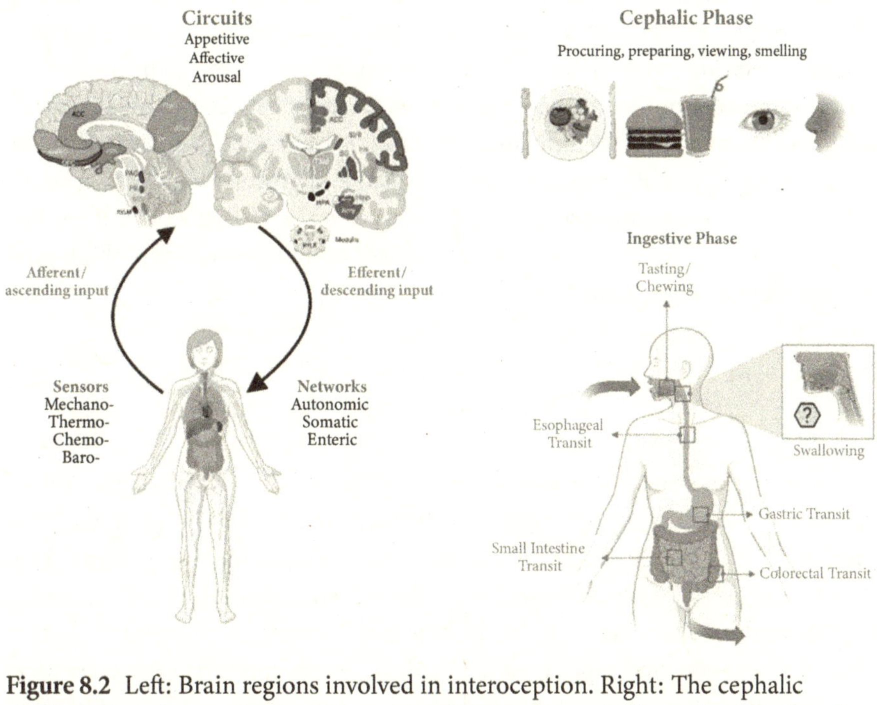

Figure 8.2 Left: Brain regions involved in interoception. Right: The cephalic and ingestive phases of eating, illustrating the gastrointestinal transit of food, and swallowing as the key checkpoint at which an ingested food stimulus produces distinct forms of interoceptive signaling in the gastrointestinal tract (described further in the text).

Adapted from Khalsa et al. (2022). Gastrointestinal interoception in eating disorders: charting a new path. *Current Psychiatry Reports*, *24*(1), 47–60. https://doi.org/10.1007/s11920-022-01318-3. Under a Creative Commons Attribution 4.0 International (CC BY 4.0); ACC: anterior cingulate cortex; Amy: amygdala; BG: basal ganglia; DMN: dorsal motor nucleus of the vagus; Hipp: hippocampus; HPA: hypothalamus and pituitary gland; Ins: insular cortex; OFC: orbitofrontal cortex; NTS: nucleus tractus solitarius; PB: parabrachial nucleus; SI/SII: primary and secondary somatosensory cortex; Thal: thalamus, vmPFC: ventromedial prefrontal cortex.

medulla (Benarroch, 1993), its role as a regulator of internal body state suggests that it exerts substantial efferent control over autonomic nervous system signaling. Thus, the CAN may be considered a key part of the efferent limb of the brain–body feedback loop that is capable of modulating interoception.

State of the Science in Eating Disorders

To survey the current status of the scientific study of interoception in eating disorders, we conducted a systematic review of the literature. Two hundred and fifty-two English Boolean search terms were utilized to evaluate major themes spanning the topics of eating disorder (i.e., anorexia nervosa, bulimia nervosa, binge-eating disorder, pica, ARFID, and rumination disorder), interoception (i.e., interocept*, visceral, cardiac, heartbeat, respiratory, esophageal, oesophageal, stomach, gastric, colon, rectal, bladder), and neurobiological (i.e., neur*, fMRI, EEG). Terms were searched on PubMed in April 2023. This search strategy was built upon the terms used in our previous systematic review (Khalsa & Lapidus, 2016) and resulted in 426 total results and 250 unique articles. Of these articles, 70 were considered to be directly relevant. Some of those deemed irrelevant did not explicitly measure or perturb interoception but spoke broadly of differences between individuals with eating disorders and healthy individuals, that, while representative of interoceptive deficits, only utilized self-report scales such as the interoceptive deficits subscale of the EDI. The following discussion thus focuses on work that explicitly probed interoception (e.g., via self-report or task-based measure) using neurobiological methodology in eating disorders.

Anorexia nervosa

There have been several previous reviews addressing the neurobiology of interoception in anorexia nervosa (AN) (for further details, see Martin et al., 2019; Simmons & DeVille, 2017). Documentation of disturbed internal perception in patients with AN dates back to the 1960s. For example, Bruch's (1962) visionary work focused on characterizing the dysfunctional sensory processing in women with AN. One of the first experimental probes of interoception in eating disorders was a groundbreaking experiment conducted by Coddington and Bruch (1970) in which small amounts of milkshake were applied directly to the stomach of participants through an ingested tube. They found that the three individuals with AN studied showed reduced detection to the delivery of the gastric perturbation relative to the 15 normal-weight individuals studied for comparison. Many studies conducted since have used less invasive approaches and a wide range of methodology including self-reports (Garner, 2004), behavioral tasks (Pollatos et al., 2008), experimental perturbation (Khalsa et al., 2015), and imaging studies (Kerr et al., 2022) to examine how women with AN sense and interpret internal bodily sensations. Generally, individuals with AN report more difficulty with interoception than healthy comparison individuals on self-report measures (for review see Martin et al., 2019). Behavioral measures of interoceptive accuracy, such as the heartbeat tapping task, also consistently reveal lower interoceptive accuracy in patients with AN compared to healthy individuals (Smith et al., 2020; Lavalley et al., 2024).

Behavioral studies have demonstrated that abnormal cardiac and respiratory interoception plays a role in the pathophysiology and neurobiology of AN. Most studies report lower interoceptive accuracy on heartbeat counting tasks in individuals with AN versus healthy individuals (Demartini et al., 2021; Fischer et al., 2016; Pollatos et al., 2008, 2016; for null results, see Lutz et al., 2019; Richard et al., 2019). Cardiac perturbation studies have also not found differences in interoceptive accuracy but identified increased cardiac intensity ratings particularly during meal anticipation, using an adrenaline-like drug called isoproterenol (Khalsa et al., 2015). Additionally, increased subjective responses to endogenous respiratory perturbation during inspiratory breath holding have differentiated individuals with AN from healthy comparisons. Fewer studies have examined behavioral measures of gastric interoception in AN. Studies have reported increased negative affect after water load tasks in women with AN (Brown et al., 2022; Kerr et al., 2022) and reduced water consumption relative to health comparisons (Brown et al., 2022). Further, a decrease in the rhythm of gastric contractions was reported after water loading in weight-restored women with AN, but not prior to weight restoration (Kerr et al., 2022). Current research using behavioral tasks therefore generally suggests that individuals with AN have abnormal interoceptive awareness, but the nature of these experiences depend upon the organ system and measures employed.

Neuroimaging studies of interoception in AN have demonstrated abnormal neural activity in patients with AN relative to health comparisons (HC). In response to perturbation of the cardiorespiratory system with isoproterenol, weight-restored women with AN displayed significant changes in resting state functional connectivity (FC) in comparison to the HC (De la Cruz et al., 2022). During this study, participants received double-blinded and randomized infusions of isoproterenol, a peripherally acting adrenaline analog, which elicits focal changes in the insular cortex in healthy (Hassanpour et al., 2018) and anxious individuals (Teed et al., 2022). Analysis of resting state FC from before versus after the perturbation revealed diminished connectivity between CAN nodes. In particular, resting state FC changes within CAN regions were correlated between the ventromedial prefrontal cortex and both anterior insula regions, and additionally, the left anterior insula was coupled with the posterior cingulate cortex (De la Cruz et al., 2022). The FC group differences between women with AN and HCs occurred in regions of the CAN and portions of networks that primarily represent the default mode network, which simplistically is thought to have a role in self-referential processing, as well as networks related to cognitive control processing and motor, somatosensory, and visual processing. These are key findings as multiple CAN regions coordinate with subcortical regions in other circuits to integrate viscerosensory input and affective information to initiate visceromotor output (Cechetto, 1987; Ledoux, 1992; Loewy & Spyer, 1990). Differences in FC in women with acute AN in comparison to HC have been previously observed in cross-sectional studies (Cha et al., 2016; Cowdrey et al., 2014; Ehrlich et al., 2015; Haynos et al., 2019; Lord et al., 2016); however, the de la Cruz and colleagues' (2022) study provided evidence of state-dependent *changes* in FC as a result of cardiorespiratory perturbation. Further, these FC changes were negatively associated with AN relevant traits, including anxiety and body image, suggesting that larger decreases in FC were related to higher trait anxiety and more disturbed perceptions of one's body. The results of this study may support other recent arguments (Sui & Gu, 2017) about the neural basis of embodied self-processing, cognitive control, and salience networks. The authors posited that increased top-down regulation in AN reflects efforts to limit exposure to anxiety producing or aversive stimuli (e.g., food) through behavioral strategies (e.g., food avoidance, restriction). They further speculated that this process would likely require coordination across numerous networks in the brain including the CAN networks, frontoparietal, motor and visual networks.

In the respiratory domain, Berner and colleagues (2018) found altered activation in women with remitted AN compared to HC during before, during, and after a breathing load task which is a task of aversive interoception. During the anticipation of an aversive breathing load task, which induces a form of dyspnea, women with remitted AN showed hypoactivation in the right posterior mid-insula, which has been implicated in prediction error related to anticipated and experienced stimuli. During and after the task women with remitted AN showed increased activation in frontal, striatal, and limbic regions which are involved in stimulus salience. Temporal patterns of activation were also different between remitted AN and HC such that women with remitted AN had elevated and steeply increasing activation during the receipt of aversive stimuli whereas the HC remained fairly steady or had only gradually increasing activation in response to aversive stimuli. Taken together, these findings suggest that women with remitted AN may be more sensitive to and have more difficulty adjusting to changes in respiratory homeostasis.

Women with remitted AN also exhibit decreased activation in the mid-insula compared to HC when asked to attend to their gastric sensations, and this neural activity pattern was associated with anxiety and eating disorder symptom severity (Kerr et al., 2022). While women with remitted AN also showed increased activity in the anterior insula compared to HC during cardiac interoception, this was not associated with clinical symptoms (Kerr et al., 2022), perhaps lending credence to the importance of studying gastrointestinal interoception in AN during the application of a relevant form of perturbation.

Functional neuroimaging studies examining neural responses to viewing food-related stimuli demonstrate abnormal neural processing of food cues compared to healthy individuals, suggesting differences in the cephalic phase of digestion (e.g., triggered by sight, smell or thoughts of food). A recent meta-analysis (Bronleigh,

Baumann, & Stapleton, 2022) detailed nine studies examining differences between HC and individuals with AN in response to viewing food related images and found several areas of differences in brain activation between groups. Specifically, areas of higher activation in AN compared to HC were found in the frontal and cingulate cortex (areas related to cognitive control), whereas hypoactivation was found in the amygdala and striatum (areas closely related to threat and reward processing) and the insula (which is related to many functions including interoception as previously discussed). Hypoactivation in AN was also exhibited in the parietal cortex, cerebellum, thalamus, parahippocampal gyrus, and lingual gyrus. Studies examining remitted AN or weight-restored patients with AN have also found differences in activation relative to HC when viewing food-related stimuli. Oberndorfer and colleagues (Oberndorfer et al., 2013) found that when compared to HC, patients with remitted AN had greater anterior insula activation when anticipating food images, but not to objects. Decreased activation in AN in the striatum and amygdala may indicate food is less rewarding to individuals with AN than HC. Further, decreased insula activity provides evidence for less interoceptive responsiveness to food stimuli in AN versus HC. Taken together, these findings suggest that abnormal neural responses to food-related cues are common across the spectrum of AN illness and recovery states, but the neural responses to the ingestion and digestion of food is an understudied area.

To date, the majority of the literature on AN has focused on cardiac interoception and on measuring perceptions of food related stimuli (e.g., food pictures). Few studies have focused on the neural processing of food digestion (i.e., once food has been swallowed, see the "Alternative Perspectives" section of this chapter) or other forms of gastrointestinal stimulation. Given that gastric sensations and other gastrointestinal functions are a key component of hunger and satiety signaling, a better understanding of the central neural processing of digestive functions may be key to understanding the pathophysiology of this disorder in greater detail (for a detailed review, see Khalsa et al., 2022).

Bulimia nervosa

Relative to AN, fewer studies have examined the neurobiological pathways of interoception in bulimia nervosa (BN; for a previous review see Klabunde, Collado, & Bohon, 2017). Those that have examined interoceptive dysfunction in BN using traditional cardiac interoception tasks show mixed findings (Klabunde et al., 2013; Pollatos & Georgiou, 2016). Some studies found no differences in interoceptive accuracy on heartbeat perception tasks in BN relative to HCs (Eshkevari et al., 2014; Pollatos & Georgiou, 2016), whereas another small study found that women with BN were less accurate in perceiving their heartbeats (Klabunde et al., 2013). At the self-report level, several studies have indicated a decrement in interoceptive awareness traits in BN in comparison to healthy individuals (Eshkevari et al., 2014; Pollatos & Georgiou, 2016).

A meta-analysis of six studies (Bronleigh, Baumann, & Stapleton, 2022) found that, when viewing food-related images, individuals with BN show higher activation in areas related to reward processing (i.e., striatum) and interoception (i.e., insula). Patients with BN also exhibited higher activation in visual processing areas such as the cuneus, lingual, and fusiform gyrus, in addition to the bilateral cerebellum. Reduced activity was noted primarily in areas implicated in cognitive control areas, such as the bilateral middle frontal gyrus, bilateral precuneus, right middle temporal gyrus and left superior temporal gyrus.

With respect to individual studies, during aversive perturbations of interoception via the delivery of inspiratory breathing loads (which induce a form of dyspnea), women with remitted BN showed increased activation compared to HC in the bilateral mid and left posterior insula, left superior frontal gyrus, dorsal anterior cingulate cortex/midcingulate, posterior cingulate cortex, bilateral putamen, and right amygdala, but no differences before or after task (Berner et al., 2019). There was also a difference in activation over the course of the task such that activation in individuals remitted from BN peaked early and decreased over breathing load before increasing again after termination of the task, whereas HCs increased activation over the task. Activation in the right amygdala during the task was associated with more self-induced vomiting. While there is less research on BN, there is sufficient evidence to suggest there is some kind of neural alterations in regard to interoception in BN. Generally, the neural pattern of these findings appears to be in an opposing direction as compared to those seen in individuals with AN, specifically related to areas of cognitive control and reward processing.

Other eating disorders and body image

The current literature is hindered by a lack of neurobiological research on interoception in a wider range of eating and feeding disorders beyond AN or BN, such as binge-eating disorder (BED), avoidant/restrictive food intake disorder (ARFID), or pica. While functional neuroimaging studies have evaluated resting state functional brain connectivity and task-based function in some of these disorders, none have examined the role of interoception. Similarly, studies that examined interoception in BED primarily did so through self-report and did not have neural measures associated with them. One noteworthy study found that, during the water load task, a transdiagnostic group of eating disorder patients reporting binge behaviors (i.e., BED and BN) drank more water than healthy controls and this was related to smaller gastric myoelectric output than in HC, potentially suggesting abnormal gastric motility signals in these patients (van Dyck et al., 2021). This was negatively related to binge episodes such that the lower the gastric myoelectric activity, the more binge eating episodes participants reported. While one could infer that such findings might be related to a reduced neural sensitivity to gastric sensations, specific studies focused on testing this hypothesis are needed.

There has been speculation that, similar to restriction of food intake in AN, the aversion to food in ARFID may be related to impaired interoceptive processes (Thomas et al., 2017). However, to date this assertion is theoretical in nature and the authors could not find any neuroimaging evidence to support this hypothesis (see Datta & Lock, 2023 for an exploratory study of cardiac interoception). Finally, studies relating to pica and interoception were based on rat models (Aguilar et al., 2020). In that study, neurons in the posterior insula cortex showed spontaneous increases in firing rate during pica behaviors (i.e., eating of non-nutritive substances, which is considered an illness behavior), and that low-frequency stimulation induced pica behaviors. The relatively few studies on this topic suggest that studies investigating the neurobiology of interoception in eating disorders such as BED, ARFID, and pica represent low-hanging fruit.

Interoception and body image: Linking external and internal misperceptions

Body image disturbance (BID) in the form of an aversive overvaluation of one's own weight and shape is a core symptom of both AN and BN (APA, 2013). Additionally, there is evidence for perceptual overestimations of body size in AN (Cash & Deagle, 1997; Farrell et al., 2005; Gardner & Brown, 2014; Mölbert et al., 2017) (but see Cornelissen et al., 2016; Mölbert et al., 2018; Phillipou et al., 2016, and for a review see Badoud & Tsakiris, 2017). Recent theoretical arguments have posited that body image perception may occur via the nervous system's faulty integration of multisensory inputs, in turn affecting perception and cognition. This is proposed to occur specifically at the integration of afferent visual stimuli (i.e., images relayed by the retina to the brain), prior cognitive schemas (i.e., how one thinks and feels about their body size and shape), and incoming or anticipated body signals (i.e., interoception). These theoretical perspectives suggest that an inability or diminished ability to accurately sense the body's physiological state causes an increased reliance and sensitivity to exteroceptive signals, especially visual signals. This leads to self-objectification or viewing one's own body as an object from the third-person perspective. As a consequence of reduced interoceptive abilities, individuals with AN and BN may have difficulty adaptively integrating external and internal signals, which could lead to an inaccurate mental representation of one's own body and ultimately body dissatisfaction (see Figure 8.3 for an illustrative model and see Choquette & Khalsa, 2025 for further detail).

In support of this proposition, several neuroimaging studies have identified inverse relationships between signaling in areas of the brain that facilitate interoceptive representation in AN and body image (De la Cruz et al., 2022; Favaro et al., 2012; Friederich et al., 2010). While examining resting state FC, there was an inverse correlation between body image disturbance and somatosensory coactivation, which may be emblematic of this processing between bodily signaling and body perception distortion (Favaro et al., 2012). Friederich and

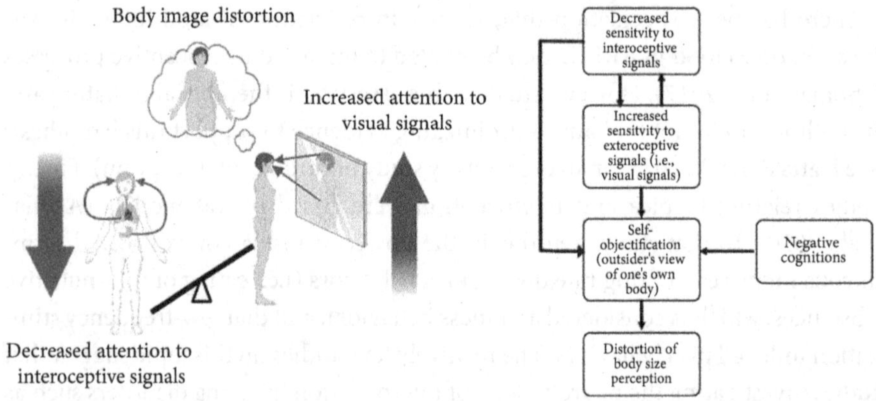

Figure 8.3 Model of body image perception disturbance in AN illustrating how impaired sensitivity to interoceptive and a heightened sensitivity to exteroceptive signals leads to distortions of perceived body size/shape in AN. Created with BioRender.com

colleagues (2010) also provided evidence of this inverse relationship such that body satisfaction score was negatively related to insula activity (higher body satisfaction scores were related to reduced right insula activity). This relationship was found only for individuals with AN, but not for healthy comparisons. Finally, in a study examining the neural response to interoceptive perturbation (discussed previously in this chapter), FC in the bilateral anterior insula, left amygdala, posterior cingulate cortex, and ventromedial prefrontal cortex were all inversely related to body image (De la Cruz et al., 2022). More generally, diminished interoception has been associated with self-objectification (Du X et al., 2003; Myers & Crowther, 2008; Tsakiris, 2013) and the susceptibility to altered views of oneself (Keizer et al., 2016; Pollatos et al., 2016; Tsakiris, Jiménez, & Costantini, 2011). The mechanistic relationship between BID and interoception has implications for treatment approaches focusing on interoception, including interoceptive exposure therapy (Boswell et al., 2019 Plasencia et al., 2019), or other more novel treatments such as reduced environmental stimulation therapy via floatation (Choquette et al., 2023) and which are discussed in a later section of this chapter.

Alternative Perspectives

No discussion of interoception is complete without acknowledging that there are varying opinions and descriptions of the definition of interoception and interoceptive awareness. This is particularly relevant for eating disorders due to the key roles played by food, eating, and digestion in these conditions. In the first introduction of the term, Sherrington (1906) included taste among the interoceptive senses, perhaps due to its relevance for conveying information on internal body states (Sherrington, 1906). But he also demarcated exteroception as pertaining to the sensitivity to stimuli emanating from outside the body (including odors), potentially complicating the picture (Berntson & Khalsa, 2021). In the years since, gustation has not always been included as an interoceptive sensation (Critchley & Garfinkel, 2017) and there is ongoing debate about the appropriate demarcation. Our view is that interoceptive processes can and do occur during the cephalic phase. Specifically, viewing food activates a conceptual representation of food ingestion in an automatic fashion that can be conscious or unconscious, resulting in activation of an interoceptive circuit focused on the anticipation of food (i.e., cephalic phase). When food is placed into the mouth to taste, it is an external object being explored by the body boundary, and thus taste is an exteroceptive process. We have suggested that the act of swallowing is an important demarcation after which a solid or liquid stimulus takes on the property of a gastrointestinal interoceptive signal (Khalsa, Berner, & Anderson, 2022). Specifically, the act of swallowing is a behavior marking the point at which the transit of the bolus (i.e., liquid or solid food) has entered the gastrointestinal tract in a unidirectional fashion for the purpose of digestion. From the perspective of predictive processing, swallowing marks the moment where anticipated ingestion can be compared with a felt ingestion at relevant interoceptive neurocircuitry.

In a recent development, some have adopted a "functionalist" argument, stating that taking a computational modeling perspective allows for a distinction between exteroception and interoception that is determined by the type of inference and associated regulatory process that is elicited by the sensory signal (Toussaint, Heinzle, & Stephan, 2024). According to this perspective, it seems possible to argue that taste could be included as an interoceptive process, given that taste activates some of the same neural structures as other forms of interoception, specifically the insula (Small, 2010) and engages cephalic representations that prepare an organism for ingestion.

A different alternative view posits that abnormal interoception is not a causal factor in the emergence of eating disorder symptoms, but rather that interoceptive deficits occur due to changes in bodily physiology as a result of starvation. However, because abnormal interoception remains even after weight is restored in patients with AN (Berner et al., 2018), this assertion is not well-supported. Rather, it seems more plausible that the development of a starvation state could lead to a perpetuating abnormality of interoception, akin to what has been referred to as an "illness scar" (Kaye, 2011). Or alternatively, such abnormalities could reflect premorbid traits that facilitate the onset of an eating disorder during certain biological and environmental conditions (e.g., puberty, prolonged dieting or physical exercise). According to this notion, developmental or predetermined trait abnormalities of interoception could cause an individual to misread their internal body signals and lead to a misperception of cues associated with meals. As a result of persistent misinterpretations of internal body state, a mindset of bodily mistrust or confusion related to internal sensations and associated affects ensues. Thus, in the context of emerging patterns of behavioral restriction, binge eating, or selective food intake (i.e., ARFID) the individual increasingly fails to make necessary associations between appetitive signals, food ingestion, and the natural resolution of homeostatic disturbances during hunger states and their termination via satiety. This leads to a self-reinforcing cycle of maladaptive behaviors that could propagate the clinical expression of an eating disorder.

It is our position that interoception influences perception and behavior via unconscious and conscious mechanisms, that both are critical to the homeostatic maintenance of healthy physiological states, and that behavioral and neural measures are necessary to optimally understand this process. However, another perspective is that conscious perceptions of interoception are a sufficient substrate for study via measures such as self-report scales or qualitative assessments. This view is often evident within the psychological literature and is certainly consistent with the clinical practice of diagnosis and treatment based on symptoms. Given that interoception is inherently a biological process, we find it difficult to see how an informed understanding of how interoceptive symptoms are produced could not include the interdisciplinary process of learning about and studying the interactions between the underlying physiological and neural systems. The advantages of an interdisciplinary approach are numerous. They include a more complete and accurate understanding of the complex systems that produce disordered eating, opportunities to hone in on latent variables that may produce a variety of illness signs and symptoms, and an ability to provide a reductive explanation for complex phenomena, including via the identification of the evolutionary building blocks of sensory perception. Thus, even though non-human animal species are not capable of verbal self-report, animal models of interoception (even those in remotely related creatures such as the octopus) may yield insights capable of informing our clinical understanding of mammalian or vertebrate interoception.

Considering that our understanding of interoception has grown with efforts to detail the complexities of these integrated systems, it is understandable that alternative views have emerged. This expanding insight builds upon more than a hundred years of neurobiological and psychological research, recognizing the intricate nature of interoception and the neural pathways that process bodily signals, both internal and external. Further debates are likely to ensue.

Emerging research

The growing study of interoception also presents a unique opportunity to integrate neuroscientific approaches with biomarker-based approaches to tracking treatment progress and relapse over the course of an individual's illness. There are now minimally invasive tools that could potentially aid with in vivo measurement or lead to advances in our understanding of how interoceptive processes change over the course of illness. These could aid the prospective assessment of relapse prediction or yield new mechanistic treatment targets for inclusion in intervention development. We will now review some practical considerations.

As mentioned earlier, much of interoception is unconscious until some kind of imbalance disrupts the homeostasis of interoceptive systems. Experimental approaches designed to create such perturbations have thus emerged as important for furthering research. Interoceptive perturbations have several advantages (Khalsa & Lapidus, 2016): they (1) allow for the investigation of interoceptive phenomenon which do not occur at baseline homeostatic states (e.g., changes in breathing, heart rate, stomach or bladder fullness, blood glucose levels); (2) actively induce variations in bodily states that enhance the detectability of subtle physiological responses (e.g., can overcome floor effects commonly observed in measurements of cardiac sensation); (3) facilitate the mechanistic manipulation of environmental context and individual expectancies, which allows for impact of perceived controllability on symptom self-reports; and (4) are often naturalistic with respect to systems physiology (e.g., manipulation of physiologically plausible hunger or thirst, or cardiac or respiratory or gastrointestinal signals).

Much of the available work on interoception in eating disorders has used self-report scales (for a meta-analysis, see Jenkinson et al., 2018). While experimental manipulation of interoception in these disorders is less common (Berner et al., 2018, 2019; De la Cruz et al., 2022; Khalsa et al., 2015), the pioneering studies done in this area have substantially enhanced our understanding of interoceptive awareness, particularly within the cardiac and respiratory domains. Because the interoceptive processes affecting individuals with eating disorders are complex, applying a more diverse range of investigational approaches may yield further valuable findings.

This is particularly true with respect to the gastrointestinal domain. For example, there are numerous opportunities to broaden the examination of neural responses to food to include direct experiences of food consumption and other sensory interactions with the gastrointestinal tract (Figure 8.2, and for a detailed review see Khalsa, Berner, & Anderson 2022). Perturbation studies of gastrointestinal interoception have strong ecological validity with respect to symptomatic reports of abdominal bloating, cramping, or premature fullness with food. Such studies have been understandably limited due to the invasive nature of such perturbation (e.g., swallowing or rectal placement of inflatable balloons or probes delivering electrical stimulation). Less invasive approaches have emerged as alternatives. For instance, the water load task involves the ingestion of water until reaching feelings of satiety or fullness (van Dyck, 2016). It is less invasive but can only be repeated once per experimental session, limiting applications of nuanced approaches such as psychophysical or computational modeling, which typically rely on larger numbers of trials to estimate perceptual parameters. The water load task is also currently limited to liquids; it does not provide information related to ingestion of solid foods. Other approaches have involved direct delivery of small amounts of swallowed nutrients such as sucrose (Frank, et al., 2008) or milkshakes (Bohon, Stice, & Spoor, 2009; Coddington & Bruch, 1970). These studies have made important contributions to our understanding of taste and nutrient ingestion in eating disorders and have helped to guide the focus of studies further toward the digestive process (Coddington & Bruch, 1970). However, additional methods are needed for further exploration of digestive tract processing in more distal regions of the gut.

In recent years, advances in both pharmacological and non-pharmacological approaches have been developed to study gastrointestinal interoception in eating disorders. Here we present some examples of these new advances and potential uses (see Table 8.1, and for a complete review see Khalsa, Berner, & Anderson, 2022). On the pharmacologic side, the development of glucagon like peptide 1 (GLP-1) agonist medications, such as semaglutide or tirzepatide (Baggio & Drucker, 2014), which substantially reduce food craving, represents a major milestone in metabolic medicine. Although these medicines are typically prescribed for achievement of blood glucose control in diabetes or for weight loss in obesity, they may be appropriate for study in certain eating disorder populations (i.e., individuals with binge-eating disorder; Richards et al., 2023) to probe the modulation of food cravings and associated neural circuitry related to interoception. However, such an approach is not advisable in individuals who have a history of engaging in prolonged caloric restriction as it may proliferate weight

Table 8.1 Novel Approaches for gastrointestinal interoception investigation in eating disorders

Method	Intended Effect
Pharmacological	
Gelesis 100 hydrogel capsule (Gelesis Inc.) (Greenway et al., 2019)	Generate feelings of fullness through increased volume and elasticity of the stomach and small intestine
Semaglutide, tirzepatide (Baggio et al., 2014)	Weight management for individuals with obesity; may impact food craving and food intake behavior.
Erythromycin (Deloose et al., 2016)	Induce gastric contractions, hunger, and food intake
Sugarbreak Resist™ Strips/Spray Gymnema sylvestre (Pickrahn et al., 2021)	Temporarily block perception of sweet taste via sucrose receptors in the tongue and stomach
Non-pharmacological	
Vibrating capsule (Vibrant Inc.) (Smith et al., 2021)	Mechanosensory stimulation of gut afferents; used to measure conscious detection and perception of sensations
SmartPill™ Motility Testing System (Medtronic Inc.) (Monti et al., 2021)	Measure pH, temperature, and pressure throughout the gastrointestinal tract; provides information on gastric emptying and transit time
High-density electrogastrogram (Carson et al., 2021)	Estimate the speed and direction of gastric slow waves after caloric stimulation
16 hour fast (Kaye et al., 2020)	Elicit hunger hormonal signaling and remove stomach contents
Gut-brain Synchrony via resting sate EGG- fMRI Rebollo et al., 2018)	Correlate activity between stomach and brain; allows for identification of the "gastric network"

reduction through reinforced avoidance of food, or potentially precipitate an eating disorder-like state (Richards & Khalsa, 2024). Erythromycin (Deloose et al., 2016), a motilin receptor agonist that stimulates gastric contractions and gastric emptying, may have utility in probing neural interoceptive networks associated with binge behaviors. The Gelesis 100 hydrogel capsule (Greenway et al., 2019) is an approach designed to support weight loss efforts when used chronically, but it represents a minimally invasive opportunity to acutely manipulate fullness states without requiring food intake. The use of a superabsorbent cellulose hydrogel matrix which expands upon contact with water allows the examination of neural processing of gut distension without the impact of caloric stimulation. Other methods may have utility in understanding the underpinnings of specific eating disorders. Finally, using an ingestible vibrating capsule, we developed a minimally invasive non-pharmacologic approach to probing the neural basis of gut sensations relevant to the symptomatology of certain eating disorders. Briefly, we found that different vibration strengths produced reliable changes in both stomach sensation and gastric-evoked brain activity (Mayeli et al., 2023). The gastric-evoked potentials showed intensity-dependent increases in amplitude such that the stronger the capsule vibration, the larger the neural response. Additionally, these neural responses were associated with subjective perception of the body, including increased stomach, breathing, and heartbeat sensations, as well as peripheral physiological responses. The amenability of these data to computational modeling revealed individual differences in novel parameters, such as the development of prior beliefs during the task and interactions with estimates of the reliability of the signals from the capsules (Smith et al., 2021). The minimally invasive and repeatable nature of the vibrating capsule is well-suited for applications in mental health settings, thus representing a substantial advance in the applicability of this interoceptive probe over existing technologies.

While not all the aforementioned methods have been applied with eating disorder populations, there is clear potential in their implementation for the advancement of our knowledge of gastrointestinal interoception in eating disorders. Future work would benefit from continued exploration of interoception using perturbation techniques, specifically, those targeted at understanding the underlying mechanism of specific gastrointestinal symptomatology that may be most relevant for eating disorders.

In addition to aiding in understanding the neural mechanisms underlying eating disorders, the inclusion of interoception in the treatment of eating disorders may provide advancements in the field. Gold standard treatments for eating disorders are enhanced cognitive behavioral therapy for eating disorders (CBT-E) (Fairburn, 2008) and family-based therapy or the Maudsley method (Lock & Le Grange, 2015); the moderate levels of efficacy suggest that additional treatment approaches are needed. More recently, treatments including interoceptive exposures have been gaining popularity in eating disorder settings (Boswell, Anderson, & Anderson, 2015; Griffen, Naumann, & Hildebrandt, 2018; Butler & Heimberg, 2020;

Zucker et al., 2019). While some studies have suggested benefits for interoceptive exposure for individuals with eating disorders (Boswell et al., 2019; Plasencia et al., 2019), the current literature is primarily based on case studies. If, as suggested by the previously discussed research, interoception is linked to eating pathology in a potentially causal manner, enhancing an individual's awareness of their internal sensations may help to improve symptomatology and prevent relapse. One novel treatment which simultaneously attenuates exteroceptive sensory input and increases awareness of interoceptive sensations is called Reduced Environmental Stimulation Therapy (REST) or floatation-REST, when delivered in a shallow aqueous pool saturated with Epsom salt (Feinstein, Khalsa, Yeh, Wohlrab, et al., 2018; Feinstein, Khalsa, Yeh, Al Zoubi, et al., 2018; Khalsa et al., 2020). This environment is suited for heightening one's attention to internal bodily states both through the reduction of external signaling and through the increased perception of cardiorespiratory sensations (Feinstein, Khalsa, Yeh, Al Zoubi, et al., 2018; Khalsa et al., 2020). Recent studies in individuals with AN have demonstrated a reduction in body dissatisfaction on the photographic figure rating scale after just one session of REST and with differences remaining at six months post intervention (Choquette et al., 2023; Khalsa et al., 2020). In addition to the effects of body image, floatation-REST has been shown to reliably produce acute reductions in anxiety in clinically anxious and depressed samples (Choquette et al., 2023; Feinstein, Khalsa, Yeh, Wohlrab, et al., 2018; Feinstein, Khalsa, Yeh, Al Zoubi, et al., 2018). Because eating disorders such AN and ARFID are characterized by high levels of comorbid anxiety that do not respond well to typical anxiolytic medications such as benzodiazepines, beta blockers, or antihistamines, this may be an adjunctive treatment of eating disorders worth exploring further.

Implications

Interoception provides an important opportunity to improve biomarker approaches to the diagnosis, monitoring, and potential treatment of conditions such as eating disorders that are characterized by abnormal internal body signaling (Khalsa & Lapidus, 2016). As reviewed in the first section of this chapter, interoception has the unique characteristic that these processes have been established across all major biological systems involved in homeostasis. These systems are well characterized within medicine and neuroscience and span genetic, cellular, neural, and systems levels. Interoception may provide a singular symptom-specific target which cuts across diagnostic categorizations for psychiatric disorders. An accurate description of the processes involved requires integrative knowledge of several disciplines that are infrequently combined including physiology, neuroscience, functional anatomy, medicine, clinical psychology, and psychiatry. While such comprehensive approaches of assessment are difficult to achieve due to the specialized nature of these disciplines, they are necessary to further the clinical applications of the science (Lane et al., 2009). Interoceptive neuroscience thus represents an area where the convergence of these distinct fields can occur to create comprehensive approaches, offering opportunities for a paradigm shift in our thinking and approaches to eating disorders.

Research into how the nervous system interprets internal signals is unveiling where cognition, reward, and internal sensory processes converge with bodily regulation, offering new perspectives on eating disorders. Leveraging perturbations of interoceptive processing, such as vibrating capsules, expanding hydrogels, motilin receptor, or GLP-1 agonist stimulation, may challenge prevailing assumptions about these disorders. Advancing our neurobiological understanding of interoception could, therefore, reshape the understanding of eating disorders, providing valuable insights into the gut–brain connection and leading to improved diagnostics and treatments.

References

Adolfi, F., Couto, B., Richter, F., Decety, J., Lopez, J., Sigman, M., Manes, F., & Ibáñez, A. (2017). Convergence of interoception, emotion, and social cognition: A twofold fMRI meta-analysis and lesion approach. *Cortex, 88*, 124–142. https://doi.org/10.1016/j.cortex.2016.12.019

Aguilar-Rivera, M., Kim, S., Coleman, T. P., Maldonado, P. E., & Torrealba, F. (2020). Interoceptive insular cortex participates in sensory processing of gastrointestinal malaise and associated behaviors. *Science Reports, 10*(1), 21642. https://doi.org/10.1038/s41598-020-78200-w

Ainley, V., & Tsakiris, M. (2013). Body conscious? Interoceptive awareness, measured by heartbeat perception, is negatively correlated with self-objectification. *PLOS ONE, 8*(2), e55568.

Al-Zubaidi, A., Iglesias, S., Stephan, K. E., Buades-Rotger, M., Heldmann, M., Nolde, J. M., Kirchner, H., Mertins, A., Jauch-Chara, K., & Münte, T. F. (2020). Effects of hunger, satiety and oral glucose on effective connectivity between hypothalamus and insular cortex. *NeuroImage, 217*, 116931. https://doi.org/10.1016/j.neuroimage.2020.116931

Alcaino, C., Farrugia, G., & Beyder, A. (2017). Mechanosensitive piezo channels in the gastrointestinal tract. *Current Topics in Membranes, 79*, 219–244. https://doi.org/10.1016/bs.ctm.2016.11.003

Andermann, M. L., & Lowell, B. B. (2017). Toward a wiring diagram understanding of appetite control. *Neuron, 95*(4), 757–778. https://doi.org/10.1016/j.neuron.2017.06.014

Avery, J. A., Liu, A. G., Ingeholm, J. E., Riddell, C. D., Gotts, S. J., & Martin, A. (2020). Taste quality representation in the human brain. *Journal of Neuroscience, 40*(5), 1042–1052. https://doi.org/10.1523/jneurosci.1751-19.2019

Badoud, D., & Tsakiris, M. (2017). From the body's viscera to the body's image: Is there a link between interoception and body image concerns? *Neuroscience & Biobehavioral Reviews, 77*, 237–246. https://doi.org/10.1016/j.neubiorev.2017.03.017

Baggio, L. L., & Drucker, D. J. (2014). Glucagon-like peptide-1 receptors in the brain: Controlling food intake and body weight. *Journal of Clinical Investigation, 124*(10), 4223–4226. https://doi.org/10.1172/JCI78371

Barrett, L. F., & Simmons, W. K. (2015). Interoceptive predictions in the brain. *Nature Reviews Neuroscience, 16*(7), 419–429. https://doi.org/10.1038/nrn3950

Benarroch, E. E. (1993). The central autonomic network: functional organization, dysfunction, and perspective. *Mayo Clinic Proceedings, 68*(10), 988–1001. https://doi.org/10.1016/s0025-6196(12)62272-1

Berner, L. A., Simmons, A. N., Wierenga, C. E., Bischoff-Grethe, A., Paulus, M. P., Bailer, U. F., Ely, A. V., & Kaye, W. H. (2018). Altered interoceptive activation before, during, and after aversive breathing load in women remitted from anorexia nervosa. *Psychological Medicine, 48*(1), 142–154. https://doi.org/10.1017/s0033291717001635

Berner, L. A., Simmons, A. N., Wierenga, C. E., Bischoff-Grethe, A., Paulus, M. P., Bailer, U. F., & Kaye, W. H. (2019). Altered anticipation and processing of aversive interoceptive experience among women remitted from bulimia nervosa. *Neuropsychopharmacology*, *44*(7), 1265–1273. https://doi.org/10.1038/s41386-019-0361-4

Berntson, G. G., & Khalsa, S. S. (2021). Neural circuits of interoception. *Trends in Neuroscience*, *44*(1), 17–28. https://doi.org/10.1016/j.tins.2020.09.011

Bohon, C., Stice, E., & Spoor, S. (2009). Female emotional eaters show abnormalities in consummatory and anticipatory food reward: A functional magnetic resonance imaging study *International Journal of Eating Disorders*, *42*(3), 210–221. https://doi.org/10.1002/eat.20615

Boswell, J. F., Anderson, L. M., & Anderson, D. A. (2015). Integration of interoceptive exposure in eating disorder treatment. *Clinical Psychology: Science and Practice*, *22*(2), 194–210.

Boswell, J. F., Anderson, L. M., Oswald, J. M., Reilly, E. E., Gorrell, S., & Anderson, D. A. (2019). A preliminary naturalistic clinical case series study of the feasibility and impact of interoceptive exposure for eating disorders. *Behavioral Research and Therapy*, *117*, 54–64. https://doi.org/10.1016/j.brat.2019.02.004

Bronleigh, M., Baumann, O., & Stapleton, P. (2022). Neural correlates associated with processing food stimuli in anorexia nervosa and bulimia nervosa: an activation likelihood estimation meta-analysis of fMRI studies. *Eating and Weight Disorders*, *27*(7), 2309–2320. https://doi.org/10.1007/s40519-022-01390-x

Brown, T. A., Perry, T. R., Kaye, W. H., & Wierenga, C. E. (2022). Pilot study of a water load test as a measure of gastric interoception in anorexia nervosa. *Eating and Weight Disorders*, *27*(6), 2223–2228. https://doi.org/10.1007/s40519-022-01376-9

Browning, K. N., Verheijden, S., & Boeckxstaens, G. E. (2017). The vagus nerve in appetite regulation, mood, and intestinal inflammation. *Gastroenterology*, *152*(4), 730–744. https://doi.org/10.1053/j.gastro.2016.10.046

Bruch, H. (1962). Perceptual and conceptual disturbances in anorexia nervosa. *Psychosomatic Medicine*, *24*, 187–194. https://doi.org/10.1097/00006842-196203000-00009

Butler, R. M., & Heimberg, R. G. (2020). Exposure therapy for eating disorders: A systematic review. *Clinical Psychology Review*, *78*, 101851. https://doi.org/10.1016/j.cpr.2020.101851

Carvalho, G. B., & Damasio, A. (2021). Interoception and the origin of feelings: A new synthesis. *Bioessays*, *43*(6), e2000261. https://doi.org/10.1002/bies.202000261

Cash, T. F., & Deagle, E. A., 3rd. (1997). The nature and extent of body-image disturbances in anorexia nervosa and bulimia nervosa: a meta-analysis. *International Journal of Eating Disorders*, *22*(2), 107–125.

Carson, D. A., O'Grady, G., Du, P., Gharibans, A. A., & Andrews, C. N. (2021). Body surface mapping of the stomach: New directions for clinically evaluating gastric electrical activity. *Neurogastroenterology & Motility*, *33*(3):e14048.

Cechetto, D. F. (1987). Central representation of visceral function. *Federation Proceedings*, *46*(1), 17–23.

Cha, J., Ide, J. S., Bowman, F. D., Simpson, H. B., Posner, J., & Steinglass, J. E. (2016). Abnormal reward circuitry in anorexia nervosa: A longitudinal, multimodal MRI study. *Human Brain Mapping*, *37*(11), 3835–3846. https://doi.org/10.1002/hbm.23279

Choquette, E. M., Flux M. C., Moseman S. E., Chappelle S., Naegele J., Upshaw V., Morton A., Paulus M. P., Feinstein J. S., & Khalsa S. S. (2023). Impact of floatation therapy on body image and anxiety in anorexia nervosa: A randomized clinical efficacy trial. *eClinicalMedicine*, 64, 102173. https://doi.org/10.1016/j.eclinm.2023.102173.

Choquette, E. M., & Khalsa, S. S. (2025). Sensing the self: The role of the insula and interoception in body image. *Current Topics in Behavior Neuroscience*, https://doi.org/10.1007/7854_2025_581

Coddington, R. D., & Bruch, H. (1970). Gastric perceptivity in normal, obese and schizophrenic subjects. *Psychosomatics*, *11*(6), 571–579. https://doi.org/10.1016/s0033-3182(70)71578-8

Cornelissen, K. K., Cornelissen, P. L., Hancock, P. J., & Tovée, M. J. (2016). Fixation patterns, not clinical diagnosis, predict body size over-estimation in eating disordered women and healthy controls. *International Journal of Eating Disorders*, *49*(5), 507–518. https://doi.org/10.1002/eat.22505

Coste, B., Mathur, J., Schmidt, M., Earley, T. J., Ranade, S., Petrus, M. J., Dubin, A. E., & Patapoutian, A. (2010). Piezo1 and Piezo2 are essential components of distinct mechanically activated cation channels. *Science*, *330*(6000), 55–60. https://doi.org/10.1126/science.1193270

Cowdrey, F. A., Filippini, N., Park, R. J., Smith, S. M., & McCabe, C. (2014). Increased resting state functional connectivity in the default mode network in recovered anorexia nervosa. *Human Brain Mapping*, *35*(2), 483–491. https://doi.org/10.1002/hbm.22202

Craig, A. D. (2002). How do you feel? Interoception: the sense of the physiological condition of the body. *Nature Reviews Neuroscience*, *3*(8), 655–666. http://www.ncbi.nlm.nih.gov/entrez/query.fcgi?cmd=Retrieve&db=PubMed&dopt=Citation&list_uids=12154366

Critchley, H. D., & Garfinkel, S. N. (2017). Interoception and emotion. *Current Opinion in Psychology*, *17*, 7–14. https://doi.org/10.1016/j.copsyc.2017.04.020

Critchley, H. D., & Harrison, N. A. (2013). Visceral influences on brain and behavior. *Neuron*, *77*(4), 624–638. https://doi.org/10.1016/j.neuron.2013.02.008

Critchley, H. D., Wiens, S., Rotshtein, P., Öhman, A., & Dolan, R. J. (2004). Neural systems supporting interoceptive awareness. *Nature Neuroscience*, *7*(2), 189–195. https://doi.org/10.1038/nn1176

Dalghi, M. G., Ruiz, W. G., Clayton, D. R., Montalbetti, N., Daugherty, S. L., Beckel, J. M., Carattino, M. D., & Apodaca, G. (2021). Functional roles for PIEZO1 and PIEZO2 in urothelial mechanotransduction and lower urinary tract interoception. *JCI Insight*, *6*(19). https://doi.org/10.1172/jci.insight.152984

Datta, N., & Lock, J. D. (2023). Exploration of interoceptive capabilities in avoidant/restrictive food intake disorder and anorexia nervosa. *Journal of Eating Disorders*, *11*(1), 189. https://doi.org/10.1186/s40337-023-00914-9

De la Cruz, F., Teed, A. R., Lapidus, R. C., Upshaw, V., Schumann, A., Paulus, M. P., Bär, K.-J., & Khalsa, S. S. (2022). Central autonomic network alterations in anorexia nervosa following peripheral adrenergic stimulation. *Biological Psychiatry: Cognitive Neuroscience and Neuroimaging*, 8(7), 720–730. https://doi.org/10.1016/j.bpsc.2022.12.009

Deloose, E., Vos, R., Janssen, P., Van den Bergh, O., Van Oudenhove, L., Depoortere, I., & Tack, J. (2016). The motilin receptor agonist erythromycin stimulates hunger and food intake through a cholinergic pathway. *American Journal of Clinical Nutrition*, *103*(3), 730–737. https://doi.org/10.3945/ajcn.115.113456

Demartini, B., Goeta, D., Marchetti, M., Bertelli, S., Anselmetti, S., Cocchi, A., Ischia, M., & Gambini, O. (2021). The effect of a single yoga class on interoceptive accuracy in patients affected by anorexia nervosa and in healthy controls: a pilot study. *Eating and Weight Disorders*, *26*(5), 1427–1435. https://doi.org/10.1007/s40519-020-00950-3

APA. (2013). Diagnostic and Statistical Manual of Mental Disorders: DSM-5. American Psychiatric Association.

Du, X., Li, Q., Xiang, G., Xiao, M., Liu, X., Chen, X., Ding, C., & Chen, H. (2023). The relationship between brain neural correlates, self-objectification, and interoceptive sensibility. *Behavioural Brain Research*, *439*, 114227. https://doi.org/10.1016/j.bbr.2022.114227

Ehrlich, S., Lord, A. R., Geisler, D., Borchardt, V., Boehm, I., Seidel, M., Ritschel, F., Schulze, A., King, J. A., Weidner, K., Roessner, V., & Walter, M. (2015). Reduced functional connectivity in the thalamo-insular subnetwork in patients with acute anorexia nervosa. *Human Brain Mapping*, *36*(5), 1772–1781. https://doi.org/10.1002/hbm.22736

Eshkevari, E., Rieger, E., Musiat, P., & Treasure, J. (2014). An investigation of interoceptive sensitivity in eating disorders using a heartbeat detection task and a self-report measure. *European Eating Disorders Review*, *22*(5), 383–388. https://doi.org/10.1002/erv.2305

Fairburn, C. G. (2008). *Cognitive behavior therapy and eating disorders*. Guilford Press.

Farrell, C., Lee, M., & Shafran, R. (2005). Assessment of body size estimation: A review. *European Eating Disorders Review*, *13*(2), 75–88. https://doi.org/10.1002/erv.622

Favaro, A., Santonastaso, P., Manara, R., Bosello, R., Bommarito, G., Tenconi, E., & Di Salle, F. (2012). Disruption of visuospatial and somatosensory functional connectivity in anorexia nervosa. *Biological Psychiatry*, *72*(10), 864–870.

Feinstein, J. S., Gould, D., & Khalsa, S. S. (2022). Amygdala-driven apnea and the chemoreceptive origin of anxiety. *Biological Psychology*, *170*, 108305. https://doi.org/10.1016/j.biopsycho.2022.108305

Feinstein, J. S., Khalsa, S. S., Yeh, H.-W.,Wohlrab, C., Simmons, W. K., Stein, M. B., & Paulus, M. P. (2018). Examining the short-term anxiolytic and antidepressant effect of Floatation-REST. *PLOS ONE*, *13*(2), e0190292. https://doi.org/10.1371/journal.pone.0190292

Feinstein, J. S., Khalsa, S. S., Yeh, H., Al Zoubi, O., Arevian, A. C., Wohlrab, C., Pantino, M. K., Cartmell, L. J., Simmons, W. K., Stein, M. B., & Paulus, M. P. (2018). The elicitation of relaxation and interoceptive awareness using floatation therapy in individuals with high anxiety sensitivity. *Biological Psychiatry: Cognitive Neuroscience and Neuroimaging*, *3*(6), 555–562. https://doi.org/10.1016/j.bpsc.2018.02.005

Fischer, D., Berberich, G., Zaudig, M., Krauseneck, T., Weiss, S., & Pollatos, O. (2016). Interoceptive processes in anorexia nervosa in the time course of cognitive-behavioral therapy: A pilot study. *Frontiers in Psychiatry*, *7*, 199. https://doi.org/10.3389/fpsyt.2016.00199

Frank, G. K. W., Oberndorfer, T. A., Simmons, A. N., Paulus, M. P., Fudge, J. L., Yang, T. T., & Kaye, W. H. (2008). Sucrose activates human taste pathways differently from artificial sweetener. *NeuroImage*, *39*(4), 1559–1569. https://doi.org/10.1016/j.neuroimage.2007.10.061

Friederich, H.-C., Brooks, S., Uher, R., Campbell, I. C., Giampietro, V., Brammer, M., Williams, S. C., Herzog, W., & Treasure, J. (2010). Neural correlates of body dissatisfaction in anorexia nervosa. *Neuropsychologia*, *48*(10), 2878–2885.

Gadsby, S. (2017). Distorted body representations in anorexia nervosa. *Conscious Cognition*, *51*, 17–33. https://doi.org/10.1016/j.concog.2017.02.015

Gardner, R. M., & Brown, D. L. (2014). Body size estimation in anorexia nervosa: A brief review of findings from 2003 through 2013. *Psychiatry Research*, *219*(3), 407–410.

Garfinkel, S. N., Seth, A. K., Barrett, A. B., Suzuki, K., & Critchley, H. D. (2015). Knowing your own heart: Distinguishing interoceptive accuracy from interoceptive awareness. *Biological Psychology*, *104*, 65–74. https://doi.org/10.1016/j.biopsycho.2014.11.004

Garner, D. M. (2004). *Eating Disorder Inventory-3. Professional manual.* Psychological Assessment Resources, Inc.

Garner, D. M., Olmstead, M. P., & Polivy, J. (1983). Development and validation of a multidimensional eating disorder inventory for anorexia nervosa and bulimia. *International Journal of Eating Disorders*, *2*(2), 15–34. https://doi.org/10.1002/1098-108X(198321)2:2<15::AID-EAT2260020203>3.0.CO;2-6

Gogolla, N. (2017). The insular cortex. *Current Biology*, *27*(12), R580–R586. https://doi.org/10.1016/j.cub.2017.05.010

Greenway, F. L., Aronne, L. J., Raben, A., Astrup, A., Apovian, C. M., Hill, J. O., Kaplan, L. M., Fujioka, K., Matejkova, E., Svacina, S., Luzi, L., Gnessi, L., Navas-Carretero, S., Alfredo Martinez, J., Still, C. D., Sannino, A., Saponaro, C., Demitri, C., Urban, L. E., . . . Heshmati, H. M. (2019). A randomized, double-blind, placebo-controlled study of gelesis100: A novel nonsystemic oral hydrogel for weight loss. *Obesity*, *27*(2), 205–216. https://doi.org/10.1002/oby.22347

Griffen, T. C., Naumann, E., & Hildebrandt, T. (2018). Mirror exposure therapy for body image disturbances and eating disorders: A review. *Clinical Psychology Review*, *65*, 163–174. https://doi.org/10.1016/j.cpr.2018.08.006

Hassanpour, M. S., Simmons, W. K., Feinstein, J. S., Luo, Q., Lapidus, R. C., Bodurka, J., Paulus, M. P., & Khalsa, S. S. (2018). The insular cortex dynamically maps changes in cardiorespiratory interoception. *Neuropsychopharmacology*, *43*(2), 426–434. https://doi.org/10.1038/npp.2017.154

Haynos, A. F., Hall, L. M. J., Lavender, J. M., Peterson, C. B., Crow, S. J., Klimes-Dougan, B., Cullen, K. R., Lim, K. O., & Camchong, J. (2019). Resting state functional connectivity of networks associated with reward and habit in anorexia nervosa. *Human Brain Mapping*, *40*(2), 652–662. https://doi.org/10.1002/hbm.24402

Jenkinson, P. M., Taylor, L., & Laws, K. R. (2018). Self-reported interoceptive deficits in eating disorders: A meta-analysis of studies using the eating disorder inventory. *Journal of Psychosomatic Research*, *110*, 38–45. https://doi.org/10.1016/j.jpsychores.2018.04.005

Kaelberer, M. M., & Bohórquez, D. V. (2018). Where the gut meets the brain. *Brain Research*, *1693*, 127. https://doi.org/10.1016/j.brainres.2018.04.039

Kaelberer, M. M., Buchanan, K. L., Klein, M. E., Barth, B. B., Montoya, M. M., Shen, X., & Bohórquez, D. V. (2018). A gut–brain neural circuit for nutrient sensory transduction. *Science*, *361*(6408). https://doi.org/10.1126/science.aat5236

Karemaker, J. M. (2022). The multibranched nerve: Vagal function beyond heart rate variability. *Biological Psychology*, *172*, 108378. https://doi.org/10.1016/j.biopsycho.2022.108378

Kaye, W. H., Wagner, A., Fudge, J. L., & Paulus, M. (2011). Neurocircuity of eating disorders. *Current Topics in Behavioral Neurosciences*, *6*, 37–57. https://doi.org/10.1007/7854_2010_85

Kaye, W. H., Wierenga, C. E., Bischoff-Grethe, A., Berner, L. A., Ely, A. V., Bailer, U. F., Paulus, M. P., & Fudge, J. L. (2020). Neural insensitivity to the effects of hunger in women remitted from anorexia nervosa. *American Journal of Psychiatry*, *177*(7), 601–610. https://doi.org/10.1176/appi.ajp.2019.19030261

Keizer, A., van Elburg, A., Helms, R., & Dijkerman, H. C. (2016). A virtual reality full body illusion improves body image disturbance in anorexia nervosa. *PLOS ONE*, *11*(10), e0163921. https://doi.org/10.1371/journal.pone.0163921

Kerr, K. L., DeVille, D. C., Moseman, S. E., & Simmons, W. K. (2022). Aberrant gastric functioning in weight-restored but not acute restricting-type anorexia nervosa: An electrogastrography study. *International Journal of Eating Disorders, 55*(10), 1384–1389. https://doi.org/10.1002/eat.23802

Khalsa, S. S., Adolphs, R., Cameron, O. G., Critchley, H. D., Davenport, P. W., Feinstein, J. S., Feusner, J. D., Garfinkel, S. N., Lane, R. D., Mehling, W. E., Meuret, A. E., Nemeroff, C. B., Oppenheimer, S., Petzschner, F. H., Pollatos, O., Rhudy, J. L., Schramm, L. P., Simmons, W. K., Stein, M. B., . . . Paulus, M. P. (2018). Interoception and mental health: A roadmap. *Biological Psychiatry: Cognitive Neuroscience and Neuroimaging, 3*(6), 501–513. https://doi.org/10.1016/j.bpsc.2017.12.004

Khalsa, S. S., Berner, L. A., & Anderson, L. M. (2022). Gastrointestinal interoception in eating disorders: Charting a new path. *Current Psychiatry Reports, 24*(1), 47–60. https://doi.org/10.1007/s11920-022-01318-3

Khalsa, S. S., Craske, M. G., Li, W., Vangala, S., Strober, M., & Feusner, J. D. (2015). Altered interoceptive awareness in anorexia nervosa: Effects of meal anticipation, consumption and bodily arousal. *International Journal of Eating Disorders, 48*(7), 889–897.

Khalsa, S. S., & Lapidus, R. C. (2016). Can interoception improve the pragmatic search for biomarkers in psychiatry? *Frontiers in Psychiatry, 7*, 121. https://doi.org/10.3389/fpsyt.2016.00121

Khalsa, S. S., Moseman, S. E., Yeh, H.-W., Upshaw, V., Persac, B., Breese, E., Lapidus, R. C., Chappelle, S., Paulus, M. P., & Feinstein, J. S. (2020). Reduced environmental stimulation in anorexia nervosa: An early-phase clinical trial [original research]. *Frontiers in Psychology, 11*. https://doi.org/10.3389/fpsyg.2020.567499

Klabunde, M., Acheson, D. T., Boutelle, K. N., Matthews, S. C., & Kaye, W. H. (2013). Interoceptive sensitivity deficits in women recovered from bulimia nervosa. *Eating Behaviors, 14*(4), 488–492. https://doi.org/10.1016/j.eatbeh.2013.08.002

Klabunde, M., Collado, D., & Bohon, C. (2017). An interoceptive model of bulimia nervosa: A neurobiological systematic review. *Journal of Psychiatric Research, 94*, 36–46. https://doi.org/10.1016/j.jpsychires.2017.06.009

Lane, R. D., Waldstein, S. R., Critchley, H. D., Derbyshire, S. W., Drossman, D. A., Wager, T. D., Schneiderman, N., Chesney, M. A., Jennings, J. R., Lovallo, W. R., Rose, R. M., Thayer, J. F., & Cameron, O. G. (2009). The rebirth of neuroscience in psychosomatic medicine, Part II: Clinical applications and implications for research. *Psychosomatic Medicine, 71*(2), 135–151. https://doi.org/10.1097/PSY.0b013e318198a11f

Lapidus, R. C., Puhl, M., Kuplicki, R., Stewart, J. L., Paulus, M. P., Rhudy, J. L., Feinstein, J. S., & Khalsa, S. S. (2020). Heightened affective response to perturbation of respiratory but not pain signals in eating, mood, and anxiety disorders. *PLOS ONE, 15*(7), e0235346. https://doi.org/10.1371/journal.pone.0235346

Lavalley, C. A., Hakimi, N., Taylor, S., Kuplicki, R., Forthman, K. L., Stewart, J. L., Paulus, M. P., Khalsa, S. S., & Smith, R. (2024). Transdiagnostic failure to adapt interoceptive precision estimates across affective, substance use, and eating disorders: A replication and extension of previous results. *Biological Psychiatry, 191*, 108825. https://doi.org/10.1016/j.biopsycho.2024.108825

Ledoux, J. E. (1992). Emotion and the amygdala. In J. P. Aggleton (Ed.), The amygdala: Neurobiological aspects of emotion, memory, and mental dysfunction (pp. 339–351). Wiley-Liss.

Liu, W. W., & Bohórquez, D. V. (2022). The neural basis of sugar preference. *Nature Reviews Neuroscience, 23*(10), 584–595. https://doi.org/10.1038/s41583-022-00613-5

Livneh, Y., & Andermann, M. L. (2021). Cellular activity in insular cortex across seconds to hours: Sensations and predictions of bodily states. *Neuron, 109*(22), 3576–3593. https://doi.org/10.1016/j.neuron.2021.08.036

Livneh, Y., Ramesh, R. N., Burgess, C. R., Levandowski, K. M., Madara, J. C., Fenselau, H., Goldey, G. J., Diaz, V. E., Jikomes, N., Resch, J. M., Lowell, B. B., & Andermann, M. L. (2017). Homeostatic circuits selectively gate food cue responses in insular cortex. *Nature, 546*(7660), 611–616. https://doi.org/10.1038/nature22375

Livneh, Y., Sugden, A. U., Madara, J. C., Essner, R. A., Flores, V. I., Sugden, L. A., Resch, J. M., Lowell, B. B., & Andermann, M. L. (2020). Estimation of current and future physiological states in insular cortex. *Neuron, 105*(6), 1094–1111.e1010. https://doi.org/10.1016/j.neuron.2019.12.027

Lock, J., & Le Grange, D. (2015). *Treatment manual for anorexia nervosa: A family-based approach*. Guilford.

Loewy, A. D., & Spyer, K. M. (1990). Central regulation of autonomic functions.

Lord, A., Ehrlich, S., Borchardt, V., Geisler, D., Seidel, M., Huber, S., Murr, J., & Walter, M. (2016). Brain parcellation choice affects disease-related topology differences increasingly from global to local network levels. *Psychiatry Research: Neuroimaging, 249*, 12–19. https://doi.org/10.1016/j.pscychresns.2016.02.001

Lutz, A. P. C., Schulz, A., Voderholzer, U., Koch, S., van Dyck, Z., & Vögele, C. (2019). Enhanced cortical processing of cardio-afferent signals in anorexia nervosa. *Clinical Neurophysiology, 130*(9), 1620–1627. https://doi.org/10.1016/j.clinph.2019.06.009

Marshall, J. M. (1994). Peripheral chemoreceptors and cardiovascular regulation. *Physiological Reviews, 74*(3), 543–594. https://doi.org/10.1152/physrev.1994.74.3.543

Martin, E., Dourish, C. T., Rotshtein, P., Spetter, M. S., & Higgs, S. (2019). Interoception and disordered eating: A systematic review. *Neuroscience & Biobehavioral Reviews, 107*, 166–191. https://doi.org/10.1016/j.neubiorev.2019.08.020

Mayeli, A., Al Zoubi, O., White, E. J., Chappelle, S., Kuplicki, R., Morton, A., Bruce, J., Smith, R., Feinstein, J. S., Bodurka, J., Paulus, M. P., & Khalsa, S. S. (2023). Parieto-occipital ERP indicators of gut mechanosensation in humans. *Nature Communications, 14*(1), 3398. https://doi.org/10.1038/s41467-023-39058-4

Mehling, W. E., Price, C., Daubenmier, J. J., Acree, M., Bartmess, E., & Stewart, A. (2012). The multidimensional assessment of interoceptive awareness (MAIA). *PLOS ONE, 7*(11), e48230. https://doi.org/10.1371/journal.pone.0048230

Min, S., Oh, Y., Verma, P., Whitehead, S. C., Yapici, N., Van Vactor, D., Suh, G. S., & Liberles, S. (2021). Control of feeding by Piezo-mediated gut mechanosensation in Drosophila. *Elife, 10*. https://doi.org/10.7554/eLife.63049

Mölbert, S. C., Klein, L., Thaler, A., Mohler, B. J., Brozzo, C., Martus, P., Karnath, H.-O., Zipfel, S., & Giel, K. E. (2017). Depictive and metric body size estimation in anorexia nervosa and bulimia nervosa: A systematic review and meta-analysis. *Clinical Psychology Review, 57*, 21–31. https://doi.org/10.1016/j.cpr.2017.08.005

Mölbert, S. C., Thaler, A., Mohler, B. J., Streuber, S., Romero, J., Black, M. J., Zipfel, S., Karnath, H. O., & Giel, K. E. (2018). Assessing body image in anorexia nervosa using biometric self-avatars in virtual reality: Attitudinal components rather than visual body size estimation are distorted. *Psychological Medicine, 48*(4), 642–653. https://doi.org/10.1017/s0033291717002008

Monti, A., Porciello, G., Panasiti, M. S., Aglioti, S. M. (2021). Gut markers of bodily self-consciousness. *bioRxiv*. 2021.03.05.434072.

Myers, T. A., & Crowther, J. H. (2008). Is self-objectification related to interoceptive awareness? An examination of potential mediating pathways to disordered eating attitudes. *Psychology of Women Quarterly, 32*(2), 172–180. https://doi.org/10.1111/j.1471-6402.2008.00421.x

Nattie, E., & Li, A. (2012). Central Chemoreceptors: Locations and Functions. In R. Terjung (Ed.), *Comprehensive Physiology* (pp. 221–254). https://doi.org/10.1002/cphy.c100083

Nord, C. L., Lawson, R. P., & Dalgleish, T. (2021). Disrupted dorsal mid-insula activation during interoception across psychiatric disorders. *American Journal of Psychiatry, 178*(8), 761–770. https://doi.org/10.1176/appi.ajp.2020.20091340

Oberndorfer, T., Simmons, A., McCurdy, D., Strigo, I., Matthews, S., Yang, T., Irvine, Z., & Kaye, W. (2013). Greater anterior insula activation during anticipation of food images in women recovered from anorexia nervosa versus controls. *Psychiatry Research, 214*(2), 132–141. https://doi.org/10.1016/j.pscychresns.2013.06.010

Paulus, M. P., & Khalsa, S. S. (2021). When you don't feel right inside: homeostatic dysregulation and the mid-insular cortex in psychiatric disorders. *American Journal of Psychiatry, 178*(8), 683–685. https://doi.org/10.1176/appi.ajp.2021.21060622

Paulus, M. P., & Stein, M. B. (2010). Interoception in anxiety and depression. *Brain Structure and Function, 214*(5), 451–463. https://doi.org/10.1007/s00429-010-0258-9

Phillipou, A., Rossell, S. L., Gurvich, C., Castle, D. J., Troje, N. F., & Abel, L. A. (2016). Body image in anorexia nervosa: Body size estimation utilising a biological motion task and eyetracking. *European Eating Disorders Review, 24*(2), 131–138. https://doi.org/10.1002/erv.2423

Pickrahn, S., Dawid, C., Babinger, T., Schmid, C., Brockhoff, A., Meyerhof, W., et al. (2021). Sensory-guided multidimensional exploration of antisweet principles from Gymnema sylvestre (Retz) schult. *Journal of Agricultural and Food Chemistry, 69*(19):5510–5527.

Pilowsky, P. M., & Goodchild, A. K. (2002). Baroreceptor reflex pathways and neurotransmitters: 10 years on. *Journal of Hypertension, 20*(9), 1675–1688. https://doi.org/10.1097/00004872-200209000-00002

Plasencia, M., Sysko, R., Fink, K., & Hildebrandt, T. (2019). Applying the disgust conditioning model of food avoidance: A case study of acceptance-based interoceptive exposure. *International Journal of Eating Disorders*, *52*(4), 473–477. https://doi.org/10.1002/eat.23045

Pollatos, O., & Georgiou, E. (2016). Normal interoceptive accuracy in women with bulimia nervosa. *Psychiatry Research*, *240*, 328–332. https://doi.org/10.1016/j.psychres.2016.04.072

Pollatos, O., Herbert, B. M., Berberich, G., Zaudig, M., Krauseneck, T., & Tsakiris, M. (2016). Atypical self-focus effect on interoceptive accuracy in anorexia nervosa [original research]. *Frontiers in Human Neuroscience*, 10. https://doi.org/10.3389/fnhum.2016.00484

Pollatos, O., Kurz, A.-L., Albrecht, J., Schreder, T., Kleemann, A. M., Schöpf, V., Kopietz, R., Wiesmann, M., & Schandry, R. (2008). Reduced perception of bodily signals in anorexia nervosa. *Eating Behaviors*, *9*(4), 381–388. https://doi.org/10.1016/j.eatbeh.2008.02.001

Rajendran, P. S., Hadaya, J., Khalsa, S. S., Yu, C., Chang, R., & Shivkumar, K. (2023). The vagus nerve in cardiovascular physiology and pathophysiology: From evolutionary insights to clinical medicine. *Seminars in Cell & Developmental Biology*, *156*(15), 190–200. https://doi.org/10.1016/j.semcdb.2023.01.001

Rebollo, I., Devauchelle, A. D., Béranger, B., Tallon-Baudry, C. (2018). Stomach-brain synchrony reveals a novel, delayed-connectivity resting-state network in humans. *eLife*. *7*, e33321.

Richard, A., Meule, A., Georgii, C., Voderholzer, U., Cuntz, U., Wilhelm, F. H., & Blechert, J. (2019). Associations between interoceptive sensitivity, intuitive eating, and body mass index in patients with anorexia nervosa and normal-weight controls. *European Eating Disorders Review*, *27*(5), 571–577. https://doi.org/10.1002/erv.2676

Richards, J., Bang, N., Ratliff, E. L., Paszkowiak, M. A., Khorgami, Z., Khalsa, S. S., & Simmons, W. K. (2023). Successful treatment of binge eating disorder with the GLP-1 agonist semaglutide: A retrospective cohort study. *Obesity Pillars*, *7*, 100080. https://doi.org/10.1016/j.obpill.2023.100080

Richards, J. R., & Khalsa, S. S. (2024). Highway to the danger zone? A cautionary account that GLP-1 receptor agonists may be too effective for unmonitored weight loss. *Obesity Reviews*, e13709. https://doi.org/10.1111/obr.13709

Riva, G., & Gaudio, S. (2012). Allocentric lock in anorexia nervosa: New evidences from neuroimaging studies. *Medical Hypotheses*, *79*(1), 113–117.

Saper, C. B. (2002). The central autonomic nervous system: conscious visceral perception and autonomic pattern generation. *Annual Review of Neuroscience*, *25*(1), 433–469. https://doi.org/10.1146/annurev.neuro.25.032502.111311

Schulz, S. M. (2016). Neural correlates of heart-focused interoception: a functional magnetic resonance imaging meta-analysis. *Philosophical Transactions of the Royal Society B: Biological Sciences*, *371*(1708). https://doi.org/10.1098/rstb.2016.0018

Seth, A. K., & Friston, K. J. (2016). Active interoceptive inference and the emotional brain. *Philosophical Transactions of the Royal Society B: Biological Sciences*, *371*(1708). https://doi.org/10.1098/rstb.2016.0007

Seth, A. K., Suzuki, K., & Critchley, H. D. (2011). An interoceptive predictive coding model of conscious presence. *Frontiers in Psychology*, *2*, 395. https://doi.org/10.3389/fpsyg.2011.00395

Sherrington, C. S. (1906). *The integrative action of the nervous system* (Vol. 35). Yale University Press.

Simmons, W. K., Avery, J. A., Barcalow, J. C., Bodurka, J., Drevets, W. C., & Bellgowan, P. (2013). Keeping the body in mind: Insula functional organization and functional connectivity integrate interoceptive, exteroceptive, and emotional awareness. *Human Brain Mapping*, *34*(11), 2944–2958. https://doi.org/10.1002/hbm.22113

Simmons, W. K., & DeVille, D. C. (2017). Interoceptive contributions to healthy eating and obesity. *Current Opinion in Psychology*, *17*, 106–112. https://doi.org/10.1016/j.copsyc.2017.07.001

Simmons, W. K., Rapuano, K. M., Kallman, S. J., Ingeholm, J. E., Miller, B., Gotts, S. J., Avery, J. A., Hall, K. D., & Martin, A. (2013). Category-specific integration of homeostatic signals in caudal but not rostral human insula. *Nature Neuroscience*, *16*(11), 1551–1552. https://doi.org/10.1038/nn.3535

Small, D. M. (2010). Taste representation in the human insula. *Brain Structure and Function*, *214*(5–6), 551–561. https://doi.org/10.1007/s00429-010-0266-9

Smith, R., Kuplicki, R., Feinstein, J. S., Forthman, K. L., Stewart, J. L., Paulus, M. P., Tulsa 1000 Investigators, & Khalsa, S. S. (2020). A Bayesian computational model reveals a failure to adapt interoceptive precision estimates across depression, anxiety, eating, and substance used disorders. *PLOS Computational Biology*, *16*, e1008484. https://doi.org/10.1371/journal.pcbi.1008484

Smith, R., Mayeli, A., Taylor, S., Al Zoubi, O., Naegele, J., & Khalsa, S. S. (2021). Gut inference: A computational modelling approach. *Biological Psychology, 164*, 108152. https://doi.org/10.1016/j.biopsycho.2021.108152

Stanghellini, G., Ballerini, M., & Mancini, M. (2019). The optical-coenaesthetic disproportion hypothesis of feeding and eating disorders in the light of neuroscience [perspective]. *Frontiers in Psychiatry*, 10. https://doi.org/10.3389/fpsyt.2019.00630

Sui, J., & Gu, X. (2017). Self as object: Emerging trends in self research. *Trends in Neuroscience, 40*(11), 643–653. https://doi.org/10.1016/j.tins.2017.09.002

Szczot, M., Pogorzala, L. A., Solinski, H. J., Young, L., Yee, P., Le Pichon, C. E., Chesler, A. T., & Hoon, M. A. (2017). Cell-type-specific splicing of Piezo2 regulates mechanotransduction. *Cell Reports, 21*(10), 2760–2771. https://doi.org/10.1016/j.celrep.2017.11.035

Taylor, E. W., Wang, T., & Leite, C. A. C. (2022). An overview of the phylogeny of cardiorespiratory control in vertebrates with some reflections on the "Polyvagal Theory." *Biological Psychology, 172*, 108382. https://doi.org/10.1016/j.biopsycho.2022.108382

Teed, A. R., Feinstein, J. S., Puhl, M., Lapidus, R. C., Upshaw, V., Kuplicki, R. T., Bodurka, J., Ajijola, O. A., Kaye, W. H., Thompson, W. K., Paulus, M. P., & Khalsa, S. S. (2022). Association of generalized anxiety disorder with autonomic hypersensitivity and blunted ventromedial prefrontal cortex activity during peripheral adrenergic stimulation: A randomized clinical trial. *JAMA Psychiatry, 79*(4), 323–332. https://doi.org/10.1001/jamapsychiatry.2021.4225

Thomas, J. J., Lawson, E. A., Micali, N., Misra, M., Deckersbach, T., & Eddy, K. T. (2017). Avoidant/restrictive food intake disorder: A three-dimensional model of neurobiology with implications for etiology and treatment. *Current Psychiatry Reports, 19*(8), 54. https://doi.org/10.1007/s11920-017-0795-5

Toussaint, B., Heinzle, J., & Stephan, K. E. (2024). A computationally informed distinction of interoception and exteroception. *Neuroscience & Biobehavioral Reviews, 159*, 105608. https://doi.org/10.1016/j.neubiorev.2024.105608

Travagli, R. A., & Anselmi, L. (2016). Vagal neurocircuitry and its influence on gastric motility. *Nature Reviews Gastroenterology & Hepatology, 13*(7), 389–401. https://doi.org/10.1038/nrgastro.2016.76

Tsakiris, M., Jiménez, A. T.-., & Costantini, M. (2011). Just a heartbeat away from one's body: Interoceptive sensitivity predicts malleability of body-representations. *Proceedings of the Royal Society B: Biological Sciences, 278*(1717), 2470–2476. https://doi.org/doi:10.1098/rspb.2010.2547

van Dyck, Z., Schulz, A., Blechert, J., Herbert, B. M., Lutz, A. P. C., & Vögele, C. (2021). Gastric interoception and gastric myoelectrical activity in bulimia nervosa and binge-eating disorder. *International Journal of Eating Disorders, 54*(7), 1106–1115. https://doi.org/10.1002/eat.23291

van Dyck, Z., Vogele, C., Blechert, J., Lutz, A. P., Schulz, A., & Herbert, B. M. (2016). The water load test as a measure of gastric interoception: Development of a two-stage protocol and application to a healthy female population. *PLOS ONE, 11*(9), e0163574. https://doi.org/10.1371/journal.pone.0163574

Veldhuizen, M. G., Albrecht, J., Zelano, C., Boesveldt, S., Breslin, P., & Lundström, J. N. (2011). Identification of human gustatory cortex by activation likelihood estimation. *Human Brain Mapping, 32*(12), 2256–2266. https://doi.org/10.1002/hbm.21188

Wang, R. L., & Chang, R. B. (2024). The coding logic of interoception. *Annual Review of Physiology, 86*, 301–327. https://doi.org/10.1146/annurev-physiol-042222-023455

Williams, E. K., Chang, R. B., Strochlic, D. E., Umans, B. D., Lowell, B. B., & Liberles, S. D. (2016). Sensory neurons that detect stretch and nutrients in the digestive system. *Cell, 166*(1), 209–221. https://doi.org/10.1016/j.cell.2016.05.011

Zanchi, D., Depoorter, A., Egloff, L., Haller, S., Mählmann, L., Lang, U. E., Drewe, J., Beglinger, C., Schmidt, A., & Borgwardt, S. (2017). The impact of gut hormones on the neural circuit of appetite and satiety: A systematic review. *Neuroscience & Biobehavioral Reviews, 80*, 457–475. https://doi.org/10.1016/j.neubiorev.2017.06.013

Zimmerman, C. A., & Knight, Z. A. (2020). Layers of signals that regulate appetite. *Current Opinions in Neurobiology, 64*, 79–88. https://doi.org/10.1016/j.conb.2020.03.007

Zucker, N. L., LaVia, M. C., Craske, M. G., Foukal, M., Harris, A. A., Datta, N., Savereide, E., & Maslow, G. R. (2019). Feeling and body investigators (FBI): ARFID division—An acceptance-based interoceptive exposure treatment for children with ARFID. *International Journal of Eating Disorders, 52*(4), 466–472. https://doi.org/10.1002/eat.22996

9

Social Cognition and Processing in Eating Disorders

Carrie McAdams and Amy Harrison

Brief Definitional Overview

Social processing: The psychological, cognitive and neural mechanisms that enable information related to oneself, other people and groups of people to be internalized and acted upon.

Communication: The behaviors that allow an individual to share their experiences with other people and groups of people and to learn from other people and groups.

Affiliation: The sense that one has positive relationships with specific other people in the world.

Self: The sense that one is an individual with agency, emotions, and an identity that is distinct in the world.

Other: A recognition that other individuals exist in the world with their own agency, emotions, and identities and can impact others.

Introduction

Social cognition refers to the internalized processing of information about social entities (oneself and others). This includes integration across sensory, emotional, and cognitive processing to generate decisions and behaviors about people. This process is highly complex. Each person interacts directly with other people within a sociocultural environment. These interactions lead to an internalization of beliefs about oneself, others, and one's social world. Positive and negative social interactions are expected to be processed differently in healthy people, allowing individuals to identify their friends and enemies. In sum, the social cognitive domain includes both an individual's ability to glean and react to information acquired through social interactions and the introspective processes when they consider their beliefs about themselves and others.

Carrie McAdams and Amy Harrison, *Social Cognition and Processing in Eating Disorders*. In: *The Handbook of the Neurobiology of Eating Disorders*. Edited by: Christina E. Wierenga and Joanna E. Steinglass, Oxford University Press.
 DOI: 10.1093/9780197675212.003.0010

Biological Framework

Social processing is a domain within the National Institute of Mental Health's (NIMH) Research Domain Organizational Criteria (RDoC), a system designed to organize experimental research in neuroscience and psychiatry. In this system, the Social Domain is divided into four constructs: Social Communication (*Communication*), Affiliation and Attachment (*Affiliation*), Perception and Understanding of Self (*Self*), and Perception and Understanding of Others (*Other*). Neural activity supporting these constructs can be measured using functional magnetic resonance imaging, electroencephalography, and eye-tracking technology.

The *Communication* construct is related to social interactions across individuals including the production and reception of facial and non-facial social information. Enhanced processing of social information related to *Communication* is observed in many sensory brain regions, such as the fusiform face area, a visual region highly specialized for facial recognition and also engaged in discerning the emotional content of a face. The language network includes neural regions within perceptual (e.g., Wernicke's area) and motor (e.g., Broca's area) regions, as well as a diverse network of areas in the temporal, parietal, and frontal lobes involved in both processing language itself as well as processing the semantic content and decision-making that occurs in relation to linguistic information (Fedorenko et al., 2024). Up to two-thirds of *Communication* between humans is non-verbal, including body language, eye-gaze, and facial expressions (Argyle & Dean, 1965). Using one's body to convey meaning and intention is a key way of emphasizing a point during social interaction and helping a person to have their needs met while also contributing to their understanding of others emotional states and intentions (Atkinson et al., 2004). The ability to express emotions in one's face in response to social and emotional stimuli is another important component of *Communication*, and it can occur both alone (e.g., watching a film that elicits a specific emotional response), or in a social context (e.g., in response to another person's emotional expression). Expressing emotion even without the presence of others allows for a congruent state between one's inner emotional experiences and their outward expression. Facial expressions can be a response to something or someone else, to convey one's own emotional state, or to emphasize one's own needs in a social context. Non-verbal behaviors are key components of efficient social interactions (Chartrand & Bargh, 1999) and can signal social affiliation (Lakin & Chartrand, 2003).

The *Affiliation* construct assesses the ability to develop connections with other people. When humans communicate and interact, emotional responses can develop, and the valence of those reactions can be used to reinforce future social interactions—such that people spend more time with people they enjoy and who enjoy them and less time with people they dislike and who may dislike them.

Affiliation and attachment thus depend on an ability to feel rewarded by the time and activity spent with specific others. Neurobiologically, reward from other people is associated with activation in subcortical structures including the ventral tegmental area, nucleus accumbens, caudate, and putamen as well as orbitofrontal cortex. Gonadal hormones (estrogen, progesterone, testosterone) and neurohormones (oxytocin, vasopressin) are also critical in the establishment of intimate and social relationships (Orsini et al., 2022). Social rewards are further modulated by neurodevelopmental stage, puberty and sex hormones, changing the importance of different types of affiliative behaviors across the lifespan (Pfeifer & Berkman, 2018). For example, young children are generally most rewarded by parental approval while adolescents prefer peer approval, and young adults prefer approval of potential intimate partners.

The *Self* and *Other* constructs of the Social Domain are related to recognition of the attributes, including agency, actions, emotions, and cognitions, of both oneself (*Self*) and others (*Other*) in the world. This includes recognition of the agency and actions of oneself and others as well as conscious self-reflection about oneself and others. Theory of mind describes knowledge of the concept that other people may have different emotions and beliefs from oneself; affective theory of mind refers to the emotions of others while cognitive theory of mind refers to the abstract concepts. People develop their own identity based on exposure to others in the world from infancy through adulthood, including how others view oneself such that each person's view of the real world is based on internalization of examples of other people. As such, processing social information about oneself and others is dependent upon *Communication* and influenced by *Affiliation.*

Neurobiologically, the default mode network is closely linked to self-reflection, with medial prefrontal cortex associated with self-relevant decision-making while the posterior cingulate and precuneus are engaged when self-reflecting about experiences (Frewen et al., 2020). Introspection about oneself and others is commonly examined with verbal appraisal paradigms ("I believe I am considerate"; "you believe I am impulsive"). A large meta-analysis has found more ventral regions of medial prefrontal cortex engaged for self-relevant stimuli while more dorsal regions are involved in other-relevant stimuli (Denny et al., 2012). Salience network regions, including the dorsal anterior cingulate and inferior frontal gyri, are activated during tasks that require mentalization as well as tasks that require decision-making in social situations. Valence, including both positive-valence systems mediating reward (e.g., putamen, caudate, and nucleus accumbens), as well as negative-valence systems (e.g., amygdala and insula) interact with the default mode network and salience network. The strength of the connections between subcortical striatal regions and frontal brain regions has been related to self-esteem in healthy young adults (Chavez & Heatherton, 2015). Such relationships are hypothesized to guide the development of positive or negative beliefs about oneself and other people (Frewen et al., 2020). The identity-value model suggests that adolescents and young adults engage in behaviors that are reinforcing of their identity because acting in a way consistent with one's identity-values creates a sense of reward, operationalized as co-activation of subcortical striatal regions with ventromedial prefrontal cortex (Berkman, Hutcherson, et al., 2017; Berkman, Livingston, et al., 2017).

Collectively, social constructs are interrelated and processed across multiple neural networks and impacted by neurohormones, environment and development (Maliske & Kanske, 2022; Orsini et al., 2022; Pfeifer & Berkman, 2018; Schurz et al., 2020). Neural activations about social information are broad, combining sensory perceptual regions with cognitive and emotional information as well as executive-function reasoning and decision-making networks (Maliske & Kanske, 2022). Specific neural regions activated vary by task demands. Perceptual or sensory regions are engaged during social activities, such as the fusiform face area to process the social or emotional content of a face, or Wernicke's area to process language. In addition, other regions may be important in the storage of semantic memories and experiences that are related to internalized social values, including the temporal pole, middle temporal gyrus, precuneus, and the temporoparietal junction. These areas may be engaged to interpret the social-emotional significance, narratives, and experiences associated with social behaviors. Midline cortical and frontal regions are typically involved in self-reflection and self-relevant decision-making, such as the medial prefrontal cortex, dorsal anterior cingulate, insula, precuneus, and the inferior frontal gyri.

State of the Science in Eating Disorders

When thinking about social processing in eating disorders, it is important to recognize that neither the biology nor the psychology is static. Biological factors may be related to genetic or trait differences that impact signaling or development of these pathways, but they could also be acutely altered based on nutritional state. Further complicating this process is that the psychological impact of having a mental illness may also change the social interactions and the environment experienced. These changes may then alter internalized beliefs about both oneself and others. Thus, consideration of age, clinical state, and history of the individual should be the norm when evaluating the social domain in eating disorders. Next, we will briefly summarize evidence suggesting alteration in social cognition and processing in eating disorders, considering relationships and key findings across studies in each construct within the Social Domain.

Communication

The *Communication* domain includes not only verbal language but also eye-gaze, body-language, and facial emotions (Argyle & Dean, 1965). Here, we will consider each area separately in relation to the state of knowledge in eating disorders.

Eye-gaze

The presence of psychopathology appears to impact individuals' use of eye-gaze with differences in the frequency and duration of fixations on key social stimuli (the eyes, nose, and mouth regions of interest) which are altered in both social anxiety disorder (Gunther et al., 2021), major depressive disorder (Suslow et al., 2020), and autistic spectrum disorder (Stuart et al., 2023). These differences have been hypothesized to result from either (1) a perception of others as social threats (as in social anxiety disorder and autistic spectrum disorder), or (2) that an absence of social reward from eye contact decreases this type of motivated behavior (as in depression).

Differences in both smooth pursuit (tracking a moving stimulus), and saccadic eye movements (rapid eye movements) have been observed in three studies considering patients with anorexia nervosa (AN) when viewing and interacting with human social stimuli (Pallanti et al., 1998; Phillipou et al., 2014; Phillipou et al., 2016). These differences suggest potential functional alterations in the neuronal circuits (e.g., the brainstem, basal ganglia, cerebellum, and multiple areas of the cerebral cortex including the dorsolateral prefrontal cortex and the anterior cingulate cortex) that control eye movements in people with AN (Kerr-Gaffney et al., 2018). In addition to those studies considering participants' interactions with disorder-salient stimuli, three studies have also examined the use of eye-gaze in relation to fixations specifically on the eye area region of interest. Watson and colleagues (2010) found that 11 women with AN demonstrated significantly reduced gaze toward the face and eyes and found it less rewarding to look at the face or eyes of others in comparison to 11 comparison women (Watson et al., 2010). Less eye contact was observed during social interactions in seven adolescents with AN relative to 12 comparison adolescents (Cipolli et al., 1989). Harrison and colleagues (2018), in a sample of 25 women with AN and 25 comparison women, found medium to large-sized reductions in the frequency and duration of eye-contact with the eye region of interest for static and moving social stimuli and with the eyes of an interlocutor during a real-life social interaction in those with AN. In addition, the group of 25 women who had recovered from AN demonstrated an intermediate profile. Importantly, autism spectrum disorder traits and anxiety symptoms were controlled for in this study, suggesting specificity in relation to eating pathology. Replication and extension of these eye-gaze studies into other types of eating psychopathology is needed.

Thus, this limited but growing literature indicates that adult women with AN show differences in their use of eye gaze, looking less at other's people's eyes. This behavior may underlie some of the social difficulties reported by this population because eye-contact is important in regulating the flow of conversation and in synchronizing social turn-taking within a social interaction (Rutter & Stephenson, 1977). A reduction in the use of this key social skill may therefore make it more difficult for people with AN to join in conversations. Further, making less eye-contact with a conversational partner may inadvertently give the impression of reduced interest and also make it more difficult for conversational partners to infer emotional states and intentions.

Body language

Emerging evidence suggests that adults and adolescents with AN may find "reading body language" and inferring the emotional state or intentions of others through their bodily cues and movements more difficult than those without AN. The Point Light Walkers Task involves viewing actors depicting these states, having been filmed in the dark with lights attached to the key joints of the body, such as elbows, hips, and head, expressing different emotional states (anger, fear, happiness, and sadness) (Johansson, 1973). Adult women with AN were less accurate than comparison women in identifying sadness, but more accurate in discriminating anger from the Point Light Walkers' movements (Zucker et al., 2013). These findings around sadness were replicated in a larger study, with 61 adults and 36 adolescents with AN tending to label sadness as a neutral emotional state unlike the 96 comparison participants (Lang et al., 2015). These data suggest that it is more difficult, particularly in the context of sadness, for people with AN to infer emotional states from others' bodily cues. These challenges in detecting sadness in others may contribute to difficulties with cognitive empathy, the ability to recognize and understand the mental states of others (Warrier et al., 2018), a process also altered in adults with AN (Kerr-Gaffney et al., 2019).

Using non-verbal communication to inform others about one's own emotional states and intentions is another aspect of social communication. Harrison (2021) investigated the ability of adults with eating disorders to use non-verbal behaviors during a real-life, social interaction that included positive, negative, and neutral topics. Reductions in the use of deictic, beat, iconic, and metaphoric gestures were observed in those with eating disorders, and this group sat more formally, and signaled less interest in their conversation partner using their posture than people without eating disorders. Those with eating disorders indicated greater anxiety through non-verbal cues such as touching their face or playing with their nails. In addition, electro-dermal activity provided a biological measure of emotional arousal during these social interactions. Those with eating disorders, regardless of the emotional valence of the topic discussed, showed significantly lower electrodermal activity than controls, suggesting that they find social interactions less arousing.

In sum, people with eating disorders may make less use of non-verbal communication tools to support social interactions. Most of the non-verbal studies examined only participants with AN, with only the last study looking at eating disorders from a transdiagnostic perspective. More data are needed to develop the understanding of this key form of social communication further, particularly involving people with experience of other eating disorders, such as binge-eating disorder (BED).

Facial emotions

A meta-analysis of six studies including adolescent and adult patients found medium-sized reductions in the expression of positive (d=0.59) and negative (d=0.58) emotions in eating disorders compared to non-eating disorder controls (Davies et al., 2016). This suggests that people with eating disorders do not communicate what they are thinking and feeling as efficiently as others and this might explain some of the social difficulties reported by patients (Harrison et al., 2014). Behaviorally, people with eating disorders also show a greater tendency to look away, or avoid looking at, the facially expressed emotional displays of others than people without eating disorders (Cardi et al., 2015). This might be because social emotional stimuli are aversive and overwhelming, and so reducing the input provides a means of regulating. However, socially, this could inadvertently indicate a lack of interest in others and reduce possible cues to understand others' feelings and intentions. One limitation of this work is that findings are limited to facially evoked emotional expressions in response to static social stimuli, such as faces, or films and, as such, do not reflect real-time social interactions. Further, these studies examined facially evoked emotional expressions in response to viewing a familiar film, potentially confounding the evoked expression with prior memories (Davies et al., 2011).

In the neural realm, early studies suggested differences in processing emotional face stimuli in the amygdala and precuneus in individuals with bulimia nervosa (BN) (Ashworth et al., 2011) and in the amygdala, fusiform gyrus, and insula among individuals with AN (Fonville et al., 2014; Leppanen et al., 2017a, 2017b). However, the largest study of facial emotion processing in both women with and recovered from AN found no whole-brain group differences; although the authors did report increased connectivity between the occipital face area and frontal regions specific for happy faces among women recovered from AN (Halls et al., 2021). More work to identify whether specific environments are associated with altered processing of facial emotions in eating disorders is needed.

Affiliation and attachment

Several lines of evidence, both psychological and biological, suggest that attachment and affiliation mechanisms may be altered in eating disorders. From a psychosocial perspective, individuals with eating disorders have smaller social networks and endorse more difficulties in relationships both with intimate partners and friendships (Arcelus et al., 2012; Lukas et al., 2022; Treasure et al., 2020; Westwood et al., 2016). One well-established behavioral paradigm, cyberball, is a ball-toss game between several players. The impact of exclusion on the participant's emotional state is examined by considering reactions after being excluded or over-included in this game. Relative to comparison women, participants with AN reported greater negative emotion when excluded (i.e., not receiving ball tosses), participants with BN reported stress when over-included (i.e., receiving the ball more times than average), and participants with BED were less stressed when they experienced over-inclusion (Meneguzzo et al., 2023). In sum, perceptions about inclusion and exclusion appear to change emotional state differently in different types of eating disorders relative to non-eating disordered cohorts.

From a biological perspective, the act of starvation reduces the levels of estrogen and oxytocin in humans (Amorim et al., 2023). Both hormones are strongly associated with affiliative social behaviors (sexual bonding, reproduction, and mothering), and changes in these hormones have been associated with differences in activation in temporal, frontal, and limbic regions of the brain (Dubol et al., 2021; Grace et al., 2018; Rappeneau & Castillo Diaz, 2024). Specifically, reductions in estrogen reduce dopamine release in the striatum in animal models (Stolzenberg & Numan, 2011; Zachry et al., 2021) and reduced estrogen during menopause in humans is associated with lower dopamine (Giannini et al., 2021). As such, the loss of estrogen as can occur during restrictive eating in many eating disorders may have acute effects on reward processing, a key component involved in forming attachments with others. Relevant to eating disorders, oxytocin is not only associated with social behavior but also related to feeding, with acute administration of oxytocin associated with decreased eating (Leslie et al., 2018).

Differences related to oxytocin processing have also been identified in individuals with AN. Genetic data support differences in the methylation of the oxytocin receptor (Kim et al., 2014; Thaler et al., 2020), while differences in oxytocin receptor polymorphisms have been associated with recovery (Acevedo et al., 2015). Altered midline neural responses during social processing in AN have also been associated with differences in oxytocin receptor polymorphisms (Sala et al., 2018). Notably, the oxytocin receptor polymorphism more common in persistent AN and associated with the brain differences in social processing (A allele of rs2254298) is also overrepresented in autistic spectrum disorder (Wilczyński et al., 2021). Methylation is a mechanism that allows changes in gene expression; changes in methylation of the oxytocin receptor has been associated with maternal care, childhood trauma, and even brain responses during social processing tasks in adults (Danoff et al., 2021). Methylation of the oxytocin receptor has also been associated with autistic spectrum disorder and impaired social traits in humans (Moerkerke et al., 2021). One recent meta-analysis found 8.8% to 24% of adult individuals with AN had a comorbid autistic spectrum disorder, and suggested that such individuals were more likely to have a prolonged course of AN (Boltri & Sapuppo, 2021).

Introspection about oneself and others

When participants with AN or BN think about themselves, differences in the use of regions within the default mode network have been reported, generally with less medial prefrontal activity during self-appraisals (McAdams et al., 2016; McAdams & Krawczyk, 2013, 2014; Xu et al., 2017). The valence of social appraisal stimuli was further considered in one study, finding reduced responses in medial prefrontal cortex, the precuneus, and inferior frontal gyri to positive self-stimuli in AN but no differences for negative self-stimuli (Mendoza et al., 2022). Interestingly, consideration of oneself in the context of other people alleviated that hypoactivation, suggesting that the act of mentalization compensates for aberrant processing of positive self-stimuli. Participants who endorsed more negative self-attributions (both healthy and patients) also engaged the insula more during direct self-reflection than during mentalization about themselves (McAdams et al., 2018). These data suggest that neural processing changes acutely during mentalization and that prior internalized beliefs about oneself may be associated with specific brain differences during self-reflection.

Neuroimaging studies of dynamic social interactions are an important next step toward a better understanding of social interactions in eating disorders. Two studies have used the trust game, a paradigm in which two people build a reciprocating relationship. Among individuals with AN, unexpectedly positive social interactions led to less activation of the precuneus and the temporoparietal junction. In individuals with BN, unexpectedly negative social interactions led to increased activations in both subcortical (striatum and amygdala) and cortical (cingulate, dorsolateral prefrontal cortex, and precuneus) regions (Luo et al., 2021). A separate study examined receipt of positive and negative social feedback in AN, finding that comparison women had more striatal and cortical activations for positive feedback while women with AN showed striatal activation after negative feedback (Via et al., 2015). Another study deployed the norm-adaptation ultimatum game, a paradigm in which participants are expected to adapt to changes in expected offers over time. Relative to comparison women, both women with and recovering from AN as well as women with BN did not adapt to changes in norms, reported less satisfaction for advantageous offers, and showed reduced orbitofrontal activations for advantageous offers but no differences for disadvantageous offers (Luo et al., 2024). In sum, social information appears to be processed differently in eating disorders, with stronger subcortical responses for negative social signals and/or weaker cortical responses for positive social signals.

Alternative Perspectives

Importantly, causality regarding how social cognitive problems promote clinical symptoms in eating disorders remains only hypothetical. Some problems in social cognition may contribute to the development of eating disorders (e.g., deficiencies in communication leading to high social anxiety) while other challenges related to social cognition may result from having had an eating disorder (e.g., being in treatment/having a mental illness reducing social interactions as a whole). Thus, the question of whether social processing is altered before an eating disorders manifests, potentially contributing to its development of eating disorders, or whether eating disorders disrupt social processing to then impair development of self-identity and social rewards remains undetermined. Determination of etiology may not be as important as recognition that this pathological cycle may contribute to maintenance of these disorders. In addition, age, illness state, and duration of illness may also impact the emergence of problems within the social domain.

Alternative perspectives also include a conceptualization that social problems are only transient features that resolve with the eating disorder. This may be true for some cases of eating disorders. Children and young adults who respond to treatment quickly may catch up in their neurodevelopmental trajectory in relation to social processing. Similarly, individuals who have completed brain development before an eating disorder begins may be less impacted in relation to long-term social functioning. Individuals with eating disorders with social cognitive disturbances could also delineate only a small subset with more severe disease or treatment-refractory courses and be related to the disease impacting neurodevelopment. This perspective seems less likely because social cognitive impairments have been reported amongst fully recovered patients with AN. The question of comorbidity with autistic spectrum disorders may also be relevant. Finally, problems expressed in the social domain may also result from problems observed in other neurobiological systems, perhaps related to learning in general or the processing of positive valence stimuli.

Sociocultural values, such as the pursuit of a thin ideal, are well-known to impact the development of eating disorders. In addition, conflict within a culture, as in the introduction of multiple alternative views also increases the risk for development of eating disorders (Becker, 2004; Becker et al., 2002). Historically, humans told stories that offered narratives about aspirational fictional characters. Before written language, people were largely exposed only to others in the context of potentially reciprocating social interactions—people in the same room as us. Today, people can access many more narratives through written, visual, and social media. This expansion of imagined possibilities about ways to exist increases the potential for internal conflicts about one's identity.

Of note, people in minority groups have a higher incidence of mental disorders, including eating disorders (Hallward et al., 2023; Parker & Harriger, 2020; Simone et al., 2020). Minority stress may increase vulnerability to eating disorder psychopathology. Minority stress approaches emphasize the role of stress-induced responses to victimization, discrimination, and internalized stigma as forms of heightened risk for psychological illnesses like eating disorders (Calzo et al., 2017). For example, several studies have demonstrated how shame, concealing one's sexual orientation, and the experience of being discriminated against increase the likelihood of eating disorder symptoms in sexual minority men and women (Bayer et al., 2017; Wang & Borders, 2017; Watson et al., 2016). Those from minority groups may be more at risk of the interpersonal difficulties described here because the experiences of being marginalized and "othered" may reduce affiliation and increase social threat. This is a vital aspect to consider in the social context of therapy, which involves the need to form a social relationship between a patient and clinician. The clinician may be from a sociodemographic group which has perpetrated discrimination and prejudice toward the patient, and with that, the patient may bring expectations of rejection, vigilance toward personal disclosures in therapy, and feeling a need to conceal important parts of their identity for fear of harm (Meyer, 2003). The impact of minority stress on interpersonal functioning in those from marginalized groups with eating disorders needs better measurement to integrate these concepts into existing models of social cognitive differences in dating disorders. As a field, efforts need to be directed toward involving these groups in research, as their experiences are not well represented in existing studies.

Implications

The data emerging in relation to communication, affiliation, self-reflection, and social interactions suggest differences in processing both positive and negative social signals in women with eating disorders. Most work has been done in AN, such that there is limited data on social processing in BN or BED. As such, we have constructed a tentative neurobiological model about social processing for restrictive eating disorders (Figure 9.1). We hypothesize that trait differences related to social communication, rewards, and anxiety may be further exacerbated by restrictive eating behaviors, potentially due to changes in estrogen and oxytocin resulting from malnutrition but also related to the low social rewards seen across multiple tasks. In addition, social experiences are often negative, perhaps due to communication difficulties and from internalized negative beliefs about self and others. The sum of these biological and environmental changes may further reduce an individual's ability to notice and internalize positive self-relevant social stimuli. This leads to a persistent, negative sense of self, including the low self-esteem and weak sense of identity common in AN. This identity problem may further impair interactions with others, with some patients being conscious of this: "I don't know who I am without my eating disorder." One important point here is that receipt of these rewards from "being who one wants to be" requires (1) an intact positive valence system to process a reward, (2) intact communication with others to understand the possibilities that one might have within their specific environment, and (3) the ability to receive and feel rewarded in response to other people.

Importantly, social cognitive function may be modifiable through interventions and is also expected to change during adolescence and young adulthood. Psychotherapy, including individual and group therapy, may be particularly important as a tool that can lead to the modification of social behaviors. For example, the tendency to blame problems on oneself rather than others or a situation is common in eating disorders (Harper et al., 2023; McAdams et al., 2015; Morrison et al., 2006; Rotenberg & Flood, 2000; Watkins et al., 2001), with both cross-sectional and longitudinal research (Harper et al., 2017) suggesting that this negative self-attribution bias changes with recovery in AN. A group art-therapy model was deployed to target social biases and interactions in women with eating disorders,

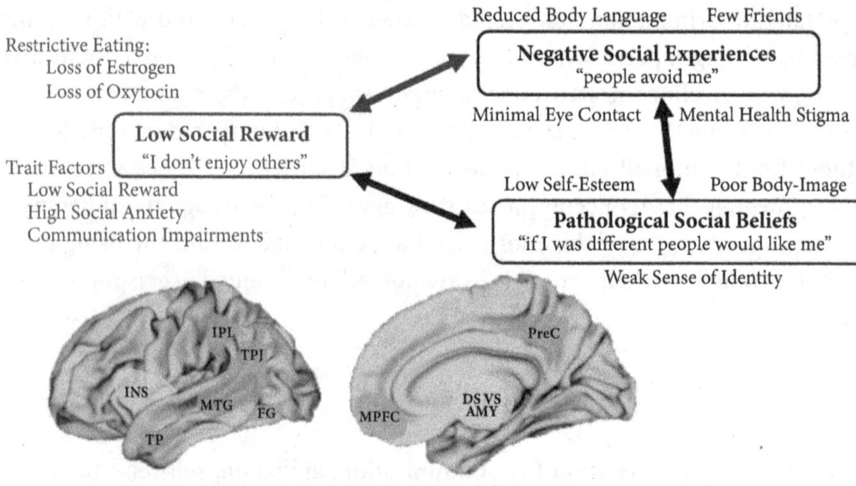

Figure 9.1 A theoretical model of how biological (low social reward), environmental (negative social experiences) and psychological (pathological social beliefs) processes may interact during a restrictive eating disorder. Neural regions that are closely associated with these processes include subcortical regions (light gray: DS, dorsal striatum; VS, ventral striatum; AMY, amygdala; INS, insula) as well as the default mode network (dark gray: MPFC, medial prefrontal cortex; PreC, precuneus; TPJ, temporoparietal junction; IPL, intraparietal lobule; MTG, medial temporal gyrus; TP, temporal pole, FG, fusiform gyrus). Default mode regions are activated during many social behaviors including analysis of body-related stimuli (IPL and TPJ), facial and eye stimuli (FG, MTG, TPJ), theory of mind (PreC, TPJ, TP), and self-reflection (MPFC, PreC).

finding improvements in self-attributions, self-esteem, and psychiatric symptoms (Hagan et al., 2021; Hunt et al., 2021). These changes occurred both acutely and persisted for four months, supporting the premise that social targets are feasible for intervention. Group therapy formats may be ideal in targeting social processes by providing a format in which multiple perspectives are explored to provide more information about social perspectives and clarity in communication with others. A better understanding of the types of social behaviors that are responsive to interventions may help to treat this aspect of eating disorders.

Similarly, social interventions that help with non-verbal communication, such as eye contact and body language, may also be helpful in treatment. There is a small literature on recovered populations who have engaged in some of the non-verbal communication and emotion recognition tasks previously discussed. With the caveat that this evidence comes from cross-sectional designs and is undoubtedly affected by various recruitment biases and the confounds of the impact of nutritional health status on the brain, this is useful work that may provide insight into how these skills can return with improved health and well-being. For example, one study compared how individuals ill with AN, recovered from AN, and comparison women (25 per group, mean age 27 years, range 18 to 55 years) interacted with the eyes of static (photos), moving (video) and real-life (in-person social interaction) social stimuli, finding impoverished responses in the ill cohort and an intermediate profile in the recovered cohort (Harrison et al., 2018). In contrast, another study compared 26 adult women (mean age 44 years, range 38 to 47 years) all of whom had recovered from adolescent-onset AN to 31 comparison women in their accuracy of recognizing basic emotions, intensity of emotional expression, response time, and visual scanning (including eye viewing) of social stimuli, observing no differences in any social-emotional construct (Dinkler et al., 2019). In this last study, six participants with AN also had a diagnosis of autism spectrum disorder and this subset did find recognizing low-intensity emotions in others more challenging. In concert, these studies suggest that the age of onset, duration of illness, comorbidities, and age of symptom remission may need to be considered when measuring social cognition in eating disorders.

In sum, many studies suggest there are impairments in social cognitive processing in eating disorders, but much work remains. Specifically, more research is needed in binge-spectrum eating disorders, men, adolescent populations, longitudinally, and in relation to illness-recovery state. Social cognitive research may offer novel psychotherapeutic targets and guide the use of adjunctive interventions for specific subpopulations of eating disorders. Understanding whether social cognitive differences are related to other cognitive or behavioral features present in eating disorders or are related to specific types of comorbidities is needed. Many fundamental questions about how neurobiological, psychological, and environmental factors within the social cognitive domain impact the development, maintenance, and recovery from eating disorders remain unanswered.

References

Acevedo, S. F., Valencia, C., Lutter, M., & McAdams, C. J. (2015). Severity of eating disorder symptoms related to oxytocin receptor polymorphisms in anorexia nervosa. *Psychiatry Research*, *228*(3), 641–648. https://doi.org/10.1016/j.psychres.2015.05.040

Amorim, T., Khiyami, A., Latif, T., & Fazeli, P. K. (2023). Neuroendocrine adaptations to starvation. *Psychoneuroendocrinology*, *157*, 106365. https://doi.org/10.1016/j.psyneuen.2023.106365

Arcelus, J., Yates, A., & Whiteley, R. (2012). Romantic relationships, clinical and sub-clinical eating disorders: a review of the literature. *Sexual and Relationship Therapy*, *27*(2), 147–161. https://doi.org/10.1080/14681994.2012.696095

Argyle, M., & Dean, J. (1965). Eye-contact, distance and affiliation. *Sociometry*, *8*, 289–304.

Ashworth, F., Pringle, A., Norbury, R., Harmer, C. J., Cowen, P. J., & Cooper, M. J. (2011). Neural response to angry and disgusted facial expressions in bulimia nervosa. *Psychological Medicine*, *41*(11), 2375–2384. https://doi.org/10.1017/S0033291711000626

Atkinson, A. P., Dittrich, W. H., Gemmell, A. J., & Young, A. W. (2004). Emotion perception from dynamic and static body expressions in point-light and full-light displays. *Perception*, *33*(6), 717–746. https://doi.org/10.1068/p5096

Bayer, V., Robert-Mccomb, J. J., Clopton, J. R., & Reich, D. A. (2017). Investigating the influence of shame, depression, and distress tolerance on the relationship between internalized homophobia and binge eating in lesbian and bisexual women. *Eating Behaviors*, *24*, 39–44. https://doi.org/10.1016/j.eatbeh.2016.12.001

Becker, A. E. (2004). Television, disordered eating, and young women in Fiji: Negotiating body image and identity during rapid social change. *Culture, Medicine, and Psychiatry*, *28*(4), 533–559. http://www.ncbi.nlm.nih.gov/pubmed/15847053

Becker, A. E., Burwell, R. A., Gilman, S. E., Herzog, D. B., & Hamburg, P. (2002). Eating behaviours and attitudes following prolonged exposure to television among ethnic Fijian adolescent girls. *British Journal of Psychiatry, 180*, 509–514. http://www.ncbi.nlm.nih.gov/pubmed/12042229

Berkman, E. T., Hutcherson, C. A., Livingston, J. L., Kahn, L. E., & Inzlicht, M. (2017). Self-control as value-based choice. *Current Directions in Psychological Science, 26*(5), 422–428. https://doi.org/10.1177/0963721417704394

Berkman, E. T., Livingston, J. L., & Kahn, L. E. (2017). The identity-value model of self-regulation: Integration, extension, and open questions. *Psychological Inquiry, 28*(2–3), 157–164. https://doi.org/10.1080/1047840X.2017.1343069

Boltri, M., & Sapuppo, W. (2021). Anorexia nervosa and autism spectrum disorder: A systematic review. *Psychiatry Research, 306*, 114271. https://doi.org/10.1016/j.psychres.2021.114271

Calzo, J. P., Blashill, A. J., Brown, T. A., & Argenal, R. L. (2017). Eating disorders and disordered weight and shape control behaviors in sexual minority populations. *Current Psychiatry Reports, 19*(8), 49. https://doi.org/10.1007/s11920-017-0801-y

Cardi, V., Corfield, F., Leppanen, J., Rhind, C., Deriziotis, S., Hadjimichalis, A., Hibbs, R., Micali, N., & Treasure, J. (2015). Emotional Processing, Recognition, Empathy and Evoked Facial Expression in Eating Disorders: An Experimental Study to Map Deficits in Social Cognition. *PloS one, 10*(8), e0133827. https://doi.org/10.1371/journal.pone.0133827

Chartrand, T. L., & Bargh, J. A. (1999). The chameleon effect: The perception–behavior link and social interaction. *Journal of Personality and Social Psychology, 76*(6), 893–910. https://doi.org/10.1037//0022-3514.76.6.893

Chavez, R. S., & Heatherton, T. F. (2015). Multimodal frontostriatal connectivity underlies individual differences in self-esteem. *Social Cognitive and Affective Neuroscience, 10*(3), 364–370. https://doi.org/10.1093/scan/nsu063

Cipolli, C., Sancini, M., Tuozzi, G., Bolzani, R., Mutinelli, P., Flamigni, C., & Porcu, E. (1989). Gaze and eye-contact with anorexic adolescents. *British Journal of Medical Psychology, 62 (Pt4)*, 365–369. https://doi.org/10.1111/j.2044-8341.1989.tb02846.x

Danoff, J. S., Connelly, J. J., Morris, J. P., & Perkeybile, A. M. (2021). An epigenetic rheostat of experience: DNA methylation of OXTR as a mechanism of early life allostasis. *Comprehensive Psychoneuroendocrinology, 8*, 100098. https://doi.org/10.1016/j.cpnec.2021.100098

Davies, H., Schmidt, U., Stahl, D., & Tchanturia, K. (2011). Evoked facial emotional expression and emotional experience in people with anorexia nervosa. *International Journal of Eating Disorders, 44*(6), 531–539. https://doi.org/10.1002/eat.20852

Davies, H., Wolz, I., Leppanen, J., Fernandez-Aranda, F., Schmidt, U., & Tchanturia, K. (2016). Facial expression to emotional stimuli in non-psychotic disorders: A systematic review and meta-analysis. *Neuroscience & Biobehavioral Reviews, 64*, 252–271. https://doi.org/10.1016/j.neubiorev.2016.02.015

Denny, B. T., Kober, H., Wager, T. D., & Ochsner, K. N. (2012). A meta-analysis of functional neuroimaging studies of self- and other judgments reveals a spatial gradient for mentalizing in medial prefrontal cortex [Comparative Study Meta-Analysis Research Support, NIH, Extramural Research Support, US Government, Non-PHS]. *Journal of Cognitive Neuroscience, 24*(8), 1742–1752. https://doi.org/10.1162/jocn_a_00233

Dinkler, L., Rydberg Dobrescu, S., Rastam, M., Gillberg, I. C., Gillberg, C., Wentz, E., & Hadjikhani, N. (2019). Visual scanning during emotion recognition in long-term recovered anorexia nervosa: An eye-tracking study. *International Journal of Eating Disorders, 52*(6), 691–700. https://doi.org/10.1002/eat.23066

Dubol, M., Epperson, C. N., Sacher, J., Pletzer, B., Derntl, B., Lanzenberger, R., Sundstrom-Poromaa, I., & Comasco, E. (2021). Neuroimaging the menstrual cycle: A multimodal systematic review. *Frontiers in Neuroendocrinology, 60*, 100878. https://doi.org/10.1016/j.yfrne.2020.100878

Fedorenko, E., Ivanova, A. A., & Regev, T. I. (2024). The language network as a natural kind within the broader landscape of the human brain. *Nature Reviews Neuroscience.* https://doi.org/10.1038/s41583-024-00802-4

Fonville, L., Giampietro, V., Surguladze, S., Williams, S., & Tchanturia, K. (2014). Increased BOLD signal in the fusiform gyrus during implicit emotion processing in anorexia nervosa. *Neuroimage: Clinical, 4*, 266–273. https://doi.org/10.1016/j.nicl.2013.12.002

Frewen, P., Schroeter, M. L., Riva, G., Cipresso, P., Fairfield, B., Padulo, C., Kemp, A. H., Palaniyappan, L., Owolabi, M., Kusi-Mensah, K., Polyakova, M., Fehertoi, N., D'Andrea, W., Lowe, L., & Northoff,

G. (2020). Neuroimaging the consciousness of self: Review, and conceptual-methodological framework. *Neuroscience & Biobehavioral Reviews, 112*, 164–212. https://doi.org/10.1016/j.neubiorev.2020.01.023

Giannini, A., Caretto, M., Genazzani, A. R., & Simoncini, T. (2021). Neuroendocrine changes during menopausal transition. *Endocrines, 2*(4), 405–416. https://doi.org/10.3390/endocrines2040036

Grace, S. A., Rossell, S. L., Heinrichs, M., Kordsachia, C., & Labuschagne, I. (2018). Oxytocin and brain activity in humans: A systematic review and coordinate-based meta-analysis of functional MRI studies. *Psychoneuroendocrinology, 96*, 6–24. https://doi.org/10.1016/j.psyneuen.2018.05.031

Gunther, V., Kropidlowski, A., Schmidt, F. M., Koelkebeck, K., Kersting, A., & Suslow, T. (2021). Attentional processes during emotional face perception in social anxiety disorder: A systematic review and meta-analysis of eye-tracking findings. *Progress in Neuro-Psychopharmacology & Biological Psychiatry, 111*, 110353. https://doi.org/10.1016/j.pnpbp.2021.110353

Hagan, W. S., Mericle, S., Hunt, B. J., Harper, J. A., Palka, J. M., Pelfrey, S., & McAdams, C. J. (2021). Qualitative patient experiences from the self-blame and perspective-taking intervention for eating disorders. *Journal of Eating Disorders, 9*(1), 127. https://doi.org/10.1186/s40337-021-00483-9

Halls, D., Leslie, M., Leppanen, J., Sedgewick, F., Surguladze, S., Fonville, L., Lang, K., Simic, M., Nicholls, D., Williams, S., & Tchanturia, K. (2021). The emotional face of anorexia nervosa: The neural correlates of emotional processing. *Human Brain Mapping, 42*(10), 3077–3087. https://doi.org/10.1002/hbm.25417

Hallward, L., Nagata, J. M., Rodgers, R. F., & Ganson, K. T. (2023). Examination of eating disorder psychopathology across sexual and gender identities among a Canadian sample. *International Journal of Eating Disorders, 56*(3), 604–615. https://doi.org/10.1002/eat.23872

Harper, J. A., Brodrick, B., Van Enkevort, E., & McAdams, C. J. (2017). Neuropsychological and cognitive correlates of recovery in anorexia nervosa. *European Eating Disorders Review, 25*(6), 491–500. https://doi.org/10.1002/erv.2539

Harper, J. A., Palka, J. M., & McAdams, C. J. (2023). Interpersonal attribution bias and social evaluation in adolescent eating disorders. *European Eating Disorders Review, 31*(2), 258–270. https://doi.org/10.1002/erv.2954

Harrison, A. (2021). Experimental investigation of non-verbal communication in eating disorders. *Psychiatry Research, 297*, 113732. https://doi.org/10.1016/j.psychres.2021.113732

Harrison, A., Mountford, V. A., & Tchanturia, K. (2014). Social anhedonia and work and social functioning in the acute and recovered phases of eating disorders. *Psychiatry Research, 218*(1–2), 187–194. https://doi.org/10.1016/j.psychres.2014.04.007

Harrison, A., Watterson, S. V., & Bennett, S. D. (2018). An experimental investigation into the use of eye-contact in social interactions in women in the acute and recovered stages of anorexia nervosa. *International Journal of Eating Disorders, 52*(1), 61–70. https://doi.org/10.1002/eat.22993

Hunt, B. J., Smith Hagan, W., Pelfrey, S., Mericle, S., Harper, J. A., Palka, J. M., & McAdams, C. (2021). Pilot data from the self-blame and perspective-taking intervention for eating disorders. *Journal of Behavioral and Cognitive Therapy, 31*(1), 57–66. https://doi.org/10.1016/j.jbct.2020.11.002

Johansson, G. (1973). Visual perception of biological motion and a model for its analysis. *Perception & Psychophysics, 14*(2), 201–211. https://doi.org/10.3758/bf03212378

Kerr-Gaffney, J., Harrison, A., & Tchanturia, K. (2018). Eye-tracking research in eating disorders: A systematic review. *International Journal of Eating Disorders*. https://doi.org/10.1002/eat.22998

Kerr-Gaffney, J., Harrison, A., & Tchanturia, K. (2019). Cognitive and affective empathy in eating disorders: A systematic review and meta-analysis. *Frontiers in Psychiatry, 10*, 102. https://doi.org/10.3389/fpsyt.2019.00102

Kim, Y. R., Kim, J. H., Kim, M. J., & Treasure, J. (2014). Differential methylation of the oxytocin receptor gene in patients with anorexia nervosa: a pilot study [Research Support, Non-US Government]. *PLOS ONE, 9*(2), e88673. https://doi.org/10.1371/journal.pone.0088673

Lakin, J. L., & Chartrand, T. L. (2003). Using nonconscious behavioral mimicry to create affiliation and rapport. *Psychological Science, 14*(4), 334–339. https://doi.org/10.1111/1467-9280.14481

Lang, K., Dapelo, M. M., Khondoker, M., Morris, R., Surguladze, S., Treasure, J., & Tchanturia, K. (2015). Exploring emotion recognition in adults and adolescents with anorexia nervosa using a body motion paradigm. *European Eating Disorders Review, 23*(4), 262–268. https://doi.org/10.1002/erv.2358

Leppanen, J., Cardi, V., Paloyelis, Y., Simmons, A., Tchanturia, K., & Treasure, J. (2017a). Blunted neural response to implicit negative facial affect in anorexia nervosa. *Biological Psychology, 128*, 105–111. https://doi.org/10.1016/j.biopsycho.2017.07.010

Leppanen, J., Cardi, V., Paloyelis, Y., Simmons, A., Tchanturia, K., & Treasure, J. (2017b). FMRI study of neural responses to implicit infant emotion in anorexia nervosa. *Frontiers in Psychology, 8*, 780. https://doi.org/10.3389/fpsyg.2017.00780

Leslie, M., Silva, P., Paloyelis, Y., Blevins, J., & Treasure, J. (2018). A systematic review and quantitative meta-analysis of oxytocin's effects on feeding. *Journal of Neuroendocrinology, 30*(8). https://doi.org/10.1111/jne.12584

Lukas, L., Buhl, C., Schulte-Korne, G., & Sfarlea, A. (2022). Family, friends, and feelings: The role of relationships to parents and peers and alexithymia in adolescents with anorexia nervosa. *Journal of Eating Disorders, 10*(1), 143. https://doi.org/10.1186/s40337-022-00661-3

Luo, Y., Mendoza, C., Pelfrey, S., Lohrenz, T., Gu, X., Montague, P. R., & McAdams, C. J. (2021). Elevated neurobehavioral responses to negative social interactions in women with bulimia nervosa. *Biological Psychiatry: Cognitive Neuroscience and Neuroimaging, 7*(7), 696–705. https://doi.org/10.1016/j.bpsc.2021.01.011

Luo, Y., Pluta, D., Brodrick, B. B., Palka, J. M., McCoy, J., Lohrenz, T., Gu, X., Vannucci, M., Montague, P. R., & McAdams, C. J. (2024). Diminished adaptation, satisfaction, and neural responses to advantageous social signals in anorexia nervosa and bulimia nervosa. *Biological Psychiatry: Cognitive Neuroscience and Neuroimaging, 9*(3), 305–313. https://doi.org/10.1016/j.bpsc.2023.10.010

Maliske, L., & Kanske, P. (2022). The social connectome—Moving toward complexity in the study of brain networks and their interactions in social cognitive and affective neuroscience. *Frontiers in Psychiatry, 13*, 845492. https://doi.org/10.3389/fpsyt.2022.845492

McAdams, C. J., Harper, J. A., & Van Enkevort, E. (2018). Mentalization and the left inferior frontal gyrus and insula. *European Eating Disorders Reviews, 26*(3), 265–271. https://doi.org/10.1002/erv.2580

McAdams, C. J., Jeon-Slaughter, H., Evans, S., Lohrenz, T., Montague, P. R., & Krawczyk, D. C. (2016). Neural differences in self-perception during illness and after weight-recovery in anorexia nervosa. *Social Cognitive and Affective Neuroscience, 11*(11), 1823–1831. https://doi.org/10.1093/scan/nsw092

McAdams, C. J., & Krawczyk, D. C. (2013). Neural responses during social and self-knowledge tasks in bulimia nervosa. *Frontiers in Psychiatry, 4*, 103. https://doi.org/10.3389/fpsyt.2013.00103

McAdams, C. J., & Krawczyk, D. C. (2014). Who am I? How do I look? Neural differences in self-identity in anorexia nervosa. *Social Cognitive and Affective Neuroscience, 9*(1), 12–21. https://doi.org/10.1093/scan/nss093

McAdams, C. J., Lohrenz, T., & Montague, P. R. (2015). Neural responses to kindness and malevolence differ in illness and recovery in women with anorexia nervosa. *Human Brain Mapping, 36*(12), 5207–5219. https://doi.org/10.1002/hbm.23005

Mendoza, C. J., Palka, J. M., Pelfrey, S. E., Hunt, B. J., Krawczyk, D. C., & McAdams, C. J. (2022). Neural processes related to negative self-concept in adult and adolescent anorexia nervosa. *European Eating Disorders Review, 30*(1), 23–35. https://doi.org/10.1002/erv.2867

Meneguzzo, P., Meregalli, V., Collantoni, E., Cardi, V., Tenconi, E., & Favaro, A. (2023). Virtual rejection and overinclusion in eating disorders: An experimental investigation of the impact on emotions, stress perception, and food attitudes. *Nutrients, 15*(4). https://doi.org/10.3390/nu15041021

Meyer, I. H. (2003). Prejudice, social stress, and mental health in lesbian, gay, and bisexual populations: Conceptual issues and research evidence. *Psychological Bulletin, 129*(5), 674–697. https://doi.org/10.1037/0033-2909.129.5.674

Moerkerke, M., Bonte, M.-L., Daniels, N., Chubar, V., Alaerts, K., Steyaert, J., & Boets, B. (2021). Oxytocin receptor gene (OXTR) DNA methylation is associated with autism and related social traits—A systematic review. *Research in Autism Spectrum Disorders, 85*. https://doi.org/10.1016/j.rasd.2021.101785

Morrison, T., Waller, G., & Lawson, R. (2006). Attributional style in the eating disorders. *Journal of Nervous and Mental Disease, 194*(4), 303–305. https://doi.org/10.1097/01.nmd.0000208114.79179.7e

Orsini, C. A., Brown, T. E., Hodges, T. E., Alonso-Caraballo, Y., Winstanley, C. A., & Becker, J. B. (2022). Neural mechanisms mediating sex differences in motivation for reward: Cognitive bias, food, gambling, and drugs of abuse. *Journal of Neuroscience, 42*(45), 8477–8487. https://doi.org/10.1523/JNEUROSCI.1378-22.2022

Pallanti, S., Quercioli, L., Zaccara, G., Ramacciotti, A. B., & Arnetoli, G. (1998). Eye movement abnormalities in anorexia nervosa. *Psychiatry Research, 78*(1–2), 59–70. https://doi.org/10.1016/s0165-1781(97)00139-x

Parker, L. L., & Harriger, J. A. (2020). Eating disorders and disordered eating behaviors in the LGBT population: A review of the literature. *Journal of Eating Disorders, 8*, 51. https://doi.org/10.1186/s40337-020-00327-y

Pfeifer, J. H., & Berkman, E. T. (2018). The development of self and identity in adolescence: Neural evidence and implications for a value-based choice perspective on motivated behavior. *Child Development Perspectives, 12*(3), 158–164. https://doi.org/10.1111/cdep.12279

Phillipou, A., Rossell, S. L., Castle, D. J., Gurvich, C., & Abel, L. A. (2014). Square wave jerks and anxiety as distinctive biomarkers for anorexia nervosa. *Investigative Ophthalmology & Visual Science, 55*(12), 8366–8370. https://doi.org/10.1167/iovs.14-15807

Phillipou, A., Rossell, S. L., Gurvich, C., Hughes, M. E., Castle, D. J., Nibbs, R. G., & Abel, L. A. (2016). Saccadic eye movements in anorexia nervosa. *PLOS ONE, 11*(3), e0152338. https://doi.org/10.1371/journal.pone.0152338

Rappeneau, V., & Castillo Diaz, F. (2024). Convergence of oxytocin and dopamine signalling in neuronal circuits: Insights into the neurobiology of social interactions across species. *Neuroscience & Biobehavioral Reviews, 161*, 105675. https://doi.org/10.1016/j.neubiorev.2024.105675

Rotenberg, K. J., & Flood, D. (2000). Dietary restraint, attributional styles for eating, and preloading effects. *Eating Behaviors, 1*(1), 63–78. http://www.ncbi.nlm.nih.gov/pubmed/15001068

Rutter, D. R., & Stephenson, G. M. (1977). The role of visual communication in synchronising conversation. *European Journal of Social Psychology, 7*, 29–37.

Sala, M., Han, K., Acevedo, S., Krawczyk, D. C., & McAdams, C. J. (2018). Oxytocin receptor polymorphism decreases midline neural activations to social stimuli in anorexia nervosa. *Frontiers in Psychology, 9*, 2183. https://doi.org/10.3389/fpsyg.2018.02183

Schurz, M., Maliske, L., & Kanske, P. (2020). Cross-network interactions in social cognition: A review of findings on task related brain activation and connectivity. *Cortex, 130*, 142–157. https://doi.org/10.1016/j.cortex.2020.05.006

Simone, M., Askew, A., Lust, K., Eisenberg, M. E., & Pisetsky, E. M. (2020). Disparities in self-reported eating disorders and academic impairment in sexual and gender minority college students relative to their heterosexual and cisgender peers. *International Journal of Eating Disorders, 53*(4), 513–524. https://doi.org/10.1002/eat.23226

Stolzenberg, D. S., & Numan, M. (2011). Hypothalamic interaction with the mesolimbic DA system in the control of the maternal and sexual behaviors in rats. *Neuroscience & Biobehavioral Reviews, 35*(3), 826–847. https://doi.org/10.1016/j.neubiorev.2010.10.003

Stuart, N., Whitehouse, A., Palermo, R., Bothe, E., & Badcock, N. (2023). eye gaze in autism spectrum disorder: A review of neural evidence for the eye avoidance hypothesis. *Journal of Autism and Developmental Disorders, 53*(5), 1884–1905. https://doi.org/10.1007/s10803-022-05443-z

Suslow, T., Husslack, A., Kersting, A., & Bodenschatz, C. M. (2020). Attentional biases to emotional information in clinical depression: A systematic and meta-analytic review of eye tracking findings. *Journal of Affective Disorders, 274*, 632–642. https://doi.org/10.1016/j.jad.2020.05.140

Thaler, L., Brassard, S., Booij, L., Kahan, E., McGregor, K., Labbe, A., Israel, M., & Steiger, H. (2020). Methylation of the OXTR gene in women with anorexia nervosa: Relationship to social behavior. *European Eating Disorders Review, 28*(1), 79–86. https://doi.org/10.1002/erv.2703

Treasure, J., Willmott, D., Ambwani, S., Cardi, V., Clark Bryan, D., Rowlands, K., & Schmidt, U. (2020). Cognitive interpersonal model for anorexia nervosa revisited: The perpetuating factors that contribute to the development of the severe and enduring illness. *Journal of Clinical Medicine, 9*(3). https://doi.org/10.3390/jcm9030630

Via, E., Soriano-Mas, C., Sanchez, I., Forcano, L., Harrison, B. J., Davey, C. G., Pujol, J., Martinez-Zalacain, I., Menchon, J. M., Fernandez-Aranda, F., & Cardoner, N. (2015). Abnormal social reward responses in anorexia nervosa: An fMRI study. *PLOS ONE, 10*(7), e0133539. https://doi.org/10.1371/journal.pone.0133539

Wang, S. B., & Borders, A. (2017). Rumination mediates the associations between sexual minority stressors and disordered eating, particularly for men. *Eating and Weight Disorders—Studies on Anorexia Bulimia and Obesity, 22*(4), 699–706. https://doi.org/10.1007/s40519-016-0350-0

Warrier, V., Toro, R., Chakrabarti, B., the iPSYCH_Broad Autism Group, Borglum, A. D., Grove, J., the 23andMe Research Team, Hinds, D. A., Bourgeron, T., & Baron-Cohen, S. (2018). Genome-wide analyses of self-reported empathy: Correlations with autism, schizophrenia, and anorexia nervosa. *Translational Psychiatry, 8*(1), 35. https://doi.org/10.1038/s41398-017-0082-6

Watkins, J. A., Sargent, R. G., Miller, P. M., Ureda, J. R., Drane, W. J., & Richler, D. L. (2001). A study of the attribution style, self-efficacy, and dietary restraint in female binge and non-binge eaters. *Eating and Weight Disorders, 6*(4), 188–196. http://www.ncbi.nlm.nih.gov/pubmed/11808814

Watson, K. K., Werling, D. M., Zucker, N. L., & Platt, M. L. (2010). Altered social reward and attention in anorexia nervosa. *Frontiers in Psychology, 1*, 36. https://doi.org/10.3389/fpsyg.2010.00036

Watson, L. B., Velez, B. L., Brownfield, J., & Flores, M. J. (2016). Minority stress and bisexual women's disordered eating: The role of maladaptive coping. *Counseling Psychologist, 44*(8), 1158–1186. https://doi.org/10.1177/0011000016669233

Westwood, H., Lawrence, V., Fleming, C., & Tchanturia, K. (2016). Exploration of friendship experiences, before and after illness onset in females with anorexia nervosa: A qualitative study. *PLOS ONE, 11*(9), e0163528. https://doi.org/10.1371/journal.pone.0163528

Wilczyński, K., Cichoń, L., Auguściak-Duma, A., Sieroń, A., & Janas-Kozik, M. (2021). Association between single nucleotide polymorphisms in oxytocin and vasopressin receptor genes and symptom severity of autism spectrum disorder—Preliminary study. *European Psychiatry, 64*(S1), S83–S84. https://doi.org/10.1192/j.eurpsy.2021.250

Xu, J., Harper, J. A., Van Enkevort, E. A., Latimer, K., Kelley, U., & McAdams, C. J. (2017). Neural activations are related to body-shape, anxiety, and outcomes in adolescent anorexia nervosa. *Journal of Psychiatric Research, 87*, 1–7. https://doi.org/10.1016/j.jpsychires.2016.12.005

Zachry, J. E., Nolan, S. O., Brady, L. J., Kelly, S. J., Siciliano, C. A., & Calipari, E. S. (2021). Sex differences in dopamine release regulation in the striatum. *Neuropsychopharmacology, 46*(3), 491–499. https://doi.org/10.1038/s41386-020-00915-1

Zucker, N., Moskovich, A., Bulik, C. M., Merwin, R., Gaddis, K., Losh, M., Piven, J., Wagner, H. R., & LaBar, K. S. (2013). Perception of affect in biological motion cues in anorexia nervosa [Research Support, NIH, Extramural]. *The International Journal of Eating Disorders, 46*(1), 12–22. https://doi.org/10.1002/eat.22062

10

Inhibitory Control in Binge-Type Eating Disorders

Valentina Cardi and Natalia Lawrence

Brief Definitional Overview

Inhibitory control: A key component of executive function that is essential for flexible, goal-directed behavior. It enables individuals to suppress attention, thoughts, and actions that are inappropriate, irrelevant, or suboptimal, such as urges to eat energy-dense foods when trying to maintain a healthy diet (Verbruggen et al., 2014a; Bari and Robbins, 2013).

Response inhibition: A behavioral index of inhibitory control that involves the inhibition of a planned response ("action restraint") or the inhibition of an already initiated action ("action cancellation") (Schachar et al., 2007).

Introduction

Weak inhibitory control has been associated with the loss of control over eating seen in people with binge-type eating disorders (Carr et al., 2021; Giel et al., 2017; Steward & Berner 2020). Weak inhibitory control is not specific to eating disorders; it has also been implicated in attention deficit/hyperactivity disorder, obsessive-compulsive disorder, substance use disorder, and mood disorders (Bari & Robbins, 2013; Verbruggen & Logan, 2008; Wright et al., 2014). Furthermore, it is a key component of self-regulation, which is associated with diverse health, financial, and interpersonal outcomes (Moffat et al., 2011; Tangney et al., 2004). In view of its importance, there have been considerable efforts to develop interventions that improve inhibitory control, and some of these will be considered in the context of treating eating disorders (see the "Implications" section of this chapter). Whilst individual differences in inhibitory control (and executive function more broadly) are highly heritable (Friedman et al., 2008), interventions that aim to boost inhibitory control, or compensate for poor inhibitory control, show some promising effects in helping individuals regulate their eating behavior.

Valentina Cardi and Natalia Lawrence, *Inhibitory Control in Binge-Type Eating Disorders*. In: *The Handbook of the Neurobiology of Eating Disorders*. Edited by: Christina E. Wierenga and Joanna E. Steinglass, Oxford University Press.
 DOI: 10.1093/9780197675212.003.0011

Measurement of inhibitory control

Inhibitory control can be assessed using self-report questionnaires, and some of these have shown associations with binge eating, such as attentional and motor impulsivity on the Barratt Impulsiveness scale (Meule & Platte, 2015; Oliva et al., 2019; Rosval et al., 2006), and negative urgency (the tendency to act rashly when distressed) on the Urgency-Premeditation-Perseverance-Sensation Seeking-Positive Urgency (UPPS-P) impulsive behavior scale (Anestis et al., 2009; Fischer et al., 2012; Kelly et al., 2014). However, inhibitory control is more commonly measured objectively using computerized reaction time tasks such as the go/no-go and stop-signal tasks. Although inhibitory control is involved in performance on a range of tests of executive function (Friedman et al., 2008), the go/no-go and stop-signal tasks are specifically used to measure response inhibition (although attention and response selection are also involved) (Verbruggen et al., 2014a).

The go/no-go task requires participants to respond to some stimuli (e.g., press a key for arrows pointing to the left) and to inhibit responses to others (e.g., do not press anything for arrows pointing to the right). Poor inhibitory control ability is indexed by a higher proportion of unsuccessful inhibitions on "no-go" trials. The stop-signal task requires participants to respond to all stimuli (e.g., press with your left index finger for a left-pointing arrow and press with your right index finger for a right-pointing arrow) except when a stop-signal is presented after a variable delay. The stop-signal can be visual or auditory and the delay of its onset is often calibrated (from a starting delay of ~250 ms) according to performance, becoming shorter with unsuccessful stop responses (which makes stopping easier), and longer with successful stops. The stop-signal task enables the measurement of the latency and efficacy of the stop process via estimation of a "stop-signal reaction time" (Verbruggen & Logan, 2008). Both the go/no-go and stop-signal tasks include a majority of "go" trials to elicit a prepotent response tendency and to place greater demands on inhibition during stop trials. However, they involve partly dissociable forms of response inhibition; the go/no-go task measures the inhibition of a planned response ("action restraint") whereas the stop-signal task measures the inhibition of an already initiated action ("action cancellation") (Schachar et al., 2007). Deficits in both tasks have been associated with eating disorders, with more consistent impairments in bulimia nervosa (BN) (Steward & Berner, 2020; Wu et al., 2013) and several positive, albeit more mixed findings in binge-eating disorder (BED) (Carr et al., 2021; Giel et al., 2017).

Response inhibition is conceptualized as a "race" between the competing "go" and "stop" processes, which the latter must win for successful inhibition to occur (Verbruggen & Logan, 2008). The likelihood of stopping is therefore influenced by the strength and speed of the "go" response, which tends to be greater for stimuli that are associated with rewarding outcomes and previous go responses, such as palatable, energy-dense food (Bianco et al., 2023; Meule et al., 2014). There are individual differences in the motivating properties of food, with those at risk of binge-type eating disorders showing enhanced attentional bias (attention capture), neural and behavioral reward responses, and motor excitation (preparedness to respond) in response to food (Giel et al., 2017; Treasure et al., 2018; Wonderlich et al., 2021). It is important to examine both general and food-specific inhibitory control in eating disorders because abnormalities may point to different underlying mechanisms and targets for intervention (e.g., deficient stopping ability in the former vs. increased food reward in the latter). It is also useful to examine measures of other types of impulsivity that are more sensitive to food reward than response inhibition, such as increased delayed discounting (tendency not to delay gratification). Evidence suggests that increased delay discounting (preference for immediate vs. delayed gratification) may be more consistently observed than deficient response inhibition in BED, whereas both may be a feature of BN (Carr et al., 2021; Steward & Berner, 2020; Wu et al., 2013). However, both deficient response inhibition and increased food incentive value have also been associated with overeating and obesity (Stice et al., 2016) and more studies in samples matched for body mass index (BMI) are needed to confirm whether these are a particular feature of BED and BN (Carr et al., 2021; Grant & Chamberlain, 2020; Veit et al., 2021).

A further important distinction should be made between the typical view of inhibitory control as a voluntary "top-down" process of executive function, mediated by the prefrontal cortex (Miller & Cohen, 2001), and more automatic, stimulus-driven, "bottom-up" forms of response inhibition (Verbruggen et al., 2014b). The latter can be achieved when certain stimuli are repeatedly associated with stop responses, such that this becomes the default or automatic response (Verbruggen & Logan, 2008). While most studies showing deficient inhibitory control in eating disorders have measured "top-down" response inhibition, intervention studies vary in whether they aim to strengthen "top-down" inhibitory control (e.g., via general cognitive training tasks) or build "bottom-up" inhibitory responses (e.g., via training associative inhibition to certain food images) (Chami et al., 2020). The former tends to show poor generalization to real-world behavior, but the latter shows promise in reducing eating disorder symptoms, including binge eating and the overvaluation of palatable foods (see the "Implications" section of this chapter).

Biological Framework

The stopping process, which is estimated to occur within 220 ms of a stop signal, activates a well-established cortico-thalamic neural network that results in the suppression of motor responses (Hannah & Aron, 2021). Early activation of the right inferior frontal cortex (rIFC, pars opercularis) and the pre-supplementary motor area (pre-SMA) within 120 ms of the stop signal is followed by a global suppression of the primary motor cortex (within 140ms), via interconnecting subcortical motor regions (the subthalamic nucleus, basal ganglia, and thalamus; for a detailed description, see Hannah & Aron, 2021).

Performance on response inhibition tasks more broadly (i.e., go/no-go and stop-signal tasks) has been associated with activation in frontostriatal networks—in the left and right inferior and middle frontal gyri, right superior frontal gyrus, anterior cingulate cortex, anterior insula, subthalamic nucleus, pre-SMA, and dorsal aspects of the striatum (Aron, 2011; Steward & Berner, 2020). There have been limited neuroimaging studies of response inhibition in binge-type eating disorders, but several findings using a range of neuroimaging modalities suggest reduced activity in frontostriatal networks during action restraint on no-go trials. Reduced activation in the right dorsolateral prefrontal cortex (DLPFC) during food-related no-go trials, measured using MEG and functional near-infrared spectroscopy, was reported in women with overweight/obesity and BED relative to those without BED (Hege et al., 2015; Veit et al., 2021). Similar findings have emerged from studies using functional magnetic resonance imaging (fMRI), showing decreased right PFC (middle frontal gyrus) and putamen activation during food and non-food no-go trials in normal-weight participants with versus without binge eating (Oliva et al., 2019). More frequent binge eating in women with BN has also been associated with reduced activation, relative to controls, during non-food no-go trials in the dorsal striatum and sensorimotor cortex (Skunde et al., 2016). Similarly, age-dependent decreases in PFC activation (left middle frontal gyrus and subgenual cingulate cortex) to non-food no-go stimuli has been seen in people with BN relative to healthy controls (Dreyfuss et al., 2017). In contrast, PFC activation was increased during food-specific stop trials (but decreased during no-go trials) in Oliva and colleagues' (2019) study of normal weight participants with binge eating. Similarly, increased medial prefrontal cortex and anterior cingular cortex activation during failed response inhibition (stop signal task) at age 14 was associated with the development of binging and purging at ages 16 to 19 (Bartholdy et al., 2019). In addition to altered brain function, those developing binge eating and purging had changes in brain structure (grey matter volume) in basal ganglia, prefrontal, and cingulate cortex regions, including some that are implicated in inhibitory control (Zhang et al., 2021). Therefore, while findings are broadly consistent with the idea that people with binge eating show abnormalities in neural mechanisms underlying response inhibition, particularly in the prefrontal cortex, the specific nature of these changes may vary depending on age- and task-related factors.

State of the Science in Eating Disorders

Inhibitory control difficulties have been most typically investigated in forms of eating disorders characterized by episodes of binge eating. This means that most observational, experimental, and clinical studies have focused on the examination of inhibitory control in patients with BN or BED. Perhaps unsurprisingly, it is difficult to find a high level of concordance across studies, due to clinical heterogeneity of the selected samples (e.g., patients with or without compensatory behaviors, with or without comorbidities with other impulsivity-related disorders, such as substance abuse, and at different stages of recovery), the large variety of assessment methods (e.g., self-report questionnaires, computerized cognitive or neuropsychological tasks), the poor concordance between these methods (Claes et al., 2006; Lijffijt et al., 2004; Wu et al., 2013) and the multiple processes which interact to determine inhibitory control performances (e.g., behavioral and cognitive inhibition). In this section, the evidence related to inhibitory control task performance will be mostly summarized from the highest quality types of publications, namely those of studies using meta-analytic procedures, systematic reviews, or randomized controlled trials.

The systematic review and meta-analysis by Wu and colleagues (2013) is one of the earliest attempts to summarize the neuropsychological evidence of inhibitory control across the spectrum of binge-type eating disorders (encompassing the diagnoses of BN, BED, and anorexia nervosa of the binge/purge subtype [AN-BP]) and to quantitatively estimate the size of these difficulties in patients compared to individuals with no eating disorders. Most of the studies included had been conducted with female patients with BN (N=20 vs. N=3 in anorexia nervosa and N=2 in BED) and differed in the extent to which they described comorbidities with other disorders, enrollment into treatment and use of medication. Seventeen of the 25 studies failed to find impairments in general inhibitory control; however, the meta-analysis highlighted that patients had overall poorer inhibitory control compared to controls (this result was significant and associated with a small effect size). The effect size for inhibitory control deficits was higher in AN-BP than BN. Twelve studies investigated inhibitory control toward disease-relevant stimuli (food/eating, shape/weight) and all had been conducted in patients with BN. Inhibitory control deficits toward food/eating stimuli and weight and shape were significant (medium effect size) in people with BN compared to controls and were significantly larger than those toward general stimuli. Similar findings were reported in later and broader reviews of neurocognitive and executive functioning, including inhibitory control, across the spectrum of eating disorders (Hirst et al., 2017; Smith, Mason et al., 2018). Hirst and colleagues (2017) reviewed the evidence related to executive functioning in people with anorexia nervosa (AN) or BN relative to healthy controls and found that overall executive functioning was significantly lower for all diagnostic groups compared to controls (Hirst et al., 2017). These difficulties were greater in people with BN compared to AN, leading to the hypothesis that patients with AN might strengthen inhibitory control through repeated practice of inhibiting eating behavior (Hirst, et al., 2017).

A year later, Smith and colleagues (2018) summarized the evidence on executive functioning from 28 systematic and meta-analytic reviews, nine of which had focused on the examination of inhibitory control, in adults with binge eating compared to normal weight controls or participants with obesity. In line with Wu and colleagues (2013), greater deficits in inhibitory control were found in response to disorder-relevant stimuli in patients with BED or BN, whereas many studies did not find convincing evidence that patients with BED had poorer general inhibitory control compared to individuals whose weight was in the normal weight or obese range. This synthesis of systematic reviews and meta-analyses concluded that stronger efforts should be made to consider potential confounding variables, such as general psychopathology, nutritional and weight status, duration of illness and developmental stage, tasks and stimuli variability, relationships between neurocognitive domains and between neurocognition and affective processing when examining inhibitory control in eating disorders. Similar conclusions to explain inconsistent findings were described in a later systematic review of impulsivity in clinical or subclinical samples of people with binge-eating episodes (Waltmann et al., 2021).

In line with the quest for more research into patient-, task-, or construct-related variables to explain findings on inhibitory control, more recent studies were published examining these. Miranda-Olivos and colleagues (2021) investigated how inhibitory control is associated with patients' clinical characteristics and found that longer duration of illness (over five years for restrictive AN, 12 years for AN-BP, and 15 years for BN or BED) was associated with a greater risk for impaired performance in inhibitory control tasks (Miranda-Olivos et al., 2021). Smith and colleagues (2019) examined fluctuations and intra-individual variability in inhibitory control to test whether these moderated the associations between negative affect and binge-eating episodes. Women experiencing binge-eating episodes were asked to complete 10-day ecological momentary assessments (i.e., they were asked to provide answers to electronic surveys administered several times a day), including a daily ambulatory go/no-go task. Individuals with poorer inhibitory control toward food cues had a higher likelihood of binge eating during the study. However, in people with binge eating or subthreshold BED and no compensatory behaviors, levels of inhibitory control were not related to the probability of binge eating. On the contrary, for those with compensatory behaviors (people with BN or people with AN-BP), higher negative affect was related to higher probability of binge eating on days characterized by lower inhibitory control toward food cues. This study was the first to investigate how fluctuations in individuals' self-regulatory capacity and negative affect interact in predicting binge eating and how these interactions change across the eating disorder spectrum. However, it only measured inhibitory control once a day and therefore could not disentangle the direction of the relationship between these variables. Recently, an integrated model to explain the onset and maintenance of binge eating has been proposed, based on the interaction between affect, reward, and cognition (Schaefer et al., 2023). This model proposes that negative affect in the moment is likely to increase the reward value of palatable foods, especially when eating is expected to result in affect improvement. Increased food reward would then augment the risk for binge eating especially when inhibitory control is low. To date, these hypotheses remain untested and are likely to find answers through studies examining multiple variables over time, in the laboratory as well as in ecologically relevant contexts.

As part of these investigations, it would be relevant to examine inhibitory control at mealtimes or snack times, with the overall goal to highlight to what extent what is found in response to food pictures translates into real life behaviors. In a study by Berner and colleagues (2022), patients with BN were instructed to complete two inhibitory control tasks, one requiring inhibiting consummatory behavior (i.e., drinking a palatable fruit shake) and one requiring to inhibit button pressing. Women with BN had overall greater inhibitory control difficulties on both tasks, compared to healthy women. Those with greater loss of control over eating and those who felt a stronger urge to binge during the task also demonstrated reduced activation of the prefrontal cortex during eating-related inhibition (Berner et al., 2022).

Overall, the investigation of inhibitory control across the spectrum of eating disorders is moving from lab-based studies toward the integration of lab-based evaluations with ecological momentary paradigms that examine inhibitory control in relation to affective, cognitive, and motivation variables. Individual patterns of relationships are likely to shape the development and implementation of personalized interventions which might be triggered in real time, and in patients' own environments, at times when inhibitory control is weaker and likely to constitute a risk factor for unhelpful eating behaviors, such as binge eating.

Implications

Based on plausible deficits in food-specific inhibitory control toward food stimuli in patients experiencing binge-eating episodes, it has been hypothesized that computerized or mobile-based trainings to remediate these difficulties might be of benefit in reducing loss of control over eating and perceived food-related reward (i.e., liking of highly palatable foods). A systematic review of the effect of food-related inhibitory control training on eating behavior or weight change (Turton et al., 2016), found that inhibitory control trainings produced a small- to medium-sized reduction in food intake, compared to a control condition. The reviewed studies included computer tasks that trained "bottom-up" inhibitory responses to specific food images. Surprisingly, at the time when the review was conducted, studies in clinical populations had not been published and therefore findings referred to non-clinical samples only. Six years later, Ince and colleagues (2021) reviewed studies examining the effectiveness of treatment approaches targeting impulsivity, including inhibitory control toward food stimuli, in patients with binge eating. The review included psychotherapy, computerized cognitive training, neuromodulation, and pharmacological approaches. The effectiveness of these treatments was assessed against a control condition (other treatment or waiting list). Findings on computer-based trainings specifically indicated that although there was some evidence that these trainings increased inhibitory control, they did not appear superior to other treatment approaches in decreasing binge-eating frequency or food cravings. One hypothesis for the lack of superiority effect when food-specific inhibitory control training was compared to a condition also including some forms of food exposure was that cue exposure itself might have worked as the active ingredient of clinical change, rather than inhibitory training specifically. This hypothesis remains to be tested in trials comparing cue exposure with food-specific inhibitory control trainings.

Our own research groups have tested food-specific inhibitory control training in patients with BN or BED over a series of pilot randomized controlled trials. In the first study, patients were allocated to computer-based food-specific inhibitory control training or general (non-food) inhibitory control training (Chami et al., 2020). The conditions included, respectively, a food or general goal planning intervention. The recruitment, retention, and adherence rates that had been pre-set were met and binge-eating frequency, eating disorder psychopathology, and food reward value (i.e., food liking) decreased in both groups, which was maintained at follow-up, with a larger effect size for the food-specific condition. In the second study (Keeler et al., 2022), patients with binge-eating episodes were randomized to receive an app-based, food-specific inhibitory control training (tailored to their own hard-to-resist/binge foods) in addition to treatment as usual or to treatment as usual alone. Again, the feasibility parameters were met or exceeded, and findings indicated that both groups reduced binge-eating frequency with greater improvements in secondary outcomes (food liking and eating disorder psychopathology) in the training condition. A third trial was conducted in Italy in a community sample of individuals who self-reported binge-eating symptoms (Cardi et al., 2022). Participants were randomly allocated to the app-based, food-specific inhibitory control training or waiting list. This trial also confirmed the pre-specified feasibility criteria and indicated that those in the training condition reported lower food-related reward (food liking), lower perceived hunger, and lower levels of depressive symptoms compared to the control condition, although no changes in eating behavior were found between conditions (Cardi et al., 2022).

All together these studies replicate the finding that it is possible to train food-specific inhibitory control in patients with binge-type eating disorders and that computerized or mobile app trainings are associated with some clinical benefit. However, similarly to other forms of clinical interventions for eating disorders (e.g., psychotherapy, pharmacotherapy), it is becoming increasingly apparent that more than one therapeutic strategy might be needed at the same time to target the same or similarly implicated mechanisms of the illness. An example of such approaches with regard to inhibitory control training is the ACCElect pilot randomized controlled trial (Giel et al., 2023). This study tested six sessions of food-specific inhibitory control combined with transcranial direct current stimulation (tDCS) of the right dorsolateral prefrontal cortex in patients with BED. The experimental condition was tested against a sham stimulation on reductions in the frequency of binge-eating episodes four weeks after the end of treatment (Giel et al., 2023). Findings indicated that the frequency of binge eating reduced more in the experimental condition, a change which was maintained over time (Giel et al., 2023).

The findings of these pilot randomized controlled trials will need to be replicated and expanded in larger randomized controlled trials of inhibitory control training, along with further elucidation of underlying mechanisms. Indeed, although it may be hard to believe that repeatedly practicing a manual stop response on a computer keyboard in response to images of food can translate into reduced food intake, there is accumulating evidence of high levels of generalizability from the stopping of manual responses to a range of real-world actions, including speech and gait (Hannah & Aron, 2021), perhaps due to the global suppression of motor responding that is involved in response inhibition.

Alternative Perspectives

The findings summarized so far seem to point toward the existence of food-specific inhibitory control difficulties in forms of eating disorders characterized by loss of control over eating. Despite this overall agreement, several questions remain unanswered and will require further experimental testing. Some of these questions, and some tentative answers from different perspectives, are discussed next.

How do different aspects of cognitive control (beyond inhibitory control) vary across the eating disorders spectrum?

Cognitive control is an umbrella term which encompasses different abilities, such as those used to inhibit motor responses, to switch between different sets of rules to complete tasks, and to allocate attention and update working memory. These abilities are variously implicated in the maintenance of different forms of eating disorders (e.g., Wonderlich et al., 2021). For example, cognitive flexibility seems to be impaired in AN (Smith, Mason, et al., 2018; see also Chapter 11), whereas mixed findings have been highlighted in BN, with some studies finding intact cognitive flexibility-related abilities (e.g., Abber et al., 2022). Similarly, AN has been associated with features compatible with increased cognitive control (e.g., perfectionism, obsessionality), whereas binge eating has been associated with lower cognitive control (Wonderlich et al., 2021). Visuospatial abilities have shown some degree of impairment in AN, but not BN (Degortes et al., 2016). These findings indicate a large heterogeneity in the performance of various constructs of cognitive control (including, and beyond inhibitory control) in patients with different types of eating disorders. Overall, they seem to point toward the presence of different cognitive profiles across subgroups of patients characterized by restrictive eating and weight loss or normal weight (and above) and episodes of overeating.

How does inhibitory control relate to affective processing?

As highlighted in recent models of eating disorders and by findings from ecological momentary assessments, it is likely that inhibitory control performance changes over time and across situations, and that it triggers the onset and/or maintenance of binge-eating symptoms through its complex relationship with affective processes, including reward sensitivity. A recent study by Murray and colleagues (2023) investigated the interaction within and between areas of the brain associated with cognitive functioning and reward perception in pre-adolescents with BED and found a widespread dysconnectivity between the nodes of these networks, replicating what was found in adults with BED (Haynos et al., 2021). It is possible that a disrupted synergy between cognitive control and reward-related brain areas contributes to the maintenance of binge-eating symptoms.

Furthermore, women with loss of control over eating report higher impulsivity, especially under negative mood (Racine et al., 2015), and patients with binge eating report both greater impulsivity and emotion regulation difficulties compared to controls (Leehr et al., 2018). Interestingly, not all negative emotions seem to be associated with poorer inhibitory control. Indeed, a study by Brassard and colleagues (2023) found that the emotion of disgust (and contamination-based disgust, in particular) is associated with greater behavioral inhibition. The findings of these studies highlight the complexity of the processes that might co-occur to explain inhibitory control difficulties in patients with eating disorders; examples of these are negative affect and the use of unhelpful emotion regulation strategies. This evidence thus strengthens the importance of developing more complex theoretical models of maintaining mechanisms, to inform the development of novel hypotheses and treatments.

To what extent could inhibitory control be explained by psychiatric disorders comorbid with binge-type eating disorders?

Depression is highly comorbid with BED (66%; Udo et al., 2019) and is also associated with response inhibition deficits (Wright et al., 2014). Impulse-control disorders, such as attention-deficit/hyperactivity disorder, oppositional defiant disorder, and conduct disorder, are also prevalent in BN and BED, and may contribute to the observed abnormalities in inhibitory control (Hudson et al., 2007; Yao et al., 2019). Indeed, recent evidence suggests that structural brain abnormalities associated with impulse-control disorders at age 14, such as reduced frontal and cingulate cortex grey matter volume, are associated with the development of binge eating and purging, and depression at ages 16 to 19 (Zhang et al., 2021).

These neural risk factors may therefore underlie the deficits in inhibitory control that are common to BN, BED, and comorbid disorders and lack specificity for a certain diagnosis or symptoms.

Do inhibitory control deficits constitute vulnerability factors or consequences of binge-type eating disorders?

Longitudinal studies are best placed to clarify whether inhibitory control deficits precede or rather follow the onset of binge-eating symptoms. Data from a large European cohort study (the IMAGEN study; Bartholdy et al., 2019) were used to investigate whether neural activity associated with motor inhibitory control at age 14 could predict those who develop binge eating and/or purging symptoms at age 16. Findings indicated that increased recruitment of the medial prefrontal cortex during failures to inhibit preceded symptom development and could be considered a biomarker for the future development of abnormal eating behaviors. This is interesting because adolescents did not show a different performance in inhibitory control, but just a different neural response during failed inhibitory control. In line with this finding, negative urgency, a construct of impulsivity, seemed to predict the onset of binge-eating symptoms in school children in combination with negative affect (Pearson et al., 2015). These studies seem to suggest that inhibitory control deficits might precede and contribute to the vulnerability to develop binge-type eating disorders. This possibility is consistent with the aforementioned high heritability of inhibitory control (Friedman et al., 2008).

Conclusions

Despite a large heterogeneity of methods, constructs, and participant variables, the literature seems to indicate that changes in inhibitory control might be implicated in eating disorders, both toward general and disorder-specific stimuli. Inhibitory control difficulties toward non-illness related stimuli might precede the development of eating disorders, as well as the development of comorbid disorders, such as those marked by high trait impulsivity. Weak inhibitory control toward food or disorder-specific stimuli may be more specifically associated with binge-eating symptoms and may develop over time. The integration of multimodal assessment methods in the laboratory, as well as the use of more ecologically valid strategies over time are likely to provide helpful information to predict inhibitory control difficulties in the moment and trigger the use of more helpful strategies. Similarly, the development of complex theoretical models that consider several individual-level variables, such as cognitive, motivational, and emotional processes might provide a useful perspective to improve the science around inhibitory control in psychiatric disorders.

References

Abber, S. R., Forman, E. M., Wierenga, C. E., & Manasse, S. M. (2022). Intact general and food-specific task-switching abilities in bulimia-spectrum eating disorders. *Eating Behaviors, 46*, 101636. https://doi.org/10.1016/j.eatbeh.2022.101636

Anestis, M. D., Smith, A. R., Fink, E. L., & Joiner, T. E. (2009). Dysregulated eating and distress: Examining the specific role of negative urgency in a clinical sample. *Cognitive Therapy and Research, 33*, 390–397. https://doi.org/10.1007/s10608-008-9201-2

Aron, A. R. (2011). From reactive to proactive and selective control: Developing a richer model for stopping inappropriate responses. *Biological Psychiatry 69*, e55–e68.

Bari, A., & Robbins, T. W. (2013). Inhibition and impulsivity: Behavioral and neural basis of response control. *Progress in Neurobiology, 108*, 44–79.

Bartholdy, S., O'Daly, O. G., Campbell, I. C., Banaschewski, T., Barker, G., Bokde, A. L. W., Bromberg, U., Büchel, C., Quinlan, E. B., Desrivières, S., Flor, H., Frouin, V., Garavan, H., Gowland, P., Heinz, A., Ittermann, B., Martinot, J. L., Paillère Martinot, M. L., Nees, F., Orfanos, D. P., . . . IMAGEN Consortium. (2019). Neural correlates of failed inhibitory control as an early marker of disordered eating in adolescents. *Biological Psychiatry, 85*(11), 956–965. https://doi.org/10.1016/j.biopsych.2019.01.027

Berner, L. A., Winter, S. R., Ayaz, H., Shewokis, P. A., Izzetoglu, M., Marsh, R., Nasser, J. A., Matteucci, A. J., & Lowe, M. R. (2022). Altered prefrontal activation during the inhibition of eating responses in women with bulimia nervosa. *Psychological Medicine*, 53(8), 3580–3590. https://doi.org/10.1017/S0033291722000198

Bianco, V., Veniero, D., D'Acunto, A., Koch, G., & Picazio, S. (2023) Challenging inhibitory control with high- and low-calorie food: A behavioural and TMS study. *Frontiers in Nutrition, 10*, 1016017. https://doi.org/10.3389/fnut.2023.1016017

Brassard, S. L., Laliberte, M., MacKillop, J., & Balodis, I. M. (2023). Disgust sensitivity and behavioural inhibitory systems in binge eating disorder: Associations with eating pathology. *Eating and Weight Disorders, 28*(15), 15. https://doi.org/10.1007/s40519-023-01544-5

Cardi, V., Meregalli, V., Di Rosa, E., Derrigo, R., Faustini, C., Keeler, J. L., Favaro, A., Treasure, J., & Lawrence, N. (2022). A community-based feasibility randomized controlled study to test food-specific inhibitory control training in people with disinhibited eating during COVID-19 in Italy. *Eating and Weight Disorders, 27*(7), 2745–2757. https://doi.org/10.1007/s40519-022-01411-9

Carr, M. M., Wiedemann, A. A., Macdonald-Gagnon, G., & Potenza, M. N. (2021). Impulsivity and compulsivity in binge eating disorder: A systematic review of behavioral studies. *Progress in Neuro-Psychopharmacology and Biological Psychiatry, 110*, 110318. https://doi.org/10.1016/j.pnpbp.2021.110318

Chami, R., Cardi, V., Lawrence, N., Macdonald, P., Rowlands, K., Hodsoll, J., & Treasure, J. (2020). Targeting binge eating in bulimia nervosa and binge eating disorder using inhibitory control training and implementation intentions: A feasibility trial. *Psychological Medicine*, 52(5), 874–883. https://doi.org/10.1017/S0033291720002494

Claes, L., Nederkoorn, C., Vandereycken, W., Guerrieri, R., & Vertommen, H. (2006). Impulsiveness and lack of inhibitory control in eating disorders. *Eating Behaviors, 7*: 196–203.

Degortes, D., Tenconi, E., Santonastaso, P., & Favaro, A. (2016). Executive functioning and visuospatial abilities in bulimia nervosa with or without a previous history of anorexia nervosa. *European Eating Disorders Review, 24*(2):139–146. https://doi.org/10.1002/erv.2430.

Dreyfuss, M. F. W., Riegel, M. L., Pedersen, G. A., Cohen, A. O., Silverman, M. R., Dyke, J. P.,Mayer, L. E. S.,Walsh, B. T.,Casey, B. J., & Broft, A. I. (2017) Patients with bulimia nervosa do not show typical neurodevelopment of cognitive control under emotional influences. *Psychiatry Research. Neuroimaging, 266*, 59–65. https://doi.org/10.1016/j.pscychresns.2017.05.001

Fischer, S., Settles, R., Collins, B., Gunn, R., Smith, G. T. (2012). The role of negative urgency and expectancies in problem drinking and disordered eating: Testing a model of comorbidity in pathological and at-risk samples. *Psychology of Addictive Behaviors, 26*, 112–123. http://dx.doi.org/10.1037/a0023460.

Friedman, N. P., Miyake, A., Young, S. E., DeFries, J. C., Corley, R. P., & Hewitt, J. K. (2008). Individual differences in executive functions are almost entirely genetic in origin. *Journal of Experimental Psychology: General, 137*(2), 201–225. https://doi.org/10.1037/0096-3445.137.2.201

Giel, K., Teufel, M., Junne, F., Zipfel, S., & Schag, K. (2017). Food-related impulsivity in obesity and binge eating disorder—A systematic update of the evidence. *Nutrients, 9*(11), 1170. http://dx.doi.org/10.3390/nu9111170

Giel, K. E., Schag, K., Max, S. M., Martus, P., Zipfel, S., Fallgatter, A. J., & Plewnia, C. (2023). Inhibitory control training enhanced by transcranial direct current stimulation to reduce binge eating episodes: Findings from the randomized phase II ACCElect trial. *Psychotherapy and Psychosomatics*, *92*(2), 101–112. https://doi.org/10.1159/000529117.

Grant, J. E., & Chamberlain, S. R. (2020). Neurocognitive findings in young adults with binge eating disorder. *International Journal of Psychiatry in Clinical Practice*, *24*(1), 71–76.

Haynos, A. F., Camchong, J., Pearson, C. M., Lavender, J. M., Mueller, B. A., Peterson, C. B., Specker, S., Raymond, N., & Lim, K. O. (2021). Resting-state hypoconnectivity of reward networks in binge eating disorders. *Cerebral Cortex*, *31*(5), 2494–2504.

Hannah, R., & Aron, A. R. (2021). Towards real-world generalizability of a circuit for action-stopping. *Nature Reviews Neuroscience*, *22*(9), 538–552.

Hege, M. A., Stingl, K. T., Kullmann, S., Schag, K., Giel, K. E., Zipfel, S., & Preissl, H. (2015). Attentional impulsivity in binge eating disorder modulates response inhibition performance and frontal brain networks. *International Journal of Obesity*, *39*, 353–360. https://doi.org/10.1038/ijo.2014.99

Hirst, R., Beard, C., Colby, K., Quittner, Z., Mills, B., & Lavender, J. (2017). Anorexia nervosa and bulimia nervosa: A meta-analysis of executive functioning. *Neuroscience & Biobehavior Reviews*, *83*, 678–690. https://doi.org/10.1016/j.neubiorev.2017.08.011.

Hudson, J. I., Hiripi, E., Pope, H. G. Jr., & Kessler, R. C. (2007). The prevalence and correlates of eating disorders in the National Comorbidity Survey Replication. *Biological Psychiatry*, *61*, 348–358.

Ince, B., Schlatter, J., Max, S., Plewnia, C., Zipfel, S., Giel, K. E., & Schag, K. (2021). Can we change binge eating behaviour by interventions addressing food-related impulsivity? A systematic review. *Journal of Eating Disorders*, *9*(1), 38. https://doi.org/10.1186/s40337-021-00384-x

Keeler, J. L., Chami, R., Cardi, V., Hodsoll, J., Bonin, E., MacDonald, P., Treasure, J., & Lawrence, N. (2022). App-based food-specific inhibitory control training as an adjunct to treatment as usual in binge-type eating disorders: A feasibility trial. *Appetite*, *168*. https://doi.org/10.1016/J.APPET.2021.105788

Kelly, N. R., Cotter, E. W., & Mazzeo, S. E. (2014). Examining the role of distress tolerance and negative urgency in binge eating behavior among women. *Eating Behaviors*, *15*(3), 483–489, https://doi.org/10.1016/j.eatbeh.2014.06.012

Leehr, E. J., Schag, K., Dresler, T., Grosse-Wentrup, M., Hautzinger, M., Fallgatter, A. J., Zipfel, S., Giel, K. E., & Ehlis, A. C. (2018). Food specific inhibitory control under negative mood in binge eating disorder: Evidence from a multimethod approach. *International Journal of Eating Disorders*, *51*(2), 112–123. https://doi.org/10.1002/eat.22818

Lijffijt, M., Bekker, E. M., Quik, E. H., Bakker, J., Kenemans, J. L., & Verbaten, M. N. (2004). Differences between low and high trait impulsivity are not associated with differences in inhibitory motor control. *Journal of Attention Disorders*, *8*: 25–32.

Meule, A., Lutz, A. P., Krawietz, V., Stützer, J., Vögele, C., & Kübler, A. (2014). Food-cue affected motor response inhibition and self-reported dieting success: a pictorial affective shifting task. *Frontiers in Psychology*, *5*, 216.

Meule, A., & Platte, P. (2015). Facets of impulsivity interactively predict body fat and binge eating in young women. *Appetite*, *87*, 352–357.

Miller, E. K. & Cohen, J. D. (2001). An integrative theory of prefrontal cortex function. *Annual Review of Neuroscience*, *24*, 167–202.

Miranda-Olivos, R., Testa, G., Lucas, I., Sánchez, I., Sánchez-González, J., Granero, R., Jiménez-Murcia, S., & Fernández-Aranda, F. (2021). Clinical factors predicting impaired executive functions in eating disorders: The role of illness duration. *Journal of Psychiatric Research*, *144*, 87–95. https://doi.org/10.1016/j.jpsychires.2021.09.042

Moffitt, T. E., Arseneault, L., Belsky, D., Dickson, N., Hancox, R. J., Harrington, H., Houts, R., Poulton, R., Roberts, B. W., Ross, S., Sears, M. R., Thomson, W. M., & Caspi, A. (2011). A gradient of childhood self-control predicts health, wealth, and public safety. *Proceedings of the National Academy of Sciences USA*, *108*(7), 2693–2698. https://doi.org/10.1073/pnas.1010076108

Murray, S. B.,Alba, C.,Duval, C. J.,Nagata, J. M.,Cabeen, R. P.,Lee, D. J.,Toga, A. W.,Siegel, S. J., & Jann, K. (2023). Aberrant functional connectivity between reward and inhibitory control networks in pre-adolescent binge eating disorder. *Psychological Medicine*, *18*, 1–10. https://doi.org/10.1017/S0033291722000514

Oliva, R., Morys, F., Horstmann, A., Castiello, U., & Begliomini, C. (2019). The impulsive brain: neural underpinnings of binge eating behavior in normal weight adults. *Appetite*, *136*, 33–49. https://doi.org/10.1016/j.appet.2018.12.043

Pearson, C. M., Zapolski, T. C. B., & Smith, G. T. (2015). A longitudinal test of impulsivity and depression pathways to early binge eating onset. *International Journal of Eating Disorders*, *48*(2), 230–237. https://doi.org/10.1002/eat.22277

Racine, S. E., Burt, S. A., Keel, P. K., Sisk, C. L., Neale, M. C., Boker, S., & Klump, K. L. (2015). Examining associations between negative urgency and key components of objective binge episodes. *International Journal of Eating Disorders*, *48*(5), 527–531. https://doi.org/10.1002/eat.22412

Rosval, L., Steiger, H., Bruce, K., Israel, M., Richardson, J., & Aubut, M. (2006). Impulsivity in women with eating disorders: Problem of response inhibition, planning, or attention? *International Journal of Eating Disorders*, *39*, 590–593. https://doi.org/10.1002/eat.20296

Schachar, R.,Logan, G. D.,Robaey, P.,Chen, S.,Ickowicz, A., & Barr, C. (2007). Restraint and cancellation: Multiple inhibition deficits in attention deficit hyperactivity disorder *Journal of Abnormal Child Psychology*, *35*, 229–238.

Schaefer, L. M., Forester, G., Dvorak, R. D., Steinglass, J., & Wonderlich, S. A. (2023). Integrating aspects of affect, reward, and cognition to develop more comprehensive models of binge-eating pathology. *International Journal of Eating Disorders*, 56(8), 1502–1510. https://doi.org/10.1002/eat.23971

Skunde, M., Walther, S., Simon, J. J., Wu, M., Bendszus, M., Herzog, W., & Friederich, H. C. (2016). Neural signature of behavioural inhibition in women with bulimia nervosa. *Journal of Psychiatry Neuroscience*, *41*, E69–E78. https://doi.org/10.1503/jpn.150335

Smith, K. E., Mason, T. B., Crosby, R. D., Engel, S. G., & Wonderlich, S. A. (2019). A multimodal, naturalistic investigation of relationships between behavioral impulsivity, affect, and binge eating. *Appetite*, *136*, 50–57. https://doi.org/10.1016/j.appet.2019.01.014

Smith, K. E., Mason, T. B., Johnson, J. S., Lavender, J. M., & Wonderlich, S. A. (2018). A systematic review of reviews of neurocognitive functioning in eating disorders: The state-of-the-literature and future directions. *International Journal of Eating Disorders*, *51*(8), 798–821. https://doi.org/10.1002/eat.22929

Steward, T., & Berner, L.A. (2020). The neurobiological basis of executive function alterations in binge eating populations. In G. Frank &L. Berner (Eds.), *Binge eating*, 137–152. Springer. https://doi.org/10.1007/978-3-030-43562-2_10

Stice, E., Lawrence, N. S., Kemps, E., & Veling, H. (2016). Training motor responses to food: A novel treatment for obesity targeting implicit processes. *Clinical Psychology Review*, *49*, 16–27.

Tangney, J. P., Baumeister, R. F., & Boone, A. L. (2004). High self-control predicts good adjustment, less pathology, better grades, and interpersonal success. *Journal of Personality*, *72*(2), 271–324.

Treasure, J., Leslie, M., Chami, R., & Fernández-Aranda, F. (2018). Are trans diagnostic models of eating disorders fit for purpose? A consideration of the evidence for food addiction. *European Eating Disorders Review*, 26, 83–91. https://doi.org/10.1002/erv.2578

Turton, R., Bruidegom, K., Cardi, V., Hirsch, C. R., & Treasure, J. (2016). Novel methods to help develop healthier eating habits for eating and weight disorders: A systematic review and meta-analysis. *Neuroscience & Biobehavioral Reviews*, *61*, 132–155.

Udo, T., Bitley, S., & Grilo, C.M. (2019). Suicide attempts in US adults with lifetime DSM-5 eating disorders. *BMC Medicine*, *17* (1), 1–13.

Veit, R., Schag, K., Schopf, E., Borutta, M., Kreutzer, J., Ehlis, A. C., Zipfel, S., Giel, K. E., Preissl, H., & Kullmann, S. (2021). Diminished prefrontal cortex activation in patients with binge eating disorder associates with trait impulsivity and improves after impulsivity-focused treatment based on a randomized controlled IMPULS trial. *NeuroImage: Clinical*, *30*, 102679.

Verbruggen, F., Best, M., Bowditch, W. A., Stevens, T., & McLaren, I. P. (2014b). The inhibitory control reflex. *Neuropsychologia*, *65*, 263–278.

Verbruggen, F., & Logan, G. D. (2008). Response inhibition in the stop-signal paradigm. *Trends in Cognitive Sciences*, *12*, 418–424. https://doi.org/10.1016/j.tics.2008.07.005

Verbruggen, F., McLaren, I. P. L., & Chambers, C. D. (2014a). Banishing the control homunculi in studies of action control and behavior change. *Perspectives on Psychological Science*, *9*, 497–524.

Waltmann, M., Herzog, N., Horstmann, A., & Deserno, L. (2021). Loss of control over eating: A systematic review of task based research into impulsive and compulsive processes in binge eating. *Neuroscience & Biobehavioral Reviews*, *129*, 330–350. https://doi.org/10.1016/j.neubiorev.2021.07.016.

Wonderlich, J. A., Bershad, M., & Steinglass, J. E. (2021). Exploring neural mechanisms related to cognitive control, reward, and affect in eating disorders: A narrative review of FMRI studies. *Neuropsychiatric Disease and Treatment*, 17, 2053–2062.

Wu, M., Giel, K. E., Skunde, M., Schag, K., Rudofsky, G., de Zwaan, M., Zipfel, S., Herzog, W., & Friederich, H.-C. (2013). Inhibitory control and decision making under risk in bulimia nervosa and binge-eating disorder. *International Journal of Eating Disorders*, *46*, 721–728. https://doi.org/10.1002/eat.22143

Wright, L., Lipszyc, J., Dupuis, A., Thayapararajah, S.W., & Schachar, R., 2014. Response inhibition and psychopathology: A meta-analysis of go/no-go task performance. *Journal of Abnormal Psychology*, *123*(2), 429.

Yao, S., Kuja-Halkola, R., Martin, J., Lu, Y., Lichtenstein, P., Norring, C., Birgegård, A., Yilmaz, Z., Hübel, C., Watson, H., Baker, J., Almqvist, C., Eating Disorders Working Group of the Psychiatric Genomics Consortium, Thornton, L. M., Magnusson, P. K., Bulik, C. M., & Larsson, H. (2019). Associations between attention-deficit/hyperactivity disorder and various eating disorders: A Swedish nationwide population study using multiple genetically informative approaches. *Biological Psychiatry*, *86*, 577–586.

Zhang, Z., Robinson, L., Jia, T., Quinlan, E. B., Tay, N., Chu, C., Barker, E. D., Banaschewski, T., Barker, G. J., Bokde, A. L. W., Flor, H., Grigis, A., Garavan, H., Gowland, P., Heinz, A., Ittermann, B., Martinot, J. L., Stringaris, A., Penttilä, J., van Noort, B., Desrivières, S. (2021). Development of disordered eating behaviors and comorbid depressive symptoms in adolescence: Neural and psychopathological predictors. *Biological Psychiatry*, *90*(12), 853–862. https://doi.org/10.1016/j.biopsych.2020.06.003

11

Cognitive Flexibility in Eating Disorders

Andrea Phillipou and Stephanie Miles

Brief Definitional Overview

Cognitive flexibility: The ability to effectively adapt to changes in the environment and/or changing task demands by selectively altering one's thoughts, responses, and/or behaviors (Deák, 2003; Diamond, 2013; Scott, 1962). Cognitive flexibility is an encompassing term which includes set-shifting and task-switching.

Set-shifting: Shifting between different mental sets or rules (Ionescu, 2012). For example, sorting food according to its color versus sorting the same food according to its calorie content. In this example, although the sorting rule has changed and a shift is required in how items are sorted, the overall task (sorting the food) had remained the same.

Task-switching: Switching between several different tasks which each have unique instructions (Badre & Wagner, 2006; Dajani & Uddin, 2015). For example, an experiment using a letter/number stimulus (e.g., 6H) that has trials where the participant must indicate if the number is greater than five and other trials where the participant needs to identify if the letter is a vowel or a consonant.

Introduction

The term cognitive flexibility refers to the ability to adapt to changes in the environment or changing task demands. Cognitive flexibility is a core executive function used in everyday life which is fundamental to changing our perspectives, re-evaluating our thoughts and beliefs, and adjusting to change (Diamond, 2013). Impaired cognitive flexibility has been suggested as a transdiagnostic factor for several mental illnesses (Grant & Chamberlain, 2023) and may be a feature of eating disorders.

From rigid thoughts and perceptions about body size and weight to inflexible rules around exercise and the types, amount, calorie content, and time that food is consumed, cognitive inflexibility appears to be characteristic of the thoughts, cognitions, and behaviors present in individuals with eating disorders.

Andrea Phillipou and Stephanie Miles, *Cognitive Flexibility in Eating Disorders*. In: *The Handbook of the Neurobiology of Eating Disorders*. Edited by: Christina E. Wierenga and Joanna E. Steinglass, Oxford University Press.
 DOI: 10.1093/9780197675212.003.0012

While black-and-white thinking and inflexible behaviors are often considered hallmark features of eating disorders themselves, particularly anorexia nervosa (AN), they also present in other areas of life, such as rituals around daily routines. The rigidity and inflexibility present can be particularly apparent in relation to treatment in eating disorders, whereby individuals with eating disorders can sometimes be reluctant to seek or commit to treatment because the illness can persuade individuals that the eating disorder is not a problem or that it serves an important function (e.g., feeling safe). Within treatment, inflexibility can also present as challenges in exploring alternative and more adaptive coping strategies, as well as a reluctance to change behaviors. Rigidity and inflexibility are often met by frustration from loved ones and treatment teams but are also generally recognized by the individual with the eating disorder themselves.

This chapter will begin with a brief overview of some of the most frequently used tasks measuring cognitive flexibility in eating disorder research, followed by a summary of the neurobiological framework underpinning performance on cognitive flexibility tasks. Next, the current state of the literature will be presented for AN, as well as for the other eating disorders. This chapter will present both research which has included objective neurocognitive tasks to evaluate cognitive flexibility and research which has used subjective self-report questionnaires to assess cognitive flexibility. Finally, this chapter will discuss the implications of gaining a better understanding of cognitive inflexibility in eating disorders.

Measurement of cognitive flexibility

Although there is dispute on how cognitive flexibility is best assessed (Dennis & Vander Wal, 2010; Stedal & Dahlgren, 2015), objective neurocognitive tasks assessing set-shifting are the most widely used method (Johnco et al., 2014), particularly the Wisconsin Cart Sorting Test (WCST) and the Trail Making Test (TMT). The WCST (Grant & Berg, 1948; Heaton, 1981) requires a participant to sort cards according to visual features using examiner feedback to determine the current sorting rule; after a predetermined number of correct sorts, the sorting rule changes without notice and the participant needs to once again use trial and error to learn how to correctly sort the cards. The number of perseverative responses (repetitive responses to ambiguous and non-ambiguous cards on the basis of an incorrect rule) and perseverative errors (perseverative responses to non-ambiguous cards) are typically used as measures of cognitive flexibility (Miles et al., 2021). The TMT (Reitan, 1958) and its iterations (Delis et al., 2001; Delis et al., 2004) requires a participant to first quickly draw a line connecting irregularly placed numbers in numerical order (Part A) and then draw a line between alternating numbers and letters in ascending sequence (i.e., 1, A, 2, B, 3, C, etc.; Part B). Part A is considered to be a baseline assessment of motor speed, working memory, and visuospatial processing and is often subtracted from Part B scores to provide an independent evaluation of cognitive flexibility. The time taken to complete the task and the number of errors made can be used as indicators of cognitive flexibility.

In addition to the WCST and TMT, the Brixton Spatial Anticipation Test (Burgess & Shallice, 1997) is another commonly used visuospatial task which requires a participant to identify and predict sequences. Participants are presented with a simple image of 10 circles across two lines. One circle is shaded, and the task requires the participant to predict which circle will be shaded in the next stimulus. Similar to the WCST, the pattern changes suddenly and participants need to adapt and determine the new sequence. The total number of incorrect responses is used as a measure of cognitive flexibility.

Like other cognitive tasks, performance on these assessments relies on many executive and non-executive processes (e.g., attention, visuospatial scanning, motor movements, learning, and memory), and therefore does not measure cognitive flexibility in isolation (i.e., the task impurity problem). In an attempt to better isolate cognitive flexibility from other executive functions, task-switching paradigms have been developed. In a typical task-switching experiment, participants are required to switch between different tasks or to repeat the same task over several trials. Responses tend to be slower and less accurate on trials that require a participant to switch tasks versus repeat trials, reflecting a cognitive cost referred to as a switch cost (Monsell, 2003). Greater switch costs are thought to reflect poorer cognitive flexibility.

Recently, subjective self-report questionnaires have also been used in some studies to assess cognitive flexibility in people with eating disorders. Self-report assessments are typically comprised of questions that ask about instances of cognitive flexibility or rigidity in everyday life and are responded to using a Likert-type scale. Questions are typically designed to evaluate both behaviors and thinking styles (e.g., "I like to look at difficult situations from many different angles," "sudden changes make me distressed"). The Cognitive Flexibility Scale (CFS) by Martin and Rubin (1995) assesses the aspects of cognitive flexibility that are required for effective communication, including awareness of communication alternatives, willingness to adapt to situations, and self-efficacy in being flexible (Dennis & Vander Wal, 2010; Martin & Rubin, 1995). The Cognitive Flexibility Inventory (CFI) is a brief self-report questionnaire designed to assess an individual's ability to create alternative explanations and solutions for difficult situations (Dennis & Vander Wal, 2010). Other self-report assessments of cognitive flexibility include the cognitive and behavioral shift subscales of the Behaviour Rating Inventory of Executive Functioning (BRIEF), the Detail and Flexibility Questionnaire, and the childhood rigidity and adulthood rigidity subscale of the EATATE Lifetime Diagnostic Interview. Whilst these scales evaluate cognitive flexibility in everyday life, one scale, the Eating Disorder Flexibility Index (Dahlgren et al., 2019) also enquires about eating disorder-specific cognitive flexibility (e.g., "before I can eat, the food has to be plated in a certain way," "I get distressed if I gain weight, no matter what I weigh"). Generally, in these self-report questionnaires a lower score is indicative of poorer cognitive flexibility.

Biological Framework

Cognitive flexibility is a higher-order executive function that relies on a number of cognitive processes. In lab-based experiments, cognitive flexibility involves attention, working memory, inhibition, and decision making (Dajani & Uddin, 2015; Logue & Gould, 2014). As such, the neural networks underlying cognitive flexibility are complex, and brain regions relied on to perform such tasks can vary between different paradigms. Although functional magnetic resonance imaging (fMRI) studies have contributed to a greater understanding of the neurobiological mechanisms involved in cognitive flexibility, research involving fMRI is limited to focusing on tasks that can be implemented within the environment of the MRI scanner, such as computerized tasks requiring responses to be made via a button box. Overall, research shows that cognitive flexibility tasks such as the WCST rely heavily on frontal brain regions, but that cognitive flexibility is likely to involve a broad network of brain areas (Anderson et al., 1991; Mountain & Snow, 1993).

Findings from healthy individuals performing the WCST have indicated that a complex network of brain regions are involved in performing the task, predominantly involving the prefrontal cortex (Buchsbaum et al., 2005; Konishi et al., 1998; Lie et al., 2006; Monchi et al., 2001; Nagahama et al., 2001; Nyhus & Barceló, 2009), but also inferior parietal regions and the anterior cingulate cortex (Buchsbaum et al., 2005; Lie et al., 2006; Monchi et al., 2001; Nagahama et al., 2001). In particular, the dorsolateral prefrontal cortex (DLPFC) has been consistently implicated in performing the WCST (Lie et al., 2006; Monchi et al., 2001; Nagahama et al., 2001). Despite various different types of task-switching tasks being employed across studies, a similar network of frontoparietal brain areas has also been implicated in task-switching paradigms (Kim et al., 2012).

State of the Science in Eating Disorders

Cognitive flexibility in anorexia nervosa

A small body of research has considered if or how cognitive flexibility may relate to eating disorder symptoms in AN. Poor cognitive flexibility has been suggested as an influential factor in the maintenance of AN symptoms and treatment resistance (Lang et al., 2014; Tchanturia et al., 2013; Treasure & Schmidt, 2013). Some research has found associations between cognitive flexibility task performance and body mass index (BMI), illness duration, and/or eating disorder symptoms (Berchio et al., 2023; Duriez et al., 2021; Sternheim et al., 2022); but other studies have not supported these relationships (Miles, Nedeljkovic, Sumner, et al., 2022; Miranda-Olivos et al., 2021; Roberts et al., 2010; Rößner et al., 2017; Tchanturia et al., 2011).

Cognitive flexibility in acute anorexia nervosa

The vast majority of cognitive flexibility research in eating disorders has focused on cognitive flexibility in people who have a current diagnosis of AN ("acute AN"). However, the findings of this body of research have been inconsistent. For the WCST, although many studies have found that adults with acute AN make significantly more perseverative responses and perseverative errors than healthy controls (HCs) (Aloi et al., 2015; Buzzichelli et al., 2018; Nakazato et al., 2010), several other studies have not found significant group differences (Giel et al., 2012; Lao-Kaim et al., 2015; Paslakis et al., 2019; Pignatti & Bernasconi, 2013). For the TMT, findings are also mixed (Abbate-Daga et al., 2011; Collantoni et al., 2023; Giel et al., 2021; Sternheim et al., 2022; Tenconi et al., 2010). The inconsistent findings for the WCST and TMT across the literature could be attributed to several factors including, but not limited to, differences in task administration (computerized vs. pen-and-paper), variations in the outcome variables reported, small sample sizes, and illness duration differences between studies. In research using visuospatial cognitive flexibility tasks, such as the Brixton Spatial Anticipation Test, the findings have been more consistent. Compared to HCs, adults with AN have been shown to make more errors (indicating poorer visuospatial cognitive flexibility), with medium to very large effect sizes reported (Konstantakopoulos et al., 2011; Lounes et al., 2011; Tchanturia et al., 2004). For tasks that target verbal aspects of cognitive flexibility (e.g., verbal fluency tasks requiring shifts between producing unique words starting with different letters), no significant group difference in task performance have been found between adults with acute AN and HCs (Konstantakopoulos et al., 2011; Nikendei et al., 2011; Pignatti & Bernasconi, 2013). Taken together, the literature to date suggests that adults with acute AN may experience difficulties in some aspects of cognitive flexibility (e.g., visuospatial), but the literature is either inconsistent in other aspects (e.g., WCST and TMT) or not evident in some cognitive flexibility domains (e.g., verbal). In adolescent samples, however, findings are much more consistent and the literature suggests that adolescents with acute AN do not significantly differ to HCs in performance on a range of cognitive flexibility tasks including the TMT, WCST, and verbal fluency (Andrés-Perpiña et al., 2011; Berchio et al., 2023; Castro-Fornieles et al., 2019; Lozano-Serra et al., 2014; McAnarney et al., 2011), suggesting that poorer performance in adults may be attributed to psychological and/or biological changes with increased illness length.

The neurobiological underpinnings of cognitive flexibility task performance have been of interest in the AN literature. Decreased activation within the anterior cingulate-striato-thalamic network among individuals with AN during a visual target detection set-shifting task has been reported; however, increased activation in the frontoparietal network indicative of greater cognitive effort and supervisory control has also been found (Zastrow et al., 2009). Similarly, findings of increased frontoparietal network activity in AN has also been reported using the WCST (Lao-Kaim et al., 2015). Other studies have reported reduced activity in the prefrontal cortex in individuals with AN on the WCST (Sato et al., 2013), as well as reduced activity in other regions, such as the posterior cingulate (Berchio et al., 2023). Other studies have failed to find any group differences between AN and HC on brain activity during the WCST (Bohon et al., 2020). Similar to behavioral findings of cognitive flexibility in AN, fMRI findings have also yielded inconsistent results making it difficult to gain an understanding of the neurobiological underpinnings that may be contributing to any differences in individuals with AN.

Cognitive flexibility in weight-restored anorexia nervosa

A very small body of research has investigated cognitive flexibility in people who are weight-restored from AN but experience ongoing eating disorder symptoms; findings are inconsistent with some studies finding significant differences from HCs and others reporting no differences (Bohon et al., 2020; Bühren et al., 2012; Castro-Fornieles et al., 2019; Tenconi et al., 2010). Differences in study designs and participant characteristics (e.g., age, illness duration, weight-restoration duration) may have contributed to the inconsistency in findings across the literature. In both longitudinal and cross-sectional research, significant differences between people with acute AN and people who are weight-restored from AN have not been found for a variety of tasks including the WCST (Bühren et al., 2012; Talbot et al., 2015); however, only a very small number of papers exist comparing illness stages thereby limiting our understanding of how cognitive flexibility may differ between illness states.

Cognitive flexibility in recovered anorexia nervosa

Research suggests that there may be no group differences between adults who have fully recovered from AN (i.e., are weight-restored and do not experience eating disorder symptoms) and HCs on certain cognitive flexibility tasks such as the TMT or verbal fluency tasks (Ely et al., 2016; Nakazato et al., 2010; Nikendei et al., 2011; Roberts et al., 2010; Tchanturia et al., 2004; Tenconi et al., 2010). Results for other cognitive flexibility tasks, such as the WCST and other visuospatial tasks, have been mixed with some studies finding group differences and others not reporting any group differences (Nakazato et al., 2010; Roberts et al., 2010; Talbot et al., 2015; Tchanturia et al., 2004). Statistical limitations (e.g., small sample sizes, unequal group sizes) and/or variations in participant characteristics (e.g., illness duration, recovery duration) may contribute to the inconsistency in findings across different studies. Furthermore, a handful of cross-sectional studies have investigated cognitive flexibility in adults recovered from AN compared to adults with acute AN, reporting no significant differences in task performance (Collantoni et al., 2023; Danner et al., 2012; Tenconi et al., 2010).

Cognitive flexibility in other eating disorders

While there has been significant interest in understanding potential issues with cognitive flexibility in individuals with AN, there has been much less research interest in the other eating disorders, such as bulimia nervosa (BN) and binge-eating disorder (BED). Unlike AN, which can be associated with rigid rules around food and eating, BN and BED are characterized by binge-eating episodes in which individuals feel as if they are losing control of their eating. As such, BN and BED are more often linked to impulsivity and problems with inhibition (see Chapter 10), rather than cognitive inflexibility. There is, however, a small body of literature on cognitive flexibility in BN and BED. There have been some reports of poor cognitive flexibility depending on the specific task used in BN, specifically set-shifting tasks such as the CatBat task (a task which involves filling in missing letters from a short story) (Tchanturia et al., 2004), the Haptic Illusion Task (a size-weight illusion task using wooden balls) (Tchanturia et al., 2004), the WCST (Miranda-Olivos et al., 2021; Tchanturia et al., 2012), and the TMT (Vall & Wade, 2015). However, other studies have not found differences using other cognitive flexibility tasks, including certain types of task-switching and set-shifting tasks (Abber et al., 2022; Galimberti et al., 2012), the TMT (Tchanturia et al., 2004), and the Brixton Spatial Anticipation Test (Tchanturia et al., 2004; Tchanturia et al., 2011). The findings in BED are somewhat more consistent with a lack of cognitive flexibility deficits found across different tasks such as the WCST (Dingemans et al., 2019), TMT (Dingemans et al., 2019; Duchesne et al., 2010; Kittel et al., 2017; Wollenhaupt et al., 2019), intra/extra-dimensional shift task (a visual discrimination task) (Grant & Chamberlain, 2020), and verbal fluency tasks (Eneva et al., 2017).

Alternate Perspectives

While the literature suggests that performance on cognitive flexibility tasks may not be impaired in individuals with BED, the findings suggest that differences may be present in individuals with AN and BN; however, the literature is inconsistent, particularly for those in the acute state of AN where findings are quite mixed. Further, as performance on cognitive flexibility tasks does not appear to differ from healthy populations among those in weight-restored or recovered states of AN, it suggests that if such deficits do exist in the acute state, that they may be related to the underweight and malnourished state rather than being a trait feature of the illness (Phillipou et al., 2018). This lack of robust findings of cognitive flexibility deficits in people with eating disorders also leads us to question how the rigidity and inflexibility we often see in individuals with eating disorders relates to brain functioning, and if we are simply not using the right tools to assess the specific types of cognitive inflexibility present in these individuals. Perhaps neurocognitive tasks of cognitive flexibility lack ecological validity. Clinically, descriptions of AN often refer to inflexible behaviors, thoughts, and rules which are specific to eating, exercise, and body image; for example, the categorization of foods as either good or bad, rules regarding mealtimes, ritualized food patterns, and a fixation on calorie-counting, intense exercise regimes, and weight loss (Aloi et al., 2015; Rößner et al., 2017; Tchanturia et al., 2013). However, these instances of inflexibility are not captured in traditional neurocognitive assessments of cognitive flexibility. Typically, neurocognitive tasks involve abstract stimuli, such as shapes, letters, or neutral words, rather than stimuli (such as food images) which may be more relevant to people with eating disorders. Neurocognitive tasks, such as the TMT and WCST, may therefore not effectively capture everyday experiences of rigidity that people with AN may experience. This poor ecological validity presents a problem for eating disorders research, as the TMT and WCST are the most commonly used assessments of cognitive flexibility (Miles et al., 2020).

Given the limitations of neurocognitive tasks for evaluating cognitive flexibility in eating disorders (i.e., poor ecological validity, the task impurity problem, etc.), some work has taken a different approach. A small body of literature now exists, specifically in AN (but not as yet in the other eating disorders), in which self-reported cognitive flexibility has been investigated. To date, most research has considered general cognitive flexibility rather than eating disorder-specific cognitive flexibility difficulties. Research has consistently demonstrated that participants with AN self-report poorer cognitive flexibility across illness states on standardized questionnaires compared to HCs (Lao-Kaim et al., 2015; Lounes et al., 2011; McAnarney et al., 2011; Miles, Nedeljkovic, & Phillipou, 2022; Sternheim et al., 2022, Miles, Nedeljkovic, Sumner, et al., 2022; Miles, Phillipou, et al., 2022). Poorer self-reported cognitive flexibility in AN has also been found to be associated with greater eating disorder symptomatology (Miles, Nedeljkovic, Sumner, et al., 2022) and poorer quality of life (Brockmeyer et al., 2022), signifying that perceived inflexibility may be associated with an individual's well-being. Scores on measures of self-reported cognitive flexibility, however, have not been found to correlate with neurocognitive assessments of cognitive flexibility in people with AN (Brockmeyer et al., 2022; Lounes et al., 2011; Miles, Nedeljkovic, Sumner, et al., 2022; Sternheim et al., 2022), suggesting that subjective and objective assessments of cognitive flexibility may be capturing different things (Howlett et al., 2023). Furthermore, rather than there being a cognitive deficit in AN, the inflexible thoughts and behaviors seen in the disorder may reflect higher order processing whereby such thoughts and behaviors are overvalued for other reasons, such as abiding by self-imposed perfectionistic standards which is a common feature of AN (Miles, Nedeljkovic, & Phillipou, 2022; Phillipou et al., 2022).

Implications

Although it remains uncertain whether deficits in cognitive flexibility do indeed exist in eating disorders and how they may relate to the illness, specific interventions targeting cognitive flexibility have been studied. Cognitive Remediation Therapy (CRT), for example, is an adjunct treatment which has been adapted for AN to improve cognitive flexibility (as well as central coherence), with the goal of preparing patients for engagement in other therapies (Baldock & Tchanturia, 2007; Fonville et al., 2014; Tchanturia et al., 2013). It is suggested that the format of CRT (neutral material which is unrelated to a patient's eating disorder; short sessions which build concentration and a sense of achievement), in addition to the attainment of skills useful to engaging in therapy and the chance to build a positive therapeutic rapport, will support a patient to begin successful treatment for their eating disorder (Baldock & Tchanturia, 2007). CRT programs include the completion of simple tasks which are designed to target cognition and self-reflection on thinking styles and the impact they may have on everyday life (Baldock & Tchanturia, 2007; Tchanturia et al., 2013). It is reasoned that practicing tasks which target cognitive flexibility will increase activation in specific brain pathways and thus cognitive flexibility may improve (Baldock & Tchanturia, 2007). Findings from a small number of studies in AN samples have suggested that CRT may be an effective program for improving performance on cognitive flexibility tasks (Brockmeyer et al., 2022; Leppanen et al., 2018; van Noort et al., 2016). Yet, other research has not supported CRT as a superior treatment for improving cognitive flexibility when compared to other adjunct therapies such as art therapy or non-specific cognitive training (Brockmeyer et al., 2022; Herbrich-Bowe et al., 2022; Sproch et al., 2019). Further, the use of neurocognitive tests to evaluate change during and after treatment may be inappropriate as neurocognitive tests are prone to practice effects (Dennis & Vander Wal, 2010). In addition, when using self-report measures of cognitive flexibility as an outcome measure of CRT, significant changes have not been reported (Genders & Tchanturia, 2010; Leppanen et al., 2018; Pretorius et al., 2012).

Overall, the proposal that there are neurocognitive deficits in cognitive flexibility in eating disorders is not well supported. While differences from healthy individuals are typically not found in those with BED, there is some suggestion that cognitive inflexibility may be present in AN and BN, but findings are inconsistent. There does, however, appear to be consistency in subjective accounts of poor cognitive flexibility in individuals with AN. In addition to methodological issues in the literature limiting our interpretations of objective cognitive flexibility task performance, neurocognitive assessments of cognitive flexibility may not tap into the specific areas of inflexibility experienced in AN or the flexibility difficulties experienced in people with AN are much more complex and span across various subtle areas of cognitive function. As individuals with AN report difficulties with cognitive flexibility despite not necessarily showing deficits in task performance, it suggests that this subjective experience may play an important role in the disorder that should be targeted with therapeutic interventions.

References

Abbate-Daga, G., Buzzichelli, S., Amianto, F., Rocca, G., Marzola, E., McClintock, S. M., & Fassino, S. (2011). Cognitive flexibility in verbal and nonverbal domains and decision making in anorexia nervosa patients: a pilot study. *BMC Psychiatry, 11*, 1–8.

Abber, S. R., Forman, E. M., Wierenga, C. E., & Manasse, S. M. (2022). Intact general and food-specific task-switching abilities in bulimia-spectrum eating disorders. *Eating Behaviors, 46*, 101636.

Aloi, M., Rania, M., Caroleo, M., Bruni, A., Palmieri, A., Cauteruccio, M. A., De Fazio, P., & Segura-García, C. (2015). Decision making, central coherence and set-shifting: a comparison between binge eating disorder, anorexia nervosa and healthy controls. *BMC Psychiatry, 15*, 6.

Anderson, S. W., Damasio, H., Jones, R. D., & Tranel, D. (1991). Wisconsin Card Sorting Test performance as a measure of frontal lobe damage. *Journal of Clinical and Experimental Neuropsychology, 13*(6), 909–922.

Andrés-Perpiña, S., Lozano-Serra, E., Puig, O., Lera-Miguel, S., Lázaro, L., & Castro-Fornieles, J. (2011). Clinical and biological correlates of adolescent anorexia nervosa with impaired cognitive profile. *European Child & Adolescent Psychiatry, 20*, 541–549.

Badre, D., & Wagner, A. D. (2006). Computational and neurobiological mechanisms underlying cognitive flexibility. *Proceedings of the National Academy of Sciences USA, 103*(18), 7186–7191.

Baldock, E., & Tchanturia, K. (2007). Translating laboratory research into practice: Foundations, functions and future of cognitive remediation therapy for anorexia nervosa. *Therapy (London), 4*(3), 285.

Berchio, C., Annen, L. C., Bouamoud, Y., & Micali, N. (2023). Temporal dynamics of cognitive flexibility in adolescents with anorexia nervosa: A high-density EEG study. *European Journal of Neuroscience, 57*(6), 962–980.

Bohon, C., Weinbach, N., & Lock, J. (2020). Performance and brain activity during the Wisconsin Card Sorting Test in adolescents with obsessive–compulsive disorder and adolescents with weight-restored anorexia nervosa. *European Child & Adolescent Psychiatry, 29*, 217–226.

Brockmeyer, T., Febry, H., Leiteritz-Rausch, A., Wünsch-Leiteritz, W., Leiteritz, A., & Friederich, H. C. (2022). Cognitive flexibility, central coherence, and quality of life in anorexia nervosa. *Journal of Eating Disorders, 10*(1), 22.

Buchsbaum, B. R., Greer, S., Chang, W. L., & Berman, K. F. (2005). Meta-analysis of neuroimaging studies of the Wisconsin Card Sorting Task and component processes. *Human Brain Mapping, 25*(1), 35–45.

Bühren, K., Mainz, V., Herpertz-Dahlmann, B., Schäfer, K., Kahraman-Lanzerath, B., Lente, C., & Konrad, K. (2012). Cognitive flexibility in juvenile anorexia nervosa patients before and after weight recovery. *Journal of Neural Transmission, 119*, 1047–1057.

Burgess, P. W., & Shallice, T. (1997). *The hayling and brixton tests*. Pearson.

Buzzichelli, S., Marzola, E., Amianto, F., Fassino, S., & Abbate-Daga, G. (2018). Perfectionism and cognitive rigidity in anorexia nervosa: Is there an association? *European Eating Disorders Review, 26*(4), 360–366.

Castro-Fornieles, J., de la Serna, E., Calvo, A., Blázquez, A., Moya, J., Lázaro, L., Andrés-Perpiñá, S., Plana, M. T., Gil, L., & Flamarique, I. (2019). Functional MRI with a set-shifting task in adolescent anorexia nervosa: A cross-sectional and follow-up study. *Neuropsychologia, 131*, 1–8.

Collantoni, E., Meregalli, V., Manara, R., Meneguzzo, P., Tenconi, E., & Favaro, A. (2023). Volume and complexity of the thalamus in anorexia nervosa: An exploratory evaluation. *European Eating Disorders Review, 31*(2), 349–359.

Dahlgren, C. L., Hage, T. W., Wonderlich, J. A., & Stedal, K. (2019). General and eating disorder specific flexibility: Development and validation of the eating disorder flexibility index (EDFLIX) questionnaire. *Frontiers in Psychology, 10*, 663.

Dajani, D. R., & Uddin, L. Q. (2015). Demystifying cognitive flexibility: Implications for clinical and developmental neuroscience. *Trends in Neuroscience, 38*(9), 571–578.

Danner, U. N., Sanders, N., Smeets, P. A., van Meer, F., Adan, R. A., Hoek, H. W., & van Elburg, A. A. (2012). Neuropsychological weaknesses in anorexia nervosa: Set-shifting, central coherence, and decision making in currently ill and recovered women. *International Journal of Eating Disorders, 45*(5), 685–694.

Deák, G. O. (2003). The development of cognitive flexibility and language abilities. *Advances in Child Development and Behavior, 31*, 273–328.

Delis, D. C., Kaplan, E., & Kramer, J. H. (2001). *Delis-Kaplan executive function system*. Pearson Assessment.

Delis, D. C., Kramer, J. H., Kaplan, E., & Holdnack, J. (2004). Reliability and validity of the Delis-Kaplan executive function system: An update. *Journal of the International Neuropsychological Society, 10*(2), 301–303.

Dennis, J. P., & Vander Wal, J. S. (2010). The cognitive flexibility inventory: Instrument development and estimates of reliability and validity. *Cognitive Therapy and Research, 34*, 241–253.

Diamond, A. (2013). Executive functions. *Annual Review of Psychology, 64*, 135–168.

Dingemans, A. E., Vanhaelen, C. B., Aardoom, J. J., & van Furth, E. F. (2019). The influence of depressive symptoms on executive functioning in binge eating disorder: A comparison of patients and non-obese healthy controls. *Psychiatry Research, 274*, 138–145.

Duchesne, M., Mattos, P., Appolinário, J. C., de Freitas, S. R., Coutinho, G., Santos, C., & Coutinho, W. (2010). Assessment of executive functions in obese individuals with binge eating disorder. *Brazilian Journal of Psychiatry, 32*(4), 381–388.

Duriez, P., Kaya Lefèvre, H., Di Lodovico, L., Viltart, O., & Gorwood, P. (2021). Increased cognitive flexibility mediates the improvement of eating disorders symptoms, depressive symptoms and level of daily life functioning in patients with anorexia nervosa treated in specialised centres. *European Eating Disorders Review, 29*(4), 600–610.

Ely, A. V., Wierenga, C. E., & Kaye, W. H. (2016). Anxiety impacts cognitive inhibition in remitted anorexia nervosa. *European Eating Disorders Review, 24*(4), 347–351.

Eneva, K. T., Arlt, J. M., Yiu, A., Murray, S. M., & Chen, E. Y. (2017). Assessment of executive functioning in binge-eating disorder independent of weight status. *International Journal of Eating Disorders, 50*(8), 942–951.

Fonville, L., Giampietro, V., Davies, H., Lounes, N., Simmons, A., Williams, S., & Tchanturia, K. (2014). Cognitive remediation, brain function and central coherence: An anorexia nervosa pilot study. *Annals of General Psychiatry, 13*(1), 1–5.

Galimberti, E., Martoni, R. M., Cavallini, M. C., Erzegovesi, S., & Bellodi, L. (2012). Motor inhibition and cognitive flexibility in eating disorder subtypes. *Progress in Neuro-Psychopharmacology and Biological Psychiatry, 36*(2), 307–312.

Genders, R., & Tchanturia, K. (2010). Cognitive remediation therapy (CRT) for anorexia in group format: a pilot study. *Eating and Weight Disorders, 15*, e234–e239.

Giel, K. E., Wittorf, A., Wolkenstein, L., Klingberg, S., Drimmer, E., Schönenberg, M., Rapp, A. M., Fallgatter, A. J., Hautzinger, M., & Zipfel, S. (2012). Is impaired set-shifting a feature of "pure" anorexia nervosa? Investigating the role of depression in set-shifting ability in anorexia nervosa and unipolar depression. *Psychiatry Research, 200*(2–3), 538–543.

Grant, D. A., & Berg, E. (1948). A behavioral analysis of degree of reinforcement and ease of shifting to new responses in a Weigl-type card-sorting problem. *Journal of Experimental Psychology, 38*(4), 404.

Grant, J. E., & Chamberlain, S. R. (2020). Neurocognitive findings in young adults with binge eating disorder. *International Journal of Psychiatry in Clinical Practice, 24*(1), 71–76.

Grant, J. E., & Chamberlain, S. R. (2023). Impaired cognitive flexibility across psychiatric disorders. *CNS Spectrums*, 28(6), 688–692.

Heaton, R. (1981). *Wisconsin card sorting test manual*, 5–57. (Revised and expanded). Psychological Assessment Resources.

Herbrich-Bowe, L., Bentz, L. K., Correll, C. U., Kappel, V., & van Noort, B. M. (2022). Randomized controlled trial of cognitive remediation therapy in adolescent inpatients with anorexia nervosa: Neuropsychological outcomes. *European Eating Disorders Review, 30*(6), 772–786.

Howlett, C. A., Miles, S., Berryman, C., Phillipou, A., & Moseley, G. L. (2023). Conflation between self-report and neurocognitive assessments of cognitive flexibility: A critical review of the Jingle Fallacy. *Australian Journal of Psychology, 75*(1), 2174684.

Ionescu, T. (2012). Exploring the nature of cognitive flexibility. *New Ideas in Psychology, 30*(2), 190–200.

Johnco, C., Wuthrich, V. M., & Rapee, R. M. (2014). Reliability and validity of two self-report measures of cognitive flexibility. *Psychological Assessment, 26(4)*, 1381.

Kim, C., Cilles, S. E., Johnson, N. F., & Gold, B. T. (2012). Domain general and domain preferential brain regions associated with different types of task switching: A meta-analysis. *Human Brain Mapping, 33*(1), 130–142.

Kittel, R., Schmidt, R., & Hilbert, A. (2017). Executive functions in adolescents with binge-eating disorder and obesity. *International Journal of Eating Disorders, 50*(8), 933–941.

Konishi, S., Nakajima, K., Uchida, I., Kameyama, M., Nakahara, K., Sekihara, K., & Miyashita, Y. (1998). Transient activation of inferior prefrontal cortex during cognitive set shifting. *Nature Neuroscience, 1*(1), 80–84.

Konstantakopoulos, G., Tchanturia, K., Surguladze, S., & David, A. (2011). Insight in eating disorders: Clinical and cognitive correlates. *Psychological Medicine, 41*(9), 1951–1961.

Lang, K., Stahl, D., Espie, J., Treasure, J., & Tchanturia, K. (2014). Set shifting in children and adolescents with anorexia nervosa: An exploratory systematic review and meta-analysis. *International Journal of Eating Disorders, 47*(4), 394–399.

Lao-Kaim, N. P., Fonville, L., Giampietro, V. P., Williams, S. C., Simmons, A., & Tchanturia, K. (2015). Aberrant function of learning and cognitive control networks underlie inefficient cognitive flexibility in anorexia nervosa: A cross-sectional fMRI study. *PLOS ONE, 10*(5), e0124027.

Leppanen, J., Adamson, J., & Tchanturia, K. (2018). Impact of cognitive remediation therapy on neurocognitive processing in anorexia nervosa. *Frontiers in Psychiatry, 9*, 96.

Lie, C.-H., Specht, K., Marshall, J. C., & Fink, G. R. (2006). Using fMRI to decompose the neural processes underlying the Wisconsin Card Sorting Test. *Neuroimage, 30*(3), 1038–1049.

Logue, S. F., & Gould, T. J. (2014). The neural and genetic basis of executive function: Attention, cognitive flexibility, and response inhibition. *Pharmacology Biochemistry and Behavior, 123*, 45–54.

Lounes, N., Khan, G., & Tchanturia, K. (2011). Assessment of cognitive flexibility in anorexia nervosa—Self-report or experimental measure? A brief report. *Journal of the International Neuropsychological Society, 17*(5), 925–928.

Lozano-Serra, E., Andrés-Perpiña, S., Lázaro-García, L., & Castro-Fornieles, J. (2014). Adolescent anorexia nervosa: Cognitive performance after weight recovery. *Journal of Psychosomatic Research, 76*(1), 6–11.

Martin, M. M., & Rubin, R. B. (1995). A new measure of cognitive flexibility. *Psychological Reports, 76*(2), 623–626.

McAnarney, E. R., Zarcone, J., Singh, P., Michels, J., Welsh, S., Litteer, T., Wang, H., & Klein, J. D. (2011). Restrictive anorexia nervosa and set-shifting in adolescents: A biobehavioral interface. *Journal of Adolescent Health, 49*(1), 99–101.

Miles, S., Gnatt, I., Phillipou, A., & Nedeljkovic, M. (2020). Cognitive flexibility in acute anorexia nervosa and after recovery: A systematic review. *Clinical Psychology Review, 81*, 101905.

Miles, S., Howlett, C. A., Berryman, C., Nedeljkovic, M., Moseley, G. L., & Phillipou, A. (2021). Considerations for using the Wisconsin Card Sorting Test to assess cognitive flexibility. *Behavior Research Methods, 53*(5), 2083–2091.

Miles, S., Nedeljkovic, M., & Phillipou, A. (2022). Can cognitive flexibility and clinical perfectionism be used to identify people with anorexia nervosa? *Journal of Clinical Medicine, 11*(7), 1954.

Miles, S., Nedeljkovic, M., Sumner, P., & Phillipou, A. (2022). Understanding self-report and neurocognitive assessments of cognitive flexibility in people with and without lifetime anorexia nervosa. *Cognitive Neuropsychiatry, 27*(5), 325–341.

Miles, S., Phillipou, A., Sumner, P., & Nedeljkovic, M. (2022). Cognitive flexibility and the risk of anorexia nervosa: An investigation using self-report and neurocognitive assessments. *Journal of Psychiatric Research, 151*, 531–538.

Miranda-Olivos, R., Testa, G., Lucas, I., Sánchez, I., Sanchez-Gonzalez, J., Granero, R., Jimenez-Murcia, S., & Fernandez-Aranda, F. (2021). Clinical factors predicting impaired executive functions in eating disorders: The role of illness duration. *Journal of Psychiatric Research, 144*, 87–95.

Monchi, O., Petrides, M., Petre, V., Worsley, K., & Dagher, A. (2001). Wisconsin Card Sorting revisited: Distinct neural circuits participating in different stages of the task identified by event-related functional magnetic resonance imaging. *Journal of Neuroscience, 21*(19), 7733–7741.

Monsell, S. (2003). Task switching. *Trends in Cognitive Sciences, 7*(3), 134–140.

Mountain, M. A., & Snow, W. G. (1993). Wisconsin Card Sorting Test as a measure of frontal pathology: A review. *Clinical Neuropsychologist, 7*(1), 108–118.

Nagahama, Y., Okada, T., Katsumi, Y., Hayashi, T., Yamauchi, H., Oyanagi, C., Konishi, J., Fukuyama, H., & Shibasaki, H. (2001). Dissociable mechanisms of attentional control within the human prefrontal cortex. *Cerebral Cortex, 11*(1), 85–92.

Nakazato, M., Hashimoto, K., Schmidt, U., Tchanturia, K., Campbell, I. C., Collier, D. A., Iyo, M., & Treasure, J. (2010). Serum glutamine, set-shifting ability and anorexia nervosa. *Annals of General Psychiatry, 9*(1), 1–8.

Nikendei, C., Funiok, C., Pfüller, U., Zastrow, A., Aschenbrenner, S., Weisbrod, M., Herzog, W., & Friederich, H.-C. (2011). Memory performance in acute and weight-restored anorexia nervosa patients. *Psychological Medicine, 41*(4), 829–838.

Nyhus, E., & Barceló, F. (2009). The Wisconsin Card Sorting Test and the cognitive assessment of prefrontal executive functions: a critical update. *Brain and Cognition, 71*(3), 437–451.

Paslakis, G., Agüera, Z., Granero, R., Sánchez, I., Riesco, N., Jiménez-Murcia, S., Fernández-García, J. C., Garrido-Sánchez, L., Tinahones, F. J., & Casanueva, F. F. (2019). Associations between neuropsychological performance and appetite-regulating hormones in anorexia nervosa and healthy controls: Ghrelin's putative role as a mediator of decision-making. *Molecular and Cellular Endocrinology, 497*, 110441.

Phillipou, A., Gurvich, C., Castle, D. J., & Rossell, S. L. (2022). Anorexia nervosa, weight restoration and biological siblings: Differences and similarities in clinical characteristics. *Australasian Psychiatry, 30*(4), 458–461.

Phillipou, A., Rossell, S. L., & Castle, D. J. (2018). Anorexia nervosa or starvation? *European Journal of Neuroscience, 48*(11), 3317–3318.

Pignatti, R., & Bernasconi, V. (2013). Personality, clinical features, and test instructions can affect executive functions in eating disorders. *Eating Behaviors, 14*(2), 233–236.

Pretorius, N., Dimmer, M., Power, E., Eisler, I., Simic, M., & Tchanturia, K. (2012). Evaluation of a cognitive remediation therapy group for adolescents with anorexia nervosa: Pilot study. *European Eating Disorders Review, 20*(4), 321–325.

Reitan, R. M. (1958). Validity of the Trail Making Test as an indicator of organic brain damage. *Perceptual and Motor Skills, 8*(3), 271–276.

Roberts, M. E., Tchanturia, K., & Treasure, J. L. (2010). Exploring the neurocognitive signature of poor set-shifting in anorexia and bulimia nervosa. *Journal of Psychiatric Research, 44*(14), 964–970.

Rößner, A., Juniak, I., van Noort, B. M., Pfeiffer, E., Lehmkuhl, U., & Kappel, V. (2017). Cognitive flexibility in juvenile anorexia nervosain relation to comorbid symptoms of depression, obsessive compulsive symptoms and duration of illness. *Zeitschrift für Kinder-und Jugendpsychiatrie und Psychotherapie*, 45(5), 371–380.

Sato, Y., Saito, N., Utsumi, A., Aizawa, E., Shoji, T., Izumiyama, M., Mushiake, H., Hongo, M., & Fukudo, S. (2013). Neural basis of impaired cognitive flexibility in patients with anorexia nervosa. *PLOS ONE, 8*(5), e61108.

Scott, W. A. (1962). Cognitive complexity and cognitive flexibility. *Sociometry, 25(4)*, 405–414. https://doi.org/10.2307/2785779

Sproch, L. E., Anderson, K. P., Sherman, M. F., Crawford, S. F., & Brandt, H. A. (2019). A randomized controlled trial of group cognitive remediation therapy for anorexia nervosa: Effects on set-shifting tasks for inpatient adults and adolescents. *International Journal of Eating Disorders, 52*(9), 1004–1014.

Stedal, K., & Dahlgren, C. L. (2015). Neuropsychological assessment in adolescents with anorexia nervosa—Exploring the relationship between self-report and performance-based testing. *Journal of Eating Disorders, 3*, 1–12.

Sternheim, L. C., van Passel, B., Dingemans, A., Cath, D., & Danner, U. N. (2022). Cognitive and experienced flexibility in patients with anorexia nervosa and obsessive compulsive disorder. *Frontiers in Psychiatry, 13*, 868921.

Talbot, A., Hay, P., Buckett, G., & Touyz, S. (2015). Cognitive deficits as an endophenotype for anorexia nervosa: An accepted fact or a need for re-examination? *International Journal of Eating Disorders, 48*(1), 15–25.

Tchanturia, K., Anderluh, M. B., Morris, R. G., Rabe-Hesketh, S., Collier, D. A., Sanchez, P., & Treasure, J. L. (2004). Cognitive flexibility in anorexia nervosa and bulimia nervosa. *Journal of the International Neuropsychological Society, 10*(4), 513–520.

Tchanturia, K., Davies, H., Roberts, M., Harrison, A., Nakazato, M., Schmidt, U., Treasure, J., & Morris, R. (2012). Poor cognitive flexibility in eating disorders: Examining the evidence using the Wisconsin Card Sorting Task. *PLOS ONE, 7*(1), e28331.

Tchanturia, K., Harrison, A., Davies, H., Roberts, M., Oldershaw, A., Nakazato, M., Stahl, D., Morris, R., Schmidt, U., & Treasure, J. (2011). Cognitive flexibility and clinical severity in eating disorders. *PLOS ONE, 6*(6), e20462.

Tchanturia, K., Lloyd, S., & Lang, K. (2013). Cognitive remediation therapy for anorexia nervosa: current evidence and future research directions. *International Journal of Eating Disorders, 46*(5), 492–495.

Tchanturia, K., Morris, R., Anderluh, M. B., Collier, D., Nikolaou, V., & Treasure, J. (2004). Set shifting in anorexia nervosa: an examination before and after weight gain, in full recovery and relationship to childhood and adult OCPD traits. *Journal of Psychiatric Research, 38*(5), 545–552.

Tenconi, E., Santonastaso, P., Degortes, D., Bosello, R., Titton, F., Mapelli, D., & Favaro, A. (2010). Set-shifting abilities, central coherence, and handedness in anorexia nervosa patients, their unaffected siblings and healthy controls: Exploring putative endophenotypes. *World Journal of Biological Psychiatry, 11*(6), 813–823.

Treasure, J., & Schmidt, U. (2013). The cognitive-interpersonal maintenance model of anorexia nervosa revisited: A summary of the evidence for cognitive, socio-emotional and interpersonal predisposing and perpetuating factors. *Journal of Eating Disorders, 1*, 1–10.

Vall, E., & Wade, T. D. (2015). Trail making task performance in inpatients with anorexia nervosa and bulimia nervosa. *European Eating Disorders Review, 23*(4), 304–311.

van Noort, B. M., Kraus, M. K. A., Pfeiffer, E., Lehmkuhl, U., & Kappel, V. (2016). Neuropsychological and behavioural short-term effects of cognitive remediation therapy in adolescent anorexia nervosa: A pilot study. *European Eating Disorders Review, 24*(1), 69–74.

Wollenhaupt, C., Wilke, L., Erim, Y., Rauh, M., Steins-Loeber, S., & Paslakis, G. (2019). The association of leptin secretion with cognitive performance in patients with eating disorders. *Psychiatry Research, 276*, 269–277.

Zastrow, A., Kaiser, S., Stippich, C., Walther, S., Herzog, W., Tchanturia, K., Belger, A., Weisbrod, M., Treasure, J., & Friederich, H.-C. (2009). Neural correlates of impaired cognitive-behavioral flexibility in anorexia nervosa. *American Journal of Psychiatry, 166*(5), 608–616.

12

Self-Regulation in Eating Disorders

Blair R. K. Shevlin, Maia A. Chester, Jessica L. Qiu, Siyi Lou, and Laura A. Berner

Brief Definitional Overview

Cognitive interference control: The ability to actively suppress or ignore irrelevant information in the service of maintaining a goal (Nigg, 2000), which is an important subprocess of attentional control (the ability to voluntarily direct attention to goal-relevant information (Quigley et al., 2017)).

Response inhibition: The ability to suppress inappropriate, automatic, or prepotent behavioral responses in support of goal-directed behavior (Masharipov et al., 2022; Verbruggen & Logan, 2008).

Delay discounting: The psychological phenomena where the subjective value of a reward declines as the delay to its receipt increases (Ainslie, 1975; Green & Myerson, 2004).

Emotion regulation: The ability to identify, manage, and control the experience and expression of emotions, both consciously and unconsciously (Rottenberg & Gross, 2003; Williams et al., 2009) to adapt to different situations and to achieve desired outcomes (Aldao et al., 2010).

Introduction

Symptoms of anorexia nervosa (AN), bulimia nervosa (BN), and binge-eating disorder (BED) involve extremes of control—ranging from prolonged periods of dietary restriction to out-of-control binge eating, purging, and other compensatory behaviors. Therefore, substantial eating disorders research using a "bottom-up" approach, as defined in this book, has focused on self-regulation. This umbrella construct is also called self-regulatory control, cognitive control, or executive control. It includes several subprocesses needed to help coordinate decisions to enact one behavior and not enact another, as well as regulate cognitions and emotional responses. Neuroimaging techniques combined with behavioral tasks have improved our understanding of the neural basis of self-regulation in healthy individuals, and applications of these approaches to individuals with eating disorders have begun to elucidate how this neural circuitry may function differently to give rise to symptoms. This chapter reviews behav-

Blair R. K. Shevlin et al., *Self-Regulation in Eating Disorders*. In: *The Handbook of the Neurobiology of Eating Disorders*. Edited by: Christina E. Wierenga and Joanna E. Steinglass, Oxford University Press.
DOI: 10.1093/9780197675212.003.0013

ioral and functional magnetic resonance imaging (fMRI) results focused on four of the most studied aspects of self-regulation in AN, BN, and BED: cognitive interference control, response inhibition, delay discounting, and emotion regulation. For each of these processes, after providing an overview of findings to date, the chapter discusses alternative perspectives, limitations, conflicting findings, and unknowns, as well as potential implications for treatment. The chapter concludes with proposals for new lines of research using new tasks and analytic techniques.

Cognitive Interference Control

Cognitive interference control is one of the most studied aspects of self-regulation in the eating disorders field. The Stroop task, the Simon Spatial Incompatibility task, and the Flanker task are commonly used to measure interference control. The Stroop task prompts participants to disregard the color of a word to read the word (e.g., the word "red" shown in a blue font). The Simon Spatial Incompatibility task requires an individual to ignore the spatial location of an arrow or a word to correctly identify the stimuli's direction. Similarly, the Flanker task requires participants to ignore the incongruent stimuli that surround a target stimulus to respond correctly to the target. Responses to incongruent trials on these tasks serve as an index of cognitive interference control.

Biological framework

Voluntary attentional control processes engage the superior frontal, inferior parietal, and superior temporal cortex (Hopfinger et al., 2000). Active interference monitoring and suppression recruits the dorsolateral prefrontal cortex (DLPFC), the ventrolateral prefrontal cortex (VLPFC), the dorsal anterior cingulate (dACC), and the parietal cortex (Blasi et al., 2006). The insula and dACC operate together in a saliency network, filtering information and directing attention toward goal-relevant stimuli (Menon & Uddin, 2010). The dorsal attention network (made of the frontal eye fields, superior parietal lobule, and intraparietal sulcus) is implicated in effortful suppression in favor of maintaining attentional focus on goal-relevant stimuli (Corbetta & Shulman, 2002; Tamber-Rosenau et al., 2018), while the ventral attention network (made of the temporoparietal junction and the ventral frontal cortex) processes stimulus-based features to switch attention to more relevant and novel information (Vossel et al., 2014). These two networks work in tandem to maintain and switch attention as needed (see Figure 12.1).

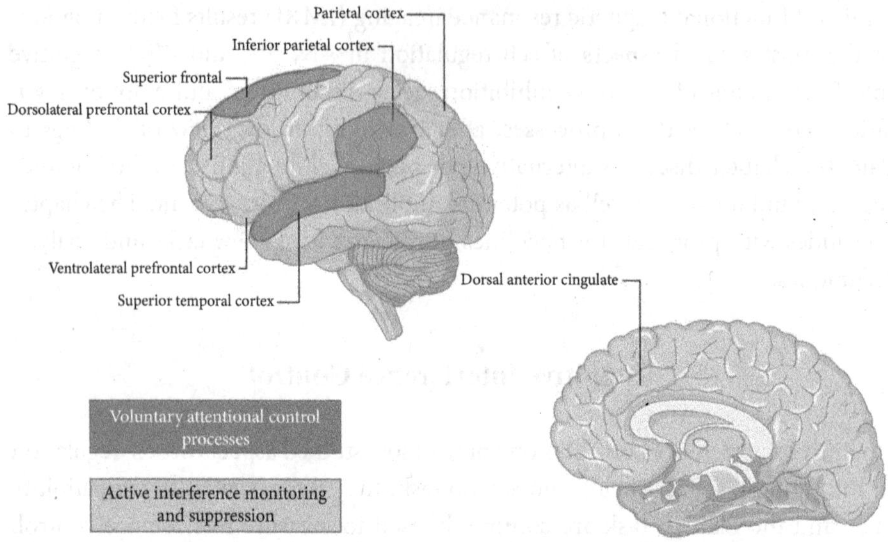

Figure 12.1 Neural circuits involved in cognitive interference control. Created with BioRender.com

State of the Science in Eating Disorders

Behavioral findings

Results from a meta-analysis of studies using mostly interference control tasks suggest that individuals with BN and the binge-eating/purging subtype of AN (AN-BP) make more errors and show pronounced slowing in reaction time on incongruent trials compared to healthy controls (Wu, Hartmann, et al., 2013). These alterations were even more pronounced in BN when tasks used disorder-specific stimuli, like pictures of food or body-related words. Generalized interference control deficits were large in AN-BP and small in BN (Wu, Hartmann, et al., 2013). In contrast, an older meta-analysis of Stroop tasks that focused on AN more broadly documented deficits only on tasks using body or weight-related stimuli (Dobson & Dozois, 2004). In BED, generalized deficits in interference control were not supported (Wu, Hartmann, et al., 2013). However, a later study found that adults with elevated body weights and loss-of-control eating, although not necessarily BED, showed deficits in traditional color-word interference (Manasse et al., 2014). In addition, more recent findings suggest that BED may be characterized by food-specific cognitive interference control deficits. Women with BED responded slower than healthy controls when presented with incongruent food stimuli during a Flanker task (Lyu et al., 2018) and exhibited more interference for food items on the n-back task (Svaldi et al., 2014). Additional research is needed to parse associations of general and food or body-specific interference control with weight status, binge-eating episode size, restriction severity, and compensatory behaviors.

Neuroimaging findings

Regardless of task performance, individuals with BED and BN seem to show reduced neural activation during interference control on tasks with general stimuli. Despite their intact behavioral performance, adults with BED performing the Stroop task had lower activation compared to weight-matched controls with no binge eating in regions implicated in self-control and interference monitoring, such as the ventromedial prefrontal cortex (VMPFC), VLPFC, and insula (Balodis et al., 2013; Duchesne et al., 2010). Two studies of women with BN found similarly reduced interference control-associated activation in the dorsal striatum, VLPFC, dACC, and parahippocampal gyrus, one in the context of impaired performance on the Simon task (Marsh et al., 2009), and one in the context of intact performance during the incongruent versus congruent target conditions of the Attention Network Task (Seitz et al., 2016). In contrast, women with BN showed impaired performance and increased activation in the DLPFC, premotor cortex, and dorsal striatum while performing a food-specific Stroop match-to-sample task (Lee et al., 2017), and individuals with AN performing a Stroop color task using weight-related words showed greater behavioral slowing on incongruent trials and increased activation of the left insula, frontal and temporal lobes and in the left middle and medial frontal gyri (Redgrave et al., 2008). Therefore, while most studies suggest that individuals with eating disorders have altered neural activation patterns during interference control tasks, the directionality of these findings has been mixed and may be task-, stimulus-type, and diagnosis-dependent.

Alternative perspective

Which components of cognitive interference control are most relevant for eating disorders?

Cognitive interference control is complex, and different tasks may elicit different aspects of the process of ignoring or suppressing competing information while also maintaining attention on a different set of information to enact a behavior (Gao et al., 2011; Svaldi et al., 2014; Yeung et al., 2020). This may be why task performance and the directionality of altered neural activation differ depending on whether disorder-relevant or general stimuli are used. To parse the different aspects of cognitive interference control and determine which components are most tightly linked to eating disorder behaviors and symptoms, eye tracking and mouse tracking may be useful in tandem with interference tasks. These methods have proven fruitful in the depression and anxiety literature (Armstrong & Olatunji, 2012). In contrast to button presses, which measure interference control in isolated moments, these tracking methods are better suited to measuring continuous attention. Because the sort of interference control needed to regulate attention away from eating disorder-related urges or cravings is presumably sustained, not intermittent, these approaches may capture alterations that are absent in brief moments but marked in the context of longer periods of time. Additional steps to improve the ecological validity of interference control tasks could include using more compelling stimuli like sounds, video clips, or smells, rather than less arousing words on a screen (Jiang & Vartanian, 2018).

Implications

As data suggest that individuals with eating disorders show deficits in the deployment of cognitive interference control when presented with disorder-relevant stimuli, Attention Bias Modification (ABM) programs may be beneficial. These computer programs train the suppression of attention toward salient stimuli and direct attention toward neutral stimuli, theoretically improving interference control for disorder-related stimuli (Kuckertz & Amir, 2015; MacLeod & Clarke, 2015). ABM may be particularly helpful for binge-spectrum eating disorders: After 10 sessions of ABM training, participants with BED and BN showed significant decreases in binge eating, lowered eating disorder symptom severity, trait food craving, and food cue reactivity (Brockmeyer et al., 2019). In another study, five sessions of ABM training were effective in reducing biases to negative social stimuli (Cardi et al., 2015). While adding an ABM intervention to inpatient programming for AN did not alter patients' attentional biases, patients with AN who completed the training experienced notable improvements in eating disorder symptom severity, depression, anxiety, and stress (Dikstein et al., 2023). Mindfulness, a method of directing thoughts toward stimuli while suppressing automatic judgments and appraisals (Greenberg et al., 2019), might also help individuals with eating disorders allocate attention away from eating-disorder-related urges and thoughts. Mindfulness practices have been shown to decrease binge eating in patients with BED (Kristeller & Hallett, 1999), decrease negative affect (Turgon et al., 2019) and body image concern in patients with BN and AN (Butryn et al., 2013), and decrease shape and weight concern, body checking, body avoidance, and anxiety in patients with AN (Dunne, 2018).

Response Inhibition

Response inhibition can be divided into reactive and proactive processes. Reactive inhibition occurs when a motor response is ceased after its initiation, while proactive inhibition occurs when a response is suppressed prior to its initiation (Meyer & Bucci, 2016; Perri, 2020; Zhang & Iwaki, 2019). Response inhibition can be divided similarly into action cancellation versus action restraint (Swick et al., 2011; Zhang et al., 2017).

Response inhibition is most commonly assessed using the stop-signal task (SST) (Verbruggen & Logan, 2008) and the go/no-go task (Simmonds et al., 2008) (see

Chapter 10). While both paradigms require subjects to respond to target stimuli and withhold responses to other stimuli, there are notable differences between them. On each trial of the SST, subjects are instructed to respond to a "go" stimulus, unless a "stop" signal occurs. The stop signal is presented in a minority of trials and with a delay after the onset of the go stimulus that varies over the course of the task (Logan et al., 2014; Verbruggen & Logan, 2008). Whereas the SST measures action cancellation (i.e., cancellation of an already initiated motor response), the go/no-go task measures action restraint (i.e., inhibition of a prepotent, but not yet initiated motor response). On go trials, subjects are required to rapidly respond to go stimuli (e.g., press a button in response to letter A) and on no-go trials, subjects must withhold responding to no-go stimuli (e.g., do not press a button in response to letter X; Aron & Poldrack, 2005; Simmonds et al., 2008; Zhang et al., 2017). As in the SST, the majority of trials are typically go-trials to increase subjects' prepotent tendency to respond (Simmonds et al., 2008).

Biological framework

Neuroimaging research in healthy individuals has implicated a bilateral frontoparietal network in response inhibition that includes the anterior insula, VLPFC, DLPFC, dorsal premotor cortex (dPMC), and bilateral intraparietal sulcus (IPS) extending into the superior parietal lobe (SPL) (Cieslik et al., 2015). The right temporoparietal junction (TPJ), the left inferior occipital gyrus, the pre-supplementary motor area (pre-SMA) extending into the dACC, and subcortical activation in the right thalamus and right caudate nucleus are also involved in response inhibition (Cieslik et al., 2015) (see Figure 12.2). Despite recognition that this common network is activated during response inhibition, withholding a response and stopping a response involve overlapping, but also distinct neural mechanisms. The go/no-go task primarily recruits frontoparietal areas (i.e., right DLPFC, right inferior parietal lobule/precuneus), whereas the SST primarily recruits cingo-opercular areas (i.e., left anterior insula, bilateral thalamus) (Swick et al., 2011). The go/no-go task elicits greater engagement of the left hemisphere, whereas the SST elicits greater engagement of the right hemisphere (Rubia et al., 2001).

State of the Science in Eating Disorders

Behavioral findings

Most studies indicate that individuals with AN-BP and BN show deficits in inhibitory control (Bruce et al., 2003; Hege et al., 2015; Wu, Giel, et al., 2013). Furthermore, some data suggest that compensatory behaviors are linked to more pronounced deficits in inhibitory control: SST deficits are larger in BN than

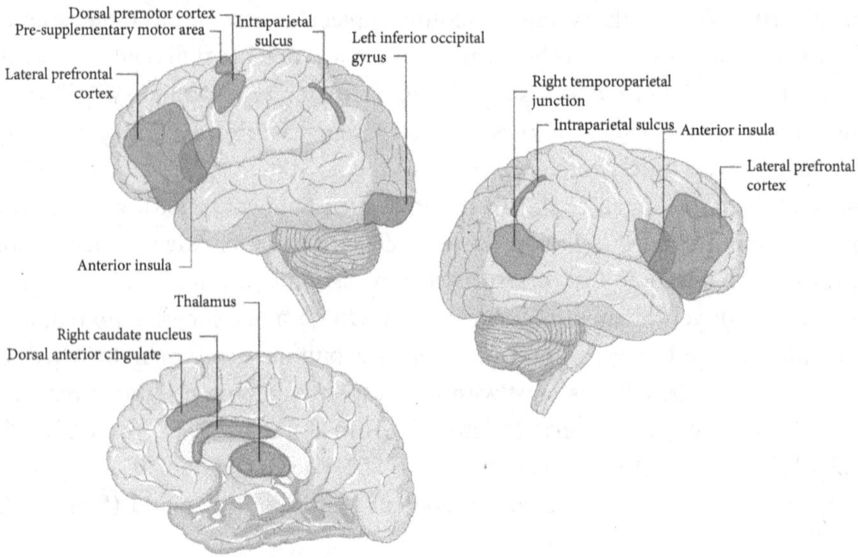

Figure 12.2 Neural circuits involved in response inhibition. Created with BioRender.com

in BED (Wu, Giel, et al., 2013) and among women with BN, individuals who misuse laxatives make more commission errors than those who do not (Bruce et al., 2003). Data from individuals with binge eating or threshold BED are more mixed, and results depend on whether food-specific tasks are used (Lavagnino et al., 2016; Manasse et al., 2016; Schag et al., 2013). Findings from studies that combine AN diagnostic subtypes or focus only on the restrictive subtype (AN-R) are similarly mixed. Although these individuals tend to report superior inhibitory control (Butler & Montgomery, 2005; Claes et al., 2006), some studies have found no differences in response inhibition performance between adolescents with AN and healthy controls (Wierenga et al., 2014), others found impaired inhibitory control in AN relative to healthy controls (Collantoni et al., 2016; Galimberti et al., 2012), and others find no difference between AN subtypes on SST task performance (Claes et al., 2006; Collantoni et al., 2016). Across eating disorder diagnoses, exposure to disorder-relevant stimuli seems to exaggerate decision-makers' predispositions. For example, response inhibition impairments in BN are even more pronounced on tasks with food stimuli (Berner et al., 2023; Wu, Giel, et al., 2013), whereas response inhibition is enhanced in the context of high-calorie versus low-calorie food stimuli in AN-R (Weinbach et al., 2020).

Neuroimaging findings

Existing literature on the neural correlates of response inhibition in eating disorders is sparse, especially for BN. Research to date suggests that more efficient activation during inhibition may play a role in dietary restriction, but that deficient or inefficient activation during response inhibition may play a role in binge eating and some compensatory behaviors. For instance, intact behavioral performance alongside reduced task-related activation in medial frontal regions (i.e., right MFG, right dorsal ACC, and left PCC) on difficult trials of the SST has been documented in adult women recovered from AN (Oberndorfer et al., 2011) and adolescent females with current AN-R (Wierenga et al., 2014). Thus, individuals with AN may require fewer neural resources to exert inhibitory control (Wierenga et al., 2014). Conversely, during go/no-go task inhibition, a mixed "binge/purge" group of adolescents, about one-third of whom were underweight, showed intact behavioral performance but increased activation in the bilateral precentral gyri, ACC, middle and superior temporal gyri, hypothalamus, and right DLPFC compared to healthy controls and adolescents with AN-R (Lock et al., 2011). These results suggest that individuals with binge eating and/or purging may require greater neural activation (i.e., compensatory brain responses) to successfully inhibit behavior.

However, similar to behavioral findings, neural correlates of response inhibition across diagnoses seem to be modulated by the salience of task stimuli. Using go/no-go tasks, one study reported that individuals with AN exhibited reduced activation of the putamen during response inhibition for food and non-food stimuli, but increased activation of the prefrontal cortex and cerebellum for physical activity stimuli (Kullmann et al., 2014). The authors speculate that physical activity places an increased demand on inhibitory control in AN. In contrast, individuals with BED and obesity demonstrate a food-specific deficit in prefrontal activation relative to controls on go/no-go task inhibition (Hege et al., 2015). A study of BN found, contrary to expectations, that more frequent binge eating was linked to reduced activation in the dorsal striatum and sensorimotor cortex during the inhibition of responses to neutral images, but not to food images (Skunde et al., 2016). Therefore, the directionality and stimulus-type specificity of response inhibition alterations remains unclear.

Alternative Perspectives

Do individuals with eating disorders over- or under-engage response inhibition circuitry?

Although it is commonly suggested that in the context of intact behavioral performance, increased brain response corresponds to greater recruitment of neural resources and decreased brain response corresponds to more efficient processing, it is also possible that the inverse is true (Wierenga et al., 2014). Decreased neural activation may indicate a failure to recruit necessary resources, a decrease in error monitoring (Wierenga et al., 2014), or a greater reliance on other brain regions (Bartholdy et al., 2016). Moreover, as behavioral findings differ across studies, and only some have directly associated brain activation and task performance metrics, the ability to draw definitive conclusions about neural patterns for response inhibition in any eating disorder remains limited. Future studies that investigate whole-brain functional connectivity during response inhibition tasks may help expand understanding of altered neural processes beyond just increased or decreased activation in particular regions (Bartholdy et al., 2016).

Which type of response inhibition matters for eating disorders?

Given the paucity of research focused on response inhibition in eating disorders, reviews, including this chapter, often combine results from the SST and the go/no-go task; however, the SST measures both cognitive and motor aspects of inhibition, whereas the motor challenge is smaller on go/no-go tasks and go/no-go commission errors arguably serve as a purer measure of the cognitive aspect of inhibition. Withholding responses before they occur (i.e., action restraint or proactive inhibition) could be most relevant for food avoidance and restrictive eating behavior. For instance, one study reported greater proactive inhibition (assessed via cued reaction time task) in participants with AN, but not those with BN or BED, compared to healthy controls (Bartholdy et al., 2016). However, the sense of loss of control over eating that characterizes binge-eating episodes can include difficulty preventing eating episodes from occurring, which may similarly result from altered action restraint. For instance, results from the Stop Signal Anticipation Task, which yields measures of both proactive and reactive inhibition, suggest that proactive inhibition may be decreased in BN (Westwater et al., 2021). On the other hand, stopping an already initiated response (i.e., action cancellation or reactive inhibition) could be most relevant for the difficulty stopping eating that characterizes binge eating. As such, both action cancellation and restraint could play a role in BN and BED. In support of this notion, individuals with non-clinical binge eating, compared to a group with no binge eating, showed no differences in task behavior, but reduced activation of the right DLPFC and putamen during go/no-go task inhibition, and increased activation of the left DLPFC during SST inhibition (Oliva et al., 2019). Thus, individuals with binge eating seem to differentially recruit frontostriatal regions to achieve successful action restraint and action cancellation. Similar studies that use directly comparable tasks within the same individuals with frank eating disorders are needed to pinpoint the specific response inhibition alterations that may contribute to specific symptoms.

Are the proper tasks being used to assess response inhibition in eating disorders?

In addition, at a neural level, there is debate about the extent to which the VLPFC, insula, and pre-SMA are necessary for response inhibition versus other related processes tapped by tasks like the go/no-go and SST (e.g., unusual or unexpected event detection; perceptual decision-making, attention, working memory; Criaud

& Boulinguez, 2013). Tasks that control for some of these factors (e.g., tasks that include an additional, rare-go stimulus that is presented as frequently as the no-go stimulus to control for the low-frequency oddball effect; Criaud & Boulinguez, 2013) have more strongly implicated the parietal cortex in response inhibition (Kolodny et al., 2017); however, to our knowledge, no published eating disorder studies of response inhibition have used these task designs. Therefore, it remains possible that neural alterations observed to date are driven by processes that support inhibition, but not inhibition itself.

Implications

Taken together, research suggests that altered frontostriatal engagement during response inhibition may contribute to eating disorders, and that response inhibition deficits may contribute to binge eating and purging. Newer medications that can enhance response inhibition and seem to have a limited impact on appetite, such as atomoxetine, may prove beneficial among individuals with binge/purge symptoms (Wilfahrt et al., 2021). Preliminary findings suggest that neurocognitive "inhibitory control training" paradigms in which individuals repeatedly practice withholding responses to disorder-relevant stimuli, may also prove fruitful for these populations (Chami et al., 2022). Non-invasive brain stimulation, such as repeated transcranial magnetic stimulation (rTMS), or neurofeedback that could further tune frontostriatal function, particularly prefrontal regulation of the striatum, may also hold promise as a treatment adjunct (Dunlop & Downar, 2017; Nitsche et al., 2008; Van den Eynde et al., 2010; Walpoth et al., 2007). However, additional research is needed to identify the optimal target, intensity, frequency, and duration of these treatments. This may prove particularly challenging for individuals with BN and those with AN-BP, who demonstrate both overcontrolled and undercontrolled eating behavior.

Delay Discounting

Self-regulatory control is also required to plan for the future and resist urges for immediate gratification. The ability to delay gratification to receive a more valuable reward in the future, or delay discounting, is one measure of this waiting-related control. Individuals who show larger decreases in reward value over time are described as having steeper discounting rates; this is reflected in a tendency to choose smaller, sooner rewards and is conceptualized as a form of decisional impulsivity (MacKillop et al., 2016). Indeed, steeper discounting rates have been found in disorders associated with impulsivity, like pathological gambling (Miedl et al., 2015), attention-deficit hyperactivity disorder (Jackson & MacKillop, 2016), and mania (Mason et al., 2012). Delay discounting can be measured using simple questionnaires with fixed questions (e.g., the Monetary Choice Questionnaire, MCQ; Kirby et al., 1999) or more elaborate tasks that adapt the presented options on each trial based on participant responses (e.g., the Delay-Discounting Task; Amlung et al., 2014). In all cases, participants make choices between a variety of smaller immediate rewards and larger delayed rewards (Lempert et al., 2019). While these tasks primarily use monetary rewards, some studies have used variants of the MCQ that present participants with delayed food rewards (Dassen et al., 2015; Hagan et al., 2021; Hendrickson et al., 2015). In all these variants, individual discounting rates (k) are commonly estimated using a hyperbolic discounting function (for a discussion of other model variants, see Green & Myerson, 2004). This parameter allows researchers to quantify the extent to which rewards are discounted as a function of their delay (see Chapter 7).

Biological framework

The processing of delayed rewards involves an expansive network of brain regions, with multiple valuation and control regions (Elton et al., 2017; Frost & McNaughton, 2017; Moreira et al., 2016; Smith et al., 2018; Volkow & Baler, 2015; Wesley & Bickel, 2014). Motivational information associated with immediate rewards increases activation in the amygdala, hippocampus, temporal lobe, insula, and ventral striatum (McClure et al., 2004, 2007; Smith et al., 2018). During a choice between immediate and delayed rewards, prefrontal regions receive both sensory inputs relayed from the junction between temporal and posterior cortices and valuation inputs from the striatum (Louie & Glimcher, 2010; see Figure 12.3). Activation in prefrontal regions associated with goal-directed behavior, such as the VMPFC and DLPFC, is thought to reflect a comparative process that weighs the trade-offs between the presented options and sends efferent signals to motor regions (Hare et al., 2014; Rodriguez et al., 2015). Notably, rTMS, cTBS, and tDCS applied to the DLPFC disrupt this comparison process and can idiosyncratically alter intertemporal choice depending on the type of stimulation (Figner et al., 2010; Shen et al., 2016; Xiong et al., 2019; Q. Zhang et al., 2023).

State of the Science in Eating Disorders

Behavioral findings

Overall, data seem to suggest that individuals with BED show increased delay discounting. However, there are several important caveats. For instance, results of a recent meta-analysis indicate that individuals with BED discount delayed rewards more steeply than healthy-weight controls (Amlung et al., 2019), but discounting rates may not reliably discriminate individuals with obesity who binge eat from

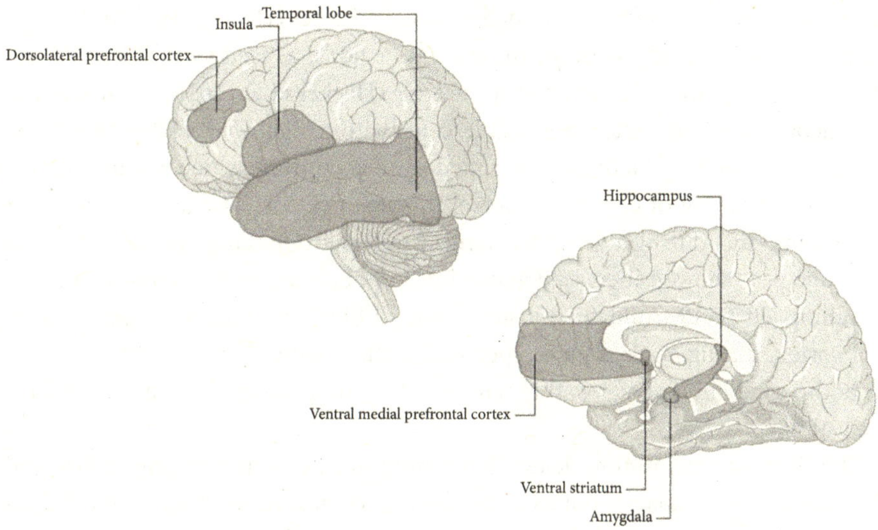

Figure 12.3 Neural circuits involved in delay discounting. Created with BioRender.com

those who do not (Stojek & MacKillop, 2017). Similarly, individuals with BN typically show greater delay discounting than healthy controls (Amlung et al., 2019). Conversely, one study found that women with full or sub-threshold BN discounted delayed food and monetary rewards less steeply than healthy controls, but they discounted food rewards more steeply than monetary rewards (Hagan et al., 2021).

In contrast to BED and BN, meta-analytic results suggest that individuals with AN discount delayed rewards less steeply than controls (Amlung et al., 2019). This behavior is consistent with the notion that increased self-regulation may contribute to the pronounced dietary restriction that characterizes the diagnosis. However, this unique pattern may be restricted to the AN-R subtype, as individuals with AN-BP have been found to discount more steeply than healthy controls in some studies (Steinglass et al., 2012; Steward et al., 2017). In addition, women remitted from BN or AN show monetary discounting rates comparable to healthy controls (Bischoff-Grethe et al., 2021; King et al., 2020; Ritschel et al., 2015; Wierenga et al., 2015), suggesting that recovery extends to more general regulatory behaviors.

Neuroimaging findings

Few studies have examined the neural underpinnings of delay discounting in eating disorders. Although one recent study of weight-recovered patients with AN found behavioral and neural patterns equivalent to those of healthy controls (King et al., 2020), other data suggest that decreased activation in control regions during delay discounting may characterize or contribute to acute AN, whereas increased activation in these regions may contribute to remission (Decker et al., 2015; Doose et al., 2020; Wierenga et al., 2015). One study found that adults with AN in a low-weight state show reduced activation in the dACC and ventral striatum during larger, later choices compared to smaller, sooner choices (Decker et al., 2015). After weight restoration, activation of these same regions, as well as the DLPFC and IPC, was greater than that of healthy controls (Decker et al., 2015). Similarly, following partial weight restoration, adolescents with AN showed a strengthening of default mode-network activation during delay discounting, which was interpreted to reflect an easing of cognitive control processes (Doose et al., 2020). Another study found that during a delay discounting task, a group remitted from AN for at least one year showed increased activation in putative cognitive control regions, including left DLPFC, bilateral insula, right VLPFC, and bilateral superior parietal cortex, during choices made specifically after eating (Wierenga et al., 2015). In both fasted and fed states, this remitted AN group showed increased DLPFC activation.

The literature examining delay discounting during neuroimaging in BN and BED is even more sparse, but existing findings do not support a role for altered activation of self-regulatory control circuitry in delay discounting in these disorders. While one study found that individuals remitted from BN showed altered neural activation in the striatum when processing immediately available rewards in fed versus fasted states, no differences were found in cognitive control regions or in association with decisions to delay rewards (Bischoff-Grethe et al., 2021). Therefore, these findings likely reflect the altered engagement of reward circuitry rather than self-regulation circuitry during delay discounting. Similarly, while steeper discounting rates and associated decreases in anterior insula activation when choosing immediate rewards over delayed rewards distinguish obese individuals from controls, these effects do not distinguish those with obesity from those with obesity and BED (Miranda-Olivos et al., 2021).

Alternative Perspective

Have delay discounting tasks measured a self-regulation process in eating disorders?

Although researchers typically interpret shallower discounting rates as reflecting self-regulatory control, specifically an ability to suppress impulsive desires (Figner et al., 2010; Hare et al., 2014; McClure et al., 2004, 2007; Peters & Büchel, 2011), an alternative perspective suggests that discounting rates actually reflect reward appraisals (Fujita, 2011; Magen et al., 2014). According to this perspective, choosing larger later rewards requires an individual to reappraise the weight they put on the immediacy of receiving a reward. This view is supported by recent work incorporating computational cognitive models, which show that individual differences in choice behavior tend to reflect variability in how rewards are appraised and biases that favor the delayed option rather than the immediate one (Zhao et al., 2019). On the other hand, other computational models that allow for both inhibitory and evaluative mechanisms find that both are needed, though inhibitory parameters better correlate with brain activation (Turner et al., 2019).

The role of the DLPFC during delay discounting is especially contentious within this debate. A major issue is that many studies base their conclusions on the reverse inference that the recruitment of DLPFC is evidence that hedonistic impulses are being successfully suppressed, without independently assessing impulsivity using other measures. However, recent work suggests that the DLPFC responds to discrepancies between choice behavior and normative goals, regardless of which goals are emphasized (Hutcherson & Tusche, 2022). Supporting this view, atrophy in dorsal regions of the prefrontal cortex impairs older adults' ability to incorporate choice-relevant information rather than their baseline preference for immediate rewards, highlighting the importance of information appraisal in delay discounting decisions (Beagle et al., 2020). From this perspective, altered DLPFC activation during delay discounting among individuals with eating disorders likely relates to how different sources of information about value are incorporated.

Developing a proper theoretical framework for contextualizing delay discounting in eating disorders will require revamped methodologies. In line with a broad call to develop new measures of intertemporal choice beyond discounting rates (Bailey et al., 2021), novel paradigms, especially those that present individuals with eating-related decisions and that incorporate food palatability (e.g., Appelhans et al., 2011), may be particularly useful. Importantly, future work focused on the role of self-regulation in intertemporal choice will need to account for the fact that time perception may be altered across eating disorders (Meneguzzo et al., 2022), likely affecting how these individuals choose to exert self-regulation to wait.

Implications

If BN and BED are characterized by steep delay discounting and AN-R is characterized by shallow delay discounting, interventions that have been shown to affect discount rates and their underlying neural circuitry may be effective. For example, preliminary data suggest that neuromodulation of the DLPFC decreases delay discounting and reduces the urge to binge eat in BN (Kekic et al., 2017). To decrease discount rates, other studies have used framing manipulations, delay exposures, delay tolerance training, and episodic future thinking (in which individuals practice imagining larger later rewards) (Rung et al., 2019). Similar interventions could be applied to target BN and BED, and perhaps the same approaches, but with an emphasis on smaller, sooner rewards or recovery-related rewards, could be helpful for AN-R.

Emotion Regulation

Acceptance, reappraisal (e.g., reinterpretation, distancing/detachment), and problem-solving are widely regarded as adaptive emotion regulation strategies, whereas rumination, avoidance, and suppression are widely regarded as maladaptive (Aldao et al., 2010). While the majority of research on emotion regulation in eating disorders relies on self-report measures, two main behavioral measures exist. In emotion regulation paradigms that are typically combined with neuroimaging (Diers et al., 2014; Ochsner et al., 2002; Walter et al., 2009), participants are presented with visual stimuli (commonly from the International Affective Picture System; Lang et al., 2005) and are instructed to either actively regulate their elicited emotion using a specific strategy taught by the experimenter or to passively view the stimuli. Participants rate the intensity of their emotion on each trial. Even with these ratings, it can be difficult to assess participants' compliance with instructions on these tasks (Demaree et al., 2006; McRae et al., 2012), so some studies simultaneously measure skin conductance as an objective measure of pre- and post-regulation arousal (e.g., Boehme et al., 2019; Steward et al., 2022). In contrast, emotional go/no-go tasks, such as the Cognitive Control Under Emotions task (CCUE; Cohen et al., 2016), provide an objective behavioral output and do not rely on individuals using an instructed cognitive strategy. However, rather than measuring emotion regulation, these tasks measure a related but slightly different construct: how emotional stimuli modulate response inhibition.

Biological framework

Explicit downregulation of negative emotions has been linked to activation of prefrontal regions (i.e., orbitofrontal cortex, DLPFC, DMPFC, VLPFC), dACC, inferior parietal cortex [IPC], bilateral anterior insula, left supplementary motor area [SMA], bilateral precuneus, and bilateral middle temporal gyrus [Beauregard et al., 2001; Buhle et al., 2014; Diekhof et al., 2011; Dolcos et al., 2011; Doré et al., 2017; Dörfel et al., 2014; Ochsner et al., 2002; Phillips et al., 2008]). During some forms of volitional emotion regulation, prefrontal regions exert a top-down inhibitory effect on the amygdala, resulting in reduced activation to aversive stimuli (Diekhof et al., 2011; Ochsner & Gross, 2005; Phillips et al., 2008). However, neuroimaging studies also suggest that different emotion regulation strategies recruit distinct neural networks. For example, detachment, expressive suppression, and distraction all recruit a right prefrontoparietal regulation network leading to reduced concurrent amygdala activation, whereas reinterpretation uniquely recruits the left VLPFC and orbitofrontal gyrus with no concurrent effect on the amygdala (Dörfel et al., 2014) (see Figure 12.4).

State of the Science in Eating Disorders

Behavioral findings

Self-report studies have consistently shown that individuals with eating disorders have limited access to adaptive emotion regulation strategies and more frequently use maladaptive strategies (Danner et al., 2014; Dingemans et al., 2017;

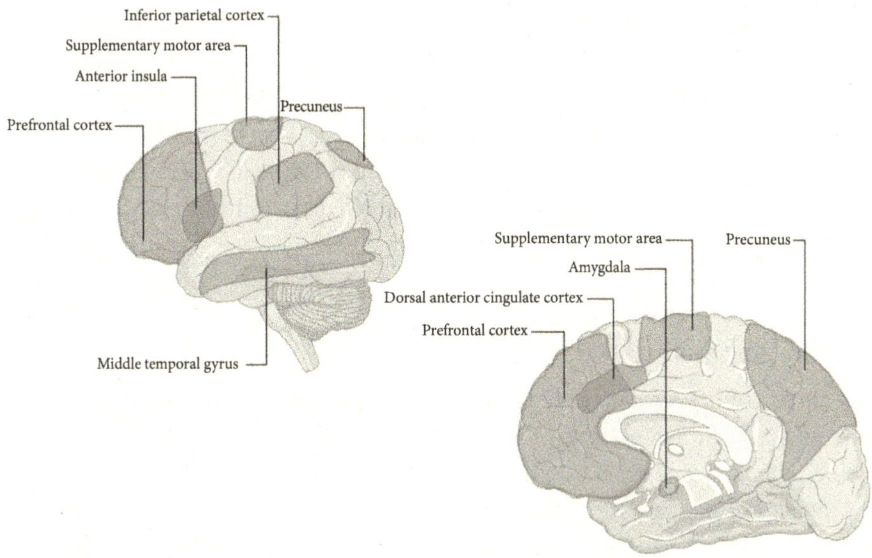

Figure 12.4 Neural circuits involved in emotion regulation. Created with BioRender.com

Lavender et al., 2015; Mallorquí-Bagué et al., 2018; Westwood et al., 2017). These difficulties in emotion regulation are trans-diagnostic and relate to symptoms (Brockmeyer et al., 2014). For example, in BN and BED, high negative affect tends to precede binge-eating episodes (Haedt-Matt & Keel, 2011; Leehr et al., 2015; Pearson, Wonderlich, et al., 2015), suggesting that binge eating may be a maladaptive emotion regulation strategy in itself. However, a systematic review and meta-analysis found that individuals with AN tend to use adaptive strategies less frequently compared to those with BN (Puttevils et al., 2021). In addition, compared with BN, BED, and AN-R, individuals with AN-BP have the greatest difficulty remaining in control of their behavior when experiencing negative emotions (Brockmeyer et al., 2019). These results suggest that AN, specifically AN-BP, may be most strongly associated with difficulties with emotional reactivity, whereas BN and BED may be more strongly linked to difficulties with emotion regulation.

Contrary to questionnaire-based results, existing data from affect ratings in emotion regulation paradigms suggest that individuals with AN do not differ from controls in their ability to downregulate their arousal or distress in response to negative affective pictures (Seidel, King, Ritschel, Boehm, Geisler, Bernardoni, Beck, et al., 2018; Steward et al., 2022). No published studies to date have used these tasks to study BN or BED. Findings from emotional go/no-go tasks have been mixed. One study reported increased commission errors in individuals with AN compared with controls, only in the context of emotionally valenced stimuli (Hildebrandt et al., 2016), another reported no task performance differences between AN, binge spectrum, and healthy control groups (Mallorquí-Bagué et al., 2020), and another reported that a mixed group of individuals with AN and BN-spectrum disorders showed increased behavioral accuracy compared with controls (Malagoli et al., 2021). Another study focused on BN found that emotional go/no-go task deficits may be developmentally dependent: individuals with BN did not show typical improvements in performance with age (Dreyfuss et al., 2017). Overall, to date, behavioral tasks have been mostly unsuccessful in capturing emotion regulation difficulties in eating disorders.

Neuroimaging findings

Only three studies to date (Seidel, King, Ritschel, Boehm, Geisler, Bernardoni, Beck, et al., 2018; Seidel, King, Ritschel, Boehm, Geisler, Bernardoni, Holzapfel, et al., 2018; Steward et al., 2022) have investigated neural correlates of emotion regulation in any eating disorder, and all have focused on AN. Two studies used the distancing strategy and found that compared to controls, individuals with AN did not show differences in ventral striatum activation when decreasing positive emotion or in amygdala activation when decreasing negative emotion (Seidel, King, Ritschel, Boehm, Geisler, Bernardoni, Beck, et al., 2018; Seidel, King, Ritschel, Boehm, Geisler, Bernardoni, Holzapfel, et al., 2018). However, adolescents with AN showed increased amygdala and DLPFC response to aversive/negative pictures during passive viewing (Seidel, King, Ritschel, Boehm, Geisler, Bernardoni, Beck, et al., 2018), indicative of increased reactivity to emotionally aversive stimuli. In contrast, another study with adult participants with AN found decreased DLPFC response and decreased coupling between the DLPFC and amygdala when individuals used the reinterpretation strategy to decrease negative emotion (Steward et al., 2022). Across studies, neural activation predicted outcome: lower ventral striatal activation during positive emotion downregulation was associated with increased body-related rumination, increased negative affect, and less weight gain (Seidel, King, Ritschel, Boehm, Geisler, Bernardoni, Beck, et al., 2018; Seidel, King, Ritschel, Boehm, Geisler, Bernardoni, Holzapfel, et al., 2018), and lower DLPFC activation during negative emotion downregulation was associated with reduced weight gain in treatment (Steward et al., 2022). Therefore, patterns of activation during attempted emotion regulation seem relevant for symptoms of AN, but the nature of this association seems to depend on the valence of the emotion, the emotion regulation strategy, and the age of the individual.

Neuroimaging research focused on emotion regulation in binge-spectrum eating disorders is even more limited. One fMRI study found that BN participants show age-dependent deficits in prefrontal cortex activation during an emotional go/no-go task compared to healthy controls (Dreyfuss et al., 2017). While these findings have implications for emotion-related processes in BN, additional research is needed to assess emotion regulation in BN and BED.

Alternative Perspectives

Do eating disorder behaviors serve an emotion regulation function?

The momentary link between negative affect and subsequent eating disorder symptoms in BN, BED, and AN is well-established. Some work using ecological momentary assessment (EMA) suggests that negative affect decreases following symptom engagement, supporting a conceptualization of eating disorder behaviors as maladaptive forms of emotion regulation partly maintained by negative reinforcement (Haedt-Matt & Keel, 2011; Leehr et al., 2015; Wonderlich et al., 2022). However, other work points to increases in negative affect or at least continued high levels of negative affect after behaviors like binge eating (Dingemans et al., 2017; Haedt-Matt & Keel, 2011). These findings undermine negative reinforcement frameworks and suggest that individuals with eating disorders may struggle to learn about the emotional outcomes of their behaviors. Some argue that inconsistent results may be related to the timing of affect ratings relative to eating disorder behaviors and the use of analytic strategies that do not consider trajectories of affect before and after behaviors (Berg et al., 2017). Future research integrating EMA with resting-state and task-based neuroimaging and psychophysiological measures like skin conductance could better evaluate how eating disorder behaviors influence emotion reactivity circuitry and whether altered emotion regulation circuit function explains the use of maladaptive emotion regulation strategies among individuals with eating disorders.

Is the primary problem with emotion regulation or discrimination?

Although self-report data strongly suggest problems with emotion regulation among individuals with eating disorders, another possibility is that these reported experiences are better understood as another manifestation of altered "bottom-up" processes, specifically interoception. Interoception, or the ability to sense the physiological condition of the body, recruits similar neural circuits to emotion regulation, is critical for successful emotion regulation, and has also been consistently found to be altered among individuals with eating disorders (Adolfi et al., 2017; Jenkinson et al., 2018; Khalsa et al., 2022; Zamariola et al., 2019; see Chapter 8). Some researchers argue that these interoceptive alterations may make it difficult for individuals with eating disorders to disentangle and learn from body signals indicating hunger and fullness from those related to emotion (Adolfi et al., 2017; Jenkinson et al., 2018; Khalsa et al., 2022; Zamariola et al., 2019). This could interfere with successful emotion identification, which is critical for the subsequent selection of an appropriate regulation strategy (Morie et al., 2022), and result in behaviors that are designed to address physiological sensations like fullness in response to physiological sensations for strong emotions. In partial support of these ideas, considerable research suggests that mistrust of body signals strongly relates to eating disorder symptom severity (Brown et al., 2017, 2020; Perry et al.,

2021), and individuals with eating disorders show elevated scores on tools that measure deficits in emotional clarity (e.g., Ruscitti et al., 2016). Additional research focused on the neural underpinnings of interoception in eating disorders could help clarify whether interventions that target interoceptive awareness or accuracy would be more effective in addressing emotion dysregulation in this population.

Implications

Neuroimaging findings in AN suggest that teaching adaptive emotion regulation strategies may be an effective intervention (Seidel, King, Ritschel, Boehm, Geisler, Bernardoni, Beck, et al., 2018). Additionally, decreasing the habitual use of suppression and increasing the use of reappraisal may be an effective treatment target for binge eating (Dingemans et al., 2017). Some existing therapies, including Integrative Cognitive-Affective Therapy (ICAT) and Dialectical Behavior Therapy (DBT), focus on helping patients develop specific skills to adaptively regulate negative emotions in lieu of binge eating (Peterson et al., 2020; Safer et al., 2009; Wonderlich et al., 2014). However, to date, these treatments have not outperformed traditional cognitive-behavioral therapy (Peterson et al., 2020; Safer et al., 2009; Wonderlich et al., 2014). If patients have difficulty effectively implementing adaptive emotion regulation skills, biologically targeted interventions like neurostimulation may enhance emotion regulation abilities (Feeser et al., 2014). However, given the mixed nature of neuroimaging findings in AN and the lack of emotion-regulation-focused neuroimaging research in BN and BED, the regions or connectivity that would be targeted, and whether the goal would be to increase or decrease activation or connectivity are not yet clear.

Limitations and Paths Forward

Overall, data seem to suggest reductions in self-regulation abilities among individuals with binge eating, and potentially enhanced or more efficient self-regulation among individuals with AN-R. However, major knowledge gaps remain. Findings across many of the constructs reviewed have been mixed, the field has yet to fully explore the latent cognitive processes that ultimately contribute to altered self-regulation in eating disorders, and the prognostic utility of self-regulation measures is still unclear. Next, we map an agenda for future research to fill these gaps.

Computational psychiatry approaches

Computational psychiatry approaches may help resolve some of the inconsistencies in behavioral and neurophysiological patterns observed in past work (see Chapter 5). Theory-driven cognitive computational models that describe the biologically feasible computations that generate behavior can offer insights into how individuals with eating disorders approach, accumulate information about, and adapt to self-regulatory control demands. For example, sequential sampling models (SSM) such as the diffusion decision model (DDM; Ratcliff & McKoon, 2008) allow for individual decision-makers to vary in their initial biases toward a specific response or in the amount of time they take to encode the stimulus or make a motor response (Myers et al., 2022; Ratcliff et al., 2016). SSMs have been applied to various self-regulation tasks, including the flanker task (Luo & Proctor, 2022; Servant & Evans, 2020), Stroop task (Bustamante et al., 2021; Fennell & Ratcliff, 2019), go/no-go task (Gomez et al., 2007; Ratcliff et al., 2018), and the SST (Logan et al., 2014; Matzke et al., 2019). In contrast to the aspects of decision-making modeled by SSMs, models based on Bayesian inference capture how individuals make predictions about the optimal level of cognitive control required in a given context and have been applied to cognitive interference control and response inhibition tasks (Jiang et al., 2014). We have recently used one such model to better understand response inhibition in remitted BN (Berner et al., 2023), and we are currently using it to study symptomatic individuals. Future applications of such models to behavioral task data, alone or in combination with fMRI, could helpfully delineate subcomponents of self-regulation across eating disorders.

Like cognitive computational models, biophysical models of neural activation and machine learning approaches also may help to resolve some of the inconsistencies in past self-regulation research findings. For example, dynamic causal modeling (DCM) can model how activation in one part of the brain influences activation in another part, and how those interactions might be modulated by a task condition (Friston et al., 2003). This approach has not yet been applied to the study of self-regulation in eating disorders, but it could allow researchers to better understand how self-regulation circuit dynamics, not just regions that make up those circuits, may be altered (He et al., 2019; Stephan et al., 2010). Similarly, machine learning approaches could be used to cluster behavior across self-regulation tasks and measures or to further determine whether classifiers based on brain and behavioral data from self-regulation tasks could accurately predict disorder risk or treatment response (Cyr et al., 2018).

Longitudinal designs

To identify optimal self-regulation-related targets for prevention efforts and targets and prognostic markers for treatment, additional longitudinal studies are needed. Some investigations of self-regulation in AN have assessed individuals before and after weight restoration (Decker et al., 2015; Doose et al., 2020). While very few studies of self-regulation in any eating disorder have adopted a developmental perspective, those studies that have yielded somewhat inconsistent findings. For example, some research has found no support for the hypothesis that self-reported impulse control deficits predicted future onset of eating disorders (Tyrka et al., 2002; Wonderlich et al., 2004); however, two other studies have found that self-reported impulsivity predicts the onset of binge eating (Pearson et al., 2012; Pearson, Zapolski, et al., 2015). Findings from the two longitudinal neuroimaging studies that have used a developmental approach have shown that increased medial frontal activation during SST stop trial errors predicts the development of binge eating and/or purging (Bartholdy et al., 2019) and that, in teens with BN, reduced cortical thickness in the right inferior frontal gyrus, a region that is implicated in multiple forms of self-regulation, persists over adolescence, even in those who achieve symptom remission (Cyr et al., 2017). The mixed nature of these findings may relate to the fact that different task-based measures of self-regulation are sometimes differentially, and often not at all, associated with self-report measures of self-regulation (e.g., Claes et al., 2006; Enticott et al., 2006). However, the majority of findings so far seem to suggest that reduced self-regulation may contribute to the development and persistence of BN symptoms into adulthood. Similarly, some preliminary data suggest that poorer inhibitory control in the context of emotion and poorer cognitive interference control predict worse outcomes after cognitive-behavioral therapy for eating disorders (Testa et al., 2022). Additionally, large studies following individuals naturalistically over development and before and after treatments could identify aspects of self-regulation that may predict outcomes or be changed by treatment. Finally, studies focused on whether altered self-regulation predicts the development and persistence of AN are needed.

References

Adolfi, F., Couto, B., Richter, F., Decety, J., Lopez, J., Sigman, M., Manes, F., & Ibáñez, A. (2017). Convergence of interoception, emotion, and social cognition: A twofold fMRI meta-analysis and lesion approach. *Cortex, 88*, 124–142. https://doi.org/10.1016/j.cortex.2016.12.019

Ainslie, G. (1975). Specious reward: A behavioral theory of impulsiveness and impulse control. *Psychological Bulletin, 82*, 463–496. https://doi.org/10.1037/h0076860

Aldao, A., Nolen-Hoeksema, S., & Schweizer, S. (2010). Emotion-regulation strategies across psychopathology: A meta-analytic review. *Clinical Psychology Review, 30*(2), 217–237. https://doi.org/10.1016/j.cpr.2009.11.004

Amlung, M., Marsden, E., Holshausen, K., Morris, V., Patel, H., Vedelago, L., Naish, K. R., Reed, D. D., & McCabe, R. E. (2019). Delay discounting as a transdiagnostic process in psychiatric disorders: A meta-analysis. *JAMA Psychiatry, 76*(11), 1176–1186. https://doi.org/10.1001/jamapsychiatry.2019.2102

Amlung, M., Sweet, L. H., Acker, J., Brown, C. L., & MacKillop, J. (2014). Dissociable brain signatures of choice conflict and immediate reward preferences in alcohol use disorders. *Addiction Biology, 19*(4), 743–753. https://doi.org/10.1111/adb.12017

Appelhans, B. M., Woolf, K., Pagoto, S. L., Schneider, K. L., Whited, M. C., & Liebman, R. (2011). Inhibiting food reward: Delay discounting, food reward sensitivity, and palatable food intake in overweight and obese women. *Obesity, 19*(11), 2175–2182. https://doi.org/10.1038/oby.2011.57

Armstrong, T., & Olatunji, B. O. (2012). Eye tracking of attention in the affective disorders: A meta-analytic review and synthesis. *Clinical Psychology Review, 32*(8), 704–723. https://doi.org/10.1016/j.cpr.2012.09.004

Aron, A. R., & Poldrack, R. A. (2005). The cognitive neuroscience of response inhibition: Relevance for genetic research in attention-deficit/hyperactivity disorder. *Biological Psychiatry, 57*(11), 1285–1292. https://doi.org/10.1016/j.biopsych.2004.10.026

Bailey, A. J., Romeu, R. J., & Finn, P. R. (2021). The problems with delay discounting: A critical review of current practices and clinical applications. *Psychological Medicine, 51*(11), 1799–1806. https://doi.org/10.1017/S0033291721002282

Balodis, I. M., Molina, N. D., Kober, H., Worhunsky, P. D., White, M. A., Sinha, R., Grilo, C. M., & Potenza, M. N. (2013). Divergent neural substrates of inhibitory control in binge eating disorder relative to other manifestations of obesity. *Obesity, 21*(2), 367–377. https://doi.org/10.1002/oby.20068

Bartholdy, S., Dalton, B., O'Daly, O. G., Campbell, I. C., & Schmidt, U. (2016). A systematic review of the relationship between eating, weight and inhibitory control using the stop signal task. *Neuroscience & Biobehavioral Reviews, 64*, 35–62. https://doi.org/10.1016/j.neubiorev.2016.02.010

Bartholdy, S., O'Daly, O. G., Campbell, I. C., Banaschewski, T., Barker, G., Bokde, A. L. W., Bromberg, U., Büchel, C., Quinlan, E. B., Desrivières, S., Flor, H., Frouin, V., Garavan, H., Gowland, P., Heinz, A., Ittermann, B., Martinot, J.-L., Paillère Martinot, M.-L., Nees, F., Orfanos, D. P., . . . IMAGEN Consortium. (2019). Neural correlates of failed inhibitory control as an early marker of disordered eating in adolescents. *Biological Psychiatry, 85*(11), 956–965. https://doi.org/10.1016/j.biopsych.2019.01.027

Beagle, A. J., Zahir, A., Borzello, M., Kayser, A. S., Hsu, M., Miller, B. L., Kramer, J. H., & Chiong, W. (2020). Amount and delay insensitivity during intertemporal choice in three neurodegenerative diseases reflects dorsomedial prefrontal atrophy. *Cortex, 124*, 54–65. https://doi.org/10.1016/j.cortex.2019.10.009

Beauregard, M., Lévesque, J., & Bourgouin, P. (2001). Neural correlates of conscious self-regulation of emotion. *Journal of Neuroscience, 21*(18), RC165–RC165. https://doi.org/10.1523/JNEUROSCI.21-18-j0001.2001

Berg, K. C., Cao, L., Crosby, R. D., Engel, S. G., Peterson, C. B., Crow, S. J., Le Grange, D., Mitchell, J. E., Lavender, J. M., Durkin, N., & Wonderlich, S. A. (2017). Negative affect and binge eating: Reconciling differences between two analytic approaches in ecological momentary assessment research. *International Journal of Eating Disorders, 50*(10), 1222–1230. https://doi.org/10.1002/eat.22770

Berner, L. A., Harlé, K. M., Simmons, A. N., Yu, A., Paulus, M. P., Bischoff-Grethe, A., Wierenga, C. E., Bailer, U. F., & Kaye, W. H. (2023). State-specific alterations in the neural computations underlying inhibitory control in women remitted from bulimia nervosa. *Molecular Psychiatry, 28*, 3055–3062. https://doi.org/10.1038/s41380-023-02063-6

Berner, L. A., Winter, S. R., Ayaz, H., Shewokis, P. A., Izzetoglu, M., Marsh, R., . . . & Lowe, M. R. (2023). Altered prefrontal activation during the inhibition of eating responses in women with bulimia nervosa. *Psychological Medicine, 53*(8), 3580–3590.

Bischoff-Grethe, A., Wierenga, C. E., Bailer, U. F., McClure, S. M., & Kaye, W. H. (2021). Satiety does not alter the ventral striatum's response to immediate reward in bulimia nervosa. *Journal of Abnormal Psychology, 130*, 862–874. https://doi.org/10.1037/abn0000712

Blasi, G., Goldberg, T. E., Weickert, T., Das, S., Kohn, P., Zoltick, B., Bertolino, A., Callicott, J. H., Weinberger, D. R., & Mattay, V. S. (2006). Brain regions underlying response inhibition and interference monitoring and suppression. *European Journal of Neuroscience, 23*(6), 1658–1664. https://doi.org/10.1111/j.1460-9568.2006.04680.x

Boehme, S., Biehl, S. C., & Mühlberger, A. (2019). Effects of differential strategies of emotion regulation. *Brain Sciences, 9*(9), article 9. https://doi.org/10.3390/brainsci9090225

Brockmeyer, T., Friederich, H.-C., Küppers, C., Chowdhury, S., Harms, L., Simmonds, J., Gordon, G., Potterton, R., & Schmidt, U. (2019). Approach bias modification training in bulimia nervosa and binge-eating disorder: A pilot randomized controlled trial. *International Journal of Eating Disorders, 52*(5), 520–529. https://doi.org/10.1002/eat.23024

Brockmeyer, T., Skunde, M., Wu, M., Bresslein, E., Rudofsky, G., Herzog, W., & Friederich, H.-C. (2014). Difficulties in emotion regulation across the spectrum of eating disorders. *Comprehensive Psychiatry, 55*(3), 565–571. https://doi.org/10.1016/j.comppsych.2013.12.001

Brown, T. A., Berner, L. A., Jones, M. D., Reilly, E. E., Cusack, A., Anderson, L. K., Kaye, W. H., & Wierenga, C. E. (2017). Psychometric evaluation and norms for the multidimensional assessment of interoceptive awareness (MAIA) in a clinical eating disorders sample. *European Eating Disorders Review, 25*(5), 411–416. https://doi.org/10.1002/erv.2532

Brown, T. A., Vanzhula, I. A., Reilly, E. E., Levinson, C. A., Berner, L. A., Krueger, A., Lavender, J. M., Kaye, W. H., & Wierenga, C. E. (2020). Body mistrust bridges interoceptive awareness and eating disorder symptoms. *Journal of Abnormal Psychology, 129*(5), 445–456. https://doi.org/10.1037/abn0000516

Bruce, K. R., Koerner, N. M., Steiger, H., & Young, S. N. (2003). Laxative misuse and behavioral disinhibition in bulimia nervosa. *International Journal of Eating Disorders, 33*(1), 92–97. https://doi.org/10.1002/eat.10116

Buhle, J. T., Silvers, J. A., Wager, T. D., Lopez, R., Onyemekwu, C., Kober, H., Weber, J., & Ochsner, K. N. (2014). Cognitive reappraisal of emotion: A meta-analysis of human neuroimaging studies. *Cerebral Cortex, 24*(11), 2981–2990. https://doi.org/10.1093/cercor/bht154

Bustamante, L., Lieder, F., Musslick, S., Shenhav, A., & Cohen, J. (2021). Learning to overexert cognitive control in a stroop task. *Cognitive, Affective, & Behavioral Neuroscience, 21*(3), 453–471. https://doi.org/10.3758/s13415-020-00845-x

Butler, G. K. L., & Montgomery, A. M. J. (2005). Subjective self-control and behavioural impulsivity coexist in anorexia nervosa. *Eating Behaviors, 6*(3), 221–227. https://doi.org/10.1016/j.eatbeh.2004.11.002

Butryn, M. L., Juarascio, A., Shaw, J., Kerrigan, S. G., Clark, V., O'Planick, A., & Forman, E. M. (2013). Mindfulness and its relationship with eating disorders symptomatology in women receiving residential treatment. *Eating Behaviors, 14*(1), 13–16. https://doi.org/10.1016/j.eatbeh.2012.10.005

Cardi, V., Esposito, M., Bird, G., Rhind, C., Yiend, J., Schifano, S., Hirsch, C., & Treasure, J. (2015). A preliminary investigation of a novel training to target cognitive biases towards negative social stimuli in anorexia nervosa. *Journal of Affective Disorders, 188*, 188–193. https://doi.org/10.1016/j.jad.2015.08.019

Chami, R., Cardi, V., Lawrence, N., MacDonald, P., Rowlands, K., Hodsoll, J., & Treasure, J. (2022). Targeting binge eating in bulimia nervosa and binge eating disorder using inhibitory control training and implementation intentions: A feasibility trial. *Psychological Medicine, 52*(5), 874–883. https://doi.org/10.1017/S0033291720002494

Cieslik, E. C., Mueller, V. I., Eickhoff, C. R., Langner, R., & Eickhoff, S. B. (2015). Three key regions for supervisory attentional control: Evidence from neuroimaging meta-analyses. *Neuroscience & Biobehavioral Reviews, 48*, 22–34. https://doi.org/10.1016/j.neubiorev.2014.11.003

Claes, L., Nederkoorn, C., Vandereycken, W., Guerrieri, R., & Vertommen, H. (2006). Impulsiveness and lack of inhibitory control in eating disorders. *Eating Behaviors, 7*(3), 196–203. https://doi.org/10.1016/j.eatbeh.2006.05.001

Cohen, A. O., Breiner, K., Steinberg, L., Bonnie, R. J., Scott, E. S., Taylor-Thompson, K., Rudolph, M. D., Chein, J., Richeson, J. A., Heller, A. S., Silverman, M. R., Dellarco, D. V., Fair, D. A., Galván, A., & Casey, B. J. (2016). When is an adolescent an adult? Assessing cognitive control in emotional and nonemotional contexts. *Psychological Science, 27*(4), 549–562. https://doi.org/10.1177/0956797615627625

Collantoni, E., Michelon, S., Tenconi, E., Degortes, D., Titton, F., Manara, R., Clementi, M., Pinato, C., Forzan, M., Cassina, M., Santonastaso, P., & Favaro, A. (2016). Functional connectivity correlates of response inhibition impairment in anorexia nervosa. *Psychiatry Research: Neuroimaging, 247*, 9–16. https://doi.org/10.1016/j.pscychresns.2015.11.008

Corbetta, M., & Shulman, G. L. (2002). Control of goal-directed and stimulus-driven attention in the brain. *Nature Reviews Neuroscience, 3*(3), article 3. https://doi.org/10.1038/nrn755

Criaud, M., & Boulinguez, P. (2013). Have we been asking the right questions when assessing response inhibition in go/no-go tasks with fMRI? A meta-analysis and critical review. *Neuroscience & Biobehavioral Reviews, 37*(1), 11–23. https://doi.org/10.1016/j.neubiorev.2012.11.003

Cyr, M., Kopala-Sibley, D. C., Lee, S., Chen, C., Stefan, M., Fontaine, M., Terranova, K., Berner, L. A., & Marsh, R. (2017). Reduced inferior and orbital frontal thickness in adolescent bulimia nervosa persists over two-year follow-up. *Journal of the American Academy of Child & Adolescent Psychiatry, 56*(10), 866–874.e7. https://doi.org/10.1016/j.jaac.2017.08.008

Cyr, M., Yang, X., Horga, G., & Marsh, R. (2018). Abnormal fronto-striatal activation as a marker of threshold and subthreshold Bulimia Nervosa. *Human Brain Mapping, 39*(4), 1796–1804. https://doi.org/10.1002/hbm.23955

Danner, U. N., Sternheim, L., & Evers, C. (2014). The importance of distinguishing between the different eating disorders (sub)types when assessing emotion regulation strategies. *Psychiatry Research, 215*(3), 727–732. https://doi.org/10.1016/j.psychres.2014.01.005

Dassen, F. C. M., Houben, K., & Jansen, A. (2015). Time orientation and eating behavior: Unhealthy eaters consider immediate consequences, while healthy eaters focus on future health. *Appetite, 91*, 13–19. https://doi.org/10.1016/j.appet.2015.03.020

Decker, J. H., Figner, B., & Steinglass, J. E. (2015). On weight and waiting: Delay discounting in anorexia nervosa pretreatment and posttreatment. *Biological Psychiatry*, *78*(9), 606–614. https://doi.org/10.1016/j.biopsych.2014.12.016

Demaree, H. A., Robinson, J. L., Pu, J., & Allen, J. J. B. (2006). Strategies actually employed during response-focused emotion regulation research: Affective and physiological consequences. *Cognition and Emotion*, *20*(8), 1248–1260. https://doi.org/10.1080/02699930500405303

Diekhof, E. K., Geier, K., Falkai, P., & Gruber, O. (2011). Fear is only as deep as the mind allows: A coordinate-based meta-analysis of neuroimaging studies on the regulation of negative affect. *NeuroImage*, *58*(1), 275–285. https://doi.org/10.1016/j.neuroimage.2011.05.073

Diers, K., Weber, F., Brocke, B., Strobel, A., & Schönfeld, S. (2014). Instructions matter: A comparison of baseline conditions for cognitive emotion regulation paradigms. *Frontiers in Psychology*, *5*, 347 https://www.frontiersin.org/journals/psychology/articles/10.3389/fpsyg.2014.00347

Dikstein, H., Gilon-Mann, T., Halevi-Yosef, R., Enoch-Levi, A., Hamdan, S., Gur, E., Haim, Y. B., Lazarov, A., Treasure, J., & Stein, D. (2023). Attention bias modification add-on to inpatient treatment for young women with anorexia nervosa—A randomized controlled trial. *European Eating Disorders Review*, *31*(2), 285–302. https://doi.org/10.1002/erv.2957

Dingemans, A., Danner, U., & Parks, M. (2017). Emotion regulation in binge eating disorder: A review. *Nutrients*, *9*(11), article 11. https://doi.org/10.3390/nu9111274

Dobson, K. S., & Dozois, D. J. A. (2004). Attentional biases in eating disorders: A meta-analytic review of Stroop performance. *Clinical Psychology Review*, *23*(8), 1001–1022. https://doi.org/10.1016/j.cpr.2003.09.004

Dolcos, F., Iordan, A. D., & Dolcos, S. (2011). Neural correlates of emotion–cognition interactions: A review of evidence from brain imaging investigations. *Journal of Cognitive Psychology*, *23*(6), 669–694. https://doi.org/10.1080/20445911.2011.594433

Doose, A., King, J. A., Bernardoni, F., Geisler, D., Hellerhoff, I., Weinert, T., Roessner, V., Smolka, M. N., & Ehrlich, S. (2020). Strengthened default mode network activation during delay discounting in adolescents with anorexia nervosa after partial weight restoration: A longitudinal fMRI study. *Journal of Clinical Medicine*, *9*(4), article 4. https://doi.org/10.3390/jcm9040900

Doré, B. P., Weber, J., & Ochsner, K. N. (2017). Neural predictors of decisions to cognitively control emotion. *Journal of Neuroscience*, *37*(10), 2580–2588. https://doi.org/10.1523/JNEUROSCI.2526-16.2016

Dörfel, D., Lamke, J.-P., Hummel, F., Wagner, U., Erk, S., & Walter, H. (2014). Common and differential neural networks of emotion regulation by detachment, reinterpretation, distraction, and expressive suppression: A comparative fMRI investigation. *NeuroImage*, *101*, 298–309. https://doi.org/10.1016/j.neuroimage.2014.06.051

Dreyfuss, M. F. W., Riegel, M. L., Pedersen, G. A., Cohen, A. O., Silverman, M. R., Dyke, J. P., Mayer, L. E. S., Walsh, B. T., Casey, B. J., & Broft, A. I. (2017). Patients with bulimia nervosa do not show typical neurodevelopment of cognitive control under emotional influences. *Psychiatry Research: Neuroimaging*, *266*, 59–65. https://doi.org/10.1016/j.pscychresns.2017.05.001

Duchesne, M., Mattos, P., Appolinário, J. C., de Freitas, S. R., Coutinho, G., Santos, C., & Coutinho, W. (2010). Assessment of executive functions in obese individuals with binge eating disorder. *Revista Brasileira De Psiquiatria*, *32*(4), 381–388. https://doi.org/10.1590/s1516-44462010000400011

Dunlop, K., & Downar, J. (2017). Ensuring that novel resting-state fMRI metrics are physiologically grounded, interpretable and meaningful (A commentary on Canna et al., 2017). *European Journal of Neuroscience*, *45*(9), 1127–1128. https://doi.org/10.1111/ejn.13560

Dunne, J. (2018). Mindfulness in anorexia nervosa: An integrated review of the literature. *Journal of the American Psychiatric Nurses Association*, *24*(2), 109–117. https://doi.org/10.1177/1078390317711250

Elton, A., Smith, C. T., Parrish, M. H., & Boettiger, C. A. (2017). Neural systems underlying individual differences in intertemporal decision-making. *Journal of Cognitive Neuroscience*, *29*(3), 467–479. https://doi.org/10.1162/jocn_a_01069

Enticott, P. G., Ogloff, J. R. P., & Bradshaw, J. L. (2006). Associations between laboratory measures of executive inhibitory control and self-reported impulsivity. *Personality and Individual Differences*, *41*(2), 285–294. https://doi.org/10.1016/j.paid.2006.01.011

Feeser, M., Prehn, K., Kazzer, P., Mungee, A., & Bajbouj, M. (2014). Transcranial direct current stimulation enhances cognitive control during emotion regulation. *Brain Stimulation*, *7*(1), 105–112. https://doi.org/10.1016/j.brs.2013.08.006

Fennell, A., & Ratcliff, R. (2019). Does response modality influence conflict? Modelling vocal and manual response Stroop interference. *Journal of Experimental Psychology: Learning, Memory, and Cognition*, *45*, 2098–2119. https://doi.org/10.1037/xlm0000689

Figner, B., Knoch, D., Johnson, E. J., Krosch, A. R., Lisanby, S. H., Fehr, E., & Weber, E. U. (2010). Lateral prefrontal cortex and self-control in intertemporal choice. *Nature Neuroscience*, *13*(5), article 5. https://doi.org/10.1038/nn.2516

Friston, K. J., Harrison, L., & Penny, W. (2003). Dynamic causal modelling. *NeuroImage*, *19*(4), 1273–1302. https://doi.org/10.1016/S1053-8119(03)00202-7

Frost, R., & McNaughton, N. (2017). The neural basis of delay discounting: A review and preliminary model. *Neuroscience & Biobehavioral Reviews*, *79*, 48–65. https://doi.org/10.1016/j.neubiorev.2017.04.022

Fujita, K. (2011). On conceptualizing self-control as more than the effortful inhibition of impulses. *Personality and Social Psychology Review*, *15*(4), 352–366. https://doi.org/10.1177/1088868311411165

Galimberti, E., Martoni, R. M., Cavallini, M. C., Erzegovesi, S., & Bellodi, L. (2012). Motor inhibition and cognitive flexibility in eating disorder subtypes. *Progress in Neuro-Psychopharmacology and Biological Psychiatry*, *36*(2), 307–312. https://doi.org/10.1016/j.pnpbp.2011.10.017

Gao, X., Wang, Q., Jackson, T., Zhao, G., Liang, Y., & Chen, H. (2011). Biases in orienting and maintenance of attention among weight dissatisfied women: An eye-movement study. *Behaviour Research and Therapy*, *49*(4), 252–259. https://doi.org/10.1016/j.brat.2011.01.009

Gomez, P., Ratcliff, R., & Perea, M. (2007). A model of the go/no-go task. *Journal of Experimental Psychology: General*, *136*(3), 389–413. https://doi.org/10.1037/0096-3445.136.3.389

Green, L., & Myerson, J. (2004). A discounting framework for choice with delayed and probabilistic rewards. *Psychological Bulletin*, *130*, 769–792. https://doi.org/10.1037/0033-2909.130.5.769

Greenberg, J., Romero, V. L., Elkin-Frankston, S., Bezdek, M. A., Schumacher, E. H., & Lazar, S. W. (2019). Reduced interference in working memory following mindfulness training is associated with increases in hippocampal volume. *Brain Imaging and Behavior*, *13*(2), 366–376. https://doi.org/10.1007/s11682-018-9858-4

Haedt-Matt, A. A., & Keel, P. K. (2011). Revisiting the affect regulation model of binge eating: A meta-analysis of studies using ecological momentary assessment. *Psychological Bulletin*, *137*(4), 660–681. https://doi.org/10.1037/a0023660

Hagan, K. E., Jarmolowicz, D. P., & Forbush, K. T. (2021). Reconsidering delay discounting in bulimia nervosa. *Eating Behaviors*, *41*, 101506. https://doi.org/10.1016/j.eatbeh.2021.101506

Hare, T., Hakimi, S., & Rangel, A. (2014). Activity in dlPFC and its effective connectivity to vmPFC are associated with temporal discounting. *Frontiers in Neuroscience*, *8*, 50. https://doi.org/10.3389/fnins.2014.00050

He, Q., Huang, X., Zhang, S., Turel, O., Ma, L., & Bechara, A. (2019). Dynamic causal modeling of insular, striatal, and prefrontal cortex activities during a food-specific go/nogo task. *Biological Psychiatry: Cognitive Neuroscience and Neuroimaging*, *4*(12), 1080–1089. https://doi.org/10.1016/j.bpsc.2018.12.005

Hege, M. A., Stingl, K. T., Kullmann, S., Schag, K., Giel, K. E., Zipfel, S., & Preissl, H. (2015). Attentional impulsivity in binge eating disorder modulates response inhibition performance and frontal brain networks. *International Journal of Obesity*, *39*(2), article 2. https://doi.org/10.1038/ijo.2014.99

Hendrickson, K. L., Rasmussen, E. B., & Lawyer, S. R. (2015). Measurement and validation of measures for impulsive food choice across obese and healthy-weight individuals. *Appetite*, *90*, 254–263. https://doi.org/10.1016/j.appet.2015.03.015

Hildebrandt, T., Grotzinger, A., & Schulz, K. (2016). Anorexia nervosa, emotional go/no-go, and the distinct effect of testosterone. *International Journal of Eating Disorders*, *49*(1), 69–76. https://doi.org/10.1002/eat.22456

Hopfinger, J. B., Buonocore, M. H., & Mangun, G. R. (2000). The neural mechanisms of top-down attentional control. *Nature Neuroscience*, *3*(3), article 3. https://doi.org/10.1038/72999

Hutcherson, C. A., & Tusche, A. (2022). Evidence accumulation, not "self-control," explains dorsolateral prefrontal activation during normative choice. *eLife*, *11*, e65661. https://doi.org/10.7554/eLife.65661

Jackson, J. N. S., & MacKillop, J. (2016). Attention-deficit/hyperactivity disorder and monetary delay discounting: A meta-analysis of case-control studies. *Biological Psychiatry: Cognitive Neuroscience and Neuroimaging*, *1*(4), 316–325. https://doi.org/10.1016/j.bpsc.2016.01.007

Jenkinson, P. M., Taylor, L., & Laws, K. R. (2018). Self-reported interoceptive deficits in eating disorders: A meta-analysis of studies using the eating disorder inventory. *Journal of Psychosomatic Research*, *110*, 38–45. https://doi.org/10.1016/j.jpsychores.2018.04.005

Jiang, J., Heller, K., & Egner, T. (2014). Bayesian modeling of flexible cognitive control. *Neuroscience & Biobehavioral Reviews, 46*, 30–43. https://doi.org/10.1016/j.neubiorev.2014.06.001

Jiang, M. Y. W., & Vartanian, L. R. (2018). A review of existing measures of attentional biases in body image and eating disorders research. *Australian Journal of Psychology, 70*(1), 3–17. https://doi.org/10.1111/ajpy.12161

Kekic, M., McClelland, J., Bartholdy, S., Boysen, E., Musiat, P., Dalton, B., Tiza, M., David, A. S., Campbell, I. C., & Schmidt, U. (2017). Single-session transcranial direct current stimulation temporarily improves symptoms, mood, and self-regulatory control in bulimia nervosa: A randomised controlled trial. *PLOS ONE, 12*(1), e0167606. https://doi.org/10.1371/journal.pone.0167606

Khalsa, S. S., Berner, L. A., & Anderson, L. M. (2022). Gastrointestinal interoception in eating disorders: Charting a new path. *Current Psychiatry Reports, 24*(1), 47–60. https://doi.org/10.1007/s11920-022-01318-3

King, J. A., Bernardoni, F., Geisler, D., Ritschel, F., Doose, A., Pauligk, S., Pásztor, K., Weidner, K., Roessner, V., Smolka, M. N., & Ehrlich, S. (2020). Intact value-based decision-making during intertemporal choice in women with remitted anorexia nervosa? An fMRI study. *Journal of Psychiatry and Neuroscience, 45*(2), 108–116. https://doi.org/10.1503/jpn.180252

Kirby, K. N., Petry, N. M., & Bickel, W. K. (1999). Heroin addicts have higher discount rates for delayed rewards than non-drug-using controls. *Journal of Experimental Psychology: General, 128*, 78–87. https://doi.org/10.1037/0096-3445.128.1.78

Kolodny, T., Mevorach, C., & Shalev, L. (2017). Isolating response inhibition in the brain: Parietal versus frontal contribution. *Cortex, 88*, 173–185. https://doi.org/10.1016/j.cortex.2016.12.012

Kristeller, J. L., & Hallett, C. B. (1999). An exploratory study of a meditation-based intervention for binge eating disorder. *Journal of Health Psychology, 4*(3), 357–363. https://doi.org/10.1177/135910539900400305

Kuckertz, J. M., & Amir, N. (2015). Attention bias modification for anxiety and phobias: Current status and future directions. *Current Psychiatry Reports, 17*(2), 9. https://doi.org/10.1007/s11920-014-0545-x

Kullmann, S., Giel, K. E., Hu, X., Bischoff, S. C., Teufel, M., Thiel, A., Zipfel, S., & Preissl, H. (2014). Impaired inhibitory control in anorexia nervosa elicited by physical activity stimuli. *Social Cognitive and Affective Neuroscience, 9*(7), 917–923. https://doi.org/10.1093/scan/nst070

Lang, P. J., Bradley, M. M., Cuthbert, B. N., & Center for the Study of Emotion and Attention. (2005). *International affective picture system* [Dataset]. APA PsycTests. https://doi.org/10.1037/t66667-000

Lavagnino, L., Arnone, D., Cao, B., Soares, J. C., & Selvaraj, S. (2016). Inhibitory control in obesity and binge eating disorder: A systematic review and meta-analysis of neurocognitive and neuroimaging studies. *Neuroscience & Biobehavioral Reviews, 68*, 714–726. https://doi.org/10.1016/j.neubiorev.2016.06.041

Lavender, J. M., Wonderlich, S. A., Engel, S. G., Gordon, K. H., Kaye, W. H., & Mitchell, J. E. (2015). Dimensions of emotion dysregulation in anorexia nervosa and bulimia nervosa: A conceptual review of the empirical literature. *Clinical Psychology Review, 40*, 111–122. https://doi.org/10.1016/j.cpr.2015.05.010

Lee, J. E., Namkoong, K., & Jung, Y.-C. (2017). Impaired prefrontal cognitive control over interference by food images in binge-eating disorder and bulimia nervosa. *Neuroscience Letters, 651*, 95–101. https://doi.org/10.1016/j.neulet.2017.04.054

Leehr, E. J., Krohmer, K., Schag, K., Dresler, T., Zipfel, S., & Giel, K. E. (2015). Emotion regulation model in binge eating disorder and obesity—A systematic review. *Neuroscience & Biobehavioral Reviews, 49*, 125–134. https://doi.org/10.1016/j.neubiorev.2014.12.008

Lempert, K. M., Steinglass, J. E., Pinto, A., Kable, J. W., & Simpson, H. B. (2019). Can delay discounting deliver on the promise of RDoC? *Psychological Medicine, 49*(2), 190–199. https://doi.org/10.1017/S0033291718001770

Lock, J., Garrett, A., Beenhakker, J., & Reiss, A. L. (2011). Aberrant brain activation during a response inhibition task in adolescent eating disorder subtypes. *American Journal of Psychiatry, 168*(1), 55–64. https://doi.org/10.1176/appi.ajp.2010.10010056

Logan, G. D., Van Zandt, T., Verbruggen, F., & Wagenmakers, E.-J. (2014). On the ability to inhibit thought and action: General and special theories of an act of control. *Psychological Review, 121*, 66–95. https://doi.org/10.1037/a0035230

Louie, K., & Glimcher, P. W. (2010). Separating value from choice: Delay discounting activity in the lateral intraparietal area. *Journal of Neuroscience, 30*(16), 5498–5507. https://doi.org/10.1523/JNEUROSCI.5742-09.2010

Luo, C., & Proctor, R. W. (2022). A diffusion model for the congruency sequence effect. *Psychonomic Bulletin & Review, 29*(6), 2034–2051. https://doi.org/10.3758/s13423-022-02119-8

Lyu, Z., Zheng, P., Lu, S., & Qin, M. (2018). Impaired conflict monitoring to food cues in women who binge eat. *Frontiers in Psychology*, 9. https://www.frontiersin.org/articles/10.3389/fpsyg.2018.02585

MacKillop, J., Weafer, J., C. Gray, J., Oshri, A., Palmer, A., & de Wit, H. (2016). The latent structure of impulsivity: Impulsive choice, impulsive action, and impulsive personality traits. *Psychopharmacology, 233*(18), 3361–3370. https://doi.org/10.1007/s00213-016-4372-0

MacLeod, C., & Clarke, P. J. F. (2015). The attentional bias modification approach to anxiety intervention. *Clinical Psychological Science, 3*, 58–78. https://doi.org/10.1177/2167702614560749

Magen, E., Kim, B., Dweck, C. S., Gross, J. J., & McClure, S. M. (2014). Behavioral and neural correlates of increased self-control in the absence of increased willpower. *Proceedings of the National Academy of Sciences, 111*(27), 9786–9791. https://doi.org/10.1073/pnas.1408991111

Malagoli, C., Cerro, P. F., Vecchiato, C., & Usai, M. C. (2021). Cognitive and emotional regulation in adolescents and young women with eating disorders. *Eating and Weight Disorders, 26*(1), 375–383. https://doi.org/10.1007/s40519-020-00859-x

Mallorquí-Bagué, N., Testa, G., Lozano-Madrid, M., Vintró-Alcaraz, C., Sánchez, I., Riesco, N., Granero, R., Perales, J. C., Navas, J. F., Megías-Robles, A., Martínez-Zalacaín, I., Veciana de Las Heras, M., Jiménez-Murcia, S., & Fernández-Aranda, F. (2020). Emotional and non-emotional facets of impulsivity in eating disorders: From anorexia nervosa to bulimic spectrum disorders. *European Eating Disorders Review, 28*(4), 410–422. https://doi.org/10.1002/erv.2734

Mallorquí-Bagué, N., Vintró-Alcaraz, C., Sánchez, I., Riesco, N., Agüera, Z., Granero, R., Jiménez-Múrcia, S., Menchón, J. M., Treasure, J., & Fernández-Aranda, F. (2018). Emotion regulation as a transdiagnostic feature among eating disorders: Cross-sectional and longitudinal approach. *European Eating Disorders Review, 26*(1), 53–61. https://doi.org/10.1002/erv.2570

Manasse, S. M., Espel, H. M., Schumacher, L. M., Kerrigan, S. G., Zhang, F., Forman, E. M., & Juarascio, A. S. (2016). Does impulsivity predict outcome in treatment for binge eating disorder? A multimodal investigation. *Appetite, 105*, 172–179. https://doi.org/10.1016/j.appet.2016.05.026

Manasse, S. M., Juarascio, A. S., Forman, E. M., Berner, L. A., Butryn, M. L., & Ruocco, A. C. (2014). Executive functioning in overweight individuals with and without loss-of-control eating. *European Eating Disorders Review, 22*(5), 373–377. https://doi.org/10.1002/erv.2304

Marsh, R., Steinglass, J. E., Gerber, A. J., Graziano O'Leary, K., Wang, Z., Murphy, D., Walsh, B. T., & Peterson, B. S. (2009). Deficient activity in the neural systems that mediate self-regulatory control in bulimia nervosa. *Archives of General Psychiatry, 66*(1), 51–63. https://doi.org/10.1001/archgenpsychiatry.2008.504

Masharipov, R., Korotkov, A., Medvedev, S., & Kireev, M. (2022). Evidence for non-selective response inhibition in uncertain contexts revealed by combined meta-analysis and Bayesian analysis of fMRI data. *Scientific Reports, 12*(1), 10137. https://doi.org/10.1038/s41598-022-14221-x

Mason, L., O'Sullivan, N., Blackburn, M., Bentall, R., & El-Deredy, W. (2012). I want it now! Neural correlates of hypersensitivity to immediate reward in hypomania. *Biological Psychiatry, 71*(6), 530–537. https://doi.org/10.1016/j.biopsych.2011.10.008

Matzke, D., Curley, S., Gong, C. Q., & Heathcote, A. (2019). Inhibiting responses to difficult choices. *Journal of Experimental Psychology: General, 148*, 124–142. https://doi.org/10.1037/xge0000525

McClure, S. M., Ericson, K. M., Laibson, D. I., Loewenstein, G., & Cohen, J. D. (2007). Time discounting for primary rewards. *Journal of Neuroscience, 27*(21), 5796–5804. https://doi.org/10.1523/JNEUROSCI.4246-06.2007

McClure, S. M., Laibson, D. I., Loewenstein, G., & Cohen, J. D. (2004). Separate neural systems value immediate and delayed monetary rewards. *Science, 306*(5695), 503–507. https://doi.org/10.1126/science.1100907

McRae, K., Ciesielski, B., & Gross, J. J. (2012). Unpacking cognitive reappraisal: Goals, tactics, and outcomes. *Emotion, 12*(2), 250–255. https://doi.org/10.1037/a0026351

Meneguzzo, P., Mancini, C., Ormitti, A., Bonello, E., & Todisco, P. (2022). Time evaluation and its accuracy in eating disorders: Differences in relation to interoceptive awareness. *Eating and Weight Disorders, 27*(7), 2551–2560. https://doi.org/10.1007/s40519-022-01394-7

Menon, V., & Uddin, L. Q. (2010). Saliency, switching, attention and control: A network model of insula function. *Brain Structure and Function, 214*(5), 655–667. https://doi.org/10.1007/s00429-010-0262-0

Meyer, H. C., & Bucci, D. J. (2016). Neural and behavioral mechanisms of proactive and reactive inhibition. *Learning & Memory, 23*(10), 504–514. https://doi.org/10.1101/lm.040501.115

Miedl, S. F., Wiswede, D., Marco-Pallarés, J., Ye, Z., Fehr, T., Herrmann, M., & Münte, T. F. (2015). The neural basis of impulsive discounting in pathological gamblers. *Brain Imaging and Behavior, 9*(4), 887–898. https://doi.org/10.1007/s11682-015-9352-1

Miranda-Olivos, R., Steward, T., Martínez-Zalacaín, I., Mestre-Bach, G., Juaneda-Seguí, A., Jiménez-Murcia, S., Fernández-Formoso, J. A., Vilarrasa, N., Heras, M. V. de las, Custal, N., Virgili, N., Lopez-Urdiales, R., Menchón, J. M., Granero, R., Soriano-Mas, C., & Fernandez-Aranda, F. (2021). The neural correlates of delay discounting in obesity and binge eating disorder. *Journal of Behavioral Addictions, 10*(3), 498–507. https://doi.org/10.1556/2006.2021.00023

Moreira, D., Pinto, M., Almeida, F., Barros, S., & Barbosa, F. (2016). Neurobiological bases of intertemporal choices: A comprehensive review. *Aggression and Violent Behavior, 26*, 1–8. https://doi.org/10.1016/j.avb.2015.11.003

Morie, K. P., Crowley, M. J., Mayes, L. C., & Potenza, M. N. (2022). The process of emotion identification: Considerations for psychiatric disorders. *Journal of Psychiatric Research, 148*, 264–274. https://doi.org/10.1016/j.jpsychires.2022.01.053

Myers, C. E., Interian, A., & Moustafa, A. A. (2022). A practical introduction to using the drift diffusion model of decision-making in cognitive psychology, neuroscience, and health sciences. *Frontiers in Psychology, 13*, 1039172. https://doi.org/10.3389/fpsyg.2022.1039172

Nigg, J. T. (2000). On inhibition/disinhibition in developmental psychopathology: Views from cognitive and personality psychology and a working inhibition taxonomy. *Psychological Bulletin, 126*(2), 220–246. https://doi.org/10.1037/0033-2909.126.2.220

Nitsche, M. A., Cohen, L. G., Wassermann, E. M., Priori, A., Lang, N., Antal, A., Paulus, W., Hummel, F., Boggio, P. S., Fregni, F., & Pascual-Leone, A. (2008). Transcranial direct current stimulation: State of the art 2008. *Brain Stimulation, 1*(3), 206–223. https://doi.org/10.1016/j.brs.2008.06.004

Oberndorfer, T. A., Kaye, W. H., Simmons, A. N., Strigo, I. A., & Matthews, S. C. (2011). Demand-specific alteration of medial prefrontal cortex response during an inhibition task in recovered anorexic women. *International Journal of Eating Disorders, 44*(1), 1–8. https://doi.org/10.1002/eat.20750

Ochsner, K. N., Bunge, S. A., Gross, J. J., & Gabrieli, J. D. E. (2002). Rethinking feelings: An fMRI study of the cognitive regulation of emotion. *Journal of Cognitive Neuroscience, 14*(8), 1215–1229. https://doi.org/10.1162/089892902760807212

Ochsner, K. N., & Gross, J. J. (2005). The cognitive control of emotion. *Trends in Cognitive Sciences, 9*(5), 242–249. https://doi.org/10.1016/j.tics.2005.03.010

Oliva, R., Morys, F., Horstmann, A., Castiello, U., & Begliomini, C. (2019). The impulsive brain: Neural underpinnings of binge eating behavior in normal-weight adults. *Appetite, 136*, 33–49. https://doi.org/10.1016/j.appet.2018.12.043

Pearson, C. M., Combs, J. L., Zapolski, T. C. B., & Smith, G. T. (2012). A longitudinal transactional risk model for early eating disorder onset. *Journal of Abnormal Psychology, 121*(3), 707–718. https://doi.org/10.1037/a0027567

Pearson, C. M., Wonderlich, S. A., & Smith, G. T. (2015). A risk and maintenance model for bulimia nervosa: From impulsive action to compulsive behavior. *Psychological Review, 122*, 516–535. https://doi.org/10.1037/a0039268

Pearson, C. M., Zapolski, T. C. B., & Smith, G. T. (2015). A longitudinal test of impulsivity and depression pathways to early binge eating onset. *International Journal of Eating Disorders, 48*(2), 230–237. https://doi.org/10.1002/eat.22277

Perri, R. L. (2020). Is there a proactive and a reactive mechanism of inhibition? Towards an executive account of the attentional inhibitory control model. *Behavioural Brain Research, 377*, 112243. https://doi.org/10.1016/j.bbr.2019.112243

Perry, T. R., Wierenga, C. E., Kaye, W. H., & Brown, T. A. (2021). Interoceptive awareness and suicidal ideation in a clinical eating disorder sample: The role of body trust. *Behavior Therapy, 52*(5), 1105–1113. https://doi.org/10.1016/j.beth.2020.12.001

Peters, J., & Büchel, C. (2011). The neural mechanisms of inter-temporal decision-making: Understanding variability. *Trends in Cognitive Sciences, 15*(5), 227–239. https://doi.org/10.1016/j.tics.2011.03.002

Peterson, C. B., Engel, S. G., Crosby, R. D., Strauman, T., Smith, T. L., Klein, M., Crow, S. J., Mitchell, J. E., Erickson, A., Cao, L., Bjorlie, K., & Wonderlich, S. A. (2020). Comparing integrative cognitive-affective therapy and guided self-help cognitive-behavioral therapy to treat binge-eating disorder using standard and naturalistic momentary outcome measures: A randomized controlled trial. *International Journal of Eating Disorders, 53*(9), 1418–1427. https://doi.org/10.1002/eat.23324

Phillips, M. L., Ladouceur, C. D., & Drevets, W. C. (2008). A neural model of voluntary and automatic emotion regulation: Implications for understanding the pathophysiology and neurodevelopment of bipolar disorder. *Molecular Psychiatry, 13*(9), article 9. https://doi.org/10.1038/mp.2008.65

Puttevils, L., Vanderhasselt, M.-A., Horczak, P., & Vervaet, M. (2021). Differences in the use of emotion regulation strategies between anorexia and bulimia nervosa: A systematic review and meta-analysis. *Comprehensive Psychiatry, 109*, 152262. https://doi.org/10.1016/j.comppsych.2021.152262

Quigley, L., Wright, C. A., Dobson, K. S., & Sears, C. R. (2017). Measuring attentional control ability or beliefs? Evaluation of the factor structure and convergent validity of the attentional control scale. *Journal of Psychopathology and Behavioral Assessment, 39*(4), 742–754. https://doi.org/10.1007/s10862-017-9617-7

Ratcliff, R., Huang-Pollock, C., & McKoon, G. (2018). Modeling individual differences in the go/no-go task with a diffusion model. *Decision, 5*, 42–62. https://doi.org/10.1037/dec0000065

Ratcliff, R., & McKoon, G. (2008). The diffusion decision model: Theory and data for two-choice decision tasks. *Neural Computation, 20*(4), 873–922. https://doi.org/10.1162/neco.2008.12-06-420

Ratcliff, R., Smith, P. L., Brown, S. D., & McKoon, G. (2016). Diffusion decision model: Current issues and history. *Trends in Cognitive Sciences, 20*(4), 260–281. https://doi.org/10.1016/j.tics.2016.01.007

Redgrave, G. W., Bakker, A., Bello, N. T., Caffo, B. S., Coughlin, J. W., Guarda, A. S., McEntee, J. E., Pekar, J. J., Reinblatt, S. P., Verduzco, G., & Moran, T. H. (2008). Differential brain activation in anorexia nervosa to fat and thin words during a stroop task. *NeuroReport, 19*(12), 1181–1185. https://doi.org/10.1097/WNR.0b013e32830a70f2

Ritschel, F., King, J. A., Geisler, D., Flohr, L., Neidel, F., Boehm, I., Seidel, M., Zwipp, J., Ripke, S., Smolka, M. N., Roessner, V., & Ehrlich, S. (2015). Temporal delay discounting in acutely ill and weight-recovered patients with anorexia nervosa. *Psychological Medicine, 45*(6), 1229–1239. https://doi.org/10.1017/S0033291714002311

Rodriguez, C. A., Turner, B. M., Zandt, T. V., & McClure, S. M. (2015). The neural basis of value accumulation in intertemporal choice. *European Journal of Neuroscience, 42*(5), 2179–2189. https://doi.org/10.1111/ejn.12997

Rottenberg, J., & Gross, J. J. (2003). When emotion goes wrong: Realizing the promise of affective science. *Clinical Psychology: Science and Practice, 10*(2), 227–232. https://doi.org/10.1093/clipsy.bpg012

Rubia, K., Russell, T., Overmeyer, S., Brammer, M. J., Bullmore, E. T., Sharma, T., Simmons, A., Williams, S. C. R., Giampietro, V., Andrew, C. M., & Taylor, E. (2001). Mapping motor inhibition: Conjunctive brain activations across different versions of go/no-go and stop tasks. *NeuroImage, 13*(2), 250–261. https://doi.org/10.1006/nimg.2000.0685

Rung, J. M., Peck, S., Hinnenkamp, J. E., Preston, E., & Madden, G. J. (2019). Changing delay discounting and impulsive choice: Implications for addictions, prevention, and human health. *Perspectives on Behavior Science, 42*(3), 397–417. https://doi.org/10.1007/s40614-019-00200-7

Ruscitti, C., Rufino, K., Goodwin, N., & Wagner, R. (2016). Difficulties in emotion regulation in patients with eating disorders. *Borderline Personality Disorder and Emotion Dysregulation, 3*(1), 3. https://doi.org/10.1186/s40479-016-0037-1

Safer, D. L., Telch, C. F., & Chen, E. Y. (2009). *Dialectical behavior therapy for binge eating and bulimia*. Guilford Press.

Schag, K., Teufel, M., Junne, F., Preissl, H., Hautzinger, M., Zipfel, S., & Giel, K. E. (2013). Impulsivity in binge eating disorder: Food cues elicit increased reward responses and disinhibition. *PLoS ONE, 8*(10), e76542. https://doi.org/10.1371/journal.pone.0076542

Seidel, M., King, J. A., Ritschel, F., Boehm, I., Geisler, D., Bernardoni, F., Beck, M., Pauligk, S., Biemann, R., Strobel, A., Goschke, T., Walter, H., Roessner, V., & Ehrlich, S. (2018). Processing and regulation of negative emotions in anorexia nervosa: An fMRI study. *NeuroImage: Clinical, 18*, 1–8. https://doi.org/10.1016/j.nicl.2017.12.035

Seidel, M., King, J. A., Ritschel, F., Boehm, I., Geisler, D., Bernardoni, F., Holzapfel, L., Diestel, S., Diers, K., Strobel, A., Goschke, T., Walter, H., Roessner, V., & Ehrlich, S. (2018). The real-life costs of emotion regulation in anorexia nervosa: A combined ecological momentary assessment and fMRI study. *Translational Psychiatry, 8*(1), article 1. https://doi.org/10.1038/s41398-017-0004-7

Seitz, J., Hueck, M., Dahmen, B., Schulte-Rüther, M., Legenbauer, T., Herpertz-Dahlmann, B., & Konrad, K. (2016). Attention network dysfunction in bulimia nervosa—An fMRI study. *PLOS ONE, 11*(9), e0161329. https://doi.org/10.1371/journal.pone.0161329

Servant, M., & Evans, N. J. (2020). A diffusion model analysis of the effects of aging in the Flanker Task. *Psychology and Aging, 35*, 831–849. https://doi.org/10.1037/pag0000546

Shen, B., Yin, Y., Wang, J., Zhou, X., McClure, S. M., & Li, J. (2016). High-definition tDCS alters impulsivity in a baseline-dependent manner. *NeuroImage, 143*, 343–352. https://doi.org/10.1016/j.neuroimage.2016.09.006

Simmonds, D. J., Pekar, J. J., & Mostofsky, S. H. (2008). Meta-analysis of go/no-go tasks demonstrating that fMRI activation associated with response inhibition is task-dependent. *Neuropsychologia, 46*(1), 224–232. https://doi.org/10.1016/j.neuropsychologia.2007.07.015

Skunde, M., Walther, S., Simon, J. J., Wu, M., Bendszus, M., Herzog, W., & Friederich, H.-C. (2016). Neural signature of behavioural inhibition in women with bulimia nervosa. *Journal of Psychiatry and Neuroscience, 41*(5), E69–E78. https://doi.org/10.1503/jpn.150335

Smith, B. J., Monterosso, J. R., Wakslak, C. J., Bechara, A., & Read, S. J. (2018). A meta-analytical review of brain activity associated with intertemporal decisions: Evidence for an anterior-posterior tangibility axis. *Neuroscience & Biobehavioral Reviews, 86*, 85–98. https://doi.org/10.1016/j.neubiorev.2018.01.005

Steinglass, J. E., Figner, B., Berkowitz, S., Simpson, H. B., Weber, E. U., & Walsh, B. T. (2012). Increased capacity to delay reward in anorexia nervosa. *Journal of the International Neuropsychological Society, 18*(4), 773–780. https://doi.org/10.1017/S1355617712000446

Stephan, K. E., Penny, W. D., Moran, R. J., den Ouden, H. E. M., Daunizeau, J., & Friston, K. J. (2010). Ten simple rules for dynamic causal modeling. *NeuroImage, 49*(4), 3099–3109. https://doi.org/10.1016/j.neuroimage.2009.11.015

Steward, T., Martínez-Zalacaín, I., Mestre-Bach, G., Sánchez, I., Riesco, N., Jiménez-Murcia, S., Fernández-Formoso, J. A., Heras, M. V. de las, Custal, N., Menchón, J. M., Soriano-Mas, C., & Fernandez-Aranda, F. (2022). Dorsolateral prefrontal cortex and amygdala function during cognitive reappraisal predicts weight restoration and emotion regulation impairment in anorexia nervosa. *Psychological Medicine, 52*(5), 844–852. https://doi.org/10.1017/S0033291720002457

Steward, T., Mestre-Bach, G., Vintró-Alcaraz, C., Agüera, Z., Jiménez-Murcia, S., Granero, R., & Fernández-Aranda, F. (2017). Delay discounting of reward and impulsivity in eating disorders: From anorexia nervosa to binge eating disorder. *European Eating Disorders Review, 25*(6), 601–606. https://doi.org/10.1002/erv.2543

Stojek, M. M. K., & MacKillop, J. (2017). Relative reinforcing value of food and delayed reward discounting in obesity and disordered eating: A systematic review. *Clinical Psychology Review, 55*, 1–11. https://doi.org/10.1016/j.cpr.2017.04.007

Svaldi, J., Schmitz, F., Trentowska, M., Tuschen-Caffier, B., Berking, M., & Naumann, E. (2014). Cognitive interference and a food-related memory bias in binge eating disorder. *Appetite, 72*, 28–36. https://doi.org/10.1016/j.appet.2013.09.014

Swick, D., Ashley, V., & Turken, U. (2011). Are the neural correlates of stopping and not going identical? Quantitative meta-analysis of two response inhibition tasks. *NeuroImage, 56*(3), 1655–1665. https://doi.org/10.1016/j.neuroimage.2011.02.070

Tamber-Rosenau, B. J., Asplund, C. L., & Marois, R. (2018). Functional dissociation of the inferior frontal junction from the dorsal attention network in top-down attentional control. *Journal of Neurophysiology, 120*(5), 2498–2512. https://doi.org/10.1152/jn.00506.2018

Testa, G., Granero, R., Misiolek, A., Vintró-Alcaraz, C., Mallorqui-Bagué, N., Lozano-Madrid, M., Heras, M. V. D. L., Sánchez, I., Jiménez-Murcia, S., & Fernández-Aranda, F. (2022). Impact of impulsivity and therapy response in eating disorders from a neurophysiological, personality and cognitive perspective. *Nutrients, 14*(23), article 23. https://doi.org/10.3390/nu14235011

Turgon, R., Ruffault, A., Juneau, C., Blatier, C., & Shankland, R. (2019). Eating disorder treatment: A systematic review and meta-analysis of the efficacy of mindfulness-based programs. *Mindfulness, 10*(11), 2225–2244. https://doi.org/10.1007/s12671-019-01216-5

Turner, B. M., Rodriguez, C. A., Liu, Q., Molloy, M. F., Hoogendijk, M., & McClure, S. M. (2019). On the neural and mechanistic bases of self-control. *Cerebral Cortex, 29*(2), 732–750. https://doi.org/10.1093/cercor/bhx355

Tyrka, A. R., Waldron, I., Graber, J. A., & Brooks-Gunn, J. (2002). Prospective predictors of the onset of anorexic and bulimic syndromes. *International Journal of Eating Disorders, 32*(3), 282–290. https://doi.org/10.1002/eat.10094

Van den Eynde, F., Claudino, A. M., Mogg, A., Horrell, L., Stahl, D., Ribeiro, W., Uher, R., Campbell, I., & Schmidt, U. (2010). Repetitive transcranial magnetic stimulation reduces cue-induced food craving in bulimic disorders. *Biological Psychiatry, 67*(8), 793–795. https://doi.org/10.1016/j.biopsych.2009.11.023

Verbruggen, F., & Logan, G. D. (2008). Response inhibition in the stop-signal paradigm. *Trends in Cognitive Sciences, 12*(11), 418–424. https://doi.org/10.1016/j.tics.2008.07.005

Volkow, N. D., & Baler, R. D. (2015). NOW vs LATER brain circuits: Implications for obesity and addiction. *Trends in Neurosciences*, *38*(6), 345–352. https://doi.org/10.1016/j.tins.2015.04.002

Vossel, S., Geng, J. J., & Fink, G. R. (2014). Dorsal and ventral attention systems: Distinct neural circuits but collaborative roles. *The Neuroscientist*, *20*(2), 150–159. https://doi.org/10.1177/1073858413494269

Walpoth, M., Hoertnagl, C., Mangweth-Matzek, B., Kemmler, G., Hinterhölzl, J., Conca, A., & Hausmann, A. (2007). Repetitive transcranial magnetic stimulation in bulimia nervosa: Preliminary results of a single-centre, randomised, double-blind, sham-controlled trial in female outpatients. *Psychotherapy and Psychosomatics*, *77*(1), 57–60. https://doi.org/10.1159/000110061

Walter, H., Kalckreuth, A. von, Schardt, D., Stephan, A., Goschke, T., & Erk, S. (2009). The temporal dynamics of voluntary emotion regulation. *PLOS ONE*, *4*(8), e6726. https://doi.org/10.1371/journal.pone.0006726

Weinbach, N., Lock, J., & Bohon, C. (2020). Superior response inhibition to high-calorie foods in adolescents with anorexia nervosa. *Behaviour Research and Therapy*, *124*, 103441. https://doi.org/10.1016/j.brat.2019.103441

Wesley, M. J., & Bickel, W. K. (2014). Remember the future II: Meta-analyses and functional overlap of working memory and delay discounting. *Biological Psychiatry*, *75*(6), 435–448. https://doi.org/10.1016/j.biopsych.2013.08.008

Westwater, M. L., Mancini, F., Gorka, A. X., Shapleske, J., Serfontein, J., Grillon, C., Ernst, M., Ziauddeen, H., & Fletcher, P. C. (2021). Prefrontal responses during proactive and reactive inhibition are differentially impacted by stress in anorexia and bulimia nervosa. *Journal of Neuroscience*, *41*(20), 4487–4499. https://doi.org/10.1523/JNEUROSCI.2853-20.2021

Westwood, H., Kerr-Gaffney, J., Stahl, D., & Tchanturia, K. (2017). Alexithymia in eating disorders: Systematic review and meta-analyses of studies using the Toronto Alexithymia Scale. *Journal of Psychosomatic Research*, *99*, 66–81. https://doi.org/10.1016/j.jpsychores.2017.06.007

Wierenga, C., Bischoff-Grethe, A., Melrose, A. J., Grenesko-Stevens, E., Irvine, Z., Wagner, A., Simmons, A., Matthews, S., Yau, W.-Y. W., Fennema-Notestine, C., & Kaye, W. H. (2014). Altered BOLD response during inhibitory and error processing in adolescents with anorexia nervosa. *PLOS ONE*, *9*(3), e92017. https://doi.org/10.1371/journal.pone.0092017

Wierenga, C. E., Bischoff-Grethe, A., Melrose, A. J., Irvine, Z., Torres, L., Bailer, U. F., Simmons, A., Fudge, J. L., McClure, S. M., Ely, A., & Kaye, W. H. (2015). Hunger does not motivate reward in women remitted from anorexia nervosa. *Biological Psychiatry*, *77*(7), 642–652. https://doi.org/10.1016/j.biopsych.2014.09.024

Wilfahrt, R. P., Wilfahrt, L. G., & Matthews Hamburg, A. (2021). Atomoxetine reduced binge/purge symptoms in a case of anorexia nervosa binge/purge type. *Clinical Neuropharmacology*, *44*(2), 68. https://doi.org/10.1097/WNF.0000000000000438

Williams, L. E., Bargh, J. A., Nocera, C. C., & Gray, J. R. (2009). The unconscious regulation of emotion: Nonconscious reappraisal goals modulate emotional reactivity. *Emotion*, *9*(6), 847–854. https://doi.org/10.1037/a0017745

Wonderlich, J. A., Crosby, R. D., Engel, S. G., Crow, S. J., Peterson, C. B., Le Grange, D., Wonderlich, S. A., & Fischer, S. (2022). Negative affect and binge eating: Assessing the unique trajectories of negative affect before and after binge-eating episodes across eating disorder diagnostic classifications. *International Journal of Eating Disorders*, *55*(2), 223–230. https://doi.org/10.1002/eat.23648

Wonderlich, S. A., Connolly, K. M., & Stice, E. (2004). Impulsivity as a risk factor for eating disorder behavior: Assessment implications with adolescents. *International Journal of Eating Disorders*, *36*(2), 172–182. https://doi.org/10.1002/eat.20033

Wonderlich, S. A., Peterson, C. B., Crosby, R. D., Smith, T. L., Klein, M. H., Mitchell, J. E., & Crow, S. J. (2014). A randomized controlled comparison of integrative cognitive-affective therapy (ICAT) and enhanced cognitive-behavioral therapy (CBT-E) for bulimia nervosa. *Psychological Medicine*, *44*(3), 543–553. https://doi.org/10.1017/S0033291713001098

Wu, M., Giel, K. E., Skunde, M., Schag, K., Rudofsky, G., de Zwaan, M., Zipfel, S., Herzog, W., & Friederich, H.-C. (2013). Inhibitory control and decision making under risk in bulimia nervosa and binge-eating disorder. *International Journal of Eating Disorders*, *46*(7), 721–728. https://doi.org/10.1002/eat.22143

Wu, M., Hartmann, M., Skunde, M., Herzog, W., & Friederich, H.-C. (2013). Inhibitory control in bulimic-type eating disorders: A systematic review and meta-analysis. *PLOS ONE*, *8*(12), e83412. https://doi.org/10.1371/journal.pone.0083412

Xiong, G., Li, X., Dong, Z., Cai, S., Huang, J., & Li, Q. (2019). Modulating activity in the prefrontal cortex changes intertemporal choice for loss: A transcranial direct current stimulation study. *Frontiers in Human Neuroscience, 13*. https://www.frontiersin.org/articles/10.3389/fnhum.2019.00167

Yeung, M. K., Lee, T. L., & Chan, A. S. (2020). Neurocognitive development of flanker and Stroop interference control: A near-infrared spectroscopy study. *Brain and Cognition, 143*, 105585. https://doi.org/10.1016/j.bandc.2020.105585

Zamariola, G., Frost, N., Van Oost, A., Corneille, O., & Luminet, O. (2019). Relationship between interoception and emotion regulation: New evidence from mixed methods. *Journal of Affective Disorders, 246*, 480–485. https://doi.org/10.1016/j.jad.2018.12.101

Zhang, F., & Iwaki, S. (2019). Common neural network for different functions: An investigation of proactive and reactive inhibition. *Frontiers in Behavioral Neuroscience*, 13. https://www.frontiersin.org/articles/10.3389/fnbeh.2019.00124

Zhang, Q., Wang, S., Zhu, Q., Yan, J., Zhang, T., Zhang, J., Jin, Z., & Li, L. (2023). The brain stimulation of DLPFC regulates choice preference in intertemporal choice self-other differences. *Behavioural Brain Research, 440*, 114265. https://doi.org/10.1016/j.bbr.2022.114265

Zhang, R., Geng, X., & Lee, T. M. C. (2017). Large-scale functional neural network correlates of response inhibition: An fMRI meta-analysis. *Brain Structure and Function, 222*(9), 3973–3990. https://doi.org/10.1007/s00429-017-1443-x

Zhao, W. J., Diederich, A., Trueblood, J. S., & Bhatia, S. (2019). Automatic biases in intertemporal choice. *Psychonomic Bulletin & Review, 26*(2), 661–668. https://doi.org/10.3758/s13423-019-01579-9

13
Visuospatial and Neuropsychological Functions in Eating Disorders

C. Alix Timko and Annabel Susanin

Brief Definitional Overview

Visuospatial functioning: The neurocognitive ability to analyze features and organize them into a whole. This functioning includes complex behaviors associated with the perception of the world, such as finding and tracking objects, judging distances, and manipulating objects.

Working memory: Memory of limited capacity in which a small number of chunks can be manipulated.

Long-term memory: Memory of potentially unlimited capacity that includes a variety of different types of memory.

Processing speed: How quickly one can complete a mental task.

Attention: How individuals manage information coming from the environment, process it, and react to it. Attention can be "grabbed" via stimuli in the environment or it can be voluntarily focused on stimuli.

Introduction

Over the last two decades, there has been increased interest in neuropsychological functioning of individuals with eating disorders. The rationale for this focus is primarily to understand disease processes and to identify potential targets for treatment. Frequently observed behaviors (e.g., rigid rule following around food, perceptual disruptions in both portion size and body image, impulsivity, control, etc.) have been identified as putative endophenotypes of eating disorders (Holliday et al., 2005; Lopez et al., 2009). Researchers have focused their efforts on examining differences amongst those with eating disorders, healthy controls, and individuals recovered from eating disorders in an attempt to demonstrate that observed behavioral impairments are evident at the neuropsychological level (i.e., those with eating disorders differ from healthy controls) and that those impairments persist outside of the illness state (i.e., are observed in those who are recovered). Broadly speaking, research indicates that there are differences (to be discussed) in

C. Alix Timko and Annabel Susanin, *Visuospatial and Neuropsychological Functions in Eating Disorders*. In: *The Handbook of the Neurobiology of Eating Disorders*. Edited by: Christina E. Wierenga and Joanna E. Steinglass, Oxford University Press.
 DOI: 10.1093/9780197675212.003.0014

the neuropsychological functioning of those with eating disorders, indicating that these differences could represent a risk factor for disease onset or for a more persistent course of illness—although caveats to this broad finding will be discussed. Nonetheless, it remains important to elucidate the neuropsychological underpinnings of disorder risk or maintenance as they may highlight key areas to target in treatment.

This chapter focuses on visuospatial and neuropsychological functions related to eating disorder behaviors in individuals with anorexia nervosa (AN) and bulimia nervosa (BN). There is a small amount of published literature focused on these functions in binge-eating disorder (BED); thus, research in this area will be summarized when possible. However, given the relative newness of avoidant/restrictive food intake disorder (ARFID) as a diagnosis, there is not enough research to include it in this chapter. Chapters 10 to 12 explore executive functioning in those with eating disorders, focusing on cognitive inflexibilities including set-shifting/cognitive flexibility and inhibitory or self-regulatory control; therefore, these concepts will not receive in-depth attention in this chapter.

Biological Framework

Neuropsychological functioning is broadly defined as mental processes and functions including the processing, storing, and use of information. It can include the integration of different systems to support thinking, attention, and memory. In this chapter, the focus will be on visuospatial functioning, memory, attention, processing speed. While discussed independently, these functions are interrelated. In the context of eating disorders, there is no single, overarching, neurobiologically based theoretical model to account for all disruptions in visuospatial and neuropsychological functioning observed—although a number of theoretical models of disorder maintenance include a neuropsychological component (e.g., Cognitive Interpersonal Maintenance Model; Schmidt & Treasure, 2006; Treasure et al., 2020; Treasure & Schmidt, 2013). The exception may be the insula model, proposed by Nunn and colleagues (Nunn et al., 2008, 2011). This model highlights how the insula serves as a hub in the brain, connecting to almost every other area and playing a role in regulating the autonomic nervous system, appetite, interoceptive awareness, amongst others. According to this hypothesis, the insula is dysfunctional and cannot facilitate communication between cortical and subcortical structures hypothesized in playing a putative role in AN (Nunn et al., 2011). However, this model has not been thoroughly examined, integrated into other models, or applied to eating disorders other than AN. Therefore, in lieu of an explication of theoretical models regarding possible disruptions in neuropsychological and visuospatial functioning, Table 13.1 summarizes the primary structures or brain circuits believed to be involved in each domain discussed in this chapter.

Table 13.1 Broad overview of brain circuits and structures implicated in neuropsychological and visuospatial functioning

Neuropsychological Construct	Structures and circuits implicated
Visuospatial functioning	Dorsal pathway through the occipitoparietal cortex to the dorsolateral prefrontal cortex (DLPFC). The dorsal pathway is linked to spatial processing, movement, and location. Networks connecting the DLPFC to the parietal cortex are implicated in attention and non-verbal working memory.
	Ventral pathway through the occipitotemporal cortex to the ventrolateral prefrontal cortex. The visual pathway is linked to perception of patterns and objects. This is implicated in global vs local processing and is related to central coherence.
	Extrastriate body area (EBA) is processed in the posterior and inferior temporal sulcus and fusiform body area (FBA). FBA is processed in the posterior fusiform gyrus. The ventral-occipital temporal system is implicated in the processing of faces (and thus social interaction).
Memory	There is a complex network for encoding, storing and retrieval of information that involves the temporal (including hippocampus) and cortical structures. The medial temporal structures are involved in storage, the prefrontal cortex is implicated in retrieval of information.
	For autobiographical memories, the medial prefrontal cortex plays a role in retrieval of the cognitive and emotional component of the memories; the lateral posterior parietal and precuneus are also activated in the retrieval of these memories.
Attention	Maintaining vigilance during tasks involves the interaction of a variety of systems/regions in the brain (most frequently the right cerebral cortex) and the brain stem.
	Processing stimuli involves either the dorsal or ventral attention system. In the dorsal attention network, stimuli are processed first by frontal eye fields then by the intraparietal sulcus/superior parietal lobe. The temporoparietal junction and the ventral frontal cortex are primarily implicated in the ventral attention system.
	Becoming aware of stimuli in the environment typically involves the connection between the midline cortex and the anterior cingulate cortex.
	Threatening stimuli are received by the amygdala and insula before moving into the dorsomedial pre-frontal cortex and the dorsal anterior cingulate. Emotional regulation moves through the ventromedial prefrontal cortex and the rostral and subgenual anterior cingulate. The ventrolateral cortex plays a role in modulating limbic activity related to attention and avoidance.
Processing speed	The parietal and temporal cortices, frontal cortex, and cerebellum may be implicated.

State of the Science in Eating Disorders

In this broad review of visuospatial and neuropsychological functioning in eating disorders, the primary focus is on research conducted in adults. Of note, most research participants in works cited were white women. The comparison group, when present, varies across studies. While some compare those with eating disorders to healthy controls, others have compared acutely ill individuals with AN to those who are weight restored or recovered (typically defined as 95% of expected body weight or median body mass index [BMI]). Research from the adolescent literature is beginning to point to the possibility that weight restoration to the median BMI is likely not sufficient for everyone, particularly those with a history of higher body weight, (Steinberg et al., 2022) and that *true* weight restoration may require returning to the pre-illness growth curve. Thus, it is possible that many adult individuals with AN classified as "weight-restored" or in recovery/remission may instead be weight and nutritionally suppressed, questioning whether findings of lingering inefficiencies/deficits in those who are weight-restored are indicative of traits that persist "into recovery" or are simply a sign of continued weight suppression. Most of the research reviewed is cross-sectional in nature and studies different aspects of neuropsychological functioning in isolation. Small sample sizes are common (Stedal et al., 2021). There is also a lack of standardization of measures employed across studies; when the same assessment tool is used, the scoring methods employed may be different. Finally, different neuropsychological domains have been studied in isolation, with a limited number of studies exploring the interactive nature of neuropsychological functioning. Across the board, whether deficits or alterations in function observed are part of general disorder etiology, a scar of the illness, or a risk factor in those with a persistent course cannot be determined. The following discussion must be interpreted through the lens of these limitations.

Visuospatial abilities

Visuospatial functioning refers to the ability to analyze features and parts and to organize them into a whole. It includes more complex behaviors associated with perception of world including finding and tracking objects, judging distances, and manipulating objects (Stiles et al., 2020). In eating disorders, most of the work in this area has focused on central coherence and perceptual errors.

Central coherence

A large focus of research on visuospatial processing in those with eating disorders has focused on deepening our understanding of central coherence. Visuospatial processing occurs at both a global and local level, with global level information typically processed first. Difficulties in global processing can interfere with processing at the local level, whereas the reverse is not true (Stiles et al., 2020). Weak central coherence refers to an overly detailed processing style wherein one struggles with processing the whole. Although weak central coherence was first observed in women with AN (Lopez, Tchanturia, Stahl, Booth, et al., 2008), its role has since been explored in other eating disorders, including BN and BED.

A smaller body of work has examined central coherence in unaffected relatives to help establish whether weak central coherence is an endophenotype for eating disorders (Lang, Treasure, et al., 2016; Teconi et al., 2010). Clinically, an overly detailed processing style can contribute to observed preoccupation with food, weight, shape, exercise, and so on. Weak central coherence is also hypothesized to contribute to body image disturbance and distorted perception of body size. In the social-cognitive realm, it may be related to difficulties in understanding the broader context of social cues contributing to interpersonal difficulties and poorer overall social functioning. From a clinical perspective, difficulty with global processing could contribute to difficulties in understanding how decisions around eating could impact longer-term decisions.

Studies investigating visuospatial or perceptual differences in eating disorders vary widely in sample size, assessment tools, and demographics. The Rey Osterrieth Complex Figure Test (ROCF) is the most commonly used assessment of weak central coherence in samples of individuals with eating disorders (Lang, Roberts, et al., 2016). In this task, individuals are asked to reproduce a complex figure by first copying it, then by immediately recalling the image, and finally by recalling the image 20 minutes later. Direct copy is the most commonly used assessment; however, delayed recall may be the most sensitive to weak central coherence (Stedal et al., 2021).

Meta-analyses provide a more robust overview of the state of the research (Fuglset, 2019; Keegan et al., 2021; Lang et al., 2014; Lang, Roberts, et al., 2016). Generally speaking, meta-analytic studies indicate that women with AN (Lang et al., 2014; Smith et al., 2018; Stedal et al., 2021) or BN (Lopez, Tchanturia, Stahl, & Treasure, 2008; Roberts et al., 2012; Smith et al., 2018) have weak central coherence compared to healthy controls, with no difference between those with restricting (AN-R) and binge/purge (AN-BP) subtype of AN (Van Autreve & Vervaet, 2015). Other research has found no evidence of weak central coherence in individuals with BN, including in those with a history of AN (Degortes et al., 2016). When comparing individuals with AN who are weight restored/recovered to those acutely ill, most studies find no differences between the groups (Fuglset, 2019), indicating that an overly detailed processing style is present in the absence of malnutrition. In contrast, some research found no difference between healthy control and weight restored individuals, highlighting that central coherence may improve with weight restoration (Fuglset, 2019; Teconi et al., 2010).

Studies have not supported links between illness related variables (length of illness, BMI, comorbid conditions) and central coherence (Keegan et al., 2021; Lang, Roberts, et al., 2016), although a recent meta-analysis did find that age and BMI were moderators—with older individuals and those with lower BMI having more impairment in visuospatial processing (Stedal et al., 2021). Of note, in a meta-analysis focused on neuropsychological functioning in individuals with severe and enduring AN, no differences were seen in central coherence between healthy controls and those with a long course of illness (Broomfield et al., 2021). Weak central coherence is hypothesized to be an endophenotype for AN and BN, and it has mostly been explored in unaffected family members of those with AN. In general, unaffected family members have weaker central coherence compared to healthy controls (Kanakam et al., 2013; Lang, Roberts, et al., 2016; Teconi et al., 2010). Data from individuals with BED are more limited and findings are equivocal. Individuals with BED have been found to have less accuracy on the ROCF than individuals with AN (Aloi et al., 2015), but they do not appear to differ from healthy controls in terms of central coherence (Keegan et al., 2021).

Perceptual errors

Research has also focused on understanding perceptual disturbances in individuals with eating disorders—typically explored in the context of body size estimation and in food portion estimation. Body image disturbance is considered a key feature of both AN and BN, and many individuals report disturbances in how they perceive their body size. This has led to the hypothesis that individuals with AN or BN may significantly differ in body size estimation from those without eating disorders (see Chapter 17). Indeed, data suggest that individuals with AN and BN typically overestimate body size, and this is more pronounced for individuals with BN (Mölbert et al., 2017). One key aspect of this question is whether the belief that an individual with an eating disorders has about their body size stems from cognitive/affective attitudes toward the body or clear perceptual differences; that is, is there a belief that the body or food portion is larger due to cognitive/affective correlates of the eating disorder or is there a perceptual difference that is supported by underlying alterations in key brain networks?

As with other areas of visuospatial functioning, assessment methods vary and fall broadly into the categories of descriptive methods (e.g., ideographic assessment of body size via mirror or photo manipulation) or metric methods (e.g., using measurement tools to reproduce the size of one's body) (Mölbert et al., 2017). Both approaches to measurement can be potentially influenced by one's attitudes about their body. Body size is more grossly overestimated when metric as opposed to descriptive methods are used, suggesting that body size misperception may be a product of cognitive/affective influences on body image instead of a true perceptual difference (Mölbert et al., 2017).

There is a limited body of work exploring the possible role of the extrastriate body area (EBA) and fusiform body area (FBA) in body perception in eating disorders. Both the EBA and the FBA are involved in processing images of the body, with the EBA processing body parts and the FBA focused on whole bodies and the relationships between body parts (Bratch et al., 2018; Esposito et al., 2018; Suchan et al., 2013). Results of studies are equivocal, with some finding differences in how individuals with eating disorders process body-related information related to healthy controls (Eshkevari et al., 2014; Suchan et al., 2013) and that this persists even after weight restoration (Eshkevari et al., 2014). The latter has led to the hypothesis that individuals with eating disorders may have a trait level of heighted attention to visual information at the cost of other perceptual data that is exacerbated during the ill state—leading to a high focus on the body (Eshkevari et al., 2014). However, other work on differences in the EBA/FBA in individuals with eating disorders has found no difference in these systems (Esposito et al., 2018). Research on body perception in BED is very limited; the EBA is hypothesized to play a role here as well, and there is some indication that processing of body image in individuals with BED is disrupted (Lewer et al., 2017).

A smaller body of work has focused on the perception of food or portion size in those with eating disorders. Individuals with AN tend to overestimate portion size and perceive food stimuli as larger than a non-food stimulus the same size (Dörsam et al., 2020; Zitron-Emanuel et al., 2022). This effect is particularly true for smaller portion sizes and when self-reported hunger levels are low (Milos et al., 2013). Individuals with BN also rated food portions as larger compared to healthy controls; however, their estimations were smaller than individuals with AN who rated the same portion sizes (Pasi et al., 2022). Despite these differences in the reported perception of portion sizes of food, individuals with AN and BN are able to correctly order portion sizes (from small to large) and are able to perceive same size food and non-food objects as equivalent—indicating that there is likely no actual underlying biologically based perceptual deficit (Dörsam et al., 2020), and that cognitive/affective processes related to the psychological aspects of the eating disorder may play a significant role in portion size estimation. For example, studies suggest that anxiety increases as portion sizes increase and individuals describe portion sizes as larger when there is an expectation that the food will need to be eaten compared to when it is not expected to be eaten (Dörsam et al., 2020). The perception of food/portion size has not been studied in BED in this similar format; however, some work has indicated that individuals with BED have a higher threshold for defining a large portion (Chao et al., 2019).

Neurocognitive abilities

Memory

There are multiple types of memory. The terms working memory and short-term memory (memory of limited capacity in which a small number of chunks are able to be manipulated), are often used interchangeably, although some memory researchers argue they are different (Aben et al., 2012). In research on memory in eating disorders, working memory is most consistently investigated and the most common term used; therefore, this type of limited capacity and active memory will be referred to as "working" memory. Long-term memory has a potentially unlimited capacity and is complex in terms of its types (including declarative and non-declarative) and the neurocircuitry involved. Broadly speaking, declarative memory focuses on facts and information, including episodic and verbal memory (Bauer & Dugan, 2020). Autobiographical memory, which is episodic and verbal in nature, refers to memories about oneself on one's life and experiences. Non-declarative memory (also referred to as procedural or implicit memory) is related to visuospatial processing and motor skills (e.g., riding a bicycle) (Bauer & Dugan, 2020). Research in memory in individuals with eating disorders has primarily focused on (1) differences in working memory in those with eating disorders versus controls, (2) examining whether verbal versus non-verbal memory is impacted in individuals with eating disorders, and (3) identifying structural or functional differences between those with and without eating disorders in brain regions associated with memory (primarily the hippocampus).

Due to the toll of perseverative rules regarding eating, perseveration about one's body, or negative ruminations on working memory and its capacity, it has been hypothesized that working memory can be impaired in individuals with eating disorders (Dahlén et al., 2022). Working memory has been investigated with a number of different tests, yielding inconsistent findings. Over the years, systematic reviews have consistently found that working memory is impaired in individuals with AN compared to healthy controls (Dahlén et al., 2022); whereas long-term memory does not seem to be impaired (Terhoeven et al., 2023). Individuals who are weight-restored or recovered tend to no longer have evidence of impaired working memory (Stedal et al., 2021). It is important to note that when reviewing results of studies on differences in memory (and other areas of neuropsychological functioning), clinical significance is rarely discussed in tandem with statistical significance. For example, in a small sample of adult women with AN, there were no differences in memory compared to healthy controls at baseline. While memory improved after medical stabilization in women with AN, it was still in the normal range. As the authors highlight, this statistically significant improvement may not have clinical or functional relevance (Rylander et al., 2020).

Some studies have reported deficits in verbal working memory compared to non-verbal memory (Dahlén et al., 2022), whereas others have found no differences (Stedal et al., 2021). Importantly, verbal and non-verbal (or visuospatial) are often not parsed in research on memory in individuals with eating disorders. Thus, equivocal findings may be a result of not reporting on these types of memory separately. When disentangled, a meta-analysis (Dahlén et al., 2022) indicated that those with AN have more impairment in verbal compared to non-verbal memory. No differences in memory have been shown between healthy controls and those with severe and enduring AN (Broomfield et al., 2021).

Other research has focused on whether individuals with AN have impaired ability to recall specific autobiographical memories; it has been hypothesized that they may be more likely to recall categories of memories or events as opposed to specific memories (Huber et al., 2015). This tendency is referred to as overgeneralized autobiographical memory. When specific, individuals with AN tend to have fewer autobiographical memories compared to healthy controls; both frequency of memories and overgeneralized memories are more pronounced in response to disorder eliciting prompts (Huber et al., 2015). Although work in this area is limited, it has been suggested that more general and less frequent autobiographical recall could serve an affect regulation function, such that recalling general as opposed to specific memories allows for the avoidance of emotions (positive and negative) associated with specific memories. In addition, overgeneralized autobiographical memory could be associated with greater inflexibility and linked to self-referential processes (Huber et al., 2015; Keeler et al., 2022; Terhoeven et al., 2023). More comprehensive studies exploring these constructs in tandem are needed. There are limited data indicating that difficulties in retrieving autobiographical memory dissipate with weight restoration (Keeler et al., 2022).

Finally, the hippocampus has received the most attention as the brain structure typically involved in memory. Overall, hippocampal volume is reduced in women with AN (Keeler et al., 2020) and this is associated with BMI but not length of illness (Collantoni et al., 2021). The reduction in volume appears to be reversible with weight restoration. Interestingly, women with AN who also engage in compulsive exercise have greater hippocampal volume than healthy controls; with weight restoration and cessation of exercise, there is a reduction of volume such that is similar to weight restored women with AN who did not exercise (Beadle et al., 2015). It remains unclear what impact, if any, this reduction would have on memory. There is greater activation in the hippocampus in response to food stimuli, although few studies have examined activation and there is a great deal of heterogeneity in the stimuli and paradigms used in the studies that did (Keeler et al., 2020). It is also important to note that the hippocampus is implicated in reward, specifically the hippocampus is part of mesocorticolimbic pathway via which dopamine modulates food reward. Thus, alterations in hippocampal volume and activation may be related to different aspect of memory and could also be a function of other systems implicated in the pathophysiology of AN.

There has been less focus on memory in individuals with BN and BED, with limited data indicating no differences in verbal and non-verbal working memory between individuals with BN and healthy controls (Smith et al., 2018). Data from individuals with BED are equivocal (Smith et al., 2018). There is some indication that those with BN and BED may have similar impairments (i.e., less frequent and overgeneral) in autobiographical memory (Laberg & Andersson, 2004; Svaldi et al., 2011).

Attention/attentional bias

Attention includes those times when one's focus is drawn to novel, unique, or relevant stimuli in our environment as well as the voluntarily direction of attention to particular stimuli to achieve certain goals or engage in certain behaviors (Rueda & Conejero, 2020). Attentional bias refers to the increased likelihood of directing attention to concern relevant versus concern irrelevant stimuli in any given situation. For eating disorders, concern relevant stimuli are typically conceptualized as food or body-related stimuli (as compared to non-concern relevant stimuli such as furniture). However, other work has focused on the attentional bias to other potentially relevant stimuli such as perceived threat via negative emotion (e.g., anxiety) or social rejection (Cardi et al., 2013). Several systematic reviews (Brooks et al., 2011; Kerr-Gaffney et al., 2018; Ralph-Nearman et al., 2019; Stojek et al., 2018; Stott et al., 2021) present conflicting information regarding the degree of attention/avoidance paid toward disease eliciting stimuli. As in other areas, the testing paradigms and stimuli used vary across studies. Unlike in other neuropsychological domains, there has been more research conducted on attentional bias toward food in BED.

The most commonly used tasks to assess attentional bias include modifications of the Stroop Task, Dot-Probe Task, and Eye Tracking (Ralph-Nearman et al., 2019; Stott et al., 2021). The modified Stroop presents both neutral (e.g., furniture) and disease salient words in a variety of colors; individuals are asked to name the color in which each word is written. Slower reading of disease salient words indicates an attention bias toward those words. In individuals with eating disorders, the modified Stroop has included both body/shape/weight and food related words. In the Dot-Probe Task, individuals view two words (neutral and disease related); after a short period, both words disappear and a dot appears in place of one of them—participants are then asked to press a button to indicate the location of the dot. A faster reaction to one type of stimulus over the other indicates a bias to that type of stimuli. Finally, eye tracking tasks measure the length of gaze on a stimulus and eye saccades, which allows for the determination of attention and avoidance. In any of these tasks, food, body, or emotional stimuli can be used (Kerr-Gaffney et al., 2018).

Overall, individuals with BN and AN have a greater (and equivalent) attentional bias toward food stimuli compared to healthy controls when measured with the modified Stroop (Brooks et al., 2011; Stott et al., 2021). However, when assessed with the dot-probe task, individuals with eating disorders have a bias away from food (depending on the specific stimuli) (Ralph-Nearman et al., 2019). Low calorie foods are avoided and there is increased vigilance for high calorie foods. Individuals with AN evidence a bias toward food initially that is followed by avoidance in eye-tracking paradigms (Stott et al., 2021). Eye-tracking studies generally support a bias for food stimuli in those with BED (Smith et al., 2018), with adults with BED having an overall longer gaze than healthy controls (Kerr-Gaffney et al., 2019).

More consistent attention to body-related stimuli in BN compared to healthy controls is observed in the modified Stroop; mixed findings exist for AN with some studies finding a bias toward body related stimuli and others not finding this in relation to healthy controls (Stott et al., 2021). When using the dot-probe task, meta-analyses suggest there is a bias away from body related stimuli or no difference in those with an eating disorder compared to healthy controls. With eye-tracking, individuals with BN tend to have a bias toward low-weight body images and away from higher-weight body images (Smith et al., 2018); whereas those with BED tend to have a bias for their own bodies compared to others. When looking at their own or other bodies, individuals with AN, BN, and BED gaze longer at body parts they deem to be unattractive (Kerr-Gaffney et al., 2019).

Attentional bias to threatening stimuli have been explored using the modified Stroop and Dot-Probe. In these studies, attention to negative emotions associated with correlates of eating disorders (e.g., social anxiety, harm avoidance, etc.) were explored. "Threatening stimuli" include negative emotional wors such as "fail" or "rejection." In the former, individuals with BED and BN have a greater bias toward threatening stimuli (Stojek et al., 2018). In the latter, individuals with BN and AN have a bias toward rejecting stimuli and away from accepting stimuli (Jáuregui-Lobera, 2013; Stojek et al., 2018).

Literature on attentional bias in eating disorders is extensive but also widely varied in terms of how studies measure attention and on which disorders they focus (Stott et al., 2021). Works cited indicate that adult women with AN and BN tend to focus longer on food-related stimuli, yet what can be inferred from these data is still ambiguous as healthy controls who are fasted also pay more attention to food related stimuli (Placanica et al., 2002). The recent increase in use of eye-tracking procedures to assess attention bias should provide more opportunities to parse out the impact of approach and avoidance motivation on attentional bias; longitudinal research could be used to track how this changes over the course of treatment and with weight restoration. It is also important to assess how attentional bias may relate to visuospatial functioning. For example, avoiding food stimuli or attending longer to certain body parts could contribute to reported under/overestimation of size.

Processing speed

Processing speed refers to taking in information (including identification or discrimination, integration) and then acting on the information or completing the task (Kramer et al., 2020). It is not frequently explored in individuals with eating disorders, even though it is related to performance on the most common task-based assessments of neuropsychological functioning. Processing speed can impact reaction time tasks, particularly if there is a decisional component involved (Ferraro et al., 2018). Across the board, individuals with eating disorders have slower processing speed than healthy controls (Diaz-Marsa et al., 2023; Stedal et al., 2021), although it is likely that this is due to malnutrition than specific disease processes. In individuals with BED, those in a higher weight body may have slower processing speed but that may be due to weight status and not BED (Eneva et al., 2017).

Summary

Visuospatial abilities and overall neuropsychological functioning have been of interest in eating disorders for several years. The goal of work in this area has primarily been to understand how individuals with an eating disorder differ from healthy controls in the acute state of illness and whether these differences are maintained once remission or weight restoration is reached. Many observed impairments have been hypothesized to be an endophenotype for eating disorders. Endophenotypes are intermediate expressions of an underlying genetic vulnerability; they occur more frequently in individuals with the disorder or illness, also occur in relatives of the affected person, and are present in the acutely ill and healthy state (Gottesman & Gould, 2003; Gould & Gottesman, 2006). Endophenotypes must also be reliably measured as their identification can inform and advance research on the inter-complexity of environment and genes (Glahn et al., 2014). Ideally, understanding differences in visuospatial and neuropsychological functioning will improve our understanding of putative endophenotypes, identify the role they may play as a risk or maintenance factor of the illness, and inform the development of novel treatment approaches.

To date, the most advanced research has been the exploration of attentional bias. Implications for increased attention toward or avoidance of stimuli can inform exposure to feared stimuli as well as possible attention bias training. However, research around neuropsychological functioning is too heterogeneous to allow for firm conclusions. The heterogeneity of assessment tools/task paradigms, small sample sizes, and narrow samples (i.e., mostly white women) results in a paucity of conclusive evidence. This, in turn, undermines our ability to generate models about the etiology and/or maintenance of eating disorders that incorporate visuospatial and neuropsychological functioning. Few studies control for age, length of illness, IQ, mood, or medication status. The heterogeneity of research is most easily assessed via meta-analyses; however, these are of mixed quality (Smith et al., 2018; Stedal et al., 2021; Stott et al., 2021). Further, it remains impossible to consider prevailing approaches to understanding neuropsychological dysfunction without fully accounting for how these disorders are inherently impacted by the confounding variable of (prolonged) malnutrition. In many cases, renourishment appears to reverse observed deficits, though longitudinal research is rare, and it is unknown whether the sample is truly remitted (i.e., if participants are truly weight restored). When impairment in visuospatial or neuropsychological functions remain after weight restoration—it cannot be determined whether these are true endophenotypes of the illness, or a scar of being acutely ill during a period of critical brain development or due to the persistent course of illness (Smith et al., 2018).

Alternative Perspective

Research on neuropsychological and visuospatial functioning in individuals with eating disorders is driven, in part, by the hypothesis that deficits in these areas are an endophenotype or risk factor for illness development. However, many participants in research studies investigating these impairments are adult women. While most studies include adults, the age of onset for eating disorders is in adolescence, a key period of brain development. The physical impact of malnutrition on the developing brain is not understood (Galler et al., 2017). Combined with the breadth of age and developmental stage of patients at onset, adult functioning (while ill or weight restored) may greatly depend on when they become ill; the course of illness (e.g., degree of weight suppression, weight cycling, presence of binging/purging), and the presence/absence of certain physical or psychological comorbidities (e.g., inflammation, anxiety). The inextricable linkage of malnutrition and eating disorder psychopathology makes it uniquely difficult to assess the visuospatial and neuropsychological underpinnings of these disorders—particularly in adults. Data from adult women may not generalize to individuals with eating disorders at younger ages or a different biological sex. Instead of focusing research on adults with the bias that any differences found are representative of an endophenotype, alternative hypotheses are that any visuospatial or neuropsychological differences observed are due to malnutrition as opposed to the eating disorder. In this case, they could be a state-based difference due to malnutrition or a scar of the illness due to onset during a critical period of brain development that worsens over the course of illness.

Research on adults with eating disorders provides information about visuospatial and neuropsychological functioning in those with a longer course of illness than what may occur or be present in individuals at diagnosis. Furthermore, in adult samples it is potentially even harder to disentangle the impact of prolonged malnutrition from the psychological conditions that are illness-specific. In the case of BN and BED, one might argue that malnutrition plays less of a role; however, women in these groups will often have periods of restriction, may be undernourished, or may be missing key macro/micronutrients during a key period of development. The deprivation of nutrients and caloric intake can impact brain organization and development in adolescents.

A shift from the assumption that any underlying differences are due to AN (as opposed to malnutrition) also requires a shift on the population we study, the goals of research, and the goals of intervention development. The adolescent brain is a developing brain. The impact of malnutrition may be akin to a brain injury. For example, there are volume changes in the brain of adolescents with AN (Seitz et al., 2016) and literature on the long-term impact of malnutrition during early development signifies that these changes can cause permanent consequences (Galler et al., 2012, 2021; Szutorisz & Hurd, 2016). Malnutrition during adolescence has the potential to pause or permanently alter a normal developmental trajectory. In the case of the latter, how the brain reorganizes could depend on what the normal developmental trajectory was (i.e., were there already weaknesses in some neuropsychological functioning, how early was white matter growth, has puberty begun), when malnutrition occurred, how acute weight loss was, and how long the brain was malnourished or undernourished. It is possible that multiple different patterns of reorganization and different degrees of integration of neuropsychological functioning could result from malnourishment. Thus, what is observed in adults may be a scar due to presence or persistence of malnutrition.

Research in neuropsychological functioning in adolescents is equivocal, raising the criticism that studying neuropsychological functioning in adolescents is not fruitful. Unfortunately, most of the work done in this area has the same pitfalls of adult samples: small sample sizes, heterogeneity in tasks and assessments, and cross-sectional design. Age is rarely controlled for though it is an important moderator (Stedal et al., 2022). Longitudinal studies of neuropsychological functioning in youth with eating disorders are rare. Given how important the timing of and length of malnutrition is in understanding the role of visuospatial and neuropsychological functioning in the context of eating disorders, longitudinal studies in youth with eating disorders are essential.

As in adults, those assigned male sex at birth are frequently excluded from research on neuropsychological functioning. When included, the samples are usually too small to examine sex differences (Timko et al., 2019). Given that there are sex differences in adolescent brain development (Beltz et al., 2020), it is important to understand how those differences interact with malnutrition and impact neuropsychological functioning in individuals with eating disorders. Elucidating sex differences could help to understand underlying risk or maintenance factors for these illnesses. As in adults, most of the work in adolescents has been in AN, with less work done in individuals with BN or BED. Likewise, including weight restored youth in studies has the same concern as with adults—weight restored is often considered to be the 50th percentile BMI; however, youth may need to restore to their growth curve (Steinberg et al., 2022), which could be above the 50th percentile BMI. If adolescents are not fully weight restored, it is likely that their neuropsychological functioning will continue to be impaired, resulting in the common presentation of illness in adults.

Summary of findings in youth

Few systematic reviews focus solely on adolescents. Importantly, mixed samples of adolescents and adults are common and have been excluded here due to difficulties in isolating the adolescent sample. Generally speaking, results from adolescent samples mirror those from adults, with the most robust evidence for weak central coherence, disruptions in memory, and attentional bias toward disease eliciting stimuli.

Visuospatial abilities

One of the more robust findings (Stedal et al., 2022) is that youth with AN have weak central coherence compared to healthy controls (Brown et al., 2018; Lang, Roberts, et al., 2016) even when weight restored (Weinbach et al., 2017); although there are a number of studies that fail to find evidence of an overly detailed processing style (Herbrich et al., 2018; Rose et al., 2014; van Noort et al., 2016) and others indicating that it normalizes with weight restoration (Lozano-Serra et al., 2014). Adolescents with BN also have lower accuracy in visuospatial abilities (Darcy et al., 2015).

Memory

Memory is impaired in youth with AN (Kjaersdam Telléus et al., 2015; Prince et al., 2022; Stedal et al., 2022), although it is hypothesized that this may be more state based (i.e., related to the impact of malnutrition as opposed to the psychological correlates of the eating disorder) and linked to lower levels of sex hormones that are present when in a malnourished state (Buehren et al., 2011). Youth with AN demonstrate increased activation in the parietal and temporal areas when engaging in a working memory task compared to healthy controls. Their performance on the task was similar, indicating that youth with AN may have to work harder to have normal functioning. Importantly, increased activation did not occur in the youth when weight restored (Castro-Fornieles et al., 2010). Overgeneralization in autobiographical memory is also present in adolescence and it appears to worsen with length of illness, indicating that some difficulties observed may be due to malnutrition and not disease processes (Bomba et al., 2014).

Attention/attentional bias

As in adults, adolescents with AN, BN, and BED have an attentional bias toward body parts deemed unattractive (Bauer et al., 2017). Attentional bias toward palatable foods is present in adolescents with loss of control eating and who are in higher weight bodies (Shank et al., 2015).

Processing speed

Processing speed is impaired in youth with AN and improves with weight restoration (Hemmingsen et al., 2021).

Implications

The exploration of visuospatial and neuropsychological functioning in those with eating disorders provides information essential to developing novel treatments and therapies, including symptom characterization, diagnostic formulation, and interventions. A goal in research focused on understanding neuropsychological functioning in eating disorders is to determine if there is an underlying endophenotype or profile that could predict outcome or inform treatment. To truly move in the direction of answering this question, efforts must focus on children and adolescents with eating disorders to parse out the impact of malnutrition from the impact of the eating disorder. It is possible that observed deficits are due solely to the short and long-term impact of malnutrition on the brain. To date, there has not been enough focus on the development and integration of different aspects of neuropsychological functioning and how they are impacted by malnourishment and undernourishment.

Any impairments in neuropsychological functioning (including aspects discussed in other chapters of this Handbook) present before illness onset are likely transdiagnostic vulnerabilities and not unique to eating disorders. In addition, it is possible that they are only a risk factor for those who will have a persistent course and are subsequently worsened by ongoing malnutrition. Focusing on adolescents and using longitudinal study designs (and considering age, pubertal status, biological sex) is the best way to answer these questions. If, indeed, much of what is observed is due to malnutrition—our focus can shift to ways to mitigate this impact (including focusing on rapid renourishment, nutritional/nutrition supplementals, adding in cognitive rehabilitation to treatment packages, etc.).

Helping individuals with eating disorders and (perhaps more importantly) their caregivers to understand the impact of an eating disorder on neuropsychological functioning could have a positive impact on treatment outcome. Educating individuals and their caregivers on the relationship between eating disorder behaviors and specific brain functions will provide insight into how and why behaviors are impacted by both malnutrition and the eating disorder. This education may be empowering to caregivers and improve their self-efficacy in helping their loved one with an eating disorder recover (Knatz et al., 2015). Understanding the complex interplay between malnutrition, eating disorders, and neuropsychological functioning may help individuals with an eating disorder and their caregiver(s) externalize the eating disorder and could serve as a motivating factor in recovery.

References

Aben, B., Stapert, S., & Blokland, A. (2012). About the distinction between working memory and short-term memory. *Frontiers in Psychology, 3*. https://doi.org/10.3389/fpsyg.2012.00301

Aloi, M., Rania, M., Caroleo, M., Bruni, A., Palmieri, A., Cauteruccio, M. A., De Fazio, P., & Segura-García, C. (2015). Decision making, central coherence and set-shifting: A comparison between binge eating disorder, anorexia nervosa and healthy controls. *BMC Psychiatry, 15*(1), 6. https://doi.org/10.1186/s12888-015-0395-z

Bauer, A., Schneider, S., Waldorf, M., Braks, K., Huber, T. J., Adolph, D., & Vocks, S. (2017). Selective visual attention towards oneself and associated state body satisfaction: An eye-tracking study in adolescents with different types of eating disorders. *Journal of Abnormal Child Psychology, 45*(8), 1647–1661. https://doi.org/10.1007/s10802-017-0263-z

Bauer, P. J., & Dugan, J. A. (2020). Memory development. In J. Rubenstein, P. Rakic, B. Chen, & K. Y. Kwan (Eds.), *Neural circuit and cognitive development* (pp. 395–412). Elsevier. https://doi.org/10.1016/B978-0-12-814411-4.00018-4

Beadle, J. N., Paradiso, S., Brumm, M., Voss, M., Halmi, K., & McCormick, L. M. (2015). Larger hippocampus size in women with anorexia nervosa who exercise excessively than healthy women. *Psychiatry Research: Neuroimaging, 232*(2), 193–199. https://doi.org/10.1016/j.pscychresns.2014.10.013

Beltz, A. M., Kelly, D. P., & Berenbaum, S. A. (2020). Sex differences in brain and behavioral development. In J. Rubenstein, P. Rakic, B. Chen, & K. Y. Kwan (Eds.), *Neural circuit and cognitive development* (pp. 585–638). Elsevier. https://doi.org/10.1016/B978-0-12-814411-4.00027-5

Bomba, M., Marfone, M., Brivio, E., Oggiano, S., Broggi, F., Neri, F., & Nacinovich, R. (2014). Autobiographical memory in adolescent girls with anorexia nervosa: Autobiographical memory in anorexic girls. *European Eating Disorders Review, 22*(6), 479–486. https://doi.org/10.1002/erv.2321

Bratch, A., Engel, S., Burton, P., & Kersten, D. (2018). The fusiform body area represents spatial relationships between pairs of body parts. *Journal of Vision, 18*(10), 408. https://doi.org/10.1167/18.10.408

Brooks, S., Prince, A., Stahl, D., Campbell, I. C., & Treasure, J. (2011). A systematic review and meta-analysis of cognitive bias to food stimuli in people with disordered eating behaviour. *Clinical Psychology Review, 31*(1), 37–51. https://doi.org/10.1016/j.cpr.2010.09.006

Broomfield, C., Stedal, K., & Touyz, S. (2021). The neuropsychological profile of severe and enduring anorexia nervosa: A systematic review. *Frontiers in Psychology, 12*, 708536. https://doi.org/10.3389/fpsyg.2021.708536

Brown, M., Loeb, K. L., McGrath, R. E., Tiersky, L., Zucker, N., & Carlin, A. (2018). Executive functioning and central coherence in anorexia nervosa: Pilot investigation of a neurocognitive endophenotype. *European Eating Disorders Review, 26*(5), 489–498. https://doi.org/10.1002/erv.2597

Buehren, K., Konrad, K., Schaefer, K., Kratzsch, J., Kahraman-Lanzerath, B., Lente, C., & Herpertz-Dahlmann, B. (2011). Association between neuroendocrinological parameters and learning and memory functions in adolescent anorexia nervosa before and after weight recovery. *Journal of Neural Transmission, 118*(6), 963–968. https://doi.org/10.1007/s00702-010-0567-4

Cardi, V., Matteo, R. D., Corfield, F., & Treasure, J. (2013). Social reward and rejection sensitivity in eating disorders: An investigation of attentional bias and early experiences. *World Journal of Biological Psychiatry, 14*(8), 622–633. https://doi.org/10.3109/15622975.2012.665479

Castro-Fornieles, J., Caldú, X., Andrés-Perpiñá, S., Lázaro, L., Bargalló, N., Falcón, C., Plana, M. T., & Junqué, C. (2010). A cross-sectional and follow-up functional MRI study with a working memory task in adolescent anorexia nervosa. *Neuropsychologia, 48*(14), 4111–4116. https://doi.org/10.1016/j.neuropsychologia.2010.10.003

Chao, A. M., Wadden, T. A., Walsh, O. A., Gruber, K. A., Alamuddin, N., Berkowitz, R. I., & Tronieri, J. S. (2019). Perceptions of a large amount of food based on binge-eating disorder diagnosis. *International Journal of Eating Disorders, 52*(7), 801–808. https://doi.org/10.1002/eat.23076

Collantoni, E., Tenconi, E., Solmi, M., Meneguzzo, P., Marzola, E., D'Agata, F., Gotti, S., Daga, G. A., Manara, R., & Favaro, A. (2021). Hippocampal volumes in anorexia nervosa at different stages of the disorder. *European Eating Disorders Review, 29*(1), 112–122. https://doi.org/10.1002/erv.2806

Dahlén, A. D., Gaudio, S., Schiöth, H. B., & Brooks, S. J. (2022). Phonological working memory is adversely affected in adults with anorexia nervosa: A systematic literature review. *Eating and Weight Disorders, 27*(6), 1931–1952. https://doi.org/10.1007/s40519-022-01370-1

Darcy, A. M., Fitzpatrick, K. K., Manasse, S. M., Datta, N., Klabunde, M., Colborn, D., Aspen, V., Stiles-Shields, C., Labuschagne, Z., Le Grange, D., & Lock, J. (2015). Central coherence in adolescents with bulimia nervosa spectrum eating disorders: Central coherence in adolescent bulimia. *International Journal of Eating Disorders, 48*(5), 487–493. https://doi.org/10.1002/eat.22340

Degortes, D., Tenconi, E., Santonastaso, P., & Favaro, A. (2016). Executive Functioning and Visuospatial Abilities in Bulimia Nervosa with or without a Previous history of anorexia nervosa: Cognitive functioning in bulimia nervosa. *European Eating Disorders Review, 24*(2), 139–146. https://doi.org/10.1002/erv.2430

Diaz-Marsa, M., Pemau, A., de la Torre-Luque, A., Vaz-Leal, F., Rojo-Moreno, L., Beato-Fernandez, L., Graell, M., Carrasco-Diaz, A., & Carrasco, J. L. (2023). Executive dysfunction in eating disorders: Relationship with clinical features. *Progress in Neuro-Psychopharmacology and Biological Psychiatry, 120*, 110649. https://doi.org/10.1016/j.pnpbp.2022.110649

Dörsam, A. F., Mack, I., Kögel, L., Zipfel, S., & Giel, K. E. (2020). How do patients with eating disorders perceive and evaluate food portion sizes? A systematic review. *European Eating Disorders Review, 28*(4), 398–409. https://doi.org/10.1002/erv.2743

Eneva, K. T., Arlt, J. M., Yiu, A., Murray, S. M., & Chen, E. Y. (2017). Assessment of executive functioning in binge-eating disorder independent of weight status. *International Journal of Eating Disorders, 50*(8), 942–951. https://doi.org/10.1002/eat.22738

Eshkevari, E., Rieger, E., Longo, M. R., Haggard, P., & Treasure, J. (2014). Persistent body image disturbance following recovery from eating disorders: Persistent body image disturbance after recovery. *International Journal of Eating Disorders, 47*(4), 400–409. https://doi.org/10.1002/eat.22219

Esposito, R., Cieri, F., di Giannantonio, M., & Tartaro, A. (2018). The role of body image and self-perception in anorexia nervosa: The neuroimaging perspective. *Journal of Neuropsychology, 12*(1), 41–52. https://doi.org/10.1111/jnp.12106

Ferraro, F. R., Kramer, R., & Weigel, S. (2018). Speed of processing time slowing in eating disorders. *Journal of General Psychology, 145*(1), 79–92. https://doi.org/10.1080/00221309.2017.1421136

Fuglset, T. S. (2019). Set-shifting, central coherence and decision-making in individuals recovered from anorexia nervosa: A systematic review. *Journal of Eating Disorders, 7*(1), 22. https://doi.org/10.1186/s40337-019-0251-5

Galler, J. R., Bringas-Vega, M. L., Tang, Q., Rabinowitz, A. G., Musa, K. I., Chai, W. J., Omar, H., Abdul Rahman, M. R., Abd Hamid, A. I., Abdullah, J. M., & Valdés-Sosa, P. A. (2021). Neurodevelopmental effects of childhood malnutrition: A neuroimaging perspective. *NeuroImage, 231*, 117828. https://doi.org/10.1016/j.neuroimage.2021.117828

Galler, J. R., Bryce, C. P., Zichlin, M. L., Fitzmaurice, G., Eaglesfield, G. D., & Waber, D. P. (2012). Infant malnutrition is associated with persisting attention deficits in middle adulthood. *Journal of Nutrition, 142*(4), 788–794. https://doi.org/10.3945/jn.111.145441

Galler, J. R., Koethe, J. R., & Yolken, R. H. (2017). Neurodevelopment: The impact of nutrition and inflammation during adolescence in low-resource settings. *Pediatrics, 139*(Supplement 1), 72–84.

Glahn, D. C., Knowles, E. E. M., McKay, D. R., Sprooten, E., Raventós, H., Blangero, J., Gottesman, I. I., & Almasy, L. (2014). Arguments for the sake of endophenotypes: Examining common misconceptions about the use of endophenotypes in psychiatric genetics. *American Journal of Medical Genetics Part B: Neuropsychiatric Genetics, 165*(2), 122–130. https://doi.org/10.1002/ajmg.b.32221

Gottesman, I. I., & Gould, T. D. (2003). The endophenotype concept in psychiatry: Etymology and strategic intentions. *American Journal of Psychiatry, 160*(4), 636–645.

Gould, T. D., & Gottesman, I. I. (2006). Psychiatric endophenotypes and the development of valid animal models. *Genes, Brain and Behavior, 5*(2), 113–119. https://doi.org/10.1111/j.1601-183X.2005.00186.x

Hemmingsen, S. D., Wesselhoeft, R., Lichtenstein, M. B., Sjögren, J. M., & Støving, R. K. (2021). Cognitive improvement following weight gain in patients with anorexia nervosa: A systematic review. *European Eating Disorders Review, 29*(3), 402–426. https://doi.org/10.1002/erv.2796

Herbrich, L., Kappel, V., van Noort, B. M., & Winter, S. (2018). Differences in set-shifting and central coherence across anorexia nervosa subtypes in children and adolescents. *European Eating Disorders Review, 26*(5), 499–507. https://doi.org/10.1002/erv.2605

Holliday, J., Tchanturia, K., Landau, S., Collier, D., & Treasure, J. (2005). Is impaired set-shifting an endophenotype of anorexia nervosa? *American Journal of Psychiatry, 162*, 2269–2275.

Huber, J., Salatsch, C., Ingenerf, K., Schmid, C., Maatouk, I., Weisbrod, M., Herzog, W., Friederich, H.-C., & Nikendei, C. (2015). Characteristics of disorder-related autobiographical memory in acute anorexia nervosa patients: Autobiographical memory in AN. *European Eating Disorders Review, 23*(5), 379–389. https://doi.org/10.1002/erv.2379

Jáuregui-Lobera, I. (2013). Neuropsychology of eating disorders: 1995–2012. *Neuropsychiatric Disease and Treatment, 9*, 415–430. https://doi.org/10.2147/NDT.S42714

Kanakam, N., Raoult, C., Collier, D., & Treasure, J. (2013). Set shifting and central coherence as neurocognitive endophenotypes in eating disorders: A preliminary investigation in twins. *World Journal of Biological Psychiatry, 14*(6), 464–475. https://doi.org/10.3109/15622975.2012.665478

Keegan, E., Tchanturia, K., & Wade, T. D. (2021). Central coherence and set-shifting between nonunderweight eating disorders and anorexia nervosa: A systematic review and meta-analysis. *International Journal of Eating Disorders, 54*(3), 229–243. https://doi.org/10.1002/eat.23430

Keeler, J. L., Peters-Gill, G., Treasure, J., Himmerich, H., Tchanturia, K., & Cardi, V. (2022). Difficulties in retrieving specific details of autobiographical memories and imagining positive future events in individuals with acute but not remitted anorexia nervosa. *Journal of Eating Disorders, 10*(1), 172. https://doi.org/10.1186/s40337-022-00684-w

Keeler, J., Patsalos, O., Thuret, S., Ehrlich, S., Tchanturia, K., Himmerich, H., & Treasure, J. (2020). Hippocampal volume, function, and related molecular activity in anorexia nervosa: A scoping review. *Expert Review of Clinical Pharmacology, 13*(12), 1367–1387. https://doi.org/10.1080/17512433.2020.1850256

Kerr-Gaffney, J., Harrison, A., & Tchanturia, K. (2018). Social anxiety in the eating disorders: A systematic review and meta-analysis. *Psychological Medicine*, 48(15), 2477–2491. https://doi.org/10.1017/S0033291718000752

Kerr-Gaffney, J., Harrison, A., & Tchanturia, K. (2019). Eye-tracking research in eating disorders: A systematic review. *International Journal of Eating Disorders, 52*(1), 3–27. https://doi.org/10.1002/eat.22998

Kjaersdam Telléus, G., Jepsen, J. R., Bentz, M., Christiansen, E., Jensen, S. O., Fagerlund, B., & Thomsen, P. H. (2015). Cognitive profile of children and adolescents with anorexia nervosa. *European Eating Disorders Review, 23*(1), 34–42.

Knatz, S., Wierenga, C. E., Murray, S. B., Hill, L., & Kaye, W. H. (2015). Neurobiologically informed treatment for adults with anorexia nervosa: A novel approach to a chronic disorder. *Dialogues in Clinical Neuroscience, 17*(2), 229–236. https://doi.org/10.31887/DCNS.2015.17.2/sknatz

Kramer, E., Koo, B., Restrepo, A., Koyama, M., Neuhaus, R., Pugh, K., Andreotti, C., & Milham, M. (2020). Diagnostic associations of processing speed in a transdiagnostic, pediatric sample. *Scientific Reports, 10*(1), 10114. https://doi.org/10.1038/s41598-020-66892-z

Laberg, S., & Andersson, G. (2004). Autobiographical memories in patients treated for bulimia nervosa. *European Eating Disorders Review, 12*(1), 34–41. https://doi.org/10.1002/erv.534

Lang, K., Lopez, C., Stahl, D., Tchanturia, K., & Treasure, J. (2014). Central coherence in eating disorders: An updated systematic review and meta-analysis. *World Journal of Biological Psychiatry, 15*(8), 586–598.

Lang, K., Roberts, M., Harrison, A., Lopez, C., Goddard, E., Khondoker, M., Treasure, J., & Tchanturia, K. (2016). Central coherence in eating disorders: A synthesis of studies using the rey osterrieth complex figure test. *PLOS ONE, 11*(11), e0165467. https://doi.org/10.1371/journal.pone.0165467

Lang, K., Treasure, J., & Tchanturia, K. (2016). Is inefficient cognitive processing in anorexia nervosa a familial trait? A neuropsychological pilot study of mothers of offspring with a diagnosis of anorexia nervosa. *World Journal of Biological Psychiatry, 17*(4), 258–265. https://doi.org/10.3109/15622975.2015.1112035

Lewer, M., Bauer, A., Hartmann, A., & Vocks, S. (2017). different facets of body image disturbance in binge eating disorder: A review. *Nutrients, 9*(12), 1294. https://doi.org/10.3390/nu9121294

Lopez, C., Tchanturia, K., Stahl, D., Booth, R., Holliday, J., & Treasure, J. (2008). An examination of the concept of central coherence in women with anorexia nervosa. *International Journal of Eating Disorders, 41*(2), 143–152.

Lopez, C., Tchanturia, K., Stahl, D., & Treasure, J. (2008). Central coherence in eating disorders: A systematic review. *Psychological Medicine, 38*(10), 1393–1404. https://doi.org/10.1017/S0033291708003486

Lopez, C., Tchanturia, K., Stahl, D., & Treasure, J. (2009). Weak central coherence in eating disorders: A step towards looking for an endophenotype of eating disorders. *Journal of Clinical and Experimental Neuropsychology, 31*(1), 117–125.

Lozano-Serra, E., Andrés-Perpiña, S., Lázaro-García, L., & Castro-Fornieles, J. (2014). Adolescent anorexia nervosa: Cognitive performance after weight recovery. *Journal of Psychosomatic Research, 76*(1), 6–11. https://doi.org/10.1016/j.jpsychores.2013.10.009

Milos, G., Kuenzli, C., Soelch, C. M., Schumacher, S., Moergeli, H., & Mueller-Pfeiffer, C. (2013). How much should I eat? Estimation of meal portions in anorexia nervosa. *Appetite, 63*, 42–47. https://doi.org/10.1016/j.appet.2012.12.016

Mölbert, S. C., Klein, L., Thaler, A., Mohler, B. J., Brozzo, C., Martus, P., Karnath, H.-O., Zipfel, S., & Giel, K. E. (2017). Depictive and metric body size estimation in anorexia nervosa and bulimia nervosa: A systematic review and meta-analysis. *Clinical Psychology Review, 57*, 21–31. https://doi.org/10.1016/j.cpr.2017.08.005

Nunn, K., Frampton, I., Fuglset, T. S., Törzsök-Sonnevend, M., & Lask, B. (2011). Anorexia nervosa and the insula. *Medical Hypotheses, 76*(3), 353–357.

Nunn, K., Frampton, I., Gordon, I., & Lask, B. (2008). The fault is not in her parents but in her insula—A neurobiological hypothesis of anorexia nervosa. *European Eating Disorders Review, 16*(5), 355–360.

Pasi, P., Piccolo, M., Kaufmann, L.-K., Martin-Soelch, C., Müller-Pfeiffer, C., & Milos, G. (2022). Estimation of meal portions in bulimia nervosa compared to anorexia nervosa and healthy controls. *Eating and Weight Disorders, 27*(7), 2665–2672. https://doi.org/10.1007/s40519-022-01410-w

Placanica, J. L., Faunce, G. J., & Soames Job, R. F. (2002). The effect of fasting on attentional biases for food and body shape/weight words in high and low eating disorder inventory scorers. *International Journal of Eating Disorders, 32*(1), 79–90. https://doi.org/10.1002/eat.10066

Prince, T., McLoughlin, L., Lagopoulos, J., Elwyn, R., & Hermens, D. F. (2022). The neural correlates of socio-cognitive factors and eating disorders in young people: A systematic review. *Journal of Psychiatric Research, 156*, 647–659. https://doi.org/10.1016/j.jpsychires.2022.10.058

Ralph-Nearman, C., Achee, M., Lapidus, R., Stewart, J. L., & Filik, R. (2019). A systematic and methodological review of attentional biases in eating disorders: Food, body, and perfectionism. *Brain and Behavior, 9*(12). https://doi.org/10.1002/brb3.1458

Roberts, M. E., Tchanturia, K., & Treasure, J. L. (2012). Is attention to detail a similarly strong candidate endophenotype for anorexia nervosa and bulimia nervosa? *World Journal of Biological Psychiatry, 0*, 1–12.

Rose, M., Frampton, I. J., & Lask, B. (2014). Central coherence, organizational strategy, and visuospatial memory in children and adolescents with anorexia nervosa. *Applied Neuropsychology: Child, 3*(4), 284–296. https://doi.org/10.1080/21622965.2013.775064

Rueda, M. R., & Conejero, A. (2020). Developing attention and self-regulation in infancy and childhood. In J. Rubenstein, P. Rakic, B. Chen, & K. Y. Kwan (Eds.), *Neural circuit and cognitive development* (pp. 505–522). Elsevier. https://doi.org/10.1016/B978-0-12-814411-4.00023-8

Rylander, M., Taylor, G., Bennett, S., Pierce, C., Keniston, A., & Mehler, P. S. (2020). Evaluation of cognitive function in patients with severe anorexia nervosa before and after medical stabilization. *Journal of Eating Disorders*, *8*(1), 35. https://doi.org/10.1186/s40337-020-00312-5

Schmidt, U., & Treasure, J. (2006). Anorexia nervosa: Valued and visible. A cognitive-interpersonal maintenance model and its implications for research and practice. *British Journal of Clinical Psychology*, *45*(3), 343–366.

Seitz, J., Herpertz-Dahlmann, B., & Konrad, K. (2016). Brain morphological changes in adolescent and adult patients with anorexia nervosa. *Journal of Neural Transmission*, *123*(8), 949–959.

Shank, L. M., Tanofsky-Kraff, M., Nelson, E. E., Shomaker, L. B., Ranzenhofer, L. M., Hannallah, L. M., Field, S. E., Vannucci, A., Bongiorno, D. M., Brady, S. M., Condarco, T., Demidowich, A., Kelly, N. R., Cassidy, O., Simmons, W. K., Engel, S. G., Pine, D. S., & Yanovski, J. A. (2015). Attentional bias to food cues in youth with loss of control eating. *Appetite*, *87*, 68–75. https://doi.org/10.1016/j.appet.2014.11.027

Smith, K. E., Mason, T. B., Johnson, J. S., Lavender, J. M., & Wonderlich, S. A. (2018). A systematic review of reviews of neurocognitive functioning in eating disorders: The state-of-the-literature and future directions. *International Journal of Eating Disorders*, *51*(8), 798–821. https://doi.org/10.1002/eat.22929

Stedal, K., Broomfield, C., Hay, P., Touyz, S., & Scherer, R. (2021). Neuropsychological functioning in adult anorexia nervosa: A meta-analysis. *Neuroscience & Biobehavioral Reviews*, *130*, 214–226. https://doi.org/10.1016/j.neubiorev.2021.08.021

Stedal, K., Scherer, R., Touyz, S., Hay, P., & Broomfield, C. (2022). Research review: Neuropsychological functioning in young anorexia nervosa: A meta-analysis. *Journal of Child Psychology and Psychiatry*, *63*(6), 616–625. https://doi.org/10.1111/jcpp.13562

Steinberg, D. M., Perry, T. R., Freestone, D., Hellner, M., Baker, J. H., & Bohon, C. (2022). Evaluating differences in setting expected body weight for children and adolescents in eating disorder treatment. *International Journal of Eating Disorders*, *56*(3), 595–603. https://doi.org/10.1002/eat.23868

Stiles, J., Akshoomoff, N. A., & Haist, F. (2020). The development of visuospatial processing. In J. Rubenstein, P. Rakic, B. Chen, & K. Y. Kwan (Eds.), *Neural circuit and cognitive development* (pp. 359–393). Elsevier. https://doi.org/10.1016/B978-0-12-814411-4.00017-2

Stojek, M., Shank, L. M., Vannucci, A., Bongiorno, D. M., Nelson, E. E., Waters, A. J., Engel, S. G., Boutelle, K. N., Pine, D. S., Yanovski, J. A., & Tanofsky-Kraff, M. (2018). A systematic review of attentional biases in disorders involving binge eating. *Appetite*, *123*, 367–389. https://doi.org/10.1016/j.appet.2018.01.019

Stott, N., Fox, J. R. E., & Williams, M. O. (2021). Attentional bias in eating disorders: A meta-review. *International Journal of Eating Disorders*, *54*(8), 1377–1399. https://doi.org/10.1002/eat.23560

Suchan, B., Bauser, D. S., Busch, M., Schulte, D., Grönemeyer, D., Herpertz, S., & Vocks, S. (2013). Reduced connectivity between the left fusiform body area and the extrastriate body area in anorexia nervosa is associated with body image distortion. *Behavioural Brain Research*, *241*, 80–85. https://doi.org/10.1016/j.bbr.2012.12.002

Svaldi, J., Ababneh, M., Trentowska, M., & Tuschen-Caffier, B. (2011). Overgeneral memory in binge eating disorder is linked to binge frequency. *Journal of Experimental Psychopathology*, *2*(1), 77–92. https://doi.org/10.5127/jep.007310

Szutorisz, H., & Hurd, Y. L. (2016). Feeding the developing brain: The persistent epigenetic effects of early life malnutrition. *Biological Psychiatry*, *80*(10), 730–732. https://doi.org/10.1016/j.biopsych.2016.08.032

Teconi, E., Santonastaso, P., Degortes, D., Bosello, R., Titton, F., Mapelli, D., & Favaro, A. (2010). Set-shifting abilities, central coherence, and handedness in anorexia nervosa patients, their unaffected siblings and healthy controls: Exploring putative endophenotypes. *World Journal of Biological Psychiatry*, *11*(6), 813–823.

Terhoeven, V., Nikendei, C., Faschingbauer, S., Huber, J., Young, K. D., Bendszus, M., Herzog, W., Friederich, H.-C., & Simon, J. J. (2023). Neurophysiological correlates of disorder-related autobiographical memory in anorexia nervosa. *Psychological Medicine*, *53*(3), 844–854. https://doi.org/10.1017/S003329172100221X

Timko, C. A., DeFilipp, L., & Dakanalis, A. (2019). Sex differences in adolescent anorexia and bulimia nervosa: beyond the signs and symptoms. *Current Psychiatry Reports*, *21*(1), 1.

Treasure, J., & Schmidt, U. (2013). The cognitive-interpersonal maintenance model of anorexia nervosa revisited: A summary of the evidence for cognitive, socio-emotional and interpersonal predisposing and perpetuating factors. *Journal of Eating Disorders*, *1*, 13.

Treasure, J., Willmott, D., Ambwani, S., Cardi, V., Clark Bryan, D., Rowlands, K., & Schmidt, U. (2020). Cognitive interpersonal model for anorexia nervosa revisited: The perpetuating factors that contribute to the development of the severe and enduring illness. *Journal of Clinical Medicine*, *9*(3), 630.

Van Autreve, S., & Vervaet, M. (2015). Are there differences in central coherence and set shifting across the subtypes of anorexia nervosa?: A systematic review. *Journal of Nervous & Mental Disease*, *203*(10), 774–780. https://doi.org/10.1097/NMD.0000000000000366

van Noort, B. M., Pfeiffer, E., Ehrlich, S., Lehmkuhl, U., & Kappel, V. (2016). Cognitive performance in children with acute early-onset anorexia nervosa. *European Child & Adolescent Psychiatry*, *25*(11), 1233–1244.

Weinbach, N., Perry, A., Sher, H., Lock, J. D., & Henik, A. (2017). Weak central coherence in weight-restored adolescent anorexia nervosa: Characteristics and remediation. *International Journal of Eating Disorders*, *50*(8), 924–932. https://doi.org/10.1002/eat.22711

Zitron-Emanuel, N., Ganel, T., Albini, E., Abbate-Daga, G., & Marzola, E. (2022). The perception of food size and food shape in anorexia nervosa. *Appetite*, *169*, 105858. https://doi.org/10.1016/j.appet.2021.105858

PART III

MANIFEST SYMPTOMS OF EATING DISORDERS ("TOP DOWN")

14

Restrictive Eating Through the Lens of Choice

Karin Foerde

Brief Definitional Overview

Restrictive eating: A reduction of food intake characterized by reduced caloric intake, in some cases to such an extent that body weight is significantly decreased and may become life threatening.

Decision making: The process of evaluating and choosing among alternative courses of action or options. It involves cognitive and neural computations and mechanisms that integrate sensory information, past experiences, and internal and/or external goals to arrive at a choice.

Introduction

Restrictive eating is a central characteristic of eating disorders and involves restriction of caloric intake, in particular calories from fat, as well as decreased diet variety (Schebendach et al., 2008). In the case of anorexia nervosa (AN), restrictive eating results in inappropriately low body weight that may even be life threatening (Mayer et al., 2012; Schebendach et al., 2012; Sysko et al., 2005). Restrictive eating patterns persist after treatment and are related to poor longer-term outcomes, with more restrictive diets related to likelihood of relapse (Schebendach et al., 2008; Schebendach et al., 2012; Steinglass et al., 2023). The neurobiology of feeding behavior has long been studied, resulting in a detailed mechanistic understanding of the neural circuits and physiology involved (Saper et al., 2002) (see Chapter 2). Yet, what appears to be a voluntary restriction of food intake among individuals with AN in the face of countervailing homeostatic drives, remains puzzling.

One recent approach to elucidating the neurobiology of restrictive eating is informed by the study of decision making. Decision making is the process of evaluating and choosing among options, relying on integration of sensory information, memories, and internal and/or external goals to arrive at a choice. Decision making is studied within many disciplines (Rangel et al., 2008; Shadlen & Kiani, 2013) and encompasses everything from low-level perceptual decisions to major life choices.

Karin Foerde *Restrictive Eating Through the Lens of Choice*. In: *The Handbook of the Neurobiology of Eating Disorders*. Edited by: Christina E. Wierenga and Joanna E. Steinglass, Oxford University Press. © Oxford University Press (2025). DOI: 10.1093/9780197675212.003.0015

Decision making among patients with eating disorders has often been examined in the context of value or feedback related learning tasks (e.g., the Iowa Gambling Task) (Adoue et al., 2015; Guillaume et al., 2015; Haynos et al., 2022) or inter-temporal choice tasks (Steinglass et al., 2017). These are valuable approaches (Haynos et al., 2022) that may illuminate general traits or dispositions toward learning and decision making with relevance for illness, but they lack a direct connection to restrictive eating per se. The focus of this chapter is on decisions about food. Interestingly, food choices have been studied extensively in healthy populations, sometimes as a convenient context within which to understand key tradeoffs between short-term enjoyment and long-term health or other benefits with application to general choice problems (e.g., Hare et al., 2009). Choosing what to eat remains, for most, a quotidian decision, but for individuals with eating disorders, it is a fraught and consequential decision, and one that must be confronted multiple times every day.

Despite the importance of food choices in eating disorders and their relevance for restrictive eating, the mechanisms of such decisions have received limited attention. However, to understand whether and how food decisions differ among individuals who persistently choose foods that are inadequate to sustain a healthy weight, emerging studies have focused specifically on food choice behavior. This approach starts simply by focusing on the proximate cause of restrictive eating—the food choices that are repeatedly made—without consideration of more distal causes of illness or why these patterns of behavior emerged in the first place. A straightforward characterization of this key restrictive eating behavior provides a good starting point for addressing more detailed questions, for example related to differences within diagnostic groups (e.g., subtypes of AN) or illness trajectories. Eating disorders are complex and likely have multifarious determinants, which may argue against reductive approaches, but a better understanding of neurobiology and mechanisms requires some simplification. Focusing on the decision process has provided a valuable lens on restrictive eating and has also given rise to novel hypotheses and directions for research and treatment.

The main neural circuitry of choice and what has been learned about food choice in eating disorders are outlined below. The latter focuses mainly on individuals with AN, who have been the primary target of this research and for whom restrictive eating is central.

Biological Framework

Neurobiology of decision making

Choices about food are unique in how often decisions must be made about what to eat and because these decisions are subject to the influence of basic homeostatic regulation associated with food intake (Enax & Weber, 2016; Rangel, 2013;

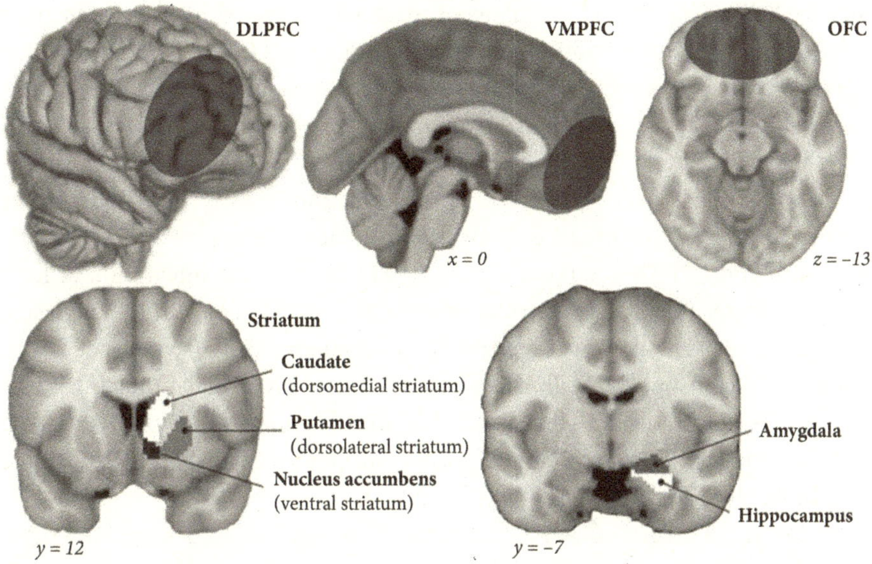

Figure 14.1 Neural circuits involved in food choices and general decision making. Dorsolateral prefrontal cortex = DLPFC; ventral medial prefrontal cortex = vmPFC; orbital frontal cortex = OFC. Locations indicated in MNI coordinates.

Wansink & Sobal, 2007). Nonetheless, there is tremendous overlap between commonly identified neural decision circuits and the circuits involved in food choices (Figure 14.1). Models of decision making generally involve multiple stages. Valuation and action selection processes are at the center, with additional processes to identify external and internal (e.g., hunger) states, evaluate the outcome of choices, and use that information to update expectations to shape future valuation and choice. Across studies in humans and animals, a set of neural regions have been shown to make somewhat distinct contributions to decision making (Hikosaka et al., 2014; Kable & Glimcher, 2009; Rangel et al., 2008).

The ventral medial prefrontal cortex (VMPFC) and ventral striatum have been implicated in representing subjective value across many studies (Bartra et al., 2013; Clithero & Rangel, 2014). The VMPFC represents value across multiple categories (e.g., food and money; although perhaps with some gradation, cf. McNamee et al., 2013), which allows comparison of options in a "common currency." This representation likely integrates information from multiple different types of computations. Inputs may come from habitual processes that slowly, through trial-and-error, have acquired a "cached" value that can rapidly and effortlessly be deployed, and are thought to depend on the dorsolateral striatum (Yin & Knowlton, 2006). By contrast, goal-directed processes that allow for more flexible consideration of current goals and context (and are slower and perhaps more effortful) are thought to involve medial PFC and dorsomedial striatum. In addition, Pavlovian processes that can be innate or learned (e.g., after illness associated with a specific food) may influence valuation and involve the amygdala, ventral striatum, and orbital frontal cortex (OFC) regions (Balleine et al., 2009; Ostlund &

Balleine, 2007). The role of memory as a source to be sampled when accumulating evidence for or against an option or to simulate imagined future outcomes, is also increasingly being considered as an important input to valuation and choice, implicating the hippocampus and medial temporal lobes (Barron et al., 2013; Biderman & Shohamy, 2021; Shadlen & Shohamy, 2016). In terms of food choices specifically, the OFC has been implicated in the valuation of food and food choices (Ballesta et al., 2020; Clithero & Rangel, 2014; Padoa-Schioppa & Assad, 2006; Plassmann et al., 2007; Suzuki et al., 2017), as well as in the integration of food related attributes (e.g., fat, sugar, vitamin content; Suzuki et al., 2017). The insula may also play a particular role in relation to food value updates (Avery et al., 2019; Balleine & Dickinson, 2000). Finally, the dorsolateral prefrontal cortex (DLPFC) is considered important for goal-directed control of choice behavior (Hare et al., 2009) and may play a role modulating valuation processes in the VMPFC (Hare et al., 2009; Hare et al., 2011; Maier et al., 2015).

Notably, the network of regions implicated broadly in decision making overlaps with regions that are repeatedly found to exhibit differential or dysfunctional engagement in individuals with eating disorders.

State of the Science in Eating Disorders

Restrictive eating as a choice—Cognitive and neural mechanisms

Among individuals with eating disorders, food choices have thus far mostly been studied in those with AN. The goal of these studies has not primarily been to examine what these individuals choose—the avoidance of calories and calories from fat has been well documented (Hadigan et al., 2000; Huse & Lucas, 1984; Mayer et al., 2012; Schebendach et al., 2019)—but rather to examine the cognitive and neural processes associated with these choices. Therefore, an important goal has been to use an experimental approach that captures restrictive eating while using functional magnetic resonance imaging (fMRI) to examine neural circuits.

To achieve this goal, the Food Choice Task (Figure 14.2) was adapted from the studies of Hare and colleagues (e.g., Hare et al., 2009) to study food choices among individuals with AN (Steinglass, Foerde, Kostro, et al., 2015). In this task, individuals are presented with a series of food images selected to represent a varied range of foods from a normal diet, rather than mainly tempting foods or diet focused items. Half of the items are low-fat foods (less than 30% of the calories from fat) and half are high-fat foods. Individuals are first asked to rate the food items for their healthiness and tastiness. Subsequently, one food item, rated as neutral on healthiness and tastiness, is selected as a reference food, and individuals are then asked to choose between that reference food item and all the other food items. To increase the likelihood of examining relevant behavior, choices can be made incentive compatible by creating a situation that encourages individuals to make choices consistent with their actual preferences. Concretely, individuals are informed that one of their

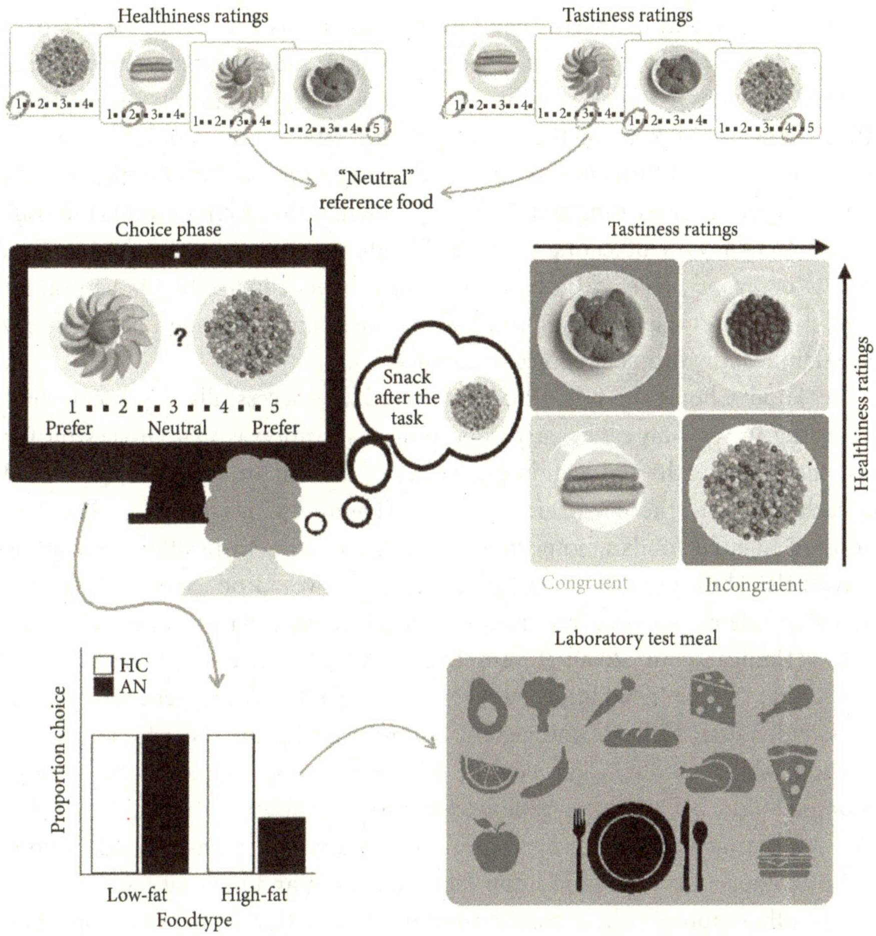

Figure 14.2 Food Choice Task. The Food Choice Task can be used to capture restrictive eating behavior. In the task, participants first rate a series of food items on their perceived Healthiness and Tastiness and a "neutral" reference food is selected for the Choice phase based on these ratings (top row). In the Choice phase, participants select whether they would prefer a snack consisting of the "neutral" reference item or a food item that changes on every trial (middle row, left). Some food items are *congruent* on Tastiness and Healthiness, potentially leading to easier decisions (middle row, right). Other food items are *incongruent* on Tastiness and Healthiness, potentially leading to decisions that may require control to resolve whether to choose based on Tastiness and Healthiness. It may require self-control to choose items of greater perceived Healthiness and lesser Tastiness, or to not choose items of lesser perceived Healthiness and greater Tastiness. Half of the food items are low fat and half are high fat (> 30% calories from fat) and the choice behavior can be quantified as the proportion of choices of the low and high-fat foods (typical pattern of results shown bottom row left). The proportion of high-fat food choices, by individuals with anorexia nervosa (AN) in particular, can be related to calories eaten in a laboratory test meal.

choices will be selected at random to determine their snack after the experimental task, thereby creating an incentive to treat each choice as if it could be realized.

One compelling reason to use a decision-making framework to study eating, is that it provides a simple starting point from which to understand restrictive eating—it focuses directly on the behavior of interest and asks people to do a simple task unmediated through task rules and strategic approaches. Another benefit to recasting restrictive eating as a decision problem is that it circumvents the issue of individuals always indicating a dislike of foods or opting for no food. Moreover, because everyone makes choices relative to a reference image that is neutral for them, it facilitates the comparison between patient and control groups that may have significantly divergent choice preferences.

The Food Choice Task has been observed to successfully capture restrictive eating in two ways. The first important observation is that choices on the task, measured as the proportion of choices of the unique food item presented on each trial over the fixed reference food (Figure 14.2), indicate low rates of choosing high-fat foods among those with AN relative to healthy comparison individuals. Thus, the task behavior reflects what would be expected based on clinical profile as has been reported across self-report, diary studies, and meal studies (Hadigan et al., 2000; Huse & Lucas, 1984; Mayer et al., 2012; Schebendach et al., 2012). In addition, choices of low-fat foods are generally similar across individuals with AN and healthy control participants (Foerde et al., 2015; Foerde et al., 2022; Steinglass, Foerde, & Kostro, 2015) suggesting that choices among AN are not due to a general response bias toward the constant reference food, and similar choice proportions for low and high-fat foods among healthy comparison women indicate that the low-fat and high-fat foods are balanced in their appeal. The second important observation is that the proportion of high-fat food choices made by individuals with AN in the task is related to how many calories they consume in a laboratory test meal (Sysko et al., 2018) (Figure 14.2). Those making fewer high-fat choices in the task also consume fewer calories in an actual meal (Foerde et al., 2015; Foerde et al., 2022). Such findings suggest that the task captures the restrictive eating pattern that it is important to understand, thereby providing a tool to examine the neural circuits involved.

To examine the neural circuits involved on the Food Choice Task, analyses of BOLD activity have focused on the striatum and VMPFC regions during the choice phase of the task. Neural correlates of choice preferences have been examined by assessing the strength of the correlation between the choice preference indicated on each trial of the choice phase and BOLD activity and comparing healthy controls and individuals with AN. Analyses focused on VMPFC regions, consistently implicated in value-based decisions (Bartra et al., 2013; Hare et al., 2009), have pointed to commonalities across groups with similar levels of engagement during choice (Foerde et al., 2015; Foerde et al., 2022). In contrast, divergence between groups has been found in analyses focused on the caudate, which has been more strongly associated with choice preferences among individuals with AN than among healthy controls, suggesting a distinct contribution of the caudate to restrictive food choices (Foerde et al., 2015; Foerde et al., 2022).

The restrictive behavioral food choice pattern has been observed across individuals with restricting and binge eating/purging subtypes of AN (Uniacke et al., 2020), as well as individuals with atypical AN (Foerde et al., 2022) and individuals with bulimia nervosa (Gianini et al., 2019). As such, the task appears to effectively capture restrictive eating aspects of eating disorders. The neural circuits have not been examined as widely as the behavioral profile and it is not known if the involvement of the caudate observed among individuals with AN may be present among those with bulimia nervosa, nor have existing neuroimaging studies been powered to examine differences between binge eating/purging subtypes. However, the link between the striatum and a core maladaptive eating behavior (Foerde et al., 2022; Lloyd et al., 2025) suggests that it may be a useful tool with which to examine restrictive eating across eating disorders.

A notable aspect of the pattern of results is that it appears to be specific for the choice phase. Group differences have not thus far been observed in the caudate during ratings of food healthiness and tastiness, suggesting that the response may not be a general one to the presence of food images (Foerde et al., 2015), consistent with other work on responses to food imagery per se (Lloyd & Steinglass, 2018). Moreover, group differences have not been observed in the nucleus accumbens or VMPFC regions reliably implicated in valuation and reward processing (Bartra et al., 2013), which may further underline the importance of choice processes specifically.

The identification of a neural region directly linked to restrictive eating has invited further attempts to probe the neural circuits of food choices using neuromodulatory approaches. A proof-of-concept study using high-frequency rTMS in a small sample of patients with AN, leveraged knowledge of frontostriatal circuits (Alexander et al., 1986; Lehéricy et al., 2004) with the aim of targeting the striatum indirectly through its connectivity with pre-frontal cortex (Muratore et al., 2021). High-frequency rTMS modulation increased the choices of high-fat foods, but not low-fat foods, relative to sham stimulation. The manipulation did not affect healthiness and tastiness ratings, pointing to the importance of the choice phase. Although there was no certainty about targeting the striatum in that study, the results support the view that frontostriatal circuits are critical for restrictive food choices.

The role of valuation in restrictive eating

Although the focus on decision making as a lens on restrictive eating has centered primarily on choices, the rating phases that precede the choice phase of the Food Choice Task may nonetheless be revelatory with respect to processes and mechanisms contributing to restrictive eating. Valuation is fundamental to choice, and it involves an individual determining the subjective value of the options before them. In the context of the Food Choice Task, this involves rating food images based on their perceived healthiness and tastiness. Although general assumptions can be made about the valuation of food items for individuals who persistently restrict their dietary intake, as is often done in a variety of tasks (Lloyd & Steinglass, 2018; Meregalli et al., 2023), such assumptions may not hold and individual ratings make it possible to learn more about valuations of a range of foods.

There are several basic questions of interest regarding valuation that can be addressed in the context of the Food Choice Task: Do individuals with AN differ from control participants in their food valuations? Do their valuations influence choice in a similar manner? Compared with controls, individuals with AN do tend to rate foods as less healthy and less tasty, and rate high-fat foods in particular as less tasty (Foerde et al., 2015; Foerde et al., 2022; Lloyd et al., 2025). This is not a surprising pattern considering illness characteristics, but it is worth noting that group differences appear modest relative to the striking difference in choices of high-fat foods. That is, individuals with AN are not simply indicating that all high-fat foods taste bad and are unhealthy, there is variability and nuance in ratings across the range of foods. Analyses examining the influence of healthiness and tastiness ratings on choices indicate that both individuals with AN and healthy controls are more likely to choose foods they rate as tastier, although this influence may be stronger among healthy controls. In contrast, healthiness influences choices much more among individuals with AN, for whom healthiness and tastiness exert similar influence on choice. In addition, the ratings of healthiness and tastiness are more correlated among individuals with AN relative to controls.

Examination of the neural representations of food attributes parallel the behavioral findings and yield similarities between patients and controls. Across both groups, healthiness and tastiness is represented in OFC regions shown to represent subjective value of food across multiple studies (Ballesta et al., 2020; Clithero & Rangel, 2014; Padoa-Schioppa & Assad, 2006; Plassmann et al., 2007; Suzuki et al., 2017). In contrast, the influence of neural representations of healthiness on food choices was stronger among individuals with AN (Xue et al., 2022). (Notably, the analyses of Xue and colleagues (2022) relied on multivariate pattern analyses, which may detect differences in representations not apparent from univariate analysis approaches typically employed [Norman et al., 2006]).

Thus, a focus on valuation in decision making adds to our understanding of food choices. Alignment between healthiness and tastiness may emerge across the lifespan (developmentally) in the population at large and can be thought of as a health promoting valuation learned over time (Lloyd et al., 2025; Van Meer et al., 2017). However, it may present a tool for over-restricting caloric intake among individuals with AN, one that may already be present earlier in illness among youth with AN (Lloyd et al., 2025).

Assessing the role of "self-control" in restrictive eating

Considering the influence of healthiness versus tastiness raises questions about self-control. In the context of AN, it should be carefully considered what can be assumed about controlled versus habitual influences on behavior. That cognitive (and neural) self-control processes are necessary or used to make certain choices cannot be assumed based on the observation of behavior that appears self-controlled. In the Food Choice Task, a "self-control" label is commonly applied to choices involving food items for which healthiness and tastiness ratings are incongruent (Figure 14.2). If a food is considered healthy and tasty or unhealthy and not tasty, it is simple to choose and not choose the food, respectively. In contrast, a food that is tasty and unhealthy or not tasty and healthy, may require more effort to determine how to weight attributes to make a choice. Moreover, which behavior requires self-control should be defined in relation to the goals of an individual. Those who are unconcerned with their food intake generally choose based on tastiness, ignoring the healthiness of food items. By contrast, those attempting to restrict caloric intake weight healthiness more, a process also reflected in differential engagement of neural processes (Hare et al., 2009). The food choices of individuals with AN generally follow this pattern, but they also differ in interesting ways.

One difference is that a greater alignment of tastiness and healthiness ratings yields fewer items for which a choice conflict (incongruence) exists. This provides one way to decrease the need for self-control processes. When confronted with a choice conflict, individuals with AN do indeed make choices that would appear consistent with implementation of self-control in that they favor healthiness. Notably, patients with AN who need to move away from a low-calorie, low-fat (normatively "healthy") diet, should make the effort toward more high-fat choices to be consistent with treatment goals. Indeed, in one study, use of "self-control" decreased after an offline rTMS treatment protocol targeting the DLPFC (Dalton et al., 2020), and in another study, decreased "self-control" use across treatment was associated with less body mass index (BMI) decline in the years after hospital discharge (Steinglass et al., 2023). Examination of the neural circuits associated with "self-control" in individuals with AN has been challenging, as the reduced number of relevant trial types have been insufficient for neuroimaging analyses. However, abnormalities in regions such as DLPFC, consistently implicated in controlled processing (Han et al., 2018), and in frontostriatal circuits more broadly, have been observed among individuals with AN across numerous studies and imaging modalities (Frank et al., 2013; Haynos et al., 2019; Lloyd et al., 2023).

Another difference relates to the time required to make "self-controlled" choices. Using "self-control" should require effort and consequently be indexed by increased response times when self-control is successfully implemented. This is what has been seen among healthy individuals, but individuals with AN showed the reverse pattern, with faster response times when "self-control" was successfully implemented (Foerde et al., 2015).

Is restrictive eating governed by habits?

What has been described above is an approach to characterizing processes involved in food choices that can be linked to actual eating, thereby allowing examination of the neural systems involved in such choices. With regard to restrictive eating, an important question concerns the nature of restrictive eating and whether it is habitual, or by contrast, goal-directed or self-controlled. It is tempting to interpret the results from neuroimaging studies in support of one view or another, but such inferences based on neuroimaging data alone are problematic due in part to difficulty mapping engagement of brain regions to cognitive processes one-to-one (Francken et al., 2022; Poldrack, 2006). While the data from the Food Choice Task and many other studies of taste and reward processing have implicated frontostriatal circuits (Frank et al., 2019; Kaye, 2008; Wierenga et al., 2015) and could be consistent with habitual behavior, alternative interpretations are also possible. Instead, it may be more useful to focus on behavior that can better inform whether habitual versus goal-directed processes are involved. Although the Food Choice Task is not designed with this purpose in mind, there are aspects of behavior measured in the task that can point to potential differences in the cognitive processes underlying behavior. For example, the pattern of response times on "self-control" trials point to more automatic deployment of choice among individuals with AN relative to HC.

Alternative Perspectives

Disturbances in basic motivational processes

A decision-making approach to understanding restrictive eating may appear to be in fundamental tension with more bottom-up approaches focused on potential disturbances in the basic motivational processes around food. Food is generally considered a primary reward, and most individuals recognize a drive toward fattier, sweeter foods, and consider them tastier. When eating becomes dysfunctional, as in the case of maladaptive, restrictive eating, a disturbance in basic motivation around food is a compelling explanation. There are several specific instantiations of these views, but two broad categories can be considered—decreased reward responses or increased aversive responses around food (or a combination).

If basic hedonic drive toward food is decreased (Kaye et al., 2020; Oberndorfer et al., 2013; Wierenga et al., 2015) and food is less rewarding to individuals with AN (Kaye, 2008; Kaye et al., 2020; Wagner et al., 2007), decreased food approach and consumptions should follow. Indeed, studies have found reduced responses to food stimuli in reward and motivation related brain circuits (Kaye et al., 2020; Keating et al., 2012; Oberndorfer et al., 2013; Wierenga et al., 2015). Conversely, other studies find increased responses to rewards and reward-related processing (Cowdrey et al., 2011; DeGuzman et al., 2017; Wagner et al., 2007). Nonetheless, general (non-food specific) disturbances in reward processing and reinforcement learning have been identified repeatedly (DeGuzman et al., 2017; Foerde & Steinglass, 2017; Haynos et al., 2022; Wierenga et al., 2022), supporting the idea that a fundamental problem with reward processing is present. A strength of this view is the more direct link to animal models in which the neurobiology and neurophysiology of eating related processes can be delineated in greater mechanistic detail (Cone et al., 2016; Duriez et al., 2019; Mequinion et al., 2015).

Another approach focuses instead on the potential aversive nature of food and measuring avoidance responses (O'Hara et al., 2015). This view does not necessarily suggest solely an automatic aversive response to high-calorie foods, but also that aversive responses to food can emerge as a result of top-down control processes due to incompatibility with the goal of restricting intake to avoid weight gain (O'Hara et al., 2015). A related idea is that disgust (Hildebrandt et al., 2015) or fear of food (Steinglass et al., 2012; Strober, 2004) plays a role in driving restrictive eating, processes that may emerge from more automatic visceral, interoceptive signals (Anderson et al., 2021; Hildebrandt et al., 2015) or as a result of association with higher level outcomes, such as being judged due to weight gain (Levinson & Williams, 2020). Findings on aversive food responses do not always match expectations (Friederich et al., 2006) and have relied in part on interpreting responses in specific brain regions to infer aversion in the absence of behavioral measures to support interpretations (Kim et al., 2012; O'Hara et al., 2015). However, avoidance processes can be challenging to study and have received more limited empirical attention than have other mechanisms. Future developments in this area may clarify the importance of such processes; for example, whether they play a greater role in some types of restrictive eating (e.g., avoidant/restrictive food intake disorder (ARFID; Menzel et al., 2019) than others (Anderson et al., 2021).

A bridge from disturbed food motivation to restrictive eating behavior

The neurobiology related to these views mostly overlap with the circuits of interest in decision making, namely frontostriatal circuits. Thus, the important discussion is centered on the exact mechanisms and processes of interest, with implications for approaches to treatment. Yet rather than truly being in tension, bottom-up approaches integrate well with the decision-making view of restrictive eating. The decision-making view can provide a connective structure between a bottom-up understanding and clinical manifestations. A strength of the decision-making approach is that it connects directly to the clinical manifestation of restrictive eating, and that observed differences in neural mechanisms are more directly linked to that manifestation. Conversely, the understanding gleaned from bottom-up approaches may fill in gaps to illuminate factors influencing predisposition to illness and tighter links with neurobiological aspects that have been examined in more detail in animal models.

The role of taste valuation in decision making can be considered as an example. While the decision approach captures that food items are deemed less rewarding (tasty) by patients, it cannot really explain why. This could be due to a general aversion to foods or a dampened reward value. Those are important distinctions that are not directly addressed by the decision-making view, in which the output in the form of a tastiness ratings may be composed of multiple distinct processes lumped together in simplified ratings. A better understanding of basic reward processing will arguably inform such thinking, as will understanding of avoidance learning and disgust. As the understanding of basic processing of the reward or aversive value of food grows, these perspectives can be integrated to refine the analyses of how these inputs to the decision process function, providing additional options to explore for interventions in the process.

Implications

An important reason to understand behavior is to be able to manipulate and change it to become more adaptive. The findings from studies of choice behavior show some promise to inform clinical practice. First, the link between restrictive eating and frontostriatal circuits has spurred the use of neuromodulation to affect these circuits. As previously noted, a pilot study using high-frequency rTMS during food choices in patients with AN, found that real rTMS, as compared to sham stimulation, led to an increase in choices of high-fat foods while leaving low-fat food choices unaffected (Muratore et al., 2021). Additionally, an offline TMS treatment protocol led to some decreases in the use of self-controlled choices (Dalton et al., 2020). Such findings will hopefully lead to further studies of neuromodulatory interventions to perturb choice mechanisms.

Second, changes in food choice behavior over the course of treatment are related to longer term outcomes (Steinglass et al., 2023). That is, the extent to which an individual can increase their choices of high-fat foods in a Food Choice Task was related to BMI in the years post hospital discharge. This points to a target behavior to change during treatment and a potential way to understand the level of support an individual may need following discharge from treatment. During inpatient treatment, eating behavior is an important focus, but free choice may be limited. In everyday life, food decisions are unique in their ubiquity and recurrence. Preparation to deal with this reality could be a useful focus to support better longer-term outcomes and bolster against relapse.

Finally, the role of valuation processes, how food healthiness and tastiness attributes are weighted, could be a focus for interventions. Manipulations to increase or decrease the focus on either attribute to shape choice are commonplace in non-clinical populations (Hare et al., 2009; Hutcherson et al., 2012; Maier et al., 2015). Among individuals with AN, the alignment between healthiness and tastiness is not absolute and the fact that both attributes contribute to choice suggests that there may be some malleability in the inputs to choice as is seen in healthy individuals (Hare et al., 2011; Hutcherson et al., 2012; Maier et al., 2015; Rramani et al., 2020; Sullivan & Huettel, 2021). Both nudging the weighting of healthiness versus tastiness in decision making, but also in unlearning (or relearning) the alignment between healthiness and tastiness are potential goals. Whether health information is overvalued (reward approach) or taste information mis/under-valued (punishment avoidance/reward non-approach), these are factors that, at least among individuals with AN, need to be disentangled and then re-evaluated to construct choices that are adaptive in light of eating goals.

Altogether, although more research is needed, current research points to the relevance of dissecting both choice itself and the processes contributing to decisions around restrictive eating to inform clinical practice.

References

Adoue, C., Jaussent, I., Olié, E., Beziat, S., Van den Eynde, F., Courtet, P., & Guillaume, S. (2015). A further assessment of decision-making in anorexia nervosa. *European Psychiatry, 30*(1), 121–127. https://doi.org/10.1016/j.eurpsy.2014.08.004

Alexander, G. E., DeLong, M. R., & Strick, P. L. (1986). Parallel organization of functionally segregated circuits linking basal ganglia and cortex. *Annual Review of Neuroscience, 9*, 357–381. https://doi.org/10.1146/annurev.ne.09.030186.002041

Anderson, L. M., Berg, H., Brown, T. A., Menzel, J., & Reilly, E. E. (2021). The role of disgust in eating disorders. *Current Psychiatry Reports, 23*(2), 4. https://doi.org/10.1007/s11920-020-01217-5

Avery, J. A., Liu, A. G., Ingeholm, J. E., Riddell, C. D., Gotts, S. J., & Martin, A. (2019). Taste quality representation in the human brain. *Journal of Neuroscience*, 40(5), 1042–1052. https://doi.org/10.1523/JNEUROSCI.1751-19.2019

Balleine, B. W., Daw, N. D., & O'Doherty, J. P. (2009). Multiple forms of value learning and the function of dopamine. In P. W. Glimcher, C. F. Camerer, E. Fehr, & R. A. Poldrack (Eds.), *Neuroeconomics: Decision making and the brain* (pp. 367–387). Academic Press.

Balleine, B. W., & Dickinson, A. (2000). The effect of lesions of the insular cortex on instrumental conditioning: Evidence for a role in incentive memory. *Journal of Neuroscience, 20*(23), 8954–8964. https://doi.org/10.1523/JNEUROSCI.20-23-08954.2000

Ballesta, S., Shi, W., Conen, K. E., & Padoa-Schioppa, C. (2020). Values encoded in orbitofrontal cortex are causally related to economic choices. *Nature, 588*(7838), 450–453. https://doi.org/10.1038/s41586-020-2880-x

Barron, H. C., Dolan, R. J., & Behrens, T. E. J. (2013). Online evaluation of novel choices by simultaneous representation of multiple memories. *Nature Neuroscience, 16*(10), 1492–1498. http://www.nature.com/neuro/journal/v16/n10/abs/nn.3515.html

Bartra, O., McGuire, J. T., & Kable, J. W. (2013). The valuation system: A coordinate-based meta-analysis of BOLD fMRI experiments examining neural correlates of subjective value. *Neuroimage, 76*, 412–427. https://doi.org/10.1016/j.neuroimage.2013.02.063

Biderman, N., & Shohamy, D. (2021). Memory and decision making interact to shape the value of unchosen options. *Nature Communications*, 1–12. https://doi.org/10.1038/s41467-021-24907-x

Clithero, J. A., & Rangel, A. (2014). Informatic parcellation of the network involved in the computation of subjective value. *Social Cognitive and Affective Neuroscience*, *9*(9), 1289–1302. https://doi.org/10.1093/scan/nst106

Cone, J. J., Fortin, S. M., McHenry, J. A., Stuber, G. D., McCutcheon, J. E., & Roitman, M. F. (2016). Physiological state gates acquisition and expression of mesolimbic reward prediction signals. *Proceedings of the National Academy of Sciences*, *113*(7), 1943–1948. https://doi.org/10.1073/pnas.1519643113

Cowdrey, F. A., Park, R. J., Harmer, C. J., & McCabe, C. (2011). Increased neural processing of rewarding and aversive food stimuli in recovered anorexia nervosa. *Biological Psychiatry*, *70*(8), 736–743. https://doi.org/10.1016/j.biopsych.2011.05.028

Dalton, B., Foerde, K., Bartholdy, S., McClelland, J., Kekic, M., Grycuk, L., Campbell, I. C., Schmidt, U., & Steinglass, J. E. (2020). The effect of repetitive transcranial magnetic stimulation on food choice-related self-control in patients with severe, enduring anorexia nervosa. *International Journal of Eating Disorders*, 53(8), 1326–1336. https://doi.org/10.1002/eat.23267

DeGuzman, M., Shott, M. E., Yang, T. T., Riederer, J., & Frank, G. K. W. (2017). Association of elevated reward prediction error response with weight gain in adolescent anorexia nervosa. *American Journal of Psychiatry*, *174*(6), 557–565. https://doi.org/10.1176/appi.ajp.2016.16060671

Duriez, P., Ramoz, N., Gorwood, P., Viltart, O., & Tolle, V. (2019). A metabolic perspective on reward abnormalities in anorexia nervosa. *Trends in Endocrinology & Metabolism*, 30(12), 915–928. https://doi.org/10.1016/j.tem.2019.08.004

Enax, L., & Weber, B. (2016). Neurobiology of food choices—between energy homeostasis, reward system, and neuroeconomics. *e-Neuroforum*, *7*, 13–22. https://doi.org/10.1007/s13295-015-0020-0

Foerde, K., Schebendach, J. E., Davis, L., Daw, N., Walsh, B. T., Shohamy, D., & Steinglass, J. E. (2022). Restrictive eating across a spectrum from healthy to unhealthy: Behavioral and neural mechanisms. *Psychological Medicine*, *52*(9), 1755–1764. https://doi.org/10.1017/S0033291720003542

Foerde, K., & Steinglass, J. E. (2017). Decreased feedback learning in anorexia nervosa persists after weight restoration. *International Journal of Eating Disorders*, *50*(4), 415–423. https://doi.org/10.1002/eat.22709

Foerde, K., Steinglass, J. E., Shohamy, D., & Walsh, B. T. (2015). Neural mechanisms supporting maladaptive food choices in anorexia nervosa. *Nature Neuroscience*, *18*(11), 1571–1573. https://doi.org/10.1038/nn.4136

Francken, J. C., Slors, M., & Craver, C. F. (2022). Cognitive ontology and the search for neural mechanisms: Three foundational problems. *Synthese*, *200*(5), 378.

Frank, G. K., Shott, M. E., Hagman, J. O., & Mittal, V. A. (2013). Alterations in brain structures related to taste reward circuitry in ill and recovered anorexia nervosa and in bulimia nervosa. *American Journal of Psychiatry*, *170*(10), 1152–1160. https://doi.org/10.1176/appi.ajp.2013.12101294

Frank, G. K. W., Shott, M. E., & DeGuzman, M. C. (2019). The neurobiology of eating disorders. *Child and Adolescent Psychiatric Clinics of North America*, *28*(4), 629–640. https://doi.org/10.1016/j.chc.2019.05.007

Friederich, H.-C., Kumari, V., Uher, R., Riga, M., Schmidt, U., Campbell, I. C., Herzog, W., & Treasure, J. (2006). Differential motivational responses to food and pleasurable cues in anorexia and bulimia nervosa: A startle reflex paradigm. *Psychological Medicine*, *36*(09), 1327–1329. https://doi.org/10.1017/S0033291706008129

Gianini, L., Foerde, K., Walsh, B. T., Riegel, M., Broft, A., & Steinglass, J. E. (2019). Negative affect, dietary restriction, and food choice in bulimia nervosa. *Eating Behaviors*, *33*, 49–54. https://doi.org/10.1016/j.eatbeh.2019.03.003

Guillaume, S., Gorwood, P., Jollant, F., Van den Eynde, F., Courtet, P., & Richard-Devantoy, S. (2015). Impaired decision-making in symptomatic anorexia and bulimia nervosa patients: A meta-analysis. *Psychological Medicine*, *45*(16), 3377–3391. https://doi.org/10.1017/S003329171500152x

Hadigan, C. M., Anderson, E. J., Miller, K. K., Hubbard, J. L., Herzog, D. B., Klibanski, A., & Grinspoon, S. K. (2000). Assessment of macronutrient and micronutrient intake in women with anorexia nervosa. *International Journal of Eating Disorders*, *28*(3), 284–292. https://doi.org/10.1002/1098-108x(200011)28:3<284::aid-eat5>3.0.co;2-g

Han, J. E., Boachie, N., Garcia-Garcia, I., Michaud, A., & Dagher, A. (2018). Neural correlates of dietary self-control in healthy adults: A meta-analysis of functional brain imaging studies. *Physiology & Behavior*, *192*, 98–108. https://doi.org/10.1016/j.physbeh.2018.02.037

Hare, T. A., Camerer, C. F., & Rangel, A. (2009). Self-control in decision-making involves modulation of the vmPFC valuation system. *Science, 324*(5927), 646–648. https://doi.org/10.1126/science.1168450

Hare, T. A., Malmaud, J., & Rangel, A. (2011). Focusing attention on the health aspects of foods changes value signals in vmPFC and improves dietary choice. *Journal of Neuroscience, 31*(30), 11077–11087. https://doi.org/papers3://publication/doi/10.1523/JNEUROSCI.6383-10.2011

Haynos, A. F., Hall, L. M. J., Lavender, J. M., Peterson, C. B., Crow, S. J., Klimes-Dougan, B., Cullen, K. R., Lim, K. O., & Camchong, J. (2019). Resting state functional connectivity of networks associated with reward and habit in anorexia nervosa. *Human Brain Mapping, 40*(2), 652–662. https://doi.org/10.1002/hbm.24402

Haynos, A. F., Widge, A. S., Anderson, L. M., & Redish, A. D. (2022). Beyond description and deficits: how computational psychiatry can enhance an understanding of decision-making in anorexia nervosa. *Current Psychiatry Reports*, 24(1), 77–87. https://doi.org/10.1007/s11920-022-01320-9

Hikosaka, O., Kim, H. F., Yasuda, M., & Yamamoto, S. (2014). Basal ganglia circuits for reward value-guided behavior. *Annual Review of Neuroscience, 37*(1), 289–306. https://doi.org/10.1146/annurev-neuro-071013-013924

Hildebrandt, T., Grotzinger, A., Reddan, M., Greif, R., Levy, I., Goodman, W., & Schiller, D. (2015). Testing the disgust conditioning theory of food-avoidance in adolescents with recent onset anorexia nervosa. *Behaviour Research and Therapy, 71*(C), 131–138. https://doi.org/10.1016/j.brat.2015.06.008

Huse, D. M., & Lucas, A. R. (1984). Dietary patterns in anorexia nervosa. *American Journal of Clinical Nutrition, 40*(2), 251–254. https://doi.org/10.1093/ajcn/40.2.251

Hutcherson, C. A., Plassmann, H., Gross, J. J., & Rangel, A. (2012). Cognitive regulation during decision making shifts behavioral control between ventromedial and dorsolateral prefrontal value systems. *Journal of Neuroscience, 32*(39), 13543–13554. https://doi.org/10.1523/JNEUROSCI.6387-11.2012

Kable, J. W., & Glimcher, P. W. (2009). The neurobiology of decision: Consensus and controversy. *Neuron, 63*(6), 733–745. https://doi.org/10.1016/j.neuron.2009.09.003

Kaye, W. (2008). Neurobiology of anorexia and bulimia nervosa. *Physiology & Behavior, 94*(1), 121–135. https://doi.org/10.1016/j.physbeh.2007.11.037

Kaye, W. H., Wierenga, C. E., Bischoff-Grethe, A., Berner, L. A., Ely, A. V., Bailer, U. F., Paulus, M. P., & Fudge, J. L. (2020). Neural insensitivity to the effects of hunger in women remitted from anorexia nervosa. *American Journal of Psychiatry, 177*(7), 601–610. https://doi.org/10.1176/appi.ajp.2019.19030261

Keating, C., Tilbrook, A. J., Rossell, S. L., Enticott, P. G., & Fitzgerald, P. B. (2012). Reward processing in anorexia nervosa. *Neuropsychologia, 50*(5), 567–575. https://doi.org/10.1016/j.neuropsychologia.2012.01.036

Kim, K. R., Ku, J., Lee, J. H., Lee, H., & Jung, Y. C. (2012). Functional and effective connectivity of anterior insula in anorexia nervosa and bulimia nervosa. *Neuroscience Letters, 521*(2), 152–157.

Lehéricy, S., Ducros, M., Van de Moortele, P.-F., Francois, C., Thivard, L., Poupon, C., Swindale, N., Ugurbil, K., & Kim, D.-S. (2004). Diffusion tensor fiber tracking shows distinct corticostriatal circuits in humans. *Annals of Neurology, 55*(4), 522–529. https://doi.org/papers3://publication/doi/10.1002/ana.20030

Levinson, C. A., & Williams, B. M. (2020). Eating disorder fear networks: Identification of central eating disorder fears. *International Journal of Eating Disorders, 53*(12), 1960–1973. https://doi.org/10.1002/eat.23382

Lloyd, E. C., Foerde, K. E., Muratore, A. F., Aw, N., Semanek, D., Steinglass, J. E., & Posner, J. (2023). Large-scale exploration of whole-brain structural connectivity in anorexia nervosa: Alterations in the connectivity of frontal and subcortical networks. *Biological Psychiatry: Cognitive Neuroscience and Neuroimaging, 8*(8), 864–873. https://doi.org/10.1016/j.bpsc.2022.06.002

Lloyd, E. C., Posner, J., Schebendach, J., Muratore, A. F., Hong, S., Ojeda, J., Rafanello, E., Steinglass, J. E., & Foerde, K. (2025). Food choice and neural reward systems in adolescents with anorexia nervosa and atypical anorexia nervosa. Journal Of Child Psychology and Psychiatry. *66*(3), 378–389. https://doi.org/10.1111/jcpp.14066

Lloyd, E. C., & Steinglass, J. E. (2018). What can food-image tasks teach us about anorexia nervosa? A systematic review. *Journal of Eating Disorders, 6*(1), 1–18. https://doi.org/10.1186/s40337-018-0217-z

Maier, S. U., Makwana, A. B., & Hare, T. A. (2015). Acute stress impairs self-control in goal-directed choice by altering multiple functional connections within the brain's decision circuits. *Neuron, 87*(3), 621–631. https://doi.org/10.1016/j.neuron.2015.07.005

Mayer, L. E., Schebendach, J., Bodell, L. P., Shingleton, R. M., & Walsh, B. T. (2012). Eating behavior in anorexia nervosa: Before and after treatment. *International Journal of Eating Disorders, 45*(2), 290–293. https://doi.org/10.1002/eat.20924

McNamee, D., Rangel, A., & O'Doherty, J. P. (2013). Category-dependent and category-independent goal-value codes in human ventromedial prefrontal cortex. *Nature Neuroscience, 16*(4), 479–485. https://doi.org/nn.3337

Menzel, J. E., Reilly, E. E., Luo, T. J., & Kaye, W. H. (2019). Conceptualizing the role of disgust in avoidant/restrictive food intake disorder: Implications for the etiology and treatment of selective eating. *International Journal of Eating Disorders, 52*(4), 462–465. https://doi.org/10.1002/eat.23006

Mequinion, M., Chauveau, C., & Viltart, O. (2015). The use of animal models to decipher physiological and neurobiological alterations of anorexia nervosa patients. *Frontiers in Endocrinol, 6*, 68. https://doi.org/10.3389/fendo.2015.00068

Meregalli, V., Tenconi, E., Cardi, V., Bonifanti, A., Meneguzzo, P., Favaro, A., & Collantoni, E. (2023). Strategic avoidance of food stimuli in patients with restrictive anorexia nervosa: An eye-tracking evaluation. *European Eating Disorders Review, 31*(6), 813–821. https://doi.org/10.1002/erv.3011

Muratore, A. F., Bershad, M., Steinglass, J. E., Foerde, K. E., Gianini, L., Broft, A., & Attia, E. (2021). Use of high-frequency repetitive transcranial magnetic stimulation to probe the neural circuitry of food choice in anorexia nervosa: A proof-of-concept study. *International Journal of Eating Disorders, 54*(11), 2031–2036. https://doi.org/10.1002/eat.23597

Norman, K. A., Polyn, S. M., Detre, G. J., & Haxby, J. V. (2006). Beyond mind-reading: Multi-voxel pattern analysis of fMRI data. *Trends in Cognitive Science, 10*(9), 424–430. https://doi.org/10.1016/j.tics.2006.07.005

O'Hara, C. B., Campbell, I. C., & Schmidt, U. (2015). A reward-centred model of anorexia nervosa: A focussed narrative review of the neurological and psychophysiological literature. *Neuroscience & Biobehavorial Reviews, 52*, 131–152. https://doi.org/10.1016/j.neubiorev.2015.02.012

Oberndorfer, T. A., Frank, G. K. W., Simmons, A. N., Wagner, A., McCurdy, D., Fudge, J. L., Yang, T. T., Paulus, M. P., & Kaye, W. H. (2013). Altered insula response to sweet taste processing after recovery from anorexia and bulimia nervosa. *American Journal of Psychiatry, 170*(10), 1143–1151. https://doi.org/10.1176/appi.ajp.2013.11111745

Ostlund, S. B., & Balleine, B. W. (2007). Orbitofrontal cortex mediates outcome encoding in Pavlovian but not instrumental conditioning. *Journal of Neuroscience, 27*(18), 4819–4825. https://doi.org/10.1523/JNEUROSCI.5443-06.2007

Padoa-Schioppa, C., & Assad, J. A. (2006). Neurons in the orbitofrontal cortex encode economic value. *Nature, 441*(7090), 223–226. https://doi.org/10.1038/nature04676

Plassmann, H., O'Doherty, J., & Rangel, A. (2007). Orbitofrontal cortex encodes willingness to pay in everyday economic transactions. *Journal of Neuroscience, 27*(37), 9984–9988. https://doi.org/10.1523/JNEUROSCI.2131-07.2007

Poldrack, R. A. (2006). Can cognitive processes be inferred from neuroimaging data?. *Trends in Cognitive Sciences, 10*(2), 59–63. https://doi.org/10.1016/j.tics.2005.12.004

Rangel, A. (2013). Regulation of dietary choice by the decision-making circuitry. *Nature Neuroscience, 16*(12), 1717–1724. https://doi.org/10.1038/nn.3561

Rangel, A., Camerer, C., & Montague, P. R. (2008). A framework for studying the neurobiology of value-based decision making [10.1038/nrn2357]. *Nature Neuroscience 9*(7), 545–556. https://doi.org/10.1038/nrn2357

Rramani, Q., Krajbich, I., Enax, L., Brustkern, L., & Weber, B. (2020). Salient nutrition labels shift peoples' attention to healthy foods and exert more influence on their choices. *Nutrition Research, 80*, 106–116. https://doi.org/10.1016/j.nutres.2020.06.013

Saper, C. B., Chou, T. C., & Elmquist, J. K. (2002). The need to feed: Homeostatic and hedonic control of eating. *Neuron, 36*(2), 199–211. https://doi.org/S0896627302009698

Schebendach, J. E., Mayer, L. E., Devlin, M. J., Attia, E., Contento, I. R., Wolf, R. L., & Walsh, B. T. (2008). Dietary energy density and diet variety as predictors of outcome in anorexia nervosa. *American Journal of Clinical Nutrition, 87*(4), 810–816. http://www.ncbi.nlm.nih.gov/entrez/query.fcgi?cmd=Retrieve&db=PubMed&dopt=Citation&list_uids=18400701

Schebendach, J., Mayer, L. E., Devlin, M. J., Attia, E., & Walsh, B. T. (2012). Dietary energy density and diet variety as risk factors for relapse in anorexia nervosa: A replication. *International Journal of Eating Disorders, 45*(1), 79–84. https://doi.org/10.1002/eat.20922

Schebendach, J. E., Uniacke, B., Walsh, B. T., Mayer, L. E. S., Attia, E., & Steinglass, J. (2019). Fat preference and fat intake in individuals with and without anorexia nervosa. *Appetite, 139*, 35–41. https://doi.org/10.1016/j.appet.2019.04.008

Shadlen, M. N., & Kiani, R. (2013). Decision making as a window on cognition. *Neuron, 80*(3), 791–806. https://doi.org/papers3://publication/doi/10.1016/j.neuron.2013.10.047

Shadlen, M. N., & Shohamy, D. (2016). Decision making and sequential sampling from memory. *Neuron, 90*(5), 927–939. https://doi.org/10.1016/j.neuron.2016.04.036

Steinglass, J., Albano, A. M., Simpson, H. B., Carpenter, K., Schebendach, J., & Attia, E. (2012). Fear of food as a treatment target: Exposure and response prevention for anorexia nervosa in an open series. *International Journal of Eating Disorders, 45*(4), 615–621. https://doi.org/10.1002/eat.20936

Steinglass, J. E., Fei, W., Foerde, K., Touzeau, C., Ruggiero, J., Lloyd, C., Attia, E., Wang, Y., & Walsh, B. T. (2023). Change in food choice during acute treatment and the effect on longer-term outcome in patients with anorexia nervosa. *Psychological Medicine*, 54(6), 1133–1141. https://doi.org/10.1017/S0033291723002933

Steinglass, J., Foerde, K., Kostro, K., Shohamy, D., & Walsh, B. T. (2015). Restrictive food intake as a choice—A paradigm for study. *International Journal of Eating Disorders, 48*(1), 59–66. https://doi.org/10.1002/eat.22345

Steinglass, J. E., Lempert, K. M., Choo, T. H., Kimeldorf, M. B., Wall, M., Walsh, B. T., Fyer, A. J., Schneier, F. R., & Simpson, H. B. (2017). Temporal discounting across three psychiatric disorders: Anorexia nervosa, obsessive compulsive disorder, and social anxiety disorder. *Depression and Anxiety, 34*(5), 463–470. https://doi.org/10.1002/da.22586

Strober, M. (2004). Pathologic fear conditioning and anorexia nervosa: On the search for novel paradigms. *International Journal of Eating Disorders, 35*(4), 504–508. https://doi.org/10.1002/eat.20029

Sullivan, N. J., & Huettel, S. A. (2021). Healthful choices depend on the latency and rate of information accumulation. *Nature Human Behavior, 5*(12), 1698–1706. https://doi.org/10.1038/s41562-021-01154-0

Suzuki, S., Cross, L., & O'Doherty, J. P. (2017). Elucidating the underlying components of food valuation in the human orbitofrontal cortex. *Nature Neuroscience, 20*(12), 1–15. https://doi.org/10.1038/s41593-017-0008-x

Sysko, R., Steinglass, J. E., Schebendach, J. E., Mayer, L. E. S., & Walsh, B. T. (2018). Rigor and reproducibility via laboratory studies of eating behavior: A focused update and conceptual review. *International Journal of Eating Disorders, 51*(7), 608–616. https://doi.org/10.1002/eat.22900

Sysko, R., Walsh, B. T., Schebendach, J., & Wilson, G. T. (2005). Eating behavior among women with anorexia nervosa. *American Journal of Clinical Nutrition, 82*(2), 296–301. https://doi.org/10.1093/ajcn.82.2.296

Uniacke, B., Slattery, R., Walsh, B. T., Shohamy, D., Foerde, K., & Steinglass, J. (2020). A comparison of food-based decision-making between restricting and binge-eating/purging subtypes of anorexia nervosa. *International Journal of Eating Disorders, 53*(10), 1751–1756. https://doi.org/10.1002/eat.23359

Van Meer, F., Van Der Laan, L. N., Viergever, M. A., Adan, R. A. H., Smeets, P. A. M., & I.Family Consortium. (2017). Considering healthiness promotes healthier choices but modulates medial prefrontal cortex differently in children compared with adults. *NeuroImage, 159*, 325–333. https://doi.org/10.1016/j.neuroimage.2017.08.007

Wagner, A., Aizenstein, H., Venkatraman, V. K., Fudge, J., May, J. C., Mazurkewicz, L., Frank, G. K., Bailer, U. F., Fischer, L., Nguyen, V., Carter, C., Putnam, K., & Kaye, W. H. (2007). Altered reward processing in women recovered from anorexia nervosa. *American Journal of Psychiatry, 164*(12), 1842–1849. https://doi.org/10.1176/appi.ajp.2007.07040575

Wansink, B., & Sobal, J. (2007). Mindless eating: The 200 daily food decisions we overlook. *Environment and Behavior, 39*(1), 106–123.

Wierenga, C. E., Bischoff-Grethe, A., Melrose, A. J., Irvine, Z., Torres, L., Bailer, U. F., Simmons, A., Fudge, J. L., McClure, S. M., Ely, A., & Kaye, W. H. (2015). Hunger does not motivate reward in women remitted from anorexia nervosa. *Biological Psychiatry, 77*(7), 642–652. https://doi.org/10.1016/j.biopsych.2014.09.024

Wierenga, C. E., Reilly, E., Bischoff-Grethe, A., Kaye, W. H., & Brown, G. G. (2022). Altered reinforcement learning from reward and punishment in anorexia nervosa: Evidence from computational modeling. *Journal of the International Neuropsychological Society, 28*(10), 1003–1015. https://doi.org/10.1017/S1355617721001326

Xue, A. M., Foerde, K., Walsh, B. T., Steinglass, J. E., Shohamy, D., & Bakkour, A. (2022). Neural representations of food-related attributes in the human orbitofrontal cortex during choice deliberation in anorexia nervosa. *Journal of Neuroscience, 42*(1), 109–120. https://doi.org/10.1523/JNEUROSCI.0958-21.2021

Yin, H. H., & Knowlton, B. J. (2006). The role of the basal ganglia in habit formation. *Nature Reviews Neuroscience, 7*, 464–476.

15

Binge Eating

Kelsey E. Hagan

Brief Definitional Overview

Binge eating: The experience of consuming an unambiguously large amount of food in a discrete period (i.e., two hours) accompanied by a subjective sense of being unable to stop eating or control what or how much is eaten (American Psychiatric Association, 2013).

Loss of control eating: The subjective experience of being unable to stop eating or control what or how much is eaten, irrespective of the amount of food consumed (World Health Organization, 2019).

Introduction

Binge eating is a transdiagnostic eating disorder symptom, and recurrent binge eating is a hallmark diagnostic criterion of binge-eating disorder (BED) and bulimia nervosa (BN), which affect 1% to 3% of the population (Stice et al., 2013; Udo & Grilo, 2018). Binge eating is prevalent and increasing among the general adult population, with 13% of Australian adults reporting a binge-eating episode within the past three months (Mitchison et al., 2017) and 40% of United States college students endorsing a binge-eating episode within the past month (Lipson & Sonneville, 2017). Adverse psychosocial and medical sequelae (Mitchison et al., 2017) and significant economic burden (Tannous et al., 2021) are associated with binge eating. More than 50% of patients with binge-eating pathology remain symptomatic or relapse after receiving first-line psychosocial and/or pharmacological treatments (Hilbert et al., 2020; Linardon, 2018; Linardon & Wade, 2018; Monteleone et al., 2022), suggesting that the core biobehavioral mechanisms of binge eating are not adequately addressed with currently available interventions.

Research examining the top-down biobehavioral mechanisms of both binge eating and subjective loss of control (LOC) eating is reviewed in this chapter. Consuming an objectively large amount of food and experiencing LOC during an eating episode are both necessary for satisfying the *Diagnostic and Statistical*

Kelsey E. Hagan, *Binge Eating*. In: *The Handbook of the Neurobiology of Eating Disorders*. Edited by: Christina E. Wierenga and Joanna E. Steinglass, Oxford University Press. © Oxford University Press (2025).
DOI: 10.1093/9780197675212.003.0016

Manual of Mental Disorders (*DSM*) binge-eating criteria. Yet, research has demonstrated that LOC is most salient to binge-eating psychopathology. For instance, independent of the amount of food consumed during an eating episode, LOC is uniquely correlated with psychosocial impairment and distress (Goldschmidt, 2017). Moreover, mental-health-related quality-of-life is similarly poor among those who experience objectively large versus subjective binge-eating episodes (Li et al., 2019). Prospective research supports the predictive validity of LOC eating and has found that up to approximately 50% of youth who experience LOC eating (regardless of size) go on to meet the criteria for an eating disorder (Hilbert et al., 2013; Tanofsky-Kraff et al., 2011). Thus, there is merit in understanding the biobehavioral mechanisms of LOC due to its centrality to binge-eating psychopathology.

Biological Framework

Broadly, applying a top-down perspective to binge eating examines how this symptom may result from the interaction of several neurobiological systems. Dominant theoretical models and decades of research have pointed to executive functioning (especially inhibitory control), cognitive processes (e.g., dietary restraint, craving), affective regulation, and reward processing (e.g., food-cue reactivity, "liking" and "wanting" food) as higher-order influences on binge eating. A neurobiological and theoretical framework for each of these influences is presented below. Further, this chapter describes what is known about each of these neurobiologically mediated influences on binge eating, with a focus on studies that have used food-related stimuli or examined eating behavior during neuroimaging, given arguments that such methods best support translational science and therapeutics for eating disorders (Walsh, 2011).

An important consideration is that the intermittent nature of binge eating poses a challenge for examining binge eating through a top-down lens, which begins with the manifest, observable symptom. Unlike food restriction, which is sustained and can be captured using an objective food-choice task administered during neuroimaging (Steinglass et al., 2015) or scanning during a fasted (restricted) state, binge eating is episodic, and LOC is subjective, and both are difficult to assess with current neurocognitive tasks during traditional neuroimaging scanning (Berner et al., 2017). To circumvent these challenges, researchers have administered palatable shakes and solutions to individuals with and without binge eating to examine neural correlates underlying consummatory behavior, but not LOC eating (e.g., Bohon & Stice, 2012; Frank et al., 2006). More recently, some have used a portable neuroimaging technology with movement tolerability called functional near-infrared spectroscopy (fNIRS) to examine prefrontal neural responses to consuming a palatable shake (Berner, Winter, et al., 2023). However, most approaches to understanding the neurobiology of binge eating have employed more passive paradigms that do not involve eating behavior.

Executive functioning: A focus on inhibitory control

Inhibitory control is the ability to successfully inhibit a response before it is initiated (proactive inhibition) or stop a response that has already been initiated (reactive inhibition). Altered inhibitory control has been proposed as a mechanism of LOC, given that LOC is characterized by a subjective sense of being unable to stop or control what or how much one is eating (Kober & Boswell, 2018; Tanofsky-Kraff et al., 2020). Traditional neurocognitive tests of inhibitory control require participants to press a button in response to certain stimuli ("go" stimuli) and withhold a button press in response to other stimuli ("no-go" stimuli, so-called go/no-go tasks) measuring proactive inhibition, or stop a response that is already underway, measuring reactive inhibition (stop-signal tasks). Among healthy individuals, go/no-go and stop-signal tasks engage the frontoparietal and cingulo-opercular control networks, and evidence suggests neurostructural alternations of regions within these networks among individuals with binge-eating pathology (Berner et al., 2018; Cyr et al., 2017).

Cognitive influences

Cognitive factors, such as attempts to restrain eating or craving, may influence how an individual approaches and engages with food, contributing to binge eating. These ideas are captured by classic theories of eating behavior and eating disorders. For instance, restraint theory suggests that dietary restraint (or dieting) contributes to reduced sensitivity to hunger and satiety cues, which may increase the propensity for binge eating (Polivy & Herman, 1985). Research supports a robust association between dietary restraint and binge eating (Elran-Barak et al., 2015; Hagan et al., 2016), but the neurobiological underpinnings of this association have yet to be fully elucidated.

Theoretical models also implicate food craving as a cognitive influence of binge eating (Jansen, 1998). Empirical work has supported this theory, finding that craving precipitates binge eating among individuals with binge-eating pathology (Chao et al., 2016; Leenaerts et al., 2023; Ng & Davis, 2013; Schaefer, Forester, Burr, et al., 2023). Food cravings in humans have also been associated with neural activation within the orbitofrontal cortex, amygdala, insula, and ventral striatum (Boswell & Kober, 2016).

Affective influences

One of the most dominant theoretical models of binge eating is the affect-regulation model (Heatherton & Baumeister, 1991), which posits that binge eating functions to (temporarily) alleviate or numb aversive affective states. Empirical support for the affect-regulation model of binge eating is robust, as decades of ecological momentary assessment research have demonstrated that self-reported increases in negative affect and decreases in positive affect increase the likelihood of subsequent binge eating and that negative affect decreases following binge eating among individuals with binge-eating pathology (Haedt-Matt & Keel, 2011). It has recently been hypothesized that the well-established link between aversive affective states and binge eating may be explained by negative affect temporarily altering neural responses to food, such that the subjective value of food increases, thereby increasing the risk for binge eating (Schaefer, Forester, Dvorak, et al., 2023). This hypothesis is supported by data suggesting that negative affect (stress) inhibits the prefrontal cortex (PFC) and engages the amygdala and striatum in humans (Arnsten, 2015), which could enhance the subjective value of food and increase the risk of binge eating.

Reward processing

The idea that reward-processing abnormalities may underlie binge eating has garnered considerable interest. For instance, it has long been posited that individuals with binge-eating pathology find food more rewarding than individuals without binge-eating pathology. Eating behavior is modulated by hypothalamic-homeostatic and mesocorticolimbic-reward circuitry (Castro et al., 2015). Mesocorticolimbic circuitry encodes "wanting" and "liking" of palatable foods (Castro et al., 2015), and, critically, wanting appears to be modulated by dopaminergic function (Berridge, 1996). In contrast, liking is postulated to be mediated by opioidergic function (Kelley et al., 2002). Researchers have theorized that alterations within this circuit and these neurotransmitters may contribute to the onset and maintenance of binge eating. Specifically, the incentive-sensitization theory of binge eating posits that persons with binge eating develop incongruencies in neural response to "wanting" and "liking" food, such that they demonstrate elevated neural response when anticipating (wanting) consumption of palatable binge foods but not when consuming (liking) binge foods (Morales & Berridge, 2020). This theory has served as a springboard for a fruitful line of inquiry investigating neural responses to food cues (wanting), as well as the development of paradigms that assess neural response to food anticipation (wanting) versus receipt (liking).

State of the Science in Eating Disorders

Inhibitory control

Meta-analytic results suggest behavioral alterations in inhibitory control on food-specific go/no-go tasks among individuals with binge-eating pathology (Schag et al., 2013; Wu, Hartmann, et al., 2013). Data on alterations in reactive inhibition to food stimuli (e.g., on the stop-signal task) are mixed (Bartholdy et al., 2016; Lavagnino et al., 2016; Wu, Giel, et al., 2013). Relatively few studies have investigated the neural correlates of inhibitory control tasks among individuals with binge eating and binge-eating pathology.

To date, one study has investigated the neural correlates of inhibitory control to food stimuli in those at risk for binge-eating pathology. This study administered food-specific versions of the go/no-go and stop-signal tasks during fMRI scanning to normal-weight adults with and without binge eating (without DSM diagnoses) (Oliva et al., 2019). Although groups did not differ in behavioral responses, they demonstrated unique neural activation patterns during response inhibition on the go/no-go and stop-signal tasks. Specifically, on no-go trials, participants with binge eating demonstrated hypoactivation of the middle frontal gyrus, precuneus, striatum (caudate, putamen), and cerebellum, and hyperactivation of occipital regions compared to those without binge eating. On stop trials in the stop-signal task, participants with binge eating demonstrated hypoactivation of the left middle frontal gyrus and cerebellum relative to those without binge eating. Findings suggest intact inhibitory control in those at risk for binge eating; however, alterations in underlying neural activation could be a herald of future behavior change and thus be a biomarker for the onset of binge-eating pathology.

The literature on the neural correlates of food-specific inhibitory control among individuals with binge-eating pathology relative to those without is somewhat mixed and has mostly focused on BN. One study found no differences in behavior and neural activation on a food-specific go/no-go task but observed hypoactivation of right sensorimotor regions and the right dorsal striatum during no-go trials on a general go/no-go task in adult women with BN compared to those without the disorder (Skunde et al., 2016). More recent work has aimed to increase the ecological validity of research on the neural correlates of inhibitory control in BN by examining attempts to inhibit eating and testing differences in inhibitory control as a function of metabolic state (i.e., fasted versus fed). Regarding the former, researchers developed a novel eating-specific go/no-go task in which participants are instructed to consume a palatable yogurt shake during go trials and inhibit consumption during no-go trials, with the assumption that this would closely approximate real-world attempts to control eating behavior (Berner, Winter, et al., 2023). Adult women with and without BN completed this novel paradigm and a general go/no-go task while wearing an fNIRS device to measure concurrent

PFC activation. Results indicated that women with BN made more commission errors (i.e., responses on no-go trials) than non-eating disorder controls on both the food-specific and general go/no-go tasks. Yet, no group differences in PFC activation during these tasks were observed. However, women who endorsed the highest sense of LOC during the eating-specific task evidenced lower bilateral ventromedial PFC and right ventrolateral PFC activation compared to controls during attempts to inhibit food consumption and lower activation in the right ventrolateral PFC activation during the eating-specific task was associated with more severe self-reported LOC eating in the entire BN sample. Together, these data suggest that insufficient engagement of prefrontal regions implicated in inhibitory control may underpin the subjective sense of LOC overeating among individuals with BN.

As mentioned, other work has tested whether inhibitory control is affected by metabolic state (being fasted for 16 hours or fed) in adult women remitted from BN and non-eating disorder controls using a counterbalanced design (Berner, Harlé, et al., 2023). In contrast to traditional approaches to analyzing stop-signal task data (i.e., sum scores), computational modeling was applied to assess how women with and without a history of BN updated their internal working models of the task to prepare to inhibit responses. Although metabolic state did not impact behavioral task performance, group by metabolic state differences in neural activation were observed. Specifically, women remitted from BN showed blunted activation in the left dorsal caudate—a brain region implicated in inhibitory control—when stop signals unexpectedly appeared, and this effect was most pronounced in women with the most frequent past binge eating. Attenuated activation of the dorsal caudate could imply difficulties with tracking signals in the environment, leading to challenges with modulating behavior, such as binge eating.

Two studies have examined the neural underpinnings of food-specific inhibitory control in adults with obesity and BED. One study found no behavioral differences on a food-specific go/no-go task between obese women with and without BED; however, women with BED showed insufficient recruitment of prefrontal regions during no-go trials during fMRI scanning (Hege et al., 2015). The second study administered a food-specific go/no-go task concurrent with fNIRS to obese adults with and without BED and normal-weight non-eating disorder controls and found similar hypoactivation of the inferior frontal gyrus and hyperactivation of the dorsolateral PFC in obese groups compared to controls during the task (Rösch et al., 2020). Thus, the limited evidence generally suggests hypoactivation of prefrontal regions during food-related inhibitory control among adults with binge-eating compared to controls; however, it is yet unclear whether these differences are specific to individuals with BED or more general to those with obesity.

Taken together, the existing literature generally suggests hypoactivation of prefrontal regions during lapses in inhibitory control on food-specific paradigms among persons with binge eating and binge-eating pathology.

Cognitive influences

Dietary restraint

One pilot study assessed the neural underpinnings of dietary restraint on eating behavior in youth with and without LOC eating by using a milkshake paradigm that allowed youth restricted versus unrestricted access to milkshakes following a week-long restriction of ice cream (Goldschmidt et al., 2018). Youth with LOC eating demonstrated higher activation of the middle frontal gyrus, cingulate gyrus, inferior frontal gyrus, and the cuneus during the milkshake paradigm compared to their unaffected counterparts; however, there were no differences in neural activation as a function of unrestricted versus restricted milkshake access. Nevertheless, findings suggest that youth who experience LOC eating may expend more cognitive effort (as evidenced by enhanced recruitment of prefrontal regions implicated in cognitive control) when eating.

Craving

Despite the promise of craving as an important top-down influence on binge eating, only one study has investigated the neural correlates of craving in binge-eating pathology (Parker et al., 2023). In this study, obese adults with and without binge eating watched videos of highly palatable food concurrent with fNIRS to assess PFC activation. Participants were instructed to crave or resist foods while viewing food-related videos. There were no significant group differences in neural activation between the binge-eating and control groups.

Considered together, there is a paucity of research investigating the influence of cognitive factors (e.g., dietary restraint and craving) on food-related paradigms administered concurrently with neuroimaging. The previously described studies employed novel paradigms with food-related stimuli and eating behavior that have high potential relevance for advancing the understanding of the neurobiology of binge eating.

Affective influences

Several studies have investigated the impact of negative affect and stress on neural responses to food and real-world binge eating among individuals with binge-eating pathology. In one study, adult women with BN completed a passive-viewing paradigm of highly palatable foods concurrent with fMRI scanning before and after completing a social stress test, and participants subsequently completed two weeks of ecological momentary assessment ratings (reporting on affect and eating disorder behaviors) (Fischer et al., 2017). After stress induction, ventromedial PFC, amygdala, and anterior cingulate cortex (ACC) activation in response to food cues in women with BN significantly decreased. Further, stress-related decreases in precuneus, dorsolateral PFC, and ACC activation to food were associated with greater increases in stress before real-world binge eating as assessed by ecological momentary assessment. Others have found that state negative affect was significantly associated with putamen, caudate, and pallidum activation during anticipated receipt of a chocolate milkshake (versus a tasteless solution)—but found no significant associations between negative affect and neural activation during milkshake receipt—in adult women with BN (Bohon & Stice, 2012). In another study, women with BED and non-eating disorder controls completed a stress induction and then completed a passive food viewing paradigm while undergoing fMRI scanning (Lyu & Jackson, 2016). Findings revealed that women with BED showed hypoactivation of the hippocampus relative to controls when viewing high-calorie food images following stress induction. Reduced hippocampal activation while viewing high-calorie food images was associated with increased chocolate consumption in a post-scan snack; however, this association was true for all participants (not just those with BED). Together, results support the hypothesis that stress inhibits prefrontal regions (which are important in regulating behavior) and increases activation within reward-related brain regions, which may enhance the subjective value of food and contribute to binge eating.

Reward processing

The question of whether neural reward circuitry responds differently to food among individuals with binge-eating pathology compared to non-eating disorder controls has garnered considerable interest. An activation likelihood estimation meta-analysis of fMRI studies found that compared to non-eating disorder controls, individuals with BN demonstrate hyperactivation within reward processing (striatum), interoceptive (insula), visual processing regions (cuneus, lingual and fusiform gyrus), and bilateral cerebellum and hypoactivation in brain regions implicated in cognitive control (PFC, ACC) and the precuneus and temporal gyrus when viewing food images (Bronleigh et al., 2022). Women with BED demonstrate hyperactivation of the medial orbitofrontal cortex while viewing palatable food images relative to non-eating disorder controls (Schienle et al., 2009). These findings from passive viewing tasks of palatable food support the hypothesis that neural substrates of food wanting are altered and reflect elevated wanting among individuals with binge-eating pathology.

To enhance the validity of research on the neurobiological underpinnings of food wanting, researchers developed a novel binge-planning paradigm that is administered concurrently with fMRI scanning (Pearson et al., 2016). In this paradigm, participants are shown food images and asked to plan a binge-eating episode by selecting food images they could later consume in private. Participants also completed a similar furniture shopping paradigm, in which they were instructed to select furniture for a new apartment. Preliminary data suggested that women with BN exhibit higher bilateral caudate and lower bilateral amygdala activation in the binge-planning task compared to the furniture selection task. Although data are preliminary, this task represents an exciting avenue for increasing the translational potential of neuroimaging research in binge eating.

Other investigations have directly tested the incentive-sensitization theory by comparing neural responses to wanting and liking food using novel paradigms. For instance, in one study, adult participants with binge-eating pathology and non-eating disorder controls completed a food-incentive delay task, adapted from the widely used monetary incentive delay task, while undergoing fMRI scanning (Simon et al., 2016). Participants could win snack points during the task, which were exchanged for food following scanning procedures. Results indicated that controls showed higher activation in the posterior cingulate cortex than individuals with binge-eating pathology during reward anticipation. However, counter to the incentive-sensitization theory, individuals with binge-eating pathology showed greater activation of the medial orbitofrontal cortex, posterior cingulate cortex, anterior medial PFC, and angular gyrus than controls during receipt of food reward (i.e., snack points). Hyperactivation of brain regions implicated in reward valuation during the liking phase of the task suggests increased hedonic processing, but not wanting, of food among individuals with binge-eating pathology, suggesting that the opioidergic system could be more involved in binge-eating pathology than previously considered.

However, results from other studies that have invoked the gustatory system with palatable shakes and tasting solutions offer variable support for this finding. For instance, compared to non-eating disorder controls, women with BN showed hypoactivation of the right anterior insula during anticipation (wanting) of a chocolate milkshake and hypoactivation of the left middle frontal gyrus, right posterior insula, right precentral gyrus, and right dorsal insula during consumption (liking) of the chocolate milkshake (Bohon & Stice, 2011). Researchers have also studied neural responses to palatable tastes (sweet and high-fat) among participants who have recovered from binge-eating pathology to avoid the potential for confounds due to altered nutritional state (i.e., extremes of hunger during periods of fasting and satiety following binge eating in BN). One study found that participants with a history of BN demonstrated lower activity in the ACC and cuneus when consuming a sweet taste (glucose) compared to controls (Frank et al., 2006). In contrast, others have found that participants remitted from BN demonstrated elevated activation of the right anterior insula during a sweet taste (sucrose) compared to non-eating disorder controls (Oberndorfer et al., 2013). Others have also tested whether metabolic state (e.g., fasted or fed) alters neural response to sweet taste (sucrose) among participants remitted from BN. Results indicated no differences in neural activation in response to sucrose as a function of metabolic state among individuals remitted from BN, which the authors suggest may represent an inability to devalue food when fed (Ely et al., 2017). However, participants remitted from BN evidenced increased activation in the left amygdala to sweet taste when fed compared to non-eating disorder controls. Concerning high-fat tastes, others have found that participants with a history of BN showed higher anterior ventral striatal response in response to tasting whipping cream compared to controls (Radeloff et al., 2014). Together, research that has experimentally examined neural response to food-related rewards suggests alterations in reward-related and prefrontal circuitry; however, the direction of these findings has been variable.

Alternative Perspectives

This chapter reviewed the existing evidence for neurobiological contributions to symptom expression among persons with binge eating, LOC eating, and binge-eating pathology, focusing on studies that used food-related stimuli or studied eating behavior. The extant literature suggests robust neural alterations in inhibitory control (and corresponding hypoactivation of the PFC) and reward processing of food stimuli. Less is known about how other higher-order processes may interact with neurobiology (and other factors) to increase vulnerability to binge eating. However, emerging work suggests that negative affect (e.g., stress) and craving are cognitive-affective influences that may play an important role in the neurobiology of binge eating.

This chapter focused on findings from studies that: (1) included food-related (vs. non-food or general) stimuli, (2) recruited samples with BN or BED, and (3) based their research around certain theoretical models (e.g., the incentive-sensitization theory of binge eating). This section highlights perspectives different than those presented above and discusses how these alternative views may or may not be integrated with those presented earlier in the chapter.

Food versus non-food stimuli

This chapter was written from the perspective that investigation of the neural correlates of binge-eating behavior will best advance science and support the development of translational therapeutics. However, top-down research on binge eating is constrained by the current lack of objective measures of LOC and binge eating compatible with neuroimaging technologies, and measurement advances are needed to improve our understanding of this behavior. In contrast, others have presented compelling arguments for examining whether reward processing and inhibitory control are altered to non-food or generally rewarding stimuli, such as money, among persons with binge-eating pathology. For example, a recently proposed illness-staging model of reward processing alterations in binge-eating pathology suggested that responses to food and non-food rewards may be initially similarly elevated among those with binge-eating pathology but that responses to food may increase and responses to non-food rewards may decrease with illness progression (Bodell & Racine, 2022). Thus, this model highlights the utility of incorporating food and non-food stimuli to understand how the valuation of different rewards shifts over time among those with binge eating.

Moreover, incorporating non-food and food stimuli may facilitate an understanding of whether top-down influences on binge eating are generally or specifically impaired, such as inhibitory control. Indeed, meta-analytic results have suggested reduced inhibitory control to non-food and food stimuli on go/no-go tasks among individuals with binge-eating pathology; however, inhibitory control deficits appear to be less pronounced in response to non-food stimuli (Wu, Hartmann, et al., 2013). Emerging work supports the utility of studying the neural underpinnings of inhibitory control to non-food stimuli among those at risk for or with binge-eating pathology. A prospective longitudinal cohort study of adolescents administered a general, non-food go/no-go paradigm during fMRI scanning to participants at age 14 and follow-up psychological measures at age 16 (Bartholdy et al., 2019). Results indicated that participants who developed binge eating at age 16 demonstrated *increased* recruitment of the ACC and medial PFC during inhibitory control lapses compared to participants who did not develop binge eating. Further, as previously described, others have found no differences in brain and behavioral responses on a food-specific go/no-go task, but observed hypoactivation of right sensorimotor regions and the right dorsal striatum during no-go trials on a general go/no-go task in adult women with BN compared to those without the disorder (Skunde et al., 2016). Another study administered a general stop-signal task and found that adult women with BN showed reduced proactive inhibition relative to non-eating disorder controls, which was accompanied by higher activation in the left dorsolateral superior frontal gyrus in women with versus without BN (Westwater et al., 2021). Reactive inhibition was intact in women with BN, and there were no differences in neural activation. This study also found that left dorsolateral superior frontal gyrus activation during proactive inhibition was positively associated with post-scan caloric intake during an *ad libitum* meal; however, this association was observed for all groups. Taken together, this example of behavioral and neural responses during food and non-food inhibitory control tasks among persons with binge-eating pathology highlights the merits of using both food and non-food stimuli in research.

Neurobiological contributions to binge eating across eating disorder diagnoses

Binge eating is a transdiagnostic symptom, occurring in BN, BED, and individuals with anorexia nervosa binge eating/purging subtype (AN-BP) who binge eat. This chapter focused on the top-down influences of binge eating in BN and BED, as the perspective of this author is that binge eating in AN-BP may be different than binge eating in BN and BED. For instance, binge eating in AN-BP may arise from a different metabolic state (chronic state of low nutrition) than binge eating in BN and BED; however, binge eating in BN often follows a period of fasting and/or restrictive eating (Elran-Barak et al., 2015). Further, emerging evidence suggests neural differences in AN-BP and BN on inhibitory control tasks and in response to tasting solutions (Oberndorfer et al., 2013; Westwater et al., 2021). However, an alternative perspective and hypothesis is that the top-down influences of binge eating are the same across low-weight and non-low-weight eating disorders.

Additionally, this chapter's presentation of top-down influences of binge eating in BED and BN assumes that neurobiological contributions to binge eating in these disorders are similar. Although recurrent engagement in binge eating is a diagnostic criterion of BED and BN, regular engagement in inappropriate compensatory behaviors is specific to BN. As such, differences in the clinical phenomenology of these disorders may differentially influence binge eating. Indeed, binge eating in BN occurs after a period of extreme caloric restriction (Zunker et al., 2011), whereas such caloric restriction would be a diagnostic rule-out for BED. Other work suggests differences in the nutritional content of binge episodes between individuals with BED and BN (Fitzgibbon & Blackman, 2000; Moraes et al., 2023). Finally, research has suggested that negative affect trajectories before and after binge eating significantly differ between individuals with BED and BN (Wonderlich et al., 2022). Taken together, there appear to be some behavioral and affective differences in binge eating between individuals with BED and BN. Thus, research that separately considers and compares the neurobiologically mediated influences of binge eating between these disorders is warranted.

Different theoretical models

Some of the research presented within this chapter was framed through the lens of dominant theories of binge eating, such as the affect regulation theory and the incentive-sensitization theory. Yet, other alternative theoretical frameworks for binge-eating pathology should be considered. For instance, results from reward processing research do not neatly align with the incentive-sensitization theory of binge eating, suggesting other models may better account for reward-related neurobiological alternations in binge eating. One such model could be the maladaptive scaling hypothesis, which posits that the subjective value of a reward is measured against an anchor, or reward that has been assigned the highest subjective value (Zald & Treadway, 2017). In the case of binge eating, highly palatable binge foods may downscale the value of typical rewards, such as money. To our knowledge, no research has empirically tested the maladaptive scaling hypothesis in binge-eating pathology, but it represents an intriguing framework for understanding binge eating.

Additionally, certain components of well-known eating disorder theories have been under-explored but could yield novel insights into the top-down mechanisms of binge-eating pathology. For example, the transdiagnostic cognitive-behavioral model of eating disorders implicates social processes in eating disorder behaviors (Fairburn, 2008), and research has found that interpersonal stress often precedes binge eating (Goldschmidt et al., 2014; Ranzenhofer et al., 2014). Moreover, emerging research suggests differences in neural processing of social information between individuals with binge-eating pathology and non-eating disorder controls (McAdams et al., 2022), but little is known about how neural differences in social processing are linked to binge-eating behavior. Nevertheless, elucidating the link between neural processing of social information and binge eating could be a fruitful avenue for enriching understanding of the top-down influences of binge eating.

Implications

The findings reviewed in this chapter have important implications for clinical practice. First, the results reinforce some techniques used in current evidence-based therapies for binge-eating pathology. For instance, findings that stress (and negative affect) may temporarily enhance the subjective value of food and risk for binge eating highlight the importance of emotion regulation and distress tolerance strategies used to modulate negative affect in dialectical behavior therapy for binge eating (Safer et al., 2009). Second, findings suggest that food-specific inhibitory control is comprised among individuals with binge-eating pathology and so support ongoing investigations of adjunctive neurocognitive inhibitory control training to reduce binge eating (Manasse et al., 2020). Third, emerging work intriguingly suggests that having recently eaten and being full (versus being in a fasted state) may make it challenging for individuals with binge-eating pathology to modulate binge-eating behavior. As such, this information could be incorporated into psychoeducation about factors that can increase vulnerability to binge eating and the management of such factors.

Although there are clinical implications of the existing research, this review highlighted three critical future directions for top-down research on binge eating to expand the clinical impact of these findings. First, the development of paradigms that can capture LOC and/or binge-eating behavior concurrent with neuroimaging is essential for pinpointing the neurobiological underpinnings of binge-eating pathology. This chapter discussed novel paradigms that measure attempts to control eating (Berner, Winter, et al., 2023) and shopping for foods to be consumed in an out-of-scanner binge-eating episode (Pearson et al., 2016). These paradigms have a high potential to refine and advance our knowledge of neural processes implicated in binge eating. However, continued research that employs these or other paradigms probing eating behavior is critically needed to elucidate our understanding of binge-eating pathology more fully and, ultimately, to create more effective treatments.

Second, most of the research reviewed here considered one or two higher-order influences on binge eating at a time and did not incorporate other factors that may influence binge eating. For instance, eating expectancies (Burr et al., 2023; Ortiz et al., 2022), perceived discrimination (Brown et al., 2022; Johnson et al., 2022), and body image concerns (Grilo et al., 2013; Stice & Van Ryzin, 2019) are some cognitive factors that have been linked to binge eating and could ostensibly increase the subjective value of food and risk of binge eating. Similarly, the impact of contextual factors, such as food insecurity and socioeconomic status, on neurobiology should be considered. Indeed, more recent theoretical models of binge-eating pathology risk and maintenance have called for increased integration of these factors into binge-eating research so that our models can be more precisely specified (Schaefer, Forester, Dvorak, et al., 2023; Tanofsky-Kraff et al., 2020).

Third, the preponderance of research on the neurobiology of binge eating to date has mostly studied adults and recruited female participants. Binge-eating pathology is often borne from an initial manifestation of LOC eating in childhood or adolescence and progresses into full-syndrome pathology in late adolescence and young adulthood (Tanofsky-Kraff et al., 2020). Characterizing the biobehavioral underpinnings of LOC eating in pediatric samples could inform precisely targeted treatments for this developmental group, and prevent the progression of LOC eating to binge-eating pathology. Additionally, although eating disorders predominantly affect girls and women, the difference is less pronounced in BED, and men have been historically understudied in eating disorders research (Swanson et al., 2011; Udo & Grilo, 2018). Given the potential roles of sex steroids on neurobiology (e.g., neural reward responses to highly palatable foods), research including men is needed to understand whether the neurobiological mechanisms are similar or different across the sexes, potentially necessitating sex-specific interventions (Culbert et al., 2021).

In conclusion, research on the neurobiological bases of binge-eating pathology is relatively nascent. However, the existing literature converges to suggest alterations in inhibitory control and reward processing brain networks that may, in concert with cognitive and contextual factors, enhance the risk and maintenance of binge-eating pathology. Additionally, exciting developments in measuring binge eating and LOC eating concurrent with neuroimaging hold promise for increasing the ecological validity of current science, advancing understanding of the neurobiology of this impairing symptom, and ultimately informing translational therapeutics.

References

American Psychiatric Association. (2013). *Diagnostic and statistical manual of mental disorders (DSM-5®)*. American Psychiatric Publishing.

Arnsten, A. F. T. (2015). Stress weakens prefrontal networks: Molecular insults to higher cognition. *Nature Neuroscience, 18*(10), 1376–1385. https://doi.org/10.1038/nn.4087

Bartholdy, S., Dalton, B., O'Daly, O. G., Campbell, I. C., & Schmidt, U. (2016). A systematic review of the relationship between eating, weight and inhibitory control using the stop signal task. *Neuroscience and Biobehavioral Reviews, 64*, 35–62. https://doi.org/10.1016/j.neubiorev.2016.02.010

Bartholdy, S., O'Daly, O. G., Campbell, I. C., Banaschewski, T., Barker, G., Bokde, A. L. W., Bromberg, U., Büchel, C., Quinlan, E. B., Desrivières, S., Flor, H., Frouin, V., Garavan, H., Gowland, P., Heinz, A., Ittermann, B., Martinot, J.-L., Paillère Martinot, M.-L., Nees, F., . . . IMAGEN Consortium. (2019). Neural correlates of failed inhibitory control as an early marker of disordered eating in adolescents. *Biological Psychiatry, 85*(11), 956–965. https://doi.org/10.1016/j.biopsych.2019.01.027

Berner, L. A., Harlé, K. M., Simmons, A. N., Yu, A., Paulus, M. P., Bischoff-Grethe, A., Wierenga, C. E., Bailer, U. F., & Kaye, W. H. (2023). State-specific alterations in the neural computations underlying inhibitory control in women remitted from bulimia nervosa. *Molecular Psychiatry, 28*(7), 3055–3062. https://doi.org/10.1038/s41380-023-02063-6

Berner, L. A., Stefan, M., Lee, S., Wang, Z., Terranova, K., Attia, E., & Marsh, R. (2018). Altered cortical thickness and attentional deficits in adolescent girls and women with bulimia nervosa. *Journal of Psychiatry & Neuroscience, 43*(3), 151–160. https://doi.org/10.1503/jpn.170070

Berner, L. A., Winter, S. R., Ayaz, H., Shewokis, P. A., Izzetoglu, M., Marsh, R., Nasser, J. A., Matteucci, A. J., & Lowe, M. R. (2023). Altered prefrontal activation during the inhibition of eating responses in women with bulimia nervosa. *Psychological Medicine, 53*(8), 3580–3590. https://doi.org/10.1017/S0033291722000198

Berner, L. A., Winter, S. R., Matheson, B. E., Benson, L., & Lowe, M. R. (2017). Behind binge eating: A review of food-specific adaptations of neurocognitive and neuroimaging tasks. *Physiology & Behavior, 176*, 59–70. https://doi.org/10.1016/j.physbeh.2017.03.037

Berridge, K. C. (1996). Food reward: Brain substrates of wanting and liking. *Neuroscience and Biobehavioral Reviews, 20*(1), 1–25. https://doi.org/10.1016/0149-7634(95)00033-b

Bodell, L. P., & Racine, S. E. (2022). A mechanistic staging model of reward processing alterations in individuals with binge-type eating disorders. *International Journal of Eating Disorders*. https://doi.org/10.1002/eat.23875

Bohon, C., & Stice, E. (2011). Reward abnormalities among women with full and subthreshold bulimia nervosa: A functional magnetic resonance imaging study. *International Journal of Eating Disorders, 44*(7), 585–595. https://doi.org/10.1002/eat.20869

Bohon, C., & Stice, E. (2012). Negative affect and neural response to palatable food intake in bulimia nervosa. *Appetite, 58*(3), 964–970. https://doi.org/10.1016/j.appet.2012.02.051

Boswell, R. G., & Kober, H. (2016). Food cue reactivity and craving predict eating and weight gain: A meta-analytic review. *Obesity Reviews, 17*(2), 159–177. https://doi.org/10.1111/obr.12354

Bronleigh, M., Baumann, O., & Stapleton, P. (2022). Neural correlates associated with processing food stimuli in anorexia nervosa and bulimia nervosa: An activation likelihood estimation meta-analysis of fMRI studies. *Eating and Weight Disorders, 27*(7), 2309–2320. https://doi.org/10.1007/s40519-022-01390-x

Brown, K. L., Graham, A. K., Perera, R. A., & LaRose, J. G. (2022). Eating to cope: Advancing our understanding of the effects of exposure to racial discrimination on maladaptive eating behaviors. *International Journal of Eating Disorders, 55*(12), 1744–1752. https://doi.org/10.1002/eat.23820

Burr, E. K., Dvorak, R. D., De Leon, A. N., Leary, A. V., Peterson, R., Schaefer, L. M., & Wonderlich, S. A. (2023). The role of eating expectancies and eating motives in the association between mood and loss-of-control eating: A national sample daily diary study. *Appetite, 180*, 106322. https://doi.org/10.1016/j.appet.2022.106322

Castro, D. C., Cole, S. L., & Berridge, K. C. (2015). Lateral hypothalamus, nucleus accumbens, and ventral pallidum roles in eating and hunger: Interactions between homeostatic and reward circuitry. *Frontiers in Systems Neuroscience, 9*, 90. https://doi.org/10.3389/fnsys.2015.00090

Chao, A. M., Grilo, C. M., & Sinha, R. (2016). Food cravings, binge eating, and eating disorder psychopathology: Exploring the moderating roles of gender and race. *Eating Behaviors, 21*, 41–47. https://doi.org/10.1016/j.eatbeh.2015.12.007

Culbert, K. M., Sisk, C. L., & Klump, K. L. (2021). A narrative review of sex differences in eating disorders: Is there a biological basis? *Clinical Therapeutics, 43*(1), 95–111. https://doi.org/10.1016/j.clinthera.2020.12.003

Cyr, M., Kopala-Sibley, D. C., Lee, S., Chen, C., Stefan, M., Fontaine, M., Terranova, K., Berner, L. A., & Marsh, R. (2017). Reduced inferior and orbital frontal thickness in adolescent bulimia nervosa persists over two-year follow-up. *Journal of the American Academy of Child and Adolescent Psychiatry, 56*(10), 866–874.e7. https://doi.org/10.1016/j.jaac.2017.08.008

Elran-Barak, R., Sztainer, M., Goldschmidt, A. B., Crow, S. J., Peterson, C. B., Hill, L. L., Crosby, R. D., Powers, P., Mitchell, J. E., & Le Grange, D. (2015). Dietary restriction behaviors and binge eating in anorexia nervosa, bulimia nervosa and binge eating disorder: Trans-diagnostic examination of the restraint model. *Eating Behaviors, 18*, 192–196. http://dx.doi.org/10.1016/j.eatbeh.2015.05.012

Ely, A. V., Wierenga, C. E., Bischoff-Grethe, A., Bailer, U. F., Berner, L. A., Fudge, J. L., Paulus, M. P., & Kaye, W. H. (2017). Response in taste circuitry is not modulated by hunger and satiety in women remitted from bulimia nervosa. *Journal of Abnormal Psychology, 126*(5), 519–530. https://doi.org/10.1037/abn0000218

Fairburn, C. G. (2008). *Cognitive behavior therapy and eating disorders.* Guilford Press.

Fischer, S., Breithaupt, L., Wonderlich, J., Westwater, M. L., Crosby, R. D., Engel, S. G., Thompson, J., Lavender, J., & Wonderlich, S. (2017). Impact of the neural correlates of stress and cue reactivity on stress related binge eating in the natural environment. *Journal of Psychiatric Research, 92*, 15–23. https://doi.org/10.1016/j.jpsychires.2017.03.017

Fitzgibbon, M. L., & Blackman, L. R. (2000). Binge eating disorder and bulimia nervosa: Differences in the quality and quantity of binge eating episodes. *International Journal of Eating Disorders, 27*(2), 238–243. https://doi.org/10.1002/(sici)1098-108x(200003)27:2<238::aid-eat12>3.0.co;2-q

Frank, G. K., Wagner, A., Achenbach, S., McConaha, C., Skovira, K., Aizenstein, H., Carter, C. S., & Kaye, W. H. (2006). Altered brain activity in women recovered from bulimic-type eating disorders after a glucose challenge: A pilot study. *International Journal of Eating Disorders, 39*(1), 76–79. https://doi.org/10.1002/eat.20210

Goldschmidt, A. B. (2017). Are loss of control while eating and overeating valid constructs? A critical review of the literature. *Obesity Reviews, 18*(4), 412–449. https://doi.org/10.1111/obr.12491

Goldschmidt, A. B., Dickstein, D. P., MacNamara, A. E., Phan, K. L., O'Brien, S., Le Grange, D., Fisher, J. O., & Keedy, S. (2018). A pilot study of neural correlates of loss of control eating in children with overweight/obesity: Probing intermittent access to food as a means of eliciting disinhibited eating. *Journal of Pediatric Psychology, 43*(8), 846–855. https://doi.org/10.1093/jpepsy/jsy009

Goldschmidt, A. B., Wonderlich, S. A., Crosby, R. D., Engel, S. G., Lavender, J. M., Peterson, C. B., Crow, S. J., Cao, L., & Mitchell, J. E. (2014). Ecological momentary assessment of stressful events and negative affect in bulimia nervosa. *Journal of Consulting and Clinical Psychology, 82*(1), 30–39. https://doi.org/10.1037/a0034974

Grilo, C. M., White, M. A., Gueorguieva, R., Wilson, G. T., & Masheb, R. M. (2013). Predictive significance of the overvaluation of shape/weight in obese patients with binge eating disorder: Findings from a randomized controlled trial with 12-month follow-up. *Psychological Medicine, 43*(6), 1335–1344. https://doi.org/10.1017/S0033291712002097

Haedt-Matt, A. A., & Keel, P. K. (2011). Revisiting the affect regulation model of binge eating: A meta-analysis of studies using ecological momentary assessment. *Psychological Bulletin, 137*(4), 660. https://doi.org/10.1037/a0023660

Hagan, K. E., Forbush, K. T., & Chen, P.-Y. (2016). Is dietary restraint a unitary or multi-faceted construct? Psychological Assessment, 29(10), 1249–1260. https://doi.org/10.1037/pas0000429.

Heatherton, T. F., & Baumeister, R. F. (1991). Binge eating as escape from self-awareness. *Psychological Bulletin, 110*, 86–108. https://doi.org/10.1037/0033-2909.110.1.86

Hege, M. A., Stingl, K. T., Kullmann, S., Schag, K., Giel, K. E., Zipfel, S., & Preissl, H. (2015). Attentional impulsivity in binge eating disorder modulates response inhibition performance and frontal brain networks. *International Journal of Obesity, 39*(2), 353–360. https://doi.org/10.1038/ijo.2014.99

Hilbert, A., Hartmann, A. S., Czaja, J., & Schoebi, D. (2013). Natural course of preadolescent loss of control eating. *Journal of Abnormal Psychology, 122*(3), 684–693. https://doi.org/10.1037/a0033330

Hilbert, A., Petroff, D., Herpertz, S., Pietrowsky, R., Tuschen-Caffier, B., Vocks, S., & Schmidt, R. (2020). Meta-analysis on the long-term effectiveness of psychological and medical treatments for binge-eating disorder. *International Journal of Eating Disorders, 53*(9), 1353–1376. https://doi.org/10.1002/eat.23297

Jansen, A. (1998). A learning model of binge eating: Cue reactivity and cue exposure. *Behaviour Research and Therapy, 36*(3), 257–272. https://doi.org/10.1016/S0005-7967(98)00055-2

Johnson, S. N., Forbush, K. T., & Swanson, T. J. (2022). The impact of discrimination on binge eating in a nationally representative sample of Latine individuals. *International Journal of Eating Disorders, 55*(8), 1120–1129. https://doi.org/10.1002/eat.23773

Kelley, A. E., Bakshi, V. P., Haber, S. N., Steininger, T. L., Will, M. J., & Zhang, M. (2002). Opioid modulation of taste hedonics within the ventral striatum. *Physiology & Behavior, 76*(3), 365–377. https://doi.org/10.1016/s0031-9384(02)00751-5

Kober, H., & Boswell, R. G. (2018). Potential psychological & neural mechanisms in binge eating disorder: Implications for treatment. *Clinical Psychology Review, 60*, 32–44. https://doi.org/10.1016/j.cpr.2017.12.004

Lavagnino, L., Arnone, D., Cao, B., Soares, J. C., & Selvaraj, S. (2016). Inhibitory control in obesity and binge eating disorder: A systematic review and meta-analysis of neurocognitive and neuroimaging studies. *Neuroscience and Biobehavioral Reviews, 68*, 714–726. https://doi.org/10.1016/j.neubiorev.2016.06.041

Leenaerts, N., Vaessen, T., Sunaert, S., Ceccarini, J., & Vrieze, E. (2023). How negative affect does and does not lead to binge eating—The importance of craving and negative urgency in bulimia nervosa. *Journal of Psychopathology and Clinical Science*. https://doi.org/10.1037/abn0000830

Li, N., Mitchison, D., Touyz, S., & Hay, P. (2019). Cross-sectional comparison of health-related quality of life and other features in people with and without objective and subjective binge eating using a general population sample. *BMJ Open, 9*(2), e024227. https://doi.org/10.1136/bmjopen-2018-024227

Linardon, J. (2018). Rates of abstinence following psychological or behavioral treatments for binge-eating disorder: Meta-analysis. *International Journal of Eating Disorders, 51*(8), 785–797. https://doi.org/10.1002/eat.22897

Linardon, J., & Wade, T. D. (2018). How many individuals achieve symptom abstinence following psychological treatments for bulimia nervosa? A meta-analytic review. *International Journal of Eating Disorders, 51*(4), 287–294. https://doi.org/10.1002/eat.22838

Lipson, S. K., & Sonneville, K. R. (2017). Eating disorder symptoms among undergraduate and graduate students at 12 U.S. colleges and universities. *Eating Behaviors, 24*, 81–88. https://doi.org/10.1016/j.eatbeh.2016.12.003

Lyu, Z., & Jackson, T. (2016). Acute stressors reduce neural inhibition to food cues and increase eating among binge eating disorder symptomatic women. *Frontiers in Behavioral Neuroscience, 10*, 188. https://doi.org/10.3389/fnbeh.2016.00188

Manasse, S. M., Lampe, E. W., Gillikin, L., Payne-Reichert, A., Zhang, F., Juarascio, A. S., & Forman, E. M. (2020). The project REBOOT protocol: Evaluating a personalized inhibitory control training as an adjunct to cognitive behavioral therapy for bulimia nervosa and binge-eating disorder. *International Journal of Eating Disorders, 53*(6), 1007–1013. https://doi.org/10.1002/eat.23225

McAdams, C. J., Efseroff, B., McCoy, J., Ford, L., & Timko, C. A. (2022). Social processing in eating disorders: Neuroimaging paradigms and research domain organizational constructs. *Current Psychiatry Reports, 24*(12), 777–788. https://doi.org/10.1007/s11920-022-01395-4

Mitchison, D., Touyz, S., González-Chica, D. A., Stocks, N., & Hay, P. (2017). How abnormal is binge eating? 18-Year time trends in population prevalence and burden. *Acta Psychiatrica Scandinavica, 136*(2), 147–155. https://doi.org/10.1111/acps.12735

Monteleone, A. M., Pellegrino, F., Croatto, G., Carfagno, M., Hilbert, A., Treasure, J., Wade, T., Bulik, C. M., Zipfel, S., Hay, P., Schmidt, U., Castellini, G., Favaro, A., Fernandez-Aranda, F., Il Shin, J., Voderholzer, U., Ricca, V., Moretti, D., Busatta, D., . . . Solmi, M. (2022). Treatment of eating disorders: A systematic meta-review of meta-analyses and network meta-analyses. *Neuroscience and Biobehavioral Reviews, 142*, 104857. https://doi.org/10.1016/j.neubiorev.2022.104857

Moraes, C. E. F. de, Antunes, M. M. L., Mourilhe, C., Sichieri, R., Hay, P., & Appolinario, J. C. (2023). Food consumption during binge eating episodes in binge eating spectrum conditions from a representative sample of a Brazilian metropolitan city. *Nutrients, 15*(7), 1573. https://doi.org/10.3390/nu15071573

Morales, I., & Berridge, K. C. (2020). "Liking" and "wanting" in eating and food reward: Brain mechanisms and clinical implications. *Physiology & Behavior, 227*, 113152. https://doi.org/10.1016/j.physbeh.2020.113152

Ng, L., & Davis, C. (2013). Cravings and food consumption in binge eating disorder. *Eating Behaviors, 14*(4), 472–475. https://doi.org/10.1016/j.eatbeh.2013.08.011

Oberndorfer, T. A., Frank, G. K. W., Simmons, A. N., Wagner, A., McCurdy, D., Fudge, J. L., Yang, T. T., Paulus, M. P., & Kaye, W. H. (2013). Altered insula response to sweet taste processing after recovery from anorexia and bulimia nervosa. *American Journal of Psychiatry, 170*(10), 1143–1151. https://doi.org/10.1176/appi.ajp.2013.11111745

Oliva, R., Morys, F., Horstmann, A., Castiello, U., & Begliomini, C. (2019). The impulsive brain: Neural underpinnings of binge eating behavior in normal-weight adults. *Appetite, 136*, 33–49. https://doi.org/10.1016/j.appet.2018.12.043

Ortiz, A. M. L., Davis, H. A., Riley, E. N., & Smith, G. T. (2022). The interaction between affective lability and eating expectancies predicts binge eating. *Eating Disorders*, *30*(3), 331–344. https://doi.org/10.1080/10640266.2021.1905449

Parker, M. N., Burton Murray, H., Piers, A. D., Muratore, A., Lowe, M. R., Manasse, S. M., Ayaz, H., & Juarascio, A. S. (2023). Prefrontal cortex activation by binge-eating status in individuals with obesity while attempting to reappraise responses to food using functional near infrared spectroscopy. *Eating and Weight Disorders*, *28*(1), 34. https://doi.org/10.1007/s40519-023-01558-z

Pearson, C. M., Chester, D. S., Powell, D., Wonderlich, S. A., & Smith, G. T. (2016). Investigating the reinforcing value of binge anticipation. *International Journal of Eating Disorders*, *49*(6), 539–541. https://doi.org/10.1002/eat.22547

Polivy, J., & Herman, C. P. (1985). Dieting and binging. A causal analysis. *The American Psychologist*, *40*(2), 193–201. https://doi.org/10.1037//0003-066x.40.2.193

Radeloff, D., Willmann, K., Otto, L., Lindner, M., Putnam, K., Leeuwen, S. V., Kaye, W. H., Poustka, F., & Wagner, A. (2014). High-fat taste challenge reveals altered striatal response in women recovered from bulimia nervosa: A pilot study. *World Journal of Biological Psychiatry*, *15*(4), 307–316. https://doi.org/10.3109/15622975.2012.671958

Ranzenhofer, L. M., Engel, S. G., Crosby, R. D., Anderson, M., Vannucci, A., Cohen, L. A., Cassidy, O., & Tanofsky-Kraff, M. (2014). Using ecological momentary assessment to examine interpersonal and affective predictors of loss of control eating in adolescent girls. *International Journal of Eating Disorders*, *47*(7), 748–757. https://doi.org/10.1002/eat.22333

Rösch, S. A., Schmidt, R., Lührs, M., Ehlis, A.-C., Hesse, S., & Hilbert, A. (2020). Evidence of fNIRS-based prefrontal cortex hypoactivity in obesity and binge-eating disorder. *Brain Sciences*, *11*(1), 19. https://doi.org/10.3390/brainsci11010019

Safer, D. L., Telch, C. F., & Chen, E. Y. (2009). *Dialectical behavior therapy for binge eating and bulimia.* Guilford Press.

Schaefer, L. M., Forester, G., Burr, E. K., Laam, L., Crosby, R. D., Peterson, C. B., Crow, S. J., Engel, S. G., Dvorak, R. D., & Wonderlich, S. A. (2023). Examining the role of craving in affect regulation models of binge eating: Evidence from an ecological momentary assessment study. *Journal of Psychopathology and Clinical Science*, *132*(6), 725–732. https://doi.org/10.1037/abn0000839

Schaefer, L. M., Forester, G., Dvorak, R. D., Steinglass, J., & Wonderlich, S. A. (2023). Integrating aspects of affect, reward, and cognition to develop more comprehensive models of binge-eating pathology. *International Journal of Eating Disorders*, *56*(8), 1502–1510. https://doi.org/10.1002/eat.23971

Schag, K., Schönleber, J., Teufel, M., Zipfel, S., & Giel, K. E. (2013). Food-related impulsivity in obesity and binge eating disorder—A systematic review. *Obesity Reviews*, *14*(6), 477–495. https://doi.org/10.1111/obr.12017

Schienle, A., Schäfer, A., Hermann, A., & Vaitl, D. (2009). Binge-eating disorder: Reward sensitivity and brain activation to images of food. *Biological Psychiatry*, *65*(8), 654–661. https://doi.org/10.1016/j.biopsych.2008.09.028

Simon, J. J., Skunde, M., Walther, S., Bendszus, M., Herzog, W., & Friederich, H.-C. (2016). Neural signature of food reward processing in bulimic-type eating disorders. *Social Cognitive and Affective Neuroscience*, *11*(9), 1393–1401. https://doi.org/10.1093/scan/nsw049

Skunde, M., Walther, S., Simon, J. J., Wu, M., Bendszus, M., Herzog, W., & Friederich, H. C. (2016). Neural signature of behavioural inhibition in women with bulimia nervosa. *Journal of Psychiatry & Neuroscience*, *41*(5), E69–78.

Steinglass, J., Foerde, K., Kostro, K., Shohamy, D., & Walsh, B. T. (2015). Restrictive food intake as a choice—A paradigm for study. *International Journal of Eating Disorders*, *48*(1), 59–66. https://doi.org/10.1002/eat.22345

Stice, E., Marti, C. N., & Rohde, P. (2013). Prevalence, incidence, impairment, and course of the proposed DSM-5 eating disorder diagnoses in an 8-year prospective community study of young women. *Journal of Abnormal Psychology*, *122*(2), 445–457. https://doi.org/10.1037/a0030679

Stice, E., & Van Ryzin, M. J. (2019). A prospective test of the temporal sequencing of risk factor emergence in the dual pathway model of eating disorders. *Journal of Abnormal Psychology*, *128*(2), 119–128. https://doi.org/10.1037/abn0000400

Swanson, S. A., Crow, S. J., Grange, D. L., Swendsen, J., & Merikangas, K. R. (2011). Prevalence and correlates of eating disorders in adolescents: Results from the national comorbidity survey replication adolescent supplement. *Archives of General Psychiatry*, *68*(7), 714–723. https://doi.org/10.1001/archgenpsychiatry.2011.22

Tannous, W. K., Hay, P., Girosi, F., Heriseanu, A. I., Ahmed, M. U., & Touyz, S. (2021). The economic cost of bulimia nervosa and binge eating disorder: A population-based study. *Psychological Medicine*, 52(16), 3924–3938. https://doi.org/10.1017/S0033291721000775

Tanofsky-Kraff, M., Schvey, N. A., & Grilo, C. M. (2020). A developmental framework of binge-eating disorder based on pediatric loss of control eating. *The American Psychologist*, *75*(2), 189–203. https://doi.org/10.1037/amp0000592

Tanofsky-Kraff, M., Shomaker, L. B., Olsen, C., Roza, C. A., Wolkoff, L. E., Columbo, K. M., Raciti, G., Zocca, J. M., Wilfley, D. E., Yanovski, S. Z., & Yanovski, J. A. (2011). A prospective study of pediatric loss of control eating and psychological outcomes. *Journal of Abnormal Psychology*, *120*(1), 108–118. https://doi.org/10.1037/a0021406

Udo, T., & Grilo, C. M. (2018). Prevalence and correlates of DSM-5–defined eating disorders in a nationally representative sample of U.S. adults. *Biological Psychiatry*, *84*(5), 345–354. https://doi.org/10.1016/j.biopsych.2018.03.014

Walsh, B. T. (2011). The importance of eating behavior in eating disorders. *Physiology & Behavior*, *104*(4), 525–529. https://doi.org/10.1016/j.physbeh.2011.05.007

Westwater, M. L., Mancini, F., Gorka, A. X., Shapleske, J., Serfontein, J., Grillon, C., Ernst, M., Ziauddeen, H., & Fletcher, P. C. (2021). Prefrontal responses during proactive and reactive inhibition are differentially impacted by stress in anorexia and bulimia nervosa. *Journal of Neuroscience*, *41*(20), 4487–4499. https://doi.org/10.1523/JNEUROSCI.2853-20.2021

Wonderlich, J. A., Crosby, R. D., Engel, S. G., Crow, S. J., Peterson, C. B., Le Grange, D., Wonderlich, S. A., & Fischer, S. (2022). Negative affect and binge eating: Assessing the unique trajectories of negative affect before and after binge-eating episodes across eating disorder diagnostic classifications. *International Journal of Eating Disorders*, *55*(2), 223–230. https://doi.org/10.1002/eat.23648

World Health Organization. (2019). *International statistical classification of diseases and related health problems* (11th ed.). World Health Organization. https://icd.who.int/

Wu, M., Giel, K. E., Skunde, M., Schag, K., Rudofsky, G., de Zwaan, M., Zipfel, S., Herzog, W., & Friederich, H.-C. (2013). Inhibitory control and decision making under risk in bulimia nervosa and binge-eating disorder. *International Journal of Eating Disorders*, *46*(7), 721–728. https://doi.org/10.1002/eat.22143

Wu, M., Hartmann, M., Skunde, M., Herzog, W., & Friederich, H. C. (2013). Inhibitory control in bulimic-type eating disorders: A systematic review and meta-analysis. *PLOS ONE*, *8*(12), e83412. https://doi.org/10.1371/journal.pone.0083412

Zald, D. H., & Treadway, M. T. (2017). Reward processing, neuroeconomics, and psychopathology. *Annual Review of Clinical Psychology*, *13*(1), 471–495. https://doi.org/10.1146/annurev-clinpsy-032816-044957

Zunker, C., Peterson, C. B., Crosby, R. D., Cao, L., Engel, S. G., Mitchell, J. E., & Wonderlich, S. A. (2011). Ecological momentary assessment of bulimia nervosa: Does dietary restriction predict binge eating? *Behaviour Research and Therapy*, *49*(10), 714–717.

16

Physical Activity and Exercise

Katherine Schaumberg, Lauren Pictor, Max Frank, and Sasha Gorrell

Brief Definitional Overview

Exercise: Intentional, structured physical activity.

Maladaptive exercise: Exercise that includes *problematic psychological sequalae* (e.g., feeling driven or compulsive; feelings of guilt when missing exercise; overreliance on exercise to manage affect and/or concerns about shape and weight, along with *life interfering symptoms* (e.g., inability to reduce exercise; exercising despite illness or injury; exercise routines interfering with work, school, or social functioning).

Life interfering symptoms: Symptoms associated with quality-of-life and/or health impacts; including limitations to social and occupational functioning.

Introduction

In the context of eating disorders, exercise presents a mental health paradox. In the general population, exercise (i.e., planned, structured physical activity) is associated with positive mental health outcomes (Chekroud et al., 2018; Deslandes et al., 2009; Vankim & Nelson, 2013) and is increasingly prescribed as a component of mental health treatment (Carek et al., 2011; Herring et al., 2010). However, during an eating disorder, exercise has a high potential to become a maladaptive behavior that demonstrates compulsive qualities and it can interfere with both quality of life and eating disorder recovery (Cook et al., 2014; Davis et al., 1997; Davis & Kaptein, 2006; Shroff et al., 2006).

Defining maladaptive exercise has led to substantial debate and myriad terminology, including compulsive exercise, obligatory exercise, compensatory exercise, exercise addiction, excessive exercise, and driven exercise, among others. While definitions of these terms and their measurement components overlap substantially (see Table 16.1 and Figure 16.1), clarification among them is occasionally necessary when synthesizing literature. This chapter uses the broad term *maladaptive exercise* unless clarifying a specific finding in which precise definition is important. While few studies have examined multiple maladaptive exercise definitions simultaneously, those that do find substantial overlap in endorsement

Katherine Schaumberg et al., *Physical Activity and Exercise*. In: *The Handbook of the Neurobiology of Eating Disorders*. Edited by: Christina E. Wierenga and Joanna E. Steinglass, Oxford University Press. © Oxford University Press (2025). DOI: 10.1093/9780197675212.003.0017

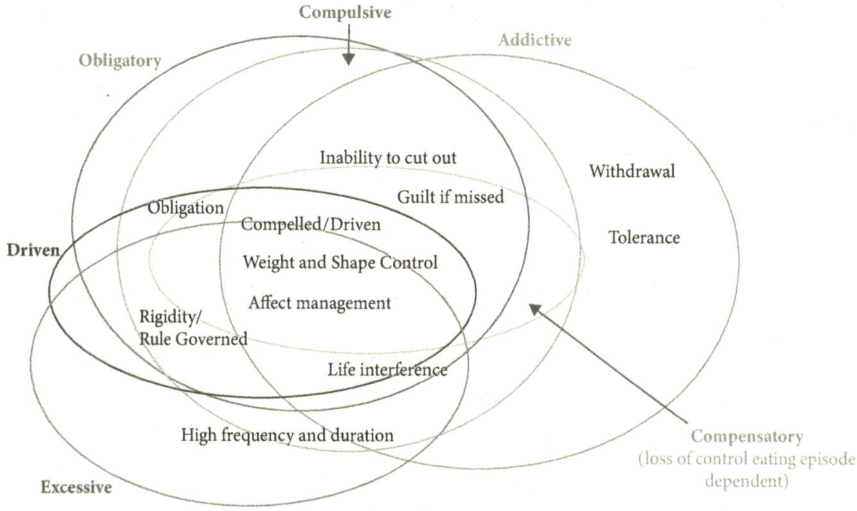

Figure 16.1 A visual aid of conceptual overlap in maladaptive exercise terminology.

of compulsive and addictive exercise, with compensatory exercise showing some distinction from other maladaptive exercise definitions (Holland et al., 2014; Scharmer et al., 2020).

Although some debate persists regarding an optimal definition of maladaptive exercise, consistent evidence indicates that some individuals can *adaptively* exercise at very high levels, which may meet frequency, intensity, and duration cutoffs that would otherwise be considered "excessive," without negative consequence (Juwono et al., 2022). Further, individuals may experience negative sequalae of maladaptive exercise even when exercise is present at moderate levels (Adkins & Keel, 2005; Young et al., 2017). Therefore, definitions of maladaptive exercise which include components assessing one's *psychological relationship with exercise* (e.g., whether exercise feels driven or compulsive; feelings of guilt when missing exercise; overreliance on exercise to manage affect and/or concerns about shape and weight) along with *life interfering symptoms* (e.g., inability to reduce exercise; exercising despite illness or injury; exercise routines interfering with work, school, or social functioning) appear to most adequately capture the predominant phenotypic presentation of maladaptive exercise in eating disorders.

Biological Framework

Basic animal and human research demonstrates that exercise can engage neurochemical pathways related to both reward promotion and threat reduction (Anderson & Shivakumar, 2013; Asmundson et al., 2013; Greenwood et al., 2012; Herring et al., 2010). Models of maladaptive exercise propose that, for individuals with eating disorders, over-engagement of these reward and threat mechanisms,

Table 16.1 Maladaptive exercise constructs

Construct	Common Measure(s) and Measure Characteristics	Example Items	Cognitive Features	Affective Features	Behavioral Features
Compensatory Exercise	Eating Disorder Examination v17.0—adapted [EDE; (Fairburn et al., 2014; Presseller et al., 2022)]: Semi-structured interview to assess symptoms associated with eating disorders; ED100K (Thornton et al., 2018): Self-reported measure that captures historical eating disorder symptoms	EDE: "When you exercised in the past month, did you exercise to control your weight, alter your shape or amount of fat, or burn off calories in direct response to a loss of control episode?" ED100K: "Have you ever used [compensatory exercise] to compensate for episodes of binge eating or over eating?"		Reduces feelings of guilt about overeating	* Occurs after an episode of overeating

Compulsive Exercise	Compulsive Exercise Test [CET; (Meyer et al., 2016)]: 24-item self-report with five subscales. Total score > 15 across subscales indicates compulsive exercise Function of Exercise Scale [FES; (DiBartolo et al., 2007)]: 16-item, self-report questionnaire that assesses motivation to exercise; the "Weight and Appearance" subscale has been shown to have positive correlations with ED symptoms Yale-Brown-Cornell Eating Disorder Scale [YBC-EDS; (Mazure et al., 1994)]: 65-item self-report about severity of symptoms with an "exercise rituals" subscale	CET: "I follow a set routine for my exercise sessions" FES: "I exercise to escape/avoid/stop bad feelings" YBC-EDS: "Need to exercise in a specific way or at a specific time"	Motivated by weight and shape control AND/OR affect regulation	Mood improvement; guilt if missed. Lack of Enjoyment Avoidance of negative affect (Withdrawal)	Exercise Rigidity Rule-Driven Behavior (Habit)b)

continued

Table 16.1 *continued*

Construct	**Common Measure(s) and Measure Characteristics**	**Example Items**	**Cognitive Features**	**Affective Features**	**Behavioral Features**
Excessive Exercise	EDE (see above) Eating Disorder Examination-Questionnaire [EDE-Q; (Fairburn & Bèglin, 1994; Luce & Crowther, 1999)]: 28-item self-report measure adapted from the EDE Eating Pathology Symptom Inventory [EPSI; (Forbush et al., 2013)]: 45-item self-report measure of current eating pathology	EDE: Over the past four weeks have you exercised as a means of controlling your weight, altering your shape or amount of fat, or burning off calories?" EDEQ: Over the past 28 days, how many times have you exercised in a "driven" or "compulsive" way as a means of controlling your weight, shape or amount of fat, or to burn off calories?" Example Item: "I felt that I needed to exercise nearly every day"	Motivated by weight and shape control		x2 Daily or almost daily; 1 hour or more
Driven Exercise	EDE; ED100K; CET (see above)	EDE: "Have you exercised even when it might interfere with other commitments or do you harm?" ED100k: "Have you ever felt compelled to exercise—like you had to do it—to control your body shape or weight?" CET: "I feel extremely guilty if I miss an exercise session"	Motivated by weight and shape control AND/OR affect regulation	Feeling "compelled" or "driven" to complete exercise	Exercise interferes with functional life activities

Exercise Addiction	Exercise Dependence Scale (EDS; Hausenblas & Downs, 2002): 21-item self-report measure on exercise dependency; scoring a 5 or 6 on 3 or more of the DSM-IV criteria for dependency indicates risk for exercise dependence	"I am unable to reduce how long I exercise"	Motivated by weight and shape control AND/OR affect regulation.	Needing to exercise more to produce a similar effect over time	Exercising more than intended Inability to reduce or cut out Interference with life activities
Obligatory Exercise	Obligatory Exercise Questionnaire (OEQ: (Pasman & Thompson, 1988): 20-item self-reported questionnaire about compelled exercise	"I sometimes feel like I don't want to exercise, but I go ahead and push myself anyway"			Exercise Rigidity Rule-Driven Behavior (Habit)

Note: Other measures of these constructs are also routinely used. Common examples of measures are provided but not meant to be exhaustive. *Endorsement required mediated by cognitive processes, may lead to exercise that is habitual and compulsive (Adams, 2009; Adams & Kirkby, 2002; Bamber et al., 2003; Bratland Sanda et al., 2011; Cook et al., 2014; Davis & Claridge, 1998; Davis & Kaptein, 2006; Guarda et al., 2015; Herring et al., 2014; Lichtenstein et al., 2017; Shroff et al., 2006).

An animal model of maladaptive exercise

Rodent research specifically suggests that free access to voluntary exercise during nutritional compromise resulting from time-restricted food access can trigger an anorexic-like syndrome. This activity-based anorexia (ABA) model is the only well-supported animal model of eating disorder onset. Changes in leptin, a hormone that modulates reward circuitry and plays a role in appetitive and satiety signaling, are specifically noted as predictive of hyperactivity (Holtkamp et al., 2003, 2006), and hypoleptinemia may be one mechanism which spurs hyperactivity in this context. Of note, female adolescent mice are particularly susceptible to experiencing ABA (Chowdhury et al., 2015), reflecting the preponderance of female (vs. male) humans who present with anorexia nervosa (AN) along with peak age of eating disorder onset. From an evolutionary psychology perspective, mechanisms of the ABA model could include that biological reinforcement of exercise is heightened during periods of starvation as a motivational effort for foraging (Adan et al., 2010), or as an attempt to raise body temperature during a starvation-induced drop in metabolism (Hillebrand et al., 2005).

Biological reinforcement of exercise

Physical activity promotes changes in the brain via increases in metabolism, oxygenation, and blood flow. Experimental research consistently demonstrates that physical activity leads to acute shifts in neurotransmitter and neurohormone availability and function across both rodents and humans. While the effects of exercise on the body are diverse, several specific effects are relevant to potential mechanisms that may give rise to and maintain patterns of maladaptive exercise. Candidate biomarkers that may play a role in these processes include leptin, brain-derived neurotrophic factor (BDNF), cortisol, endocannabinoids (eCB), serotonin (5-HT), dopamine (DA), Interleukin-6 (IL-6), epinephrine, and norepinephrine. Animal studies indicate that exercise modulates major neurotransmitters associated with a state of alertness (norepinephrine), the pleasure and reward system (DA), level of anxiety (eCB, 5-HT; Matta Mello Portugal et al., 2013), and euphoria and well-being (eCB; Dietrich & McDaniel, 2004). Basic animal and human research both support the proposition that exercise engages pathways related to both threat-reduction and reward, and an acute bout of exercise can impact peripheral concentrations of threat- and reward-related biomarkers. Evidence supporting (1) the impacts of exercise on these biomarkers and (2) connections with reward and/or threat mechanisms relevant to eating disorders are summarized in Table 16.2. While potential biological mechanisms of action to promote maladaptive exercise are largely untested in humans, leptin appears to be the strongest and most well-researched candidate biomarker at present. In addition to research supporting leptin as a mechanism of action in the ABA model (Hillebrand et al., 2008), exercise has demonstrated association with reduced plasma leptin post-exercise in a small sample with AN, but not in healthy control women (Dostalova et al., 2007). Further, plasma leptin levels have been associated with driven exercise (Ehrlich et al., 2009), and serum leptin with motor restlessness (Holtkamp et al., 2006) in AN samples. With regard to other biomarkers that may play a role in the development and maintenance of maladaptive exercise, BDNF, eCB, and cortisol currently demonstrate robust preclinical effects and evidence that exercise produces acute impacts across both animal and human samples.

Behavioral reinforcement of exercise

In addition to biological reinforcement, some research has examined exercise using behavioral reinforcement tasks and observations of exercise effects in-lab and in natural environments. Both automatic, affective processes as well as higher-order self-control can influence exercise engagement, along with the likelihood that exercise may become maladaptive.

Rewarding effects of exercise

Research investigating the rewarding effects of exercise posits that exercise may be a particularly salient reward for individuals with eating disorders, even in a context of low mood/anhedonia that is often experienced within an active eating disorder. This is believed to be due to the momentary positive affect that may spur acute bouts of exercise along with a Western cultural contextualization which supports high valuation of exercise behavior that may also shape positive-reinforcement exercise expectancies and amplify its rewarding effects (Coniglio et al., 2022). For example, a study using ecological momentary assessment in a sample of individuals with AN found that, over the course of a week, physical activity level predicted positive affect, and positive affect also predicted physical activity within the same hour and within the next hour (Karr et al., 2017). Behavioral research that has examined the willingness to work for exercise among individuals with AN additionally found that individuals with greater commitment to exercise worked harder on a progressive-ratio computer task for the opportunity to exercise as compared to those with less commitment to exercise, which persisted after weight restoration (Klein et al., 2010). This finding further highlights both (1) a high reward value of exercise reflective of willingness to work for exercise, and (2) variability

Table 16.2 Evidence supporting the impacts of exercise on candidate biomarkers and connections with reward and/or threat mechanisms relevant to eating disorders

Biomarker	Evidence of Response to Exercise	Link with Reward and/or Threat (focus on eating disorders)
Brain-derived Neurotrophic Factor	Consistent evidence that acute exercise induces changes in blood-borne BDNF: Meta-analysis (*N* = 29 studies): A bout of exercise has moderate positive effect on plasma and serum brain-derived neurotrophic factor (Hedges' g = 0.46); acute effect is potentiated by prior regular exercise training (Szuhany et al., 2015); Meta-analysis (*N* = 55 studies): concentrations of peripheral blood brain-derived neurotrophic factor are higher after acute exercise (SMD = 0.59), augmented in those with better fitness (Dinoff et al., 2017)	Expression in the mesolimbic reward system is altered in the rodent model of AN after wheel running (Ho et al., 2016) In humans, neurotrophic signaling impacts hippocampal functioning—relating to reward sensations, emotions, and mood (Kumar et al., 2019; Severinsen & Pedersen, 2020)
Cortisol	In young adults, high-intensity exercise leads to increases in cortisol after exercise compared to baseline (Guarda et al., 2015) Cortisol levels are elevated in patients with AN [e.g.,(Bailer & Kaye, 2003)] and even more so when they show high levels of driven exercise (Klein et al., 2007)	Elevated cortisol is consistently associated with threat processing, including in samples of individuals with anorexia nervosa (Guarda et al., 2015) Inpatients with anorexia nervosa show blunted reactivity to social stressors; although cortisol output was regulated with weight recovery, irregularities in hypothalamic–pituitary–adrenal (HPA) axis reactivity persisted (Schmalbach et al., 2020)
Serotonin (*5-hydroxytryptamine*)	In a recent rodent study, hyperactivity (induced by dietary restriction) was attenuated by tryptophan co-treatment (Saeed et al., 2021) and in healthy human runners, metabolomic analyses revealed that the phenylalanine, tyrosine and tryptophan biosynthesis pathway was the most relevant pathway modified, compared to controls (Tabone et al., 2021)	Prior work demonstrates associations between kynurenine metabolism and anhedonia in adolescents (Gabbay et al., 2012) and, in patients with anorexia nervosa, acute tryptophan depletion reduces reward sensitivity (Kaye et al., 2013) and reduces anxiety—even among those who are weight restored (Kaye et al., 2005)

Endocannabinoids	Acute exercise has demonstrated effects on plasma and serum measures of endocannabinoids, including in psychiatric populations (Brellenthin et al., 2017; Crombie et al., 2020; Meyer et al., 2019) Plasma AEA concentrations after exercise are associated with serum brain-derived neurotrophic factor (Heyman et al., 2012)	Rodents administered a cannabinoid antagonist or have cannabinoid receptors knocked-out reduce wheel running by 30–40% compared to controls (De Chiara et al., 2010; Dubreucq et al., 2010, 2013). This reduction relates to the *motivational* aspects of wheel running (Brellenthin et al., 2017) Wheel running is influenced by cannabinoid receptors located on GABAergic neurons in reward-processing regions such as the ventral tegmental area and striatum (De Chiara et al., 2010; Dubreucq et al., 2013). Because GABAergic neurons are co-localized with dopamine neurons in these areas, it is thought that endocannabinoid activity suppresses GABAergic output to dopamine neurons, permitting a transient increase in dopamine transmission and enhancing the biochemical reinforcement of wheel running. Exercise-induced increases in endocannabinoids are associated with central mood state improvements in human clinical and non-clinical populations (Brellenthin et al., 2017; Crombie et al., 2018, 2021; Meyer et al., 2019) and reductions in anxiety and fear ratings during a threat task (Crombie et al., 2021)
Leptin	Acute exercise was associated with reduced plasma leptin post-exercise in a small sample with anorexia nervosa, but not in healthy control women (Dostalova et al., 2007) Plasma leptin levels show association with driven exercise (Ehrlich et al., 2009) and serum leptin with motor restlessness (Holtkamp et al., 2006) in anorexia nervosa.	Leptin assists with energy homeostasis and regulation of body weight—protecting from reductions in fat-mass. Leptin also plays a role in dopaminergic reward systems, particularly in relation to suppressing food-related reward (Leinninger et al., 2009; Monteleone & Maj, 2013)
Homovanillic Acid	A bout of moderate physical activity has demonstrated impacts on plasma levels of homovanillic acid, a dopamine metabolite (Kendler et al., 1983; McMorris et al., 2008)	A pharmacological agent impacting plasma homovanillic acid is also associated with changes in brain activity when anticipating reward and loss (da Silva Alves et al., 2011) Dysfunction of dopamine reward system is implicated in addiction and eating disorders (Blum et al., 2014; O'Hara et al., 2015; Volkow et al., 2003) Anhedonia is associated with driven exercise in patients with anorexia nervosa (Davis & Woodside, 2002)

among the reinforcement value of exercise which is potentially reflective of risk for maladaptive exercise (Klein et al., 2010).

Threat-reduction effects of exercise

In addition to its rewarding effects, exercise also demonstrates substantial potential impact related to threat reduction in the context of eating disorders. Initial experience sampling studies support the notion that maladaptive exercise serves a threat-reduction effect; for example, individuals with eating disorders report reductions in negative affect post-exercise (Engel et al., 2013; Kolar et al., 2020; Reichert et al., 2020). Further, the most central eating disorder fears in a network analysis study predicted excessive exercise (but not other eating disorder behaviors) at a two-month follow-up (Levinson & Williams, 2020), suggesting the potential importance of negative reinforcement patterns to maladaptive exercise maintenance.

Potential genetic underpinnings of maladaptive exercise

Substantial differences exist in individuals' experiences of exercise, including the degree to which one finds exercise reinforcing and engages in exercise over time, and both twin and molecular genetic studies indicate that propensity for physical activity engagement is both variable and heritable (de Geus et al., 2014; Flack et al., 2019; Herring et al., 2014; Klimentidis et al., 2018). Further, high levels of physical activity are, at a genetic level, positively associated with a risk for AN (r_g = 0.17), indicating that a portion of the common-variant genetic risk that is identified with AN is shared with physical activity (associations between physical activity and other eating disorders have not yet been evaluated).

At a phenotypic level, both compulsive and addictive traits and symptoms are associated with maladaptive exercise (Davis & Kaptein, 2006; Shroff et al., 2006), with the most consistent findings indicating strong overlap between maladaptive exercise and both perfectionism and obsessive compulsive traits. These traits are often assessed concurrently; thus, it is still unclear whether premorbid obsessive-compulsive traits may give rise to the development and entrenchment of maladaptive exercise as an eating disorder develops, or whether maladaptive exercise and obsessive-compulsive symptoms may jointly influence one another during illness; however, initial genetic findings further the narrative that obsessive-compulsive disorder risk may specifically influence the likelihood of maladaptive exercise. One investigation found that, in a large, epidemiological sample of youth, maladaptive exercise was the only eating disorder behavior predicted by both an obsessive-compulsive and an AN polygenic risk score (Yilmaz et al., 2022).

Neuroanatomy

Current knowledge of the neuroanatomy underlying maladaptive exercise within eating disorders is quite limited, with no published work to-date that confirms a particular neurobiological representation of this behavior. However, theoretical discussion of maladaptive exercise in eating disorders points to neural regions associated with affect-regulation (Kolar & Gorrell, 2021), reward sensitivity (Gorrell et al., 2020, 2022), and compulsivity (Dittmer et al., 2018; Kolar et al., 2022; Meyer et al., 2011). Further, empirical evidence exists both within studies of animal models (e.g., Beeler et al., 2021; Foldi et al., 2017a, 2017b) and among human samples who have recovered from AN (e.g., O'Hara, Keyes, Renwick, Leyton, et al., 2016) that points to brain regions and processes that will inform future research efforts in this domain.

Applying neurobiological models of anorexia nervosa to exercise

When considering the neuroanatomy of restrictive eating disorders more generally, two companion models centered on striatal function, a reward-deficit model (Kaye et al., 2013; Wierenga et al., 2014) and a habit-centered model have been proposed to account for the maintenance of symptoms. Study of these models specifically in samples with AN has consistently found broad deficits in the frontostriatal network (Fladung et al., 2010; Holsen et al., 2012; Kaye et al., 2013; Steinglass & Walsh, 2016; Walsh, 2013; Wierenga et al., 2014). Here, it is proposed that in the earlier stages of illness, behavior is more goal-directed (reward-deficit model), which then transitions over time to compulsivity (habit-centered model) (Meier et al., 2020; Steinglass & Walsh, 2016; Walsh, 2013). Recent discussion of how engagement in movement might evolve across the eating disorder disease state also suggests that neural representation of this behavior might begin as more reward-related and then transition to be more habit-related over time (Melissa et al., 2020).

Neuroanatomy of exercise in animal and human research

The study of hyperactivity in rodents has robustly supported the role of mesolimbic activity and related dopamine signaling in regulating exercise behavior (Foldi et al., 2017a, 2017b), including consistent evidence that disrupting these processes can impact wheel-running activity (Klenotich et al., 2015; Verhagen et al., 2009). Recent research also suggests that some rodents might be more or less vulnerable to the ABA paradigm, suggesting that further investigations of neural mechanisms that might differentiate the two are warranted; preliminary work in this area shows that hyperdopaminergia accelerates the progression of the vulnerable phenotype (Beeler et al., 2021).

In humans, prior work also implicates both the role of habit (Tricomi et al., 2009) and reinforcement learning (Flack et al., 2021) in influencing activity levels, as well as the dopamine system more broadly in its role in impacting the drive for aerobic activity (Gorrell et al., 2022; Knab & Lightfoot, 2010). Specific to eating disorder samples, in a sample of women recovered from AN with empirical manipulation of dopamine signaling, startle potentiation was elevated in response to exercise cues but not in conditions where dopamine was experimentally depleted (O'Hara, Keyes, Renwick, Giel, et al., 2016). This finding was not replicated in another study of those recovered from AN, who were still more motivated to work for exercise in a behavioral task than healthy controls, even when dopamine was depleted (O'Hara, Keyes, Renwick, Leyton, et al., 2016). Taken together, more research is needed to determine the specific role that the striatum and other brain regions associated with reward processing and dopamine signaling may play in both initiating and maintaining exercise behavior in the context of eating disorders.

Other companion models of eating pathology draw on extensive overlap between obsessive-compulsive disorder and AN (Kaye et al., 2004; Kerr-Gaffney et al., 2018) and, specific to exercise behavior, shared anomalies in the prefrontal cortex that suggest shared underlying mechanisms (Song et al., 2021). Prior work demonstrates abnormally heightened frontal-limbic connectivity in AN (Cha et al., 2016); similarly, abnormal frontostriatal connectivity is associated with obsessive-compulsive disorder (Graybiel & Rauch, 2000), indicating a common network for compulsive behaviors across disorders. Of note, not all individuals with AN that exercise excessively show enhanced habit formation in value-based decision-making tasks (Klein et al., 2010). Therefore, whether exercise in AN can be either a form of extreme goal-directed control or a compulsive behavior—or both—may depend on the individual. Taken together, key outstanding research areas in the neurobiological study of exercise include (1) evaluating and confirming both group-level (those with vs. without eating disorders) and individual-level (among those with eating disorders) differences in reward-deficit and habit-related circuitry underlying exercise across eating disorder presentations, and (2) examining whether vulnerability to hyperactivity is present before illness onset.

State of the Science in Eating Disorders

A considerable number of individuals with eating disorders (approximately 40% to 80% of individuals with AN- and bulimia nervosa (BN)-spectrum disorders) present with maladaptive exercise (Cook et al., 2014; Davis et al., 1997; Davis & Kaptein, 2006; Shroff et al., 2006). Maladaptive exercise is an alarming and understudied eating disorder feature associated with suicidal behavior (Smith et al., 2013); poor treatment outcome, prognosis, and quality of life (Dalle Grave et al., 2008); obsessive-compulsive traits and symptoms (Davis & Kaptein, 2006; Shroff et al., 2006); anxiety (Holtkamp et al., 2004; Shroff et al., 2006); perfectionism (Shroff et al., 2006); body dissatisfaction (Brewerton et al., 1995); reward dependence (Dalle Grave et al., 2008); dietary restraint (Dalle Grave et al., 2008; Holtkamp et al., 2004); anhedonia (Davis & Woodside, 2002); and hypoleptinemia

(Holtkamp et al., 2003, 2006). Despite growing calls for action from within the eating disorder field (Cook et al., 2016; Cook & Leininger, 2017; Hausenblas et al., 2008; Hay et al., 2018) this symptom is not directly targeted in most existing eating disorder treatments. Ultimately, flexible and adaptive exercise engagement may support long-term physical and mental health, including recovery from eating disorders.

A model of maladaptive exercise

Together, current research suggests that biological responsiveness to exercise may translate to improvements in affect (either by reducing threat and/or increasing reward salience). These physiologically mediated emotional responses may be further supported by cognitive processes, which together may initiate and maintain maladaptive exercise. For a model depicting maladaptive exercise onset and maintenance, see Figure 16.2, to include potential moderators of exercise effects and to delineate specific rewarding and threat-reduction outcomes of exercise. As the field continues to move toward the development of a comprehensive model of maladaptive exercise and, ultimately, to intervention development, there are several issues of note. First, more fine-grained analysis is needed with the aim of additional precision that can lead to concrete specification of formal, testable models of maladaptive exercise behavior—moving from a verbal theory to formal, mathematical models (e.g., Millner et al., 2020). Further, as with other psychopharmacological agents, response to exercise may differ based on baseline levels of neurotransmitters, neurochemical factors, and hormones (Hill & Gorzalka, 2009), along with psychological factors, such as cognitive expectancies. We do not fully understand mechanistic factors that contribute to the substantial variability in exercise

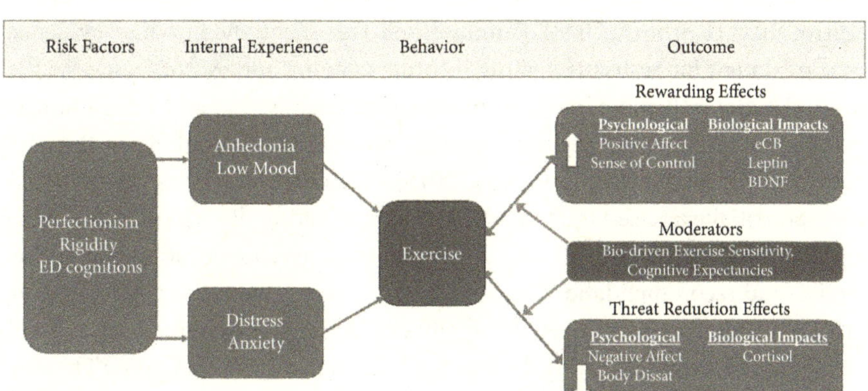

Figure 16.2 A theoretical model of maladaptive exercise.

Adapted with permission from Meyer et al. (2011). Compulsive exercise and eating disorders. *European Eating Disorders Review*. https://doi.org/10.1002/erv.1122

patterns and the presence of maladaptive exercise among those with eating disorders; for example, why some individuals present with maladaptive exercise and others do not. Greater attunement to moderators across levels of analysis (genetics, pre-exercise biomarker availability, exercise training status, exercise expectancies, neural circuitry differences, and eating disorder illness factors) may be necessary for clarifying models which account for heterogeneity of exercise-related risk across individuals and specifically target maladaptive (vs. adaptive) exercise risk. Further, biobehavioral theories contend that maladaptive exercise may serve varying primary functions, either to increase positive affect (reward), decrease negative affect (negative reinforcement), or as a rigid and compulsive (habitual) behavior. These potential functions of exercise implicate divergent neurobiological mechanisms in the development and maintenance of maladaptive exercise, which may vary across individuals, vary within individuals across time, and/or co-occur in a single behavioral instance.

Addressing maladaptive exercise in eating disorder treatment

Maladaptive exercise patterns often present early in the course of an eating disorder (Achamrah et al., 2016; Davis et al., 1997) and can mark poor treatment prognosis, suggesting that intervention strategies that directly address this symptom are essential. The most dominant treatments for eating disorders do not have specific guidance related to targeting maladaptive exercise. Enhanced Cognitive Behavioral Therapy (CBT-E), for instance, notes that exercise should be monitored and the patient should be educated about its potential effects, stating that "Unless the exercising has other functions than weight control, it generally decreases during the course of CBT-E as patients become less concerned about their eating, shape and weight," with encouragement to use more general affect management strategies to address exercise which primarily functions to reduce negative affect (Fairburn, 2008). Family-Based Treatment, the first-line, evidence-based treatment for restrictive eating disorders among adolescents, suggests that eating disorder behaviors, such as maladaptive exercise, should be minimized when they interfere with necessary weight restoration, particularly in the early stages of treatment (Lock & Le Grange, 2015). Nascent research has begun investigating potential exercise-targeted interventions in eating disorders, including an intervention for BED and BN which incorporates psychoeducation, supervised exercise, and recommendations for healthy exercise engagement (Mathisen et al., 2018, 2020), along with a targeted, cognitive behavioral intervention for compulsive exercise in restrictive eating disorders (Compulsive Exercise Activity Therapy; LEAP) (Hay et al., 2018), although neither has yet demonstrated superiority to CBT-E in targeting maladaptive exercise.

As models of maladaptive exercise are further tested and refined, treatment development can include more targeted investigation of the ways in which various psychological agents (e.g., exposure and response prevention; distress tolerance) and exercise dose (e.g., frequency, type, intensity, and duration) might be optimally incorporated into eating disorder treatment, and how prescriptions may be effectively tailored based on the function of exercise for individual patients along with their exercise-related history and risk.

Alternative Perspectives

Ethical dilemmas in exercise-related research

While there is significant interest in deepening an understanding of the psychobiology of exercise in eating disorders, particularly in the larger context of the mental health paradox that exercise behavior may pose within eating disorder treatment, some researchers advise caution in the integration of exercise into clinical research and treatment with eating disorders, which is borne from blanket recommendations of exercise abstinence for those in eating disorder recovery (Davies, 2015). Challenging this sentiment, there have been several recent calls to challenge these perceived barriers and expand research on this common eating disorder feature (Kolar & Gorrell, 2021; Touyz et al., 2017). Ultimately, a failure to advance the understanding of exercise in eating disorders and to adequately assess and address exercise behavior in treatment poses a risk to patients by perpetuating suboptimal treatment. Even if access to exercise is substantially reduced in acute treatment settings, these settings represent only a first phase of recovery for the subset of patients who access this care. Patients in free living environments are navigating ongoing choices about when, whether, and how much to exercise at different points during eating disorder recovery, with little empirical guidance. Ultimately, a recovery goal would likely include a return to adaptive activity that includes a psychologically flexible relationship with exercise, and it may even be at relatively high levels for some individuals.

Functions of exercise across eating disorders

As with many other eating disorder symptoms, most research on maladaptive exercise to date has focused on individuals diagnosed with AN. While maladaptive exercise is present across most eating disorders (except for avoidant/restrictive food intake disorder [ARFID], of which there is little data on the presence of maladaptive exercise), exercise may demonstrate different functions and associations with treatment outcome across populations. Weight preoccupation and management has been widely considered the primary function for maladaptive exercise within eating disorders, but further research related to the maintenance of maladaptive exercise has revealed additional functions (Davis et al., 1995; DiBartolo et al., 2007; Hechler et al., 2005; Schlegl et al., 2018; Taranis et al., 2011). Compulsivity, or maintaining a strict exercise schedule and experiencing guilt due to not exercising, has also been discovered as a correlate of maladaptive exercise across eating disorders (Mond et al., 2006; Taranis et al., 2011). For populations with BN specifically, an emphasis on appearance has been shown to be an important factor for exercise (Schlegl et al., 2018), while negative affect regulation is commonly seen as a function of exercise for those with restrictive eating disorders (Long et al., 1993; Meyer et al., 2016). Understanding the differing functions of exercise across eating disorders is beneficial given that improved understanding of the maintenance factors—and how to reduce them—of maladaptive exercise can better guide treatment programs for eating disorders (Meyer et al., 2016).

Implications

Given substantial heterogeneity in the presence of both adaptive and maladaptive functions of exercise across individuals, a first recommendation across eating disorder presentations includes ongoing monitoring of both patterns and functions of exercise across treatment settings. Distinguishing between adaptive and maladaptive exercise engagement may be particularly useful for both assessment and patient psychoeducation.

Further, as consistent research highlights the importance of psychological relations with exercise, interventions which seek to shape and reshape exercise expectancies may be particularly potent. One way to achieve this effectively may be to incorporate novel exercise behaviors that the patient has not engaged in previously as part of treatment, paired with an approach that challenges entrenched maladaptive cognitions related to exercise. In addition, for those who report engaging in exercise to manage negative affect, treatment might focus on diversifying affect-management strategies. Further, interventions that challenge rigidity and rules related to exercise (stopping exercise before reaching a goal, or encouraging flexibility in frequency and duration of exercise) may be useful for those who report significant rigidity in their exercise routine.

An additional recommendation includes the development of clear guidelines on both when and how to support a return to exercise during eating disorder treatment. Evidence indicates that physical activity may provide therapeutic benefit in the context of eating disorder treatment, including promoting muscle health (Rosa-Caldwell et al., 2023), preventing loss of bone density, enhanced cognitive functioning and self-regulation skills, social engagement, mood regulation, and reduction in discomfort during future eating episodes (Achamrah et al., 2016; Calogero & Pedrotty, 2004; Hausenblas et al., 2008). Further, a considerable portion of adolescents and young adults with eating disorders also participate in sports (Martinsen & Sundgot-Borgen, 2013) which, in addition to potentially enhancing risk for maladaptive exercise, can facilitate social skills and connection, motivation for recovery, and support identity development outside of an eating disorder. Finally, comorbid mood and anxiety disorders are also very common among those with eating disorders (Bühren et al., 2014), and burgeoning research indicates the benefits of exercise in the context of mental health treatment for these conditions (Asmundson et al., 2013; Carek et al., 2011; Heyman et al., 2012). Ultimately, a goal of full eating disorder recovery should include a return to adaptive exercise. To do this successfully, the field should specifically consider the training and integration of exercise professionals that may support these goals within eating disorder treatment teams, particularly for patients who have a significant history of maladaptive exercise and those who aim to engage in high levels of adaptive exercise as they progress in eating disorder recovery (e.g., athletes).

Conclusion

Exercise presents a mental health paradox and clinical conundrum in eating disorders. While exercise can promote positive mental health, it also has high potential to be a maladaptive behavior which may, in some cases, interfere with eating disorder treatment. Biobehavioral models support pharmacologic mechanisms of action that promote adaptive exercise, which may also reinforce maladaptive exercise patterns when in the fertile cognitive ground of obsessive-compulsive traits and/or weight and shape concerns. While maladaptive exercise is a common symptom of eating disorders, effective intervention and treatment methods that address exercise remain under development. Further research on the integration of adaptive exercise within eating disorder treatment and the maintenance of maladaptive exercise is necessary to inform clinical interventions. At present, monitoring and assessment of maladaptive exercise throughout treatment is recommended, with particular attention to functions of exercise (e.g., reduction of negative affect, compensatory features), which may increase intervention precision.

References

Achamrah, N., Coëffier, M., & Déchelotte, P. (2016). Physical activity in patients with anorexia nervosa. *Nutrition Reviews, 74*(5), 301–311. https://doi.org/10.1093/nutrit/nuw001

Adams, J. (2009). Understanding exercise dependence. *Journal of Contemporary Psychotherapy, 39*, 231–240.

Adams, J., & Kirkby, R. J. (2002). Excessive exercise as an addiction: A review. Addiction Research & Theory, 10(5), 415–438.

Adan, R. A. H., Hillebrand, J. J. G., Danner, U. N., Cardona Cano, S., Kas, M. J., & Verhagen, L. A. (2010). Neurobiology driving hyperactivity in activity-based anorexia. Current Topics in Behavioral Neurosciences, 6, 229–250. https://doi.org/10.1007/7854_2010_77

Adkins, E. C., & Keel, P. K. (2005). Does "excessive" or "compulsive" best describe exercise as a symptom of bulimia nervosa. *International Journal of Eating Disorders, 38*, 24–29. https://doi.org/10.1002/eat.20140

Anderson, E., & Shivakumar, G. (2013). Effects of exercise and physical activity on anxiety. *Frontiers in Psychiatry, 4*, 27.

Asmundson, G. J. G., Fetzner, M. G., DeBoer, L. B., Otto, M. W., & Smits, J. A. J. (2013). Let's get physical: A contemporary review of the anxiolytic effects of exercise for anxiety and its disorders. *Depression and Anxiety, 30*(4), 362–373. https://doi.org/10.1002/da.22043

Bailer, U. F., & Kaye, W. H. (2003). A review of neuropeptide and neuroendocrine dysregulation in anorexia and bulimia nervosa. *Current Drug Targets: CNS and Neurological Disorders, 2*(1), 53–59. https://doi.org/10.2174/1568007033338689

Bamber, D. J., Cockerill, I. M., Rodgers, S., & Carroll, D. (2003). Diagnostic criteria for exercise dependence in women. *British Journal of Sports Medicine, 37*, 393–400.

Beeler, J. A., Mourra, D., Zanca, R. M., Kalmbach, A., Gellman, C., Klein, B. Y., Ravenelle, R., Serrano, P., Moore, H., Rayport, S., Mingote, S., & Burghardt, N. S. (2021). Vulnerable and resilient phenotypes in a mouse model of anorexia nervosa. *Biological Psychiatry, 90*(12), 829–842. https://doi.org/10.1016/j.biopsych.2020.06.030

Blum, K., Thanos, P. K., & Gold, M. S. (2014). Dopamine and glucose, obesity, and reward deficiency syndrome. *Frontiers in Psychology, 5*, 919. https://doi.org/10.3389/fpsyg.2014.00919

Bratland Sanda, S., Martinsen, E. W., Rosenvinge, J. H., Rø, Ø., Hoffart, A., & Sundgot Borgen, J. (2011). Exercise dependence score in patients with longstanding eating disorders and controls: The importance of affect regulation and physical activity intensity. *European Eating Disorders Review, 19*, 249–255. https://doi.org/10.1002/erv.971/pdf

Brellenthin, A. G., Crombie, K. M., Hillard, C. J., & Koltyn, K. F. (2017). Endocannabinoid and mood responses to exercise in adults with varying activity levels. *Medicine & Science in Sports & Exercise, 49*(8), 1688–1696. https://doi.org/10.1249/MSS.0000000000001276

Brewerton, T. D., Stellefson, E. J., Hibbs, N., Hodges, E. L., & Cochrane, C. E. (1995). Comparison of eating disorder patients with and without compulsive exercising. *International Journal of Eating Disorders, 17*(4), 413–416.

Bühren, K., Schwarte, R., Fluck, F., Timmesfeld, N., Krei, M., Egberts, K., Pfeiffer, E., Fleischhaker, C., Wewetzer, C., & Herpertz-Dahlmann, B. (2014). Comorbid psychiatric disorders in female adolescents with first-onset anorexia nervosa: Comorbidity in adolescent anorexia nervosa. *European Eating Disorders Review, 22*(1), 39–44. https://doi.org/10.1002/erv.2254

Calogero, R. M., & Pedrotty, K. N. (2004). The practice and process of healthy exercise: An investigation of the treatment of exercise abuse in women with eating disorders. *Eating Disorders, 12*(4), 273–291. https://doi.org/10.1080/10640260490521352

Carek, P. J., Laibstain, S. E., & Carek, S. M. (2011). Exercise for the treatment of depression and anxiety. *International Journal of Psychiatry in Medicine, 41*(1), 15–28. https://doi.org/10.2190/PM.41.1.c

Cha, J., Ide, J. S., Bowman, F. D., Simpson, H. B., Posner, J., & Steinglass, J. E. (2016). Abnormal reward circuitry in anorexia nervosa: A longitudinal, multimodal MRI study: Abnormal Reward Circuitry in AN. *Human Brain Mapping, 37*(11), 3835–3846. https://doi.org/10.1002/hbm.23279

Chekroud, S. R., Gueorguieva, R., Zheutlin, A. B., Paulus, M., Krumholz, H. M., Krystal, J. H., & Chekroud, A. M. (2018). Association between physical exercise and mental health in 1.2 million individuals in the USA between 2011 and 2015: A cross-sectional study. *Lancet Psychiatry, 5*(9), 739–746. https://doi.org/10.1016/S2215-0366(18)30227-X

Chowdhury, T. G., Chen, Y. W., & Aoki, C. (2015). Using the activity-based anorexia rodent model to study the neurobiological basis of anorexia nervosa. *Journal of Visualized Experiments, 105*, e52927. https://doi.org/10.3791/52927

Coniglio, K. A., Cooper, M., & Selby, E. A. (2022). Behavioral reinforcement of pathological exercise in anorexia nervosa. *International Journal of Eating Disorders*, 55(2), 184–192. https://doi.org/10.1002/eat.23626

Cook, B., Hausenblas, H., & Freimuth, M. (2014). Exercise addiction and compulsive exercising: Relationship to eating disorders, substance use disorders, and addictive disorders. In In T. D. Brewerton & A. B. Dennis (Eds.), *Eating disorders, addictions, and substance use disorders* (pp. 127–144). Springer-Verlag Publishing/Springer Nature.

Cook, B., & Leininger, L. (2017). The ethics of exercise in eating disorders: Can an ethical principles approach guide the next generation of research and clinical practice? *Journal of Sport and Health Science, 6*(3), 295–298. https://doi.org/10.1016/j.jshs.2017.03.004

Cook, B., Wonderlich, S. A., Mitchell, J. E., Thompson, R., Sherman, R., & McCallum, K. (2016). Exercise in eating disorders treatment: Systematic review and proposal of guidelines. *Medicine and Science in Sports and Exercise, 48*(7), 1408–1414. https://doi.org/10.1249/MSS.0000000000000912

Crombie, K. M., Brellenthin, A. G., Hillard, C. J., & Koltyn, K. F. (2018). Psychobiological responses to aerobic exercise in individuals with posttraumatic stress disorder: Psychobiological responses to exercise in PTSD. *Journal of Traumatic Stress, 31*(1), 134–145. https://doi.org/10.1002/jts.22253

Crombie, K. M., Cisler, J. M., Hillard, C. J., & Koltyn, K. F. (2020). Aerobic exercise reduces anxiety and fear ratings to threat and increases circulating endocannabinoids in women with and without PTSD. *Mental Health and Physical Activity, 20*, 100366. https://doi.org/10.1016/j.mhpa.2020.100366

Crombie, K. M., Sartin-Tarm, A., Sellnow, K., Ahrenholtz, R., Lee, S., Matalamaki, M., Almassi, N. E., Hillard, C. J., Koltyn, K. F., Adams, T. G., & Cisler, J. M. (2021). Exercise-induced increases in Anandamide and BDNF during extinction consolidation contribute to reduced threat following reinstatement: Preliminary evidence from a randomized controlled trial. *Psychoneuroendocrinology, 132*, 105355. https://doi.org/10.1016/j.psyneuen.2021.105355

da Silva Alves, F., Schmitz, N., Figee, M., Abeling, N., Hasler, G., van der Meer, J., Nederveen, A., de Haan, L., Linszen, D., & van Amelsvoort, T. (2011). Dopaminergic modulation of the human reward system: A placebo-controlled dopamine depletion fMRI study. *Journal of Psychopharmacology, 25*(4), 538–549. https://doi.org/10.1177/0269881110367731

Dalle Grave, R., Calugi, S., & Marchesini, G. (2008). Compulsive exercise to control shape or weight in eating disorders: Prevalence, associated features, and treatment outcome. *Comprehensive Psychiatry, 49*(4), 346–352. https://doi.org/10.1016/j.comppsych.2007.12.007

Davies, R. R. (2015). The treatment of compulsive physical activity in anorexia nervosa lacks a conceptual base. *Advances in Eating Disorders: Theory, Research and Practice, 3*(1), 103–112.

Davis, C., & Claridge, G. (1998). The eating disorders as addiction: A psychobiological perspective. *Addictive Behaviors, 23*(4), 463–475.

Davis, C., & Kaptein, S. (2006). Anorexia nervosa with excessive exercise: A phenotype with close links to obsessive-compulsive disorder. *Psychiatry Research, 142*(2–3), 209–217. https://doi.org/10.1016/j.psychres.2005.11.006

Davis, C., Katzman, D. K., Kaptein, S., Kirsh, C., Brewer, H., Kalmbach, K., Olmsted, M. P., Woodside, D. B., & Kaplan, A. S. (1997). The prevalence of high-level exercise in the eating disorders: Etiological implications. *Comprehensive Psychiatry, 38*(6), 321–326.

Davis, C., Kennedy, S. H., Ralevski, E., Dionne, M., Brewer, H., Neitzert, C., & Ratusny, D. (1995). Obsessive compulsiveness and physical activity in anorexia nervosa and high-level exercising. *Journal of Psychosomatic Research, 39*(8), 967–976.

Davis, C., & Woodside, D. B. (2002). Sensitivity to the rewarding effects of food and exercise in the eating disorders. *Comprehensive Psychiatry, 43*(3), 189–194. https://doi.org/10.1053/comp.2002.32356

De Chiara, V., Errico, F., Musella, A., Rossi, S., Mataluni, G., Sacchetti, L., Siracusano, A., Castelli, M., Cavasinni, F., Bernardi, G., Usiello, A., & Centonze, D. (2010). Voluntary exercise and sucrose consumption enhance cannabinoid CB1 receptor sensitivity in the striatum. *Neuropsychopharmacology, 35*(2), 374–387. https://doi.org/10.1038/npp.2009.141

de Geus, E., Bartels, M., Kaprio, J., Lightfoot, J., & Thomis, M. (2014). Genetics of regular exercise and sedentary behaviors. *Twin Research and Human Genetics, 17*(4), 262–271. https://doi.org/10.1017/thg.2014.42

Deslandes, A., Moraes, H., Ferreira, C., Veiga, H., Silveira, H., Mouta, R., Pompeu, F. A., Coutinho, E. S., & Laks, J. (2009). Exercise and mental health: Many reasons to move. *Neuropsychobiology, 59*(4), 191–198. https://doi.org/10.1159/000223730

DiBartolo, P. M., Lin, L., Montoya, S., Neal, H., & Shaffer, C. (2007). Are there "healthy" and "unhealthy" reasons for exercise? Examining individual differences in exercise motivations using the function of exercise scale. *Journal of Clinical Sport Psychology, 1*(2), 93–120. https://doi.org/10.1123/jcsp.1.2.93

Dietrich, A., & McDaniel, W. (2004). Endocannabinoids and exercise. *British Journal of Sports Medicine, 38*(5), 536–541. https://doi.org/10.1136/bjsm.2004.011718

Dinoff, A., Herrmann, N., Swardfager, W., & Lanctôt, K. L. (2017). The effect of acute exercise on blood concentrations of brain-derived neurotrophic factor in healthy adults: A meta-analysis. *European Journal of Neuroscience, 46*(1), 1635–1646. https://doi.org/10.1111/ejn.13603

Dittmer, N., Jacobi, C., & Voderholzer, U. (2018). Compulsive exercise in eating disorders: Proposal for a definition and a clinical assessment. *Journal of Eating Disorders, 6*(1), 42. https://doi.org/10.1186/s40337-018-0219-x

Dostalova, I., Bartak, V., Papezova, H., & Nedvidkova, J. (2007). The effect of short-term exercise on plasma leptin levels in patients with anorexia nervosa. *Metabolism*, *56*(4), 497–503. https://doi.org/10.1016/j.metabol.2006.11.008

Dubreucq, S., Durand, A., Matias, I., Bénard, G., Richard, E., Soria-Gomez, E., Glangetas, C., Groc, L., Wadleigh, A., Massa, F., Bartsch, D., Marsicano, G., Georges, F., & Chaouloff, F. (2013). Ventral tegmental area cannabinoid type-1 receptors control voluntary exercise performance. *Biological Psychiatry*, *73*(9), 895–903. https://doi.org/10.1016/j.biopsych.2012.10.025

Dubreucq, S., Koehl, M., Abrous, D. N., Marsicano, G., & Chaouloff, F. (2010). CB1 receptor deficiency decreases wheel-running activity: Consequences on emotional behaviours and hippocampal neurogenesis. *Experimental Neurology*, *224*(1), 106–113. https://doi.org/10.1016/j.expneurol.2010.01.017

Ehrlich, S., Burghardt, R., Schneider, N., Broecker-Preuss, M., Weiss, D., Merle, J. V., Craciun, E. M., Pfeiffer, E., Mann, K., Lehmkuhl, U., & Hebebrand, J. (2009). The role of leptin and cortisol in hyperactivity in patients with acute and weight-recovered anorexia nervosa. *Progress in Neuro-Psychopharmacology and Biological Psychiatry*, *33*(4), 658–662. https://doi.org/10.1016/j.pnpbp.2009.03.007

Engel, S. G., Wonderlich, S. A., Crosby, R. D., Mitchell, J. E., Crow, S., Peterson, C. B., Le Grange, D., Simonich, H. K., Cao, L., & Lavender, J. M. (2013). The role of affect in the maintenance of anorexia nervosa: Evidence from a naturalistic assessment of momentary behaviors and emotion. *Journal of Abnormal Psychology*, *122*(3), 709.

Fairburn, C. (2008). *Eating disorders: The transdiagnostic view and the cognitive behavioral theory*. Guilford Press.

Fairburn, C., & Bèglin, S. J. (1994). Assessment of eating disorders: Interview or self-report questionnaire? *International Journal of Eating Disorders*, 16(4), 363–370. https://doi.org/10.1002/1098-108X(199412)16:4<363::AID-EAT2260160405>3.0.CO;2-#

Fairburn, C., Zafra, C., & Marianne, O. (2014). Eating *disorder examination* (Edition 17.0D). https://www.credo-oxford.com/pdfs/EDE_17.0D.pdf

Flack, K. D., Hays, H. M., & Moreland, J. (2021). Incentive sensitization for exercise reinforcement to increase exercise behaviors. *Journal of Health Psychology*, *26*(13), 2487–2504. https://doi.org/10.1177/1359105320914073

Flack, K. D., Pankey, C., Ufholz, K., Johnson, L., & Roemmich, J. N. (2019). Genetic variations in the dopamine reward system influence exercise reinforcement and tolerance for exercise intensity. *Behavioural Brain Research*, *375*, 112148. https://doi.org/10.1016/j.bbr.2019.112148

Fladung, A.-K., Grön, G., Grammer, K., Herrnberger, B., Schilly, E., Grasteit, S., Wolf, R. C., Walter, H., & von Wietersheim, J. (2010). A neural signature of anorexia nervosa in the ventral striatal reward system. *American Journal of Psychiatry*, *167*(2), 206–212. https://doi.org/10.1176/appi.ajp.2009.09010071

Foldi, C. J., Milton, L. K., & Oldfield, B. J. (2017a). A focus on reward in anorexia nervosa through the lens of the activity-based anorexia rodent model. *Journal of Neuroendocrinology*, *29*(10), e12479. https://doi.org/10.1111/jne.12479

Foldi, C. J., Milton, L. K., & Oldfield, B. J. (2017b). The role of mesolimbic reward neurocircuitry in prevention and rescue of the activity-based anorexia (ABA) phenotype in rats. *Neuropsychopharmacology*, *42*(12), 2292–2300. https://doi.org/10.1038/npp.2017.63

Forbush, K. T., Wildes, J. E., Pollack, L. O., Dunbar, D., Luo, J., Patterson, K., Petruzzi, L., Pollpeter, M., Miller, H., Stone, A., Bright, A., & Watson, D. (2013). Development and validation of the Eating Pathology Symptoms Inventory (EPSI). *Psychological Assessment*, *25*(3), 859–878. https://doi.org/10.1037/a0032639

Gabbay, V., Ely, B. A., Babb, J., & Liebes, L. (2012). The possible role of the kynurenine pathway in anhedonia in adolescents. *Journal of Neural Transmission*, *119*(2), 253–260. https://doi.org/10.1007/s00702-011-0685-7

Gorrell, S., Collins, A. G. E., Le Grange, D., & Yang, T. T. (2020). Dopaminergic activity and exercise behavior in anorexia nervosa. *OBM Neurobiology*, *4*(1). https://doi.org/10.21926/obm.neurobiol.2001053

Gorrell, S., Shott, M. E., & Frank, G. K. W. (2022). Associations between aerobic exercise and dopamine-related reward-processing: Informing a model of human exercise engagement. *Biological Psychology*, *171*, 108350. https://doi.org/10.1016/j.biopsycho.2022.108350

Graybiel, A. M., & Rauch, S. L. (2000). Toward a neurobiology of obsessive-compulsive disorder. *Neuron*, *28*(2), 343–347. https://doi.org/10.1016/S0896-6273(00)00113-6

Greenwood, B. N., Strong, P. V., Loughridge, A. B., Day, H. E., Clark, P. J., Mika, A., Hellwinkel, J. E., Spence, K. G., & Fleshner, M. (2012). 5-HT2C receptors in the basolateral amygdala and dorsal striatum are a novel target for the anxiolytic and antidepressant effects of exercise. *PLOS ONE, 7*(9), e46118. https://doi.org/10.1371/journal.pone.0046118

Guarda, A. S., Schreyer, C. C., Boersma, G. J., Tamashiro, K. L., & Moran, T. H. (2015). Anorexia nervosa as a motivated behavior: Relevance of anxiety, stress, fear and learning. *Physiology & Behavior, 152*(*Pt. B*), 466–472. https://doi.org/10.1016/j.physbeh.2015.04.007

Hausenblas, H. A., Cook, B. J., & Chittester, N. I. (2008). Can exercise treat eating disorders. *Exercise and Sport Sciences Reviews, 36*, 43–47.

Hausenblas, H. A., & Downs, D. S. (2002). How much is too much? The development and validation of the exercise dependence scale. *Psychology & Health, 17*(4), 387–404. https://doi.org/10.1080/08870440220000004894

Hay, P., Touyz, S., Arcelus, J., Pike, K., Attia, E., Crosby, R. D., Madden, S., Wales, J., La Puma, M., Heriseanu, A. I., Young, S., & Meyer, C. (2018). A randomized controlled trial of the compuLsive Exercise Activity TheraPy (LEAP): A new approach to compulsive exercise in anorexia nervosa. *International Journal of Eating Disorders, 51*(8), 999–1004. https://doi.org/10.1002/eat.22920

Hechler, T., Beumont, P., Marks, P., & Touyz, S. (2005). How do clinical specialists understand the role of physical activity in eating disorders? *European Eating Disorders Review, 13*(2), 125–132. https://doi.org/10.1002/erv.630

Herring, M., O'Connor, P. J., & Dishman, R. K. (2010). The effect of exercise training on anxiety symptoms among patients: A systematic review. *Archives of Internal Medicine, 170*(4), 321–331.

Herring, M., Sailors, M., & Bray, M. (2014). Genetic factors in exercise adoption, adherence and obesity. *Obesity Reviews, 15*(1), 29–39. https://doi.org/10.1111/obr.12089

Heyman, E., Gamelin, F. X., Goekint, M., Piscitelli, F., Roelands, B., Leclair, E., Di Marzo, V., & Meeusen, R. (2012). Intense exercise increases circulating endocannabinoid and BDNF levels in humans—Possible implications for reward and depression. *Psychoneuroendicrinology, 37*(6), 844–851.

Hill, M., & Gorzalka, B. (2009). The endocannabinoid system and the treatment of mood and anxiety disorders. *CNS & Neurological Disorders—Drug Targets, 8*(6), 451–458. https://doi.org/10.2174/187152709789824624

Hillebrand, J. J. G., de Rijke, C. E., Brakkee, J. H., Kas, M. J. H., & Adan, R. A. H. (2005). Voluntary access to a warm plate reduces hyperactivity in activity-based anorexia. *Physiology & Behavior, 85*(2), 151–157. https://doi.org/10.1016/j.physbeh.2005.03.017

Hillebrand, J. J. G., Kas, M. J. H., van Elburg, A. A., Hoek, H. W., & Adan, R. a. H. (2008). Leptin's effect on hyperactivity: Potential downstream effector mechanisms. *Physiology & Behavior, 94*(5), 689–695. https://doi.org/10.1016/j.physbeh.2008.04.011

Ho, E. V., Klenotich, S. J., McMurray, M. S., & Dulawa, S. C. (2016). Activity-based anorexia alters the expression of BDNF transcripts in the mesocorticolimbic reward circuit. *PLOS ONE, 11*(11), e0166756. https://doi.org/10.1371/journal.pone.0166756

Holland, L. A., Brown, T. A., & Keel, P. K. (2014). Defining features of unhealthy exercise associated with disordered eating and eating disorder diagnoses. *Psychology of Sport and Exercise, 15*(1), 116–123. https://doi.org/10.1016/j.psychsport.2013.10.005

Holsen, L. M., Lawson, E. A., Blum, J., Ko, E., Makris, N., Fazeli, P. K., Klibanski, A., & Goldstein, J. M. (2012). Food motivation circuitry hypoactivation related to hedonic and nonhedonic aspects of hunger and satiety in women with active anorexia nervosa and weight-restored women with anorexia nervosa. *Journal of Psychiatry & Neuroscience, 37*(5), 322–332. https://doi.org/10.1503/jpn.110156

Holtkamp, K., Hebebrand, J., & Herpertz-Dahlmann, B. (2004). The contribution of anxiety and food restriction on physical activity levels in acute anorexia nervosa. *International Journal of Eating Disorders, 36*(2), 163–171. https://doi.org/10.1002/eat.20035

Holtkamp, K., Herpertz-Dahlmann, B., Hebebrand, K., Mika, C., Kratzsch, J., & Hebebrand, J. (2006). Physical activity and restlessness correlate with leptin levels in patients with adolescent anorexia nervosa. *Biological Psychiatry, 60*(3), 311–313. https://doi.org/10.1016/j.biopsych.2005.11.001

Holtkamp, K., Herpertz-Dahlmann, B., Mika, C., Heer, M., Heussen, N., Fichter, M., Herpertz, S., Senf, W., Blum, W. F., Schweiger, U., Warnke, A., Ballauff, A., Remschmidt, H., & Hebebrand, J. (2003). Elevated physical activity and low leptin levels co-occur in patients with anorexia nervosa. *Journal of Clinical Endocrinology & Metabolism, 88*(11), 5169–5174. https://doi.org/10.1210/jc.2003-030569

Juwono, I. D., Tolnai, N., & Szabo, A. (2022). Exercise addiction in athletes: A systematic review of the literature. *International Journal of Mental Health and Addiction*, *20*(5), 3113–3127. https://doi.org/10.1007/s11469-021-00568-1

Karr, T. M., Cook, B., Zunker, C., Cao, L., Crosby, R. D., Wonderlich, S. A., & Mitchell, J. E. (2017). Examining physical activity and affect using objective measures: A pilot study of anorexia nervosa. *The Sport Journal*, *20*. https://thesportjournal.org/article/examining-physical-activity-and-affect-using-objective-measures-a-pilot-study-of-anorexia-nervosa/

Kaye, W. H., Bulik, C. M., Thornton, L., Barbarich, N., Masters, K., & the Price Foundation Collaborative Group. (2004). Comorbidity of anxiety disorders with anorexia and bulimia nervosa. *American Journal of Psychiatry*, *161*(12), 2215–2221. https://doi.org/10.1176/appi.ajp.161.12.2215

Kaye, W. H., Frank, G. K., Bailer, U. F., Henry, S. E., Meltzer, C. C., Price, J. C., Mathis, C. A., & Wagner, A. (2005). Serotonin alterations in anorexia and bulimia nervosa: New insights from imaging studies. *Physiology & Behavior*, *85*(1), 73–81.

Kaye, W. H., Wierenga, C. E., Bailer, U. F., Simmons, A. N., & Bischoff-Grethe, A. (2013). Nothing tastes as good as skinny feels: The neurobiology of anorexia nervosa. *Trends in Neurosciences*, *36*(2), 110–120. https://doi.org/10.1016/j.tins.2013.01.003

Kendler, K. S., Mohs, R. C., & Davis, K. L. (1983). The effects of diet and physical activity on plasma homovanillic acid in normal human subjects. *Psychiatry Research*, *8*(3), 215–223. https://doi.org/10.1016/0165-1781(83)90065-3

Kerr-Gaffney, J., Harrison, A., & Tchanturia, K. (2018). Social anxiety in the eating disorders: A systematic review and meta-analysis. *Psychological Medicine*, *48*(15), 2477–2491. https://doi.org/10.1017/S0033291718000752

Klein, D. A., Mayer, L. E. S., Schebendach, J. E., & Walsh, B. T. (2007). Physical activity and cortisol in anorexia nervosa. *Psychoneuroendocrinology*, *32*(5), 539–547. https://doi.org/10.1016/j.psyneuen.2007.03.007

Klein, D. A., Schebendach, J. E., Gershkovich, M., Bodell, L. P., Foltin, R. W., & Walsh, B. T. (2010). Behavioral assessment of the reinforcing effect of exercise in women with anorexia nervosa: Further paradigm development and data. *International Journal of Eating Disorders*, *43*(7), 611–618. https://doi.org/10.1002/eat.20758

Klenotich, S. J., Ho, E. V., McMurray, M. S., Server, C. H., & Dulawa, S. C. (2015). Dopamine D2/3 receptor antagonism reduces activity-based anorexia. *Translational Psychiatry*, *5*, e613. https://doi.org/10.1038/tp.2015.109

Klimentidis, Y. C., Raichlen, D. A., Bea, J., Garcia, D. O., Wineinger, N. E., Mandarino, L. J., Alexander, G. E., Chen, Z., & Going, S. B. (2018). Genome-wide association study of habitual physical activity in over 377,000 UK Biobank participants identifies multiple variants including CADM2 and APOE. *International Journal of Obesity*, *42*(6), 1161–1176. https://doi.org/10.1038/s41366-018-0120-3

Knab, A. M., & Lightfoot, J. T. (2010). Does the difference between physically active and couch potato lie in the dopamine system? *International Journal of Biological Sciences*, 133–150. https://doi.org/10.7150/ijbs.6.133

Kolar, D. R., & Gorrell, S. (2021). A call to experimentally study acute affect-regulation mechanisms specific to driven exercise in eating disorders. *International Journal of Eating Disorders*, *54*(3), 280–286. https://doi.org/10.1002/eat.23427

Kolar, D. R., Kaurin, A., Meule, A., Schlegl, S., Dittmer, N., & Voderholzer, U. (2022). Interpersonal, affective and compulsive features of driven exercise in anorexia nervosa. *Journal of Affective Disorders*, *307*, 53–61. https://doi.org/10.1016/j.jad.2022.03.044

Kolar, D. R., Neumayr, C., Roth, M., Voderholzer, U., Perthes, K., & Schlegl, S. (2020). Testing an emotion regulation model of physical activity in adolescents with anorexia nervosa: A pilot ecological momentary assessment. *European Eating Disorders Review*, *28*(2), 170–183. https://doi.org/10.1002/erv.2706

Kumar, A., Pareek, V., Faiq, M. A., Ghosh, S. K., & Kumari, C. (2019). Adult neurogenesis in humans: A review of basic concepts, history, current research, and clinical implications. *Innovations in Clinical Neuroscience*, *16*(5–6), 30–37.

Leinninger, G. M., Jo, Y.-H., Leshan, R. L., Louis, G. W., Yang, H., Barrera, J. G., Wilson, H., Opland, D. M., Faouzi, M. A., Gong, Y., Jones, J. C., Rhodes, C. J., Chua, S., Diano, S., Horvath, T. L., Seeley, R. J., Becker, J. B., Münzberg, H., & Myers, M. G. (2009). Leptin acts via leptin receptor-expressing lateral hypothalamic neurons to modulate the mesolimbic dopamine system and suppress feeding. *Cell Metabolism*, *10*(2), 89–98. https://doi.org/10.1016/j.cmet.2009.06.011

Levinson, C. A., & Williams, B. M. (2020). Eating disorder fear networks: Identification of central eating disorder fears. *International Journal of Eating Disorders*, 53(12), 1960–1973. https://doi.org/10.1002/eat.23382

Lichtenstein, M. B., Hinze, C. J., Emborg, B., Thomsen, F., & Hemmingsen, S. D. (2017). Compulsive exercise: Links, risks and challenges facedent. *Psychology Research and Behavioral Management, 10*, 85–95. https://doi.org/10.2147/PRBM.S113093

Lock, J., & Le Grange, D. (2015). *Treatment manual for anorexia nervosa: A family-based approach* (2nd ed.). Guildford Press.

Long, C. G., Smith, J., Midgley, M., & Cassidy, T. (1993). Over-exercising in anorexic and normal samples: Behaviour and attitudes. *Journal of Mental Health, 2*(4), 321–327. https://doi.org/10.3109/09638239309016967

Luce, K. H., & Crowther, J. H. (1999). The reliability of the eating disorder examination—Self-report questionnaire version (EDE-Q). *International Journal of Eating Disorders, 25*(3), 349–351. https://doi.org/10.1002/(SICI)1098-108X(199904)25:3<349::AID-EAT15>3.0.CO;2-M

Martinsen, M., & Sundgot-Borgen, J. (2013). Higher prevalence of eating disorders among adolescent elite athletes than controls. *Medicine & Science in Sports & Exercise, 45*(6), 1188–1197. https://doi.org/10.1249/MSS.0b013e318281a939

Mathisen, T. F., Bratland-Sanda, S., Rosenvinge, J. H., Friborg, O., Pettersen, G., Vrabel, K. A., & Sundgot-Borgen, J. (2018). Treatment effects on compulsive exercise and physical activity in eating disorders. *Journal of Eating Disorders, 6*(1), 43. https://doi.org/10.1186/s40337-018-0215-1

Mathisen, T. F., Rosenvinge, J. H., Friborg, O., Vrabel, K., Bratland-Sanda, S., Pettersen, G., & Sundgot-Borgen, J. (2020). Is physical exercise and dietary therapy a feasible alternative to cognitive behavior therapy in treatment of eating disorders? A randomized controlled trial of two group therapies. *International Journal of Eating Disorders, 53*(4), 574–585. https://doi.org/10.1002/eat.23228

Matta Mello Portugal, E., Cevada, T., Sobral Monteiro-Junior, R., Teixeira Guimarães, T., da Cruz Rubini, E., Lattari, E., Blois, C., & Camaz Deslandes, A. (2013). Neuroscience of exercise: From neurobiology mechanisms to mental health. *Neuropsychobiology, 68*(1), 1–14. https://doi.org/10.1159/000350946

Mazure, C. M., Halmi, K. A., Sunday, S. R., Romano, S. J., & Einhorn, A. M. (1994). The Yale–Brown–Cornell eating disorder scale: Development, use, reliability and validity. *Journal of Psychiatric Research, 28*(5), 425–445. https://doi.org/10.1016/0022-3956(94)90002-7

McMorris, T., Collard, K., Corbett, J., Dicks, M., & Swain, J. P. (2008). A test of the catecholamines hypothesis for an acute exercise–cognition interaction. *Pharmacology Biochemistry and Behavior, 89*(1), 106–115. https://doi.org/10.1016/j.pbb.2007.11.007

Meier, M., Kossakowski, J. J., Jones, P. J., Kay, B., Riemann, B. C., & McNally, R. J. (2020). Obsessive–compulsive symptoms in eating disorders: A network investigation. *International Journal of Eating Disorders, 53*(3), 362–371. https://doi.org/10.1002/eat.23196

Melissa, R., Lama, M., Laurence, K., Sylvie, B., Jeanne, D., Odile, V., & Nathalie, G. (2020). Physical activity in eating disorders: A systematic review. *Nutrients, 12*(1), 183. https://doi.org/10.3390/nu12010183

Meyer, C., Plateau, C. R., Taranis, L., Brewin, N., Wales, J., & Arcelus, J. (2016). The Compulsive Exercise Test: Confirmatory factor analysis and links with eating psychopathology among women with clinical eating disorders. *Journal of Eating Disorders, 4*, 22. https://doi.org/10.1186/s40337-016-0113-3

Meyer, C., Taranis, L., & Goodwin, H. (2011). Compulsive exercise and eating disorders. *European Eating Disorders Review, 19*(3), 174–189. https://doi.org/10.1002/erv.1122

Meyer, J. D., Crombie, K. M., Cook, D. B., Hillard, C. J., & Koltyn, K. F. (2019). Serum endocannabinoid and mood changes after exercise in major depressive disorder. *Medicine & Science in Sports & Exercise, 51*(9), 1909–1917. https://doi.org/10.1249/MSS.0000000000002006

Millner, A. J., Robinaugh, D. J., & Nock, M. K. (2020). Advancing the understanding of suicide: The need for formal theory and rigorous descriptive research. *Trends in Cognitive Sciences, 24*(9), 704–716. https://doi.org/10.1016/j.tics.2020.06.007

Mond, J. M., Hay, P. J., Rodgers, B., & Owen, C. (2006). An update on the definition of "excessive exercise" in eating disorders research. *International Journal of Eating Disorders, 39*, 147–153. https://doi.org/10.1002/eat.20214

Monteleone, P., & Maj, M. (2013). Dysfunctions of leptin, ghrelin, BDNF and endocannabinoids in eating disorders: Beyond the homeostatic control of food intake. *Psychoneuroendocrinology, 38*(3), 312–330. https://doi.org/10.1016/j.psyneuen.2012.10.021

O'Hara, C., Campbell, I. C., & Schmidt, U. (2015). A reward-centered model of anorexia nervosa: A focused narrative review of the neurological and psychophysiological literature. *Neuroscience & Biobehavioral Reviews, 52*, 131–152. https://doi.org/10.1016/j.neubiorev.2015.02.012

O'Hara, C., Keyes, A., Renwick, B., Giel, K., Campbell, I., & Schmidt, U. (2016). Evidence that illness-compatible cues are rewarding in women recovered from anorexia nervosa: A study of the effects of dopamine depletion on eye-blink startle responses. *PLOS ONE, 11*(10). https://doi.org/10.1371/journal.pone.0165104

O'Hara, C., Keyes, A., Renwick, B., Leyton, M., Campbell, I., & Schmidt, U. (2016). The effects of acute dopamine precursor depletion on the reinforcing value of exercise in anorexia nervosa. *PLOS ONE, 11*(1). https://doi.org/10.1371/journal.pone.0145894

Pasman, L., & Thompson, J. K. (1988). Body image and eating disturbance in obligatory runners, obligatory weightlifters, and sedentary individuals. *International Journal of Eating Disorders, 7*(6), 759–769.

Presseller, E. K., Wilkinson, M. L., Trainor, C., Lampe, E. W., & Juarascio, A. S. (2022). Self-regulation deficits moderate treatment outcomes in a clinical trial evaluating just-in-time adaptive interventions as an augmentation to cognitive-behavioral therapy for bulimia-spectrum eating disorders. *International Journal of Eating Disorders, 55*(5), 709. https://doi.org/10.1002/eat.23695

Reichert, M., Schlegel, S., Jagau, F., Timm, I., Wieland, L., Ebner-Priemer, U. W., Hartmann, A., & Zeeck, A. (2020). Mood and dysfunctional cognitions constitute within-subject antecedents and consequences of exercise in eating disorders. *Psychotherapy and Psychosomatics, 89*(2), 119–121. https://doi.org/10.1159/000504061

Rosa-Caldwell, M. E., Eddy, K. T., Rutkove, S. B., & Breithaupt, L. (2023). Anorexia nervosa and muscle health: A systematic review of our current understanding and future recommendations for study. *International Journal of Eating Disorders, 56*(3), 483–500. https://doi.org/10.1002/eat.23878

Saeed, R., Mahmood, K., Ali, S. B., & Haleem, D. J. (2021). Prevention of diet restriction induced hyperactivity but not body-weight reduction in rats co-treated with tryptophan: Relationship with striatal serotonin and dopamine metabolism and serotonin-1A auto-receptor expression. *Nutritional Neuroscience, 25*(8), 1764–1773. https://doi.org/10.1080/1028415X.2021.1901046

Scharmer, C., Gorrell, S., Schaumberg, K., & Anderson, D. (2020). Compulsive exercise or exercise dependence? Clarifying conceptualizations of exercise in the context of eating disorder pathology. *Journal of Clinical Sport Psychology, 46*, 101586.

Schlegl, S., Dittmer, N., Hoffmann, S., & Voderholzer, U. (2018). Self-reported quantity, compulsiveness and motives of exercise in patients with eating disorders and healthy controls: Differences and similarities. *Journal of Eating Disorders, 6*(1), 17. https://doi.org/10.1186/s40337-018-0202-6

Schmalbach, I., Herhaus, B., Pässler, S., Runst, S., Berth, H., Wolff-Stephan, S., & Petrowski, K. (2020). Cortisol reactivity in patients with anorexia nervosa after stress induction. *Translational Psychiatry, 10*(1), 275. https://doi.org/10.1038/s41398-020-00955-7

Severinsen, M. C. K., & Pedersen, B. K. (2020). Muscle–organ crosstalk: The emerging roles of myokines. *Endocrine Reviews, 41*(4), 594–609. https://doi.org/10.1210/endrev/bnaa016

Shroff, H., Reba, L., Thornton, L. M., Tozzi, F., Klump, K. L., Berrettini, W. H., Brandt, H., Crawford, S., Crow, S., Fichter, M. M., Goldman, D., Halmi, K. A., Johnson, C., Kaplan, A. S., Keel, P., LaVia, M., Mitchell, J., Rotondo, A., Strober, M., . . . Bulik, C. M. (2006). Features associated with excessive exercise in women with eating disorders. *International Journal of Eating Disorders, 39*(6), 454–461. https://doi.org/10.1002/eat.20247

Smith, A. R., Fink, E. L., Anestis, M. D., Ribeiro, J. D., Gordon, K. H., Davis, H., Keel, P. K., Bardone-Cone, A. M., Peterson, C. B., Klein, M. H., Crow, S., Mitchell, J. E., Crosby, R. D., Wonderlich, S. A., Le Grange, D., & Joiner, T. E. (2013). Exercise caution: Over-exercise is associated with suicidality among individuals with disordered eating. *Psychiatry Research, 206*(2–3), 246–255. https://doi.org/10.1016/j.psychres.2012.11.004

Song, W., Wang, W., Yu, S., & Lin, G. N. (2021). Dissection of the genetic association between anorexia nervosa and obsessive–compulsive disorder at the network and cellular levels. *Genes, 12*(4), 491. https://doi.org/10.3390/genes12040491

Steinglass, J. E., & Walsh, B. T. (2016). Neurobiological model of the persistence of anorexia nervosa. *Journal of Eating Disorders, 4*(1), 19. https://doi.org/10.1186/s40337-016-0106-2

Szuhany, K. L., Bugatti, M., & Otto, M. W. (2015). A meta-analytic review of the effects of exercise on brain-derived neurotrophic factor. *Journal of Psychiatric Research, 60*, 56–64. https://doi.org/10.1016/j.jpsychires.2014.10.003

Tabone, M., Bressa, C., García-Merino, J. A., Moreno-Pérez, D., Van, E. C., Castelli, F. A., Fenaille, F., & Larrosa, M. (2021). The effect of acute moderate-intensity exercise on the serum and fecal metabolomes and the gut microbiota of cross-country endurance athletes. *Scientific Reports, 11*, 3558. https://doi.org/10.1038/s41598-021-82947-1

Taranis, L., Touyz, S., & Meyer, C. (2011). Disordered eating and exercise: Development and preliminary validation of the compulsive exercise test (CET). *European Eating Disorders Review, 19*(3), 256–268. https://doi.org/10.1002/erv.1108

Thornton, L. M., Munn-Chernoff, M. A., Baker, J. H., Juréus, A., Parker, R., Henders, A. K., Larsen, J. T., Petersen, L., Watson, H. J., Yilmaz, Z., Kirk, K. M., Gordon, S., Leppä, V. M., Martin, F. C., Whiteman, D. C., Olsen, C. M., Werge, T. M., Pedersen, N. L., Kaye, W., . . . Bulik, C. M. (2018). The Anorexia Nervosa Genetics Initiative (ANGI): Overview and methods. *Contemporary Clinical Trials, 74*, 61–69. https://doi.org/10.1016/j.cct.2018.09.015

Touyz, S., Hay, P., & Noetel, M. (2017). Is the neglect of exercise in anorexia nervosa research a case of "running out" of ideas or do we need to take a "LEAP" of faith into the future. Journal of *Eating Disorders*, 5, 35. https://doi.org/10.1186/s40337-017-0157-z

Tricomi, E., Balleine, B. W., & O'Doherty, J. P. (2009). A specific role for posterior dorsolateral striatum in human habit learning. *European Journal of Neuroscience, 29*(11), 2225–2232. https://doi.org/10.1111/j.1460-9568.2009.06796.x

Vankim, N. A., & Nelson, T. F. (2013). Vigorous physical activity, mental health, perceived stress, and socializing among college students. *American Journal of Health Promotion*, 28(1), 7–15. https://doi.org/10.4278/ajhp.111101-QUAN-395

Verhagen, L. A. W., Luijendijk, M. C. M., Hillebrand, J. J. G., & Adan, R. A. H. (2009). Dopamine antagonism inhibits anorectic behavior in an animal model for anorexia nervosa. *European Neuropsychopharmacology, 19*(3), 153–160. https://doi.org/10.1016/j.euroneuro.2008.09.005

Volkow, N. D., Wang, G.-J., Maynard, L., Jayne, M., Fowler, J. S., Zhu, W., Logan, J., Gatley, S. J., Ding, Y.-S., Wong, C., & Pappas, N. (2003). Brain dopamine is associated with eating behaviors in humans. *International Journal of Eating Disorders, 33*(2), 136–142. https://doi.org/10.1002/eat.10118

Walsh, B. T. (2013). The enigmatic persistence of anorexia nervosa. *American Journal of Psychiatry, 170*(5), 477–484. https://doi.org/10.1176/appi.ajp.2012.12081074

Wierenga, C. E., Ely, A., Bischoff-Grethe, A., Bailer, U. F., Simmons, A. N., & Kaye, W. H. (2014). Are extremes of consumption in eating disorders related to an altered balance between reward and inhibition? *Frontiers in Behavioral Neuroscience*, 8, 410. https://doi.org/10.3389/fnbeh.2014.00410

Yilmaz, Z., Schaumberg, K., Halvorsen, M., Goodman, E. L., Brosof, L. C., Crowley, J. J., Anorexia Nervosa Genetics Initiative, Eating Disorders Working Group of the Psychiatric Genomics Consortium, Tourette Syndrome/Obsessive-Compulsive Disorder Working Group of the Psychiatric Genomics Consortium, Mathews, C. A., Mattheisen, M., Breen, G., Bulik, C. M., Micali, N., & Zerwas, S. C. (2022). Predicting eating disorder and anxiety symptoms using disorder-specific and transdiagnostic polygenic scores for anorexia nervosa and obsessive-compulsive disorder. *Psychological Medicine*, 53(7), 3021–3035. https://doi.org/10.1017/S0033291721005079

Young, S., Touyz, S., Meyer, C., Arcelus, J., Rhodes, P., Madden, S., Pike, K., Attia, E., Crosby, R. D., Wales, J., & Hay, P. (2017). Validity of exercise measures in adults with anorexia nervosa: The EDE, compulsive exercise test and other self-report scales. *International Journal of Eating Disorders, 50*(5), 533–541. https://doi.org/10.1002/eat.22633

17

Body Image

Jamie D. Feusner and Valentina Cazzato

Brief Definitional Overview

Body image: A multidimensional concept that includes perceptions of and attitudes toward one's own body, primarily focusing on one's physical appearance but not limited to it (Cash & Pruzinsky, 2002). This is most often divided into "perceptual" (sensory perception), cognitive, and affective factors (Cash & Deagle III, 1997; Waldman et al., 2013).

Body image disturbance: In the context of DSM-5 diagnostic criteria for anorexia nervosa, this is defined as, "Disturbance in the way in which body weight or shape is experienced, with undue influence of body weight or shape on self-evaluation or persistent lack of recognition of the seriousness of current low body weight." For bulimia nervosa, this is defined as, "Self-evaluation is unduly influenced by body shape and weight" (American Psychiatric Association, 2013).

Body size distortion: The difference between a person's perceived and actual body size (Boepple et al., 2015). In the context of eating disorders, this most often manifests as body size overestimation.

Body dissatisfaction: Negative thoughts and feelings about one's body (Grogan, 2021).

Introduction

Body image disturbance is a core feature of many eating disorders, particularly anorexia nervosa (AN) and bulimia nervosa (BN) (American Psychiatric Association, 2013). Disturbance of body image in eating disorders gained much attention when Hilde Bruch described it, in the framework of "perceptual and conceptual fields," as a pathognomonic sign in AN (Bruch, 1962). Neurobiologically, the perception of one's body, in general, is molded by reciprocal interaction between sensory perceptions of one's physical appearance, experiences based on self-observation and the reactions of others (Baker & Wertheim, 2003), and own body image representation in the brain (Vocks et al., 2010). In terms of the neurobiological contributors to body image disturbances in those with eating disorders, the field has acquired the most knowledge to date (although still incomplete) of

Jamie D. Feusner and Valentina Cazzato, *Body Image*. In: *The Handbook of the Neurobiology of Eating Disorders*.
Edited by: Christina E. Wierenga and Joanna E. Steinglass, Oxford University Press.
DOI: 10.1093/9780197675212.003.0018

the sensory-perceptual aspects. Prior to describing these aspects in eating disorders, the underlying neurophysiology and neuroanatomy of body perception in general, which includes contributions from visual perception, somatosensation, proprioception, equilibrioception, as well as their multisensory integration, will be introduced. The visual, tactile somatosensory, proprioceptive, and multisensory integration abnormalities, as well as cognitive and affective factors that may contribute to body image disturbances in individuals with eating disorders, will then be discussed. The preponderance of the research has studied these factors in AN, while much less is known in BN and other eating disorders. Current findings suggest body image disturbances in AN are not solely due to sensory-perceptual deficits or their multisensory integration in accurately representing body size but also involve a complex interplay of cognitive and emotional factors.

Biological Framework

Overview of the neural systems involved in body processing

Body perception has been proposed to depend on a "body matrix"; that is, a dynamic body-centered neural representation of a person's body and of the space around it (Moseley et al., 2012). The body matrix emerges from the flow of information across large-scale networks that link various regions of the brain (Bolognini et al., 2013; Gallace & Spence, 2014; Moseley et al., 2012). Specifically, through the connections between the posterior parietal cortex and the insular cortex, the body matrix integrates information about the body, as well as of the space directly around it, into sensory information which is centered on the body. The function of this body matrix is to preserve the integrity of the body, both physiologically and psychologically, and to adjust to alterations in our bodily structure and orientation.

Visual

Brain regions engaged in response to images of bodies differ partially from those engaged for other (non-body) images, including regions engaged in response to faces (Berlucchi & Aglioti, 2010). Visual perception of the human body selectively activates brain areas functionally located in the extrastriate body area (EBA) in the lateral occipito-temporal cortex and the fusiform body area (FBA) in the medial occipito-temporal cortex (Peelen & Downing, 2007). These two brain areas respond preferentially to visual presentation of whole bodies and single body parts (Urgesi et al., 2004) but not of faces or objects. Although the functional role played by these body-selective areas in social perception is still not clear, there is evidence that they are important in processing body form, including body shape and posture (Moro et al., 2008; Urgesi et al., 2004) and contribute to the aesthetic appreciation of human bodies (Calvo-Merino et al., 2010).

Regarding aesthetic valuation, a function of visual perception of bodies that has high evolutionary significance, support for the role of the EBA comes from two non-invasive brain stimulation studies in healthy participants (Cazzato et al., 2014, 2016) that used transcranial magnetic stimulation (TMS). TMS was delivered over the EBA and the dorsal premotor cortex while participants rated how much they liked same versus opposite-gender (virtual) human bodies. TMS over EBA affected liking judgments for opposite-gender bodies, resulting in increased aesthetic preference. However, it should be noted that TMS over EBA did not affect body weight judgments (Cazzato et al., 2014). Furthermore, women showed stronger right EBA dominance than men in body aesthetic judgments, which suggests a greater hemispheric asymmetry in women compared to men, a result which has been previously found in several studies looking at body size distortions in women (Smeets & Kosslyn, 2001). For example, unilateral presentation of self-body image in the left visual hemi-field, which is projected first to the right hemisphere, resulted in an overestimation bias in women, but not in men (Mohr et al., 2007). This suggests the role of right hemisphere areas in body image distortion in women (Aleong & Paus, 2010; Cazzato et al., 2014).

Additional neuroimaging data show that the EBA may play a role in discriminating physical attributes such as visual perspectives and body size (Carey et al., 2019). These results suggest that the role of the EBA is complex, and it may represent human bodies in a more integrative manner, which simultaneously considers multiple physical attributes of bodies. This is likely to furnish crucial information to higher brain regions responsible for making aesthetic and affective evaluations of bodies (Carey et al., 2019).

Body image concerns involve not only how the body subjectively appears to an individual but also how the person believes it appears to others. Other brain areas in addition to the EBA contribute to the understanding of the subjective and intersubjective experiences of body representations; that is, the shared understanding, perception, or interpretation of an event which involves another person. The right temporoparietal junction (TPJ), an area of the brain which is important for high-order processing of the self–other relationship (Tsakiris et al., 2008; Uddin et al., 2006) may play an active and complementary role in the complex interaction between the perceptions of one's own and other people' body (Cazzato et al., 2015).

Somatosensation

Somatosensation refers to the complex system of sensory receptors and pathways that respond to changes both at the surface of the body and within deeper tissues. This system encompasses sensations such as touch, temperature, pain, and proprioception. The skin contains numerous specialized receptors for perception of texture, pressure, vibration, pain, and itch (Johansson & Flanagan, 2009; Woolf & Ma, 2007). Research into the sense of touch has largely focused on discriminatory perception, characterizing the consequences of stimulation of a specific class of receptors, namely low-threshold mechanoreceptors found in the skin and joints. Low-threshold mechanoreceptors are innervated by myelinated Aβ afferent nerves ("Aβ" refers to the size and myelination level of these nerve fibers, with "A" denoting large diameter and "β" indicating medium myelination) which are sensory nerve fibers that enable fast conduction velocities and supporting rapid central processing. The most abundant class of skin, the hairy skin, contains proportionally fewer low-threshold mechanoreceptors and is an innervated by a class of unmyelinated low-threshold mechanosensory nerves, described as C-tactile (CT) afferents, with a conduction velocity about 50 times slower than myelinated afferents (McGlone et al., 2014). Affective touch is processed by CT-afferents (Håkan Olausson et al., 2002; McGlone et al., 2014). CT-afferents are mainly found in the hairy skin of the body and respond optimally to slow caress-like touch.

CT-afferents also constitute the peripheral physiological substrate for pleasant tactile information, given that activation of these fibers, during affective tactile interactions, is normally perceived as pleasant. Given their contribution to the hedonic value of social physical contacts, CT-afferents have been proposed to play a fundamental role in promoting social bonding and proximity seeking. Importantly, CT-afferents project to the posterior insular cortex, which is theorized to be involved in regulating the body's homeostatic balance (Craig, 2003; Håkan Olausson et al., 2002). We therefore possess a rapid "first" touch system, with clear advantages for discriminative and sensorimotor functions and in general for our survival, and a "slow" touch system with no immediate implication for survival, yet with a crucial role in promoting well-being and homeostasis.

A novel theoretical framework for the various networks involved in the many aspects of somatosensory function has been proposed, which includes several specialized routes more multimodal in nature and less independent from each other (less "informationally encapsulated") (de Haan & Dijkerman, 2020). Specifically, this model proposes the existence of a fundamental somatosensory processing unit which comprises the thalamus and the primary and secondary somatosensory areas (SI and SII). This unit, referred to as the "cylinder block," is primarily driven by somatosensory input. Within this hierarchical structure, early processing in SI (located in the anterior parietal cortex) primarily handles basic features, such as stimulus location and duration, while subsequent processing involves the detection of the direction and velocity of stimuli moving across the body surface. Higher association areas integrate these features. The connections among these components are both serial and parallel. The authors suggest that this cylinder block serves as the input for five major overlapping networks, namely haptic object recognition, action, body ownership, affective processing, and body perception. The understanding of body perception has evolved to encompass a network of various cortical regions including the EBA, the inferior parietal cortex, and the posterior insula, all of which exhibit multimodal characteristics. It is well known that body perception depends on several higher-order representations which go beyond basic somatosensory mechanisms involved in proprioception, touch, temperature, and pain. For instance, body perception can be characterized by body information which pertains to "spatial" (e.g., location of, distance between, speed of touch sensation) as well as "structural" (e.g., knowledge and awareness of the positions of body parts) properties. The processing of somatosensory information coupled with visual, vestibular, and interoceptive input leads to body awareness and body ownership, that is, the feeling that a body (or part of it) belongs to you.

Proprioception

Proprioception is defined by the sense of knowing where one's limbs and body are in space (Blanke, 2012). Proprioception contributes to body perception by providing information about limb and trunk position and movement, as well as the sense of force, effort, and heaviness (Proske & Gandevia, 2012). Receptors in the skin, muscles, and joints detect position. Afferent signals from these receptors to the brain determine the position of limbs in space (Taylor, 2009). The combination of proprioceptive information with information from other sensory modalities, such as visual, somatosensory, and equilibriosensory, creates a coherent perception of our body and its relationship to the external world (Proske & Gandevia, 2012). The purpose of proprioception is to maintain body awareness, coordinate movements, and navigate the environment effectively.

Equilibrioception (vestibular)

Equilibrioception is the sense of balance, and its primary function is likely to establish awareness of equilibrium to prevent falls. By constantly monitoring the position and movement of the body, equilibrioception provides information about spatial orientation and helps maintain an upright posture. Equilibrioception works in coordination with vision and proprioception to provide a comprehensive understanding of the body's position in space (Fuchs, 2018). Equilibrioception, distinct from proprioception, is a function of the vestibular system, which is an inner ear sensory system that relies on hair cells to detect movements and provides a sense of balance and spatial awareness (Ango & Dos Reis, 2019). Two organs in the inner ear, the sacculus and the utricle, are sensitive to gravity and linear motion, respectively. This information is conveyed to the cerebellum, which in turn coordinates it with motor movements to maintain balance and posture (Mackrous et al., 2019). Multisensory integration, particularly with visual and proprioceptive signals, occurs within the thalamus, insula, retroinsula, parietal operculum, and temporo-parietal junction, referred to as the vestibular network (Delle Monache et al., 2021; Guldin & Grüsser, 1998; Lopez & Blanke, 2011).

Multisensory integration

Multisensory integration describes how the brain integrates information from multiple senses to enhance perception (Blanke et al., 2015; Ernst & Bülthoff, 2004; Fetsch et al., 2013). Multisensory integration occurs at different levels in the brain, including at the level of individual neurons in the superior colliculus (Meredith & Stein, 1986), and cortical levels, particularly in the superior parietal cortex (Sereno & Huang, 2014). Inputs from different senses are better integrated when they occur closer together in space and time; further, the integration is more robust when the individual signals from each sensory modality are weaker; that is, no one signal strongly dominates (Blanke et al., 2015; Frassinetti et al., 2002; Stein et al., 1989; Stein & Stanford, 2008). In this way, and potentially contributing to disrupted subjective experiences of one's body, imbalanced signals from one sensory modality could disrupt the overall ability to integrate across sensory modalities, likely resulting in body size distortion.

The rubber hand illusion is an experimental paradigm that demonstrates how sight, touch, and proprioception (the sense of the relative position of one's own body parts) can be integrated to create a false sense of body ownership. In this paradigm, a rubber hand is experienced as belonging to oneself when it is viewed in an appropriate anatomical position and is stroked simultaneously with one's actual hand (Ehrsson et al., 2005). In this procedure, a participant's real hand is hidden from view, and a rubber hand is placed in front of them (Botvinick & Cohen, 1998). Both the real hand and the rubber hand are simultaneously stroked with a brush. Because the participant can see the rubber hand being stroked and feels their own hand being stroked at the same time, their brain integrates these sensations, leading to the illusion that the rubber hand is part of their body. Some participants even report feeling as though the touch they are experiencing is coming from the rubber hand itself. This illusion sheds light on the complex processes underlying body perception and has been used to explore topics like body ownership, self-awareness, and the flexibility of the brain in integrating multisensory information. The rubber hand illusion activates the ventral premotor cortex, intraparietal cortex, and cerebellum, likely reflecting the detection and integration of congruent multisensory signals (Botvinick, 2004; Ehrsson et al., 2005). This illusion is interrupted if the participant moves their hand, likely due to discrepancy between motor and sensory information.

Dynamics of bodily experience

The conscious experience of the body is updated through behavior. Already-held representations are updated with new somatosensory, proprioceptive, and visual information obtained from multiple viewpoints. This includes, for example, active comparisons by moving one's body in a mirror, changing the visual focus, and other eye gaze patterns across different body parts and the overall body (Cornelissen et al., 2009; Kerr-Gaffney et al., 2018; Laeng et al., 2014).

Selfness of body perception

Another function contributing to body processing is one that determines the "selfness" of bodily perception; that is, distinguishing if the perceived body belongs to oneself rather than to another person. Sorting of perceptual experiences into self-generated from other-generated is a feature common across many organisms (Yong, 2022). To serve this function the brain produces a duplicate of information from the motor initiation system that is compared with sensory inputs—termed "corollary discharge" (Buzsáki, 2019; Sperry, 1950; Von Holst & Mittelstaedt, 1950). This allows the brain to calculate if there is a discrepancy between what is predicted by the movement (e.g., of a body part) and what is sensed—visually or through somatosensation, proprioception, and/or equilibrioception. If there is no discrepancy, the experience is one of ownership of the body part.

Mental imagery

The capacity to explore a mentally generated image of the body, typically to interpret its characteristics and spatial properties, involves the function of mental imagery (Kosslyn, 1980). Mental imagery of own bodies is associated with activation in the EBA (mental rotation of full bodies) (Blanke et al., 2010; Perruchoud et al., 2016), TPJ, anterior parietal, premotor, superior parietal, precentral gyrus, premotor area, intraparietal sulcus, insula, and superior frontal cortex (Arzy et al., 2006; Blanke et al., 2010). Mental imagery is likely evoked in tasks aimed at quantifying the accuracy of body size estimation; these tasks typically require selecting from figure drawings or photos of bodies, or manipulating a computerized version of a body, to match the size and shape of the individual's own body in the absence of being able to simultaneously view one's own body (Gardner & Brown, 2014; Mölbert et al., 2017). Mental imagery, in general, also involves regions associated with the integration of eye movements and visual information, including the supplementary and cingulate eye fields and frontal eye fields, suggesting the role of visual search even in imagined visual imagery (Winlove et al., 2018). Mental imagery may be evoked when one spontaneously thinks about one's body. In clinical conditions involving body image disturbances, such as certain eating disorders and body dysmorphic disorder, these images may be experienced as obsessive and intrusive (Fassino & Marzola, 2018).

Summary

Body processing involves a complex interaction of sensory perceptions, self-observation, and brain representation of one's body. Body perception relies on a dynamic body-centered neural representation that integrates sensory data from various brain regions. Visual body perception activates specific brain areas, such as the EBA and the FBA, which play a role in processing body morphology and aesthetic appreciation of human bodies. The somatosensory system, proprioception, and equilibrioception also contribute to body perception, as well as multisensory integration. The brain constantly updates body representations through iterative interactions with stimuli, comparing sensory inputs to existing body representations to estimate body size and proportions.

State of the Science in Eating Disorders

Body image disturbances and body image distortion in eating disorders

Perceptual disturbances in the experience of one's body giving rise to body image distortion (inaccuracy in gauging one's body size) and evaluative body dissatisfaction including self-ideal discrepancies may contribute to body image disturbances in those with AN and BN (Cash & Brown, 1987; Cash & Deagle III, 1997; Garner & Garfinkel, 1981). Many with AN and BN misestimate that their overall body and/or body parts are larger than they are, as well as demonstrate greater body dissatisfaction, including both adults (Mölbert et al., 2017) and adolescents/children (Sattler et al., 2020).

Perceptual distortion of appearance has been studied more extensively in individuals with AN than in those with BN (Bruch, 1962; Farrell et al., 2005; Gardner & Brown, 2014; Gardner & Moncrieff, 1988; Molinari, 1995; Vitousek & Hollon, 1990). An early meta-analysis found medium-to-large effect sizes for perceptual contributions and mostly large effect sizes for attitudinal contributors to body image disturbance in individuals with AN or BN (Cash & Deagle III, 1997). Subsequent to this meta-analysis, a single study of visual perception of self and others' bodies did not find evidence of body size overestimation (Hennighausen et al., 1999). However, multiple studies of individuals with AN conducted between 2003 and 2013 showed large magnitude differences from healthy controls (HC); the most significant differences were in body part size overestimation, followed by whole-body size overestimation (reviewed in Gardner & Brown, 2014). A later meta-analysis also found evidence of overestimation of body size in individuals with AN, as well as overestimation by individuals with BN; further, body parts that are more influenced by fat deposition and other changes associated with weight gain may be more likely to be overestimated than other body parts (Mölbert et al., 2017). Thus, newer studies have more consistently found evidence for perceptual body size misestimation, whereas the older studies had more inconsistent findings. Inconsistencies in older studies may have been due to the use of analog techniques (e.g. figural drawing scales, which lacked demonstrated psychometric properties) (Gardner & Brown, 2010). In sum, the preponderance of research shows that body image distortion is a reliable finding among individuals with AN and BN.

Multiple factors may contribute to body image distortion in eating disorders. These distortions may reflect aberrancies in how the brain is creating one's internalized mental body image and may have contributions from visual perceptual, tactile/somatosensory, proprioceptive, multisensory integration, and cognitive and affective elements.

Visual perceptual distortion may underlie body image disturbances

Multiple neuropsychological studies have pointed to imbalances in global versus local processing in those with AN and those with BN, termed "weak central coherence" (Keegan et al., 2021; Lang et al., 2014; Madsen et al., 2013). Further, studies testing face and body inversion effects have corroborated the model of imbalance in global versus local processing (Groves et al., 2020; Urgesi et al., 2014). For example, using an inversion effect paradigm, which required women with AN to discriminate upright from inverted bodies, faces, and non-corporeal objects, such as houses, a study demonstrated that configural body, but not face processing, is different in those with AN than HC (Urgesi et al., 2014). Furthermore, another study provided evidence of disruption in configural processing of body stimuli in high-risk adolescents and in women recovering from body image disorders (Groves et al., 2020). Considered together, these studies suggest an unbalanced body processing style in AN that may favor a preference for detail-based processing of the human body.

Body size and shape misestimations in AN and BN may be related to brain activation and connectivity differences in body processing and visual systems (Via et al., 2018; Vocks et al., 2010). Neuroimaging studies have found reduced connectivity among individuals with AN compared with HC between the left FBA and EBA (Via et al., 2018; Vocks et al., 2010). Individuals with BN, unlike HC, did not show associations between degree of body size estimation and activation in the lateral occipital cortex nor did they activate the middle frontal gyrus during body size estimation (Mohr et al., 2011). In AN, structure and overall reduction of gray matter density in EBA was found to be negatively correlated with body size misjudgment (Suchan et al., 2010).

Using other-face and house stimuli in functional magnetic resonance imaging (fMRI) studies, reduced activity in the dorsal visual stream was observed for images conveying only global and configural information in those with (weight-restored) AN compared with HC (Li, Lai, Bohon, et al., 2015). A similar fMRI study in the same sample found, in response to viewing others' bodies, reduced neural activity in visual cortex and hyperconnectivity in dorsal visual and parietal networks in AN compared with HC (Moody et al., 2021), which was associated with appraisals of body size and appearance.

These behavioral and imaging data contribute to a model in AN (and in BN, primarily from behavioral studies to date) that the hyper-scrutiny of miniscule details could be mechanistically related to failing to "see" the appearance feature as an integrated whole, which may reflect an imbalance in global and local processing (Feusner et al., 2017). This is supported by additional imaging and electrophysiological evidence (Li, Lai, Bohon, et al., 2015; Li, Lai, Loo, et al., 2015).

Visual perception is additionally influenced by visual attention, which has important contributions from eye gaze patterns. Thus, atypical eye gaze patterns may also contribute to differences in body perception in those with eating disorders compared with HC. Several studies using eye-tracking to determine attentional biases found differences in biases toward own- or others' bodies and toward high or low body mass index bodies in AN and BN compared with HC, although with mixed findings depending on the methodology (reviewed in Stott et al., 2021). Further, studies have found abnormally short fixation duration in AN for own and others' faces, as well as short fixation duration and short saccade amplitude for others' bodies (Phillipou et al., 2015; Phillipou et al., 2016). This suggests a pattern of multiple short-duration fixations interspersed with a high number of short-distance saccades to scan multiple facial details. Saccades have been found to suppress low spatial frequency (dorsal pathway) contrast sensitivity (Burr et al., 1994). Thus, attentional allocation in conjunction with eye behaviors may have a modulatory effect on global processing.

Emotional arousal, common in those with body image disturbances when viewing or thinking about their body, may heighten local/detailed processing and further distort visual processing. Negative emotional states may contribute to visual perceptual disturbances via modulation from limbic to visual systems (Bohon et al., 2012; Lang et al., 1998). Among individuals with anxiety disorders, emotional states, particularly anxiety (highly common in those with eating disorders), have been shown to alter visual processing, enhancing detail extraction from the ventral visual system and hypervigilance to details in the environment (Pizzagalli et al., 2002; Vuilleumier et al., 2004).

Tactile somatosensation

Individuals with AN may display somatosensory impairments. These alterations are present for tactile discrimination (i.e., the ability to discriminate between sources of tactile information), but not for tactile detection (i.e., the ability to detect a tactile stimulus) (Møller, 2014). Using a measure of sensitivity to tactile pressure, such as the Von Frey Test, patients with AN did not differ from HC in detecting arm, sternum, or thigh stimulation (Keizer et al., 2012; Spitoni et al., 2015). In a Tactile Estimation Task, which asks the participant to estimate the distance between two stimuli applied to the forearm and the abdomen, patients with AN overestimated the distance between the two stimuli on the arm and abdomen as compared with HC, and higher levels of body dissatisfaction were associated with greater tactile overestimates (Keizer et al., 2011; Keizer et al., 2012). In addition, patients with AN judged horizontal tactile stimuli on the abdomen and thigh significantly wider apart than the same stimuli oriented vertically (Spitoni et al., 2015). This difference seems to persist even after treatment (Keizer et al.,

2019). Considered together, the existing research on somatosensory misperception in AN suggests that individuals with AN have poorer tactile discrimination compared to controls, specifically in those cases involving spatial discrimination, but do not differ in tactile detection. This tactile impairment seems to affect the extremities, for example, the arms and thighs, in addition to salient areas of the trunk, such as the abdomen.

Affective touch serves as a significant means of both experiencing and conveying emotions, and therefore it refers to the emotional facet of tactile sensations (McGlone et al., 2014; Håkan Olausson et al., 2002). Recent studies have provided evidence of atypical responses to gentle touch in individuals with AN, who generally report lower pleasantness to affective touch. Patients with AN perceived CT-mediated affective touch as less pleasant than HC (Crucianelli et al., 2016). Compared with HC, patients with AN rated skin stroking (across the dorsal forearm) as significantly less pleasant (Davidovic et al., 2018), also shown among individuals remitted from AN (Bischoff-Grethe et al., 2018). One study indicated that patients with AN also perceived non-affective stimulations as less pleasant than HC (Crucianelli et al., 2021), suggesting a generalized altered perception of tactile stimuli, regardless of affective nature. A more recent study reported a preserved experience of affective touch in two tasks involving both imagined and real touch experiences (Tagini et al., 2023). Top-down factors, such as the anticipation of pleasure, may also influence the experience of affective touch alongside bottom-up factors like CT sensitivity and functioning (Tagini et al., 2023; Wierenga et al., 2020). Furthermore, when observing another person receiving gentle touch (Tagini et al., 2023), those with current AN and those with remitted AN did not differ from HC in their ability to rate touch for another person (Bellard et al., 2022). However, when evaluating touch for themselves, those with AN rated pleasant touching as being less enjoyable than HC (Bellard et al., 2022). Altered responses to touch seem to occur during the anticipation (i.e., what individuals expect to be pleasant), rather than the consummatory (i.e., what individuals experience when touched). Whether individuals with AN experience a generalized altered perception of tactile stimuli, regardless of affective nature, is yet to be established. All together, these results are consistent with reports that individuals with AN typically find closeness discomforting and may contribute to difficulty maintaining close intimate relationships with a romantic partner, family, and friends (Evans & Wertheim, 1998; Fabello, 2020; Pruitt et al., 1992).

Proprioception

To date, proprioception in patients with AN has been investigated in four studies (Epstein et al., 2001; Goldzak-Kunik et al., 2012; Guardia et al., 2012; Guardia et al., 2013). In a study using two tasks, a proprioception task and a left-right orientation task, participants were asked to point to body parts as directed, in the absence of visual information (Epstein et al., 2001). No differences were found between individuals with AN and HC. In the left-right orientation task, participants were asked to point to a specific body part using a specific hand while their eyes were either open or closed. They were also asked to point at a specific part of the experimenter with a specific finger. Individuals with AN performed comparably to controls on all aspects of the left-right orientation task, but they showed poorer accuracy when pointing to specific lateralities of the experimenter's body parts (in the moderate and difficult condition). These results suggest that, in individuals with AN, the ability to localize parts of their body with and without visual information is intact.

A study using a kinesthesia task involved blindfolded participants judging the height of their hand while holding a movable vertical handle placed at varying heights (Goldzak-Kunik et al., 2012). Results indicated no discernible differences in performance between individuals with AN and controls, suggesting that the ability to estimate hand height remains intact in AN. Similarly, when spatial orientation constancy was examined with a task requiring participants to manually position a rod vertically, without visual feedback, in both upright and tilted body positions, no distinctions were observed between patients with AN and HC in the upright condition. Patients with AN differed from HC when the body was roll-tilted left or right (Guardia et al., 2012; Guardia et al., 2013).

Together, these results suggest limited differences in proprioceptive components relevant to body perception, which may contribute to body image distortions in AN.

Other sensory perception

Research using size judgments of objects (Brown et al., 2021), simple shape identification (e.g., a star, disk, egg, and heart), and weight judgments of a held object (Goldzak-Kunik et al., 2012) did not find conclusive evidence of misestimation in those with AN compared to healthy controls. However, studies of these sensory experiences are sparse, and conclusions cannot be drawn at this point.

Multisensory integration

Multisensory integration refers to the process by which the brain combines information from various sensory modalities (i.e., visual, tactile, proprioceptive, etc.) to produce a coherent perception of our body (Ehrsson, 2012; Stein & Stanford, 2008). It has been reported that individuals with eating disorders experience the rubber hand illusion more vividly than controls. One study reported that patients with AN and BN experienced the rubber hand illusion more strongly than controls. In this study, the cognitive measure (i.e., embodiment score, a subjective measure of the degree of body ownership of the rubber hand) and the perceptual measure (i.e., proprioceptive drift, a quantitative perceptual measure of the change of perceived finger location toward the rubber hand) of rubber hand illusion were found to be significantly greater in patients with eating disorders compared to HCs (Eshkevari et al., 2012). In addition, both proprioceptive drift and embodiment score correlated significantly with eating disorder psychopathology variables, including drive for thinness and body dissatisfaction in AN. A second study reported that individuals with AN demonstrated higher ownership scores than the controls in the synchronous condition but the two groups did not differ regarding proprioceptive drift (Keizer et al., 2014). Taken together, the results of these two studies seem to suggest that individuals with AN have a heightened sensitivity to visual information that may be related to an altered multisensory integration or to an impaired somatosensory information processing of the body.

Full-body illusions are experimental manipulations that create a sense of ownership over an artificial or virtual body, like the rubber hand illusion but extended to the entire body. These illusions are usually induced using virtual reality systems that provide multisensory stimuli to create a convincing experience that the participant's body is different from its actual physical form. Virtual-reality-based body swapping can decrease body size overestimation among patients with AN (Keizer et al., 2016). One study used a thin avatar to reduce overestimation in a sample of female participants with no eating disorder (Preston & Ehrsson, 2014). Another study investigated whether the embodiment of different-sized avatars could reduce body image disturbances in AN (Provenzano et al., 2019). Interpersonal multisensory stimulation (e.g., experiencing a tactile stimulation on one's own body synchronously with an observed touch at the corresponding body part on another individual's body) was applied to three different body size avatars (one reproducing participant's own perceived body, one 15% thinner and one 15% larger) presented with a first-person perspective. The authors found that whilst embodiment was stronger after synchronous interpersonal multisensory stimulation in both groups, this did not reduce body image disturbances in participants with AN. Patients with AN reported more negative emotions after embodying the largest avatar, which scaled with symptom severity. The authors interpreted these results as suggesting that the cognitive-affective component of body image is more affected than the perceptual component in AN.

Considered together, hypothetically it is possible that the results from rubber hand illusion and full-body illusion studies could be explained by an increased sensitivity to the visual component of body perception at the expense of somatosensory information processing in AN. In this way, differences between individuals with AN and HC in multisensory integration may be due to the dominance of one sensory modality (Blanke et al., 2015; Frassinetti et al., 2002; Stein et al., 1989; Stein & Stanford, 2008).

Affective and cognitive factors

The cognitive-affective component of body image disturbance in AN, which refers to thoughts, beliefs, and emotions associated with one's body, including dissatisfaction, preoccupation, and anxiety related to body shape and weight is also highly important to the understanding of this complex disorder. Several studies consistently report that individuals with AN often perceive their bodies as larger than they are and that this misperception includes not only a distorted perceptual representation but also a distorted cognitive-affective representation of the body. Body dissatisfaction is an essential feature of AN and refers to the negative evaluative thoughts and feelings related to one's body. This dissatisfaction is often associated with the drive for thinness (Stice & Shaw, 2002). Notably, the affective component of body image disturbance includes the emotional responses to body shape and appearance. In AN and BN, this often includes feelings of shame, guilt, and anxiety related to the body (Fox & Power, 2009). Further, research has shown that individuals with eating disorders have cognitive biases in processing body-related information, showing selective attention and memory for weight-related stimuli (Jansen et al., 2005).

Overall, current evidence suggests that patients' belief of being "too fat" is not only due to perceptual differences in representing own-body weight and dimensions accurately but also to a wide range of interrelated cognitive and emotional factors. Most of the evidence points to those with AN having distortion in evaluating their own body more than showing altered body representation for others, suggesting either own-body-specific sensory perceptual differences and/or strong contributions of self-related cognitive-affective factors. There are notable exceptions to this, however; for example, aberrant neural activation has been observed for others' bodies, others' faces, and objects (houses) (Li, Lai, Bohon, et al., 2015; Li, Lai, Loo, et al., 2015; Moody et al., 2021), and the body inversion effect task that used others' bodies (Groves et al., 2020; Urgesi et al., 2014). In sum, cognitive and affective features (e.g., drive for thinness and fear of weight gain) play a strong role in driving body image distortions (Frank & Treasure, 2016; Hagman et al., 2015; Mölbert et al., 2018).

Alternative Perspectives

Body image distortion is not central to the pathophysiology of eating disorders

While body image distortion is common in eating disorders and is a component of diagnostic criteria for AN, it is important to note that not all individuals with eating disorders experience it. According to DSM-5, individuals may meet criteria for AN if they have either "disturbance in the way in which one's body weight or shape is experienced" or "undue influence of body weight or shape on self-evaluation, or denial of the seriousness of the current low body weight" (American Psychiatric Association, 2013), the latter two possibilities not, therefore, requiring that someone has body image distortion (inaccurate estimation of one's body size or shape). The DSM-5 criteria for BN do not specify disturbances in the way one's body weight or shape is experienced, but rather, "self-evaluation is unduly influenced by body shape and weight." Similar to DSM-5, IDC-11's criteria for AN state, "Low body weight is overvalued and central to the person's self-evaluation, or the person's body weight or shape is inaccurately perceived to be normal or even excessive" (World Health Organization, 2004). ICD-11's criteria for BN mention, "excessive preoccupation with body weight or shape," but does not mention body image. Thus, based on the current way that AN and BN are clinically diagnosed, body image distortion is not a necessary feature.

Body image distortion in those with eating disorders is solely due to cognitive and affective factors and not perceptual factors

A key disputed issue in the field is whether body image distortion such as size misestimation in those with eating disorders is due to one or more fundamental perceptual deficits or if the cognitive and emotional components of body image (i.e., body dissatisfaction) are the drivers (Hennighausen et al., 1999) (Brown et al., 2021; Cash & Deagle III, 1997; Goldzak-Kunik et al., 2012). Discourse in the field around this topic has often been that *either* primary sensory perceptual disturbances ("bottom-up") *or* cognitive and affective factors ("top-down") cause body image distortions. This way of conceptualizing subjective perceptual experiences is that "top-down" systems act on "bottom-up" systems; an extrinsic stimulus arrives through a "bottom-up" (primary sensory) system, which is accompanied by a "top-down" (prefrontal and/or limbic system—cognitive and affective—or directed attention) reaction to the stimulus. An alternative framework is that the brain is a self-organized system whose pre-existing connectivity and dynamics are central to subjective experiences (reviewed in Buzsáki, 2019). In this theory, pre-existing intrinsic dynamic patterns constantly create internal simulations, including computations that are separate from the environment (Buzsáki & Tingley, 2023). Thus, conscious perceptual experiences in any given moment are mainly determined by pre-existing, intrinsic neural patterns such, as those linked with visual memories, and these are influenced by a combination of (a) external stimuli (e.g., visual stimuli of one's body) integrated with proprioception, somatosensory, and equilibrioceptive signals, and (b) cognitions and affect. Further, this is a dynamic process that, under normal conditions, is regularly updated from recursive interactions with the external environment, for example when trying on clothing or viewing oneself in the mirror. Hypothetically, for example, distortions in one's body image might occur if internal intrinsic patterns are excessively rigid and resistant to updating from new extrinsic information (e.g., one's body should visually appear thinner after their weight has dropped). In this way, prior memory contributions are not updated by new visual and somatosensory information or from cognitive knowledge that one's body weight is much lower than it previously was. In this framework, it is the internal, intrinsic neural connectivity and dynamics that are central; these may or may not be updated by sensory perceptual and/or cognitive and affective factors.

This supports a more nuanced and less dichotomous formulation of the cognitive/affective versus perceptual question regarding body image distortion. In this framework, one may ask *to what degree* a conscious experience of body image distortion may be due to intrinsic patterns that are, or were, influenced by aberrant sensory perceptual factors and/or have failed to dynamically update, and *to what degree* the intrinsic patterns are, or were, influenced by cognitive, affective, and memory systems. Adding further nuance is the possibility that different combinations of these factors could operate in different individuals, and different factors might operate at different times in the same individual. In sum, a less dichotomous framework for body image distortion in those with eating disorders is that, hypothetically, it may be a function of intrinsic neural patterns that are influenced to different degrees by cognitive and affective factors and misfunctioning sensory-perceptual systems, and this could be variable person-to-person and even moment-to-moment (Eshkevari et al., 2014; Garfinkel et al., 1978; Zanetti et al., 2013).

Body image distortion in those with eating disorders is primarily a function of socio-cultural norms, particularly as conveyed through social media

Effects of social media

A great deal of research effort has been directed toward understanding the sociocultural factors that play a role in the development and maintenance of body image disturbance and eating disorders. Internalization of media ideals (Thompson & Stice, 2001), negative verbal feedback (i.e., teasing), and elevated appearance comparison tendencies are all sociocultural factors which have been identified as potentially affecting an individual's perception of their own body, and subsequently their eating behavior. Within the theoretical framework of the Tripartite Influence model (Thompson et al., 1999), peers, parents, and media influences are three primary variables that may form the basis for later development of body image and eating dysfunction. In addition, the model proposes that internalization of societal ideals of appearance and heightened appearance comparison tendencies may also mediate disturbed body image and eating problems. These mediating variables are also hypothesized to lead to body image and eating outcomes. Social media have become a central element of the lives of young people around the world.

Evidence suggests that social media play a significant role in the development of eating and weight disorders, potentially exacerbating symptoms in individuals with existing conditions. Social media use, particularly on platforms like Facebook, may worsen symptoms and prolong the course of eating disorders, especially in women (Ali et al., 2022; Tan et al., 2016). Moreover, individuals with high levels of eating disorder symptoms are more likely to engage in problematic internet use (Rodgers et al., 2013). The mechanisms behind these effects are not fully understood, but one possible explanation is the phenomenon of "upward" social comparison, wherein individuals compare themselves unfavorably to others they perceive as more attractive, such as models or celebrities. This comparison can lead to body dissatisfaction and increase the risk of developing eating disorders. Overall, current social media usage appears to contribute to increased vulnerability to eating disorders by fostering body dissatisfaction and the desire for thinness (Jiotsa et al., 2021).

While at present a causative role of social media for ED cannot be provided, taken together current evidence suggests that body dissatisfaction may be partially mediated by inappropriate use of social media seeking social comparison with disturbed eating and other behaviors and their cognitive and affective counterparts, as well as sensory perceptual abnormalities. It should be noted that while social media messages are widespread, only a small portion of individuals are influenced to the extent that they meet clinical diagnosis thresholds.

In the future, longitudinal methods of investigation could be used to identify who is most susceptible to the influences of social media and the direction of relationships between social media use frequency, behavioral/cognitive/affective factors, perceptual abnormalities, with body dissatisfaction.

Implications

Body image disturbance is a critical feature of body image disorders

Disrupted experience of body size and shape is a core characteristic of body image disorders including, anorexia nervosa, other eating disorders, and body dysmorphic disorder (American Psychiatric Association, 2013). Body image dissatisfaction predicts the adoption of dieting and restrictive eating behaviors, which can be precursors to the development and persistence of eating disorders, and in that way may serve as a risk factor for the development of certain eating disorders, such as AN (Beato-Fernández et al., 2004; Jacobi et al., 2004). Further, body image disturbance predicts symptom severity and as a psychopathological feature is one of the last to change during the recovery process. Additionally, it has the potential to contribute to treatment discontinuation. Body image disturbance in AN is associated with emotional distress and can lead to time-consuming checking behaviors, such as mirror-checking and body-weighing, and (often dangerous) behaviors such as restricting calories and excessive exercise (Hoek, 2006).

Body image disturbance—A transdiagnostic phenomenon?

Although not classified as an eating disorder, body dysmorphic disorder (BDD) is a psychiatric disorder also characterized by distortion of body image. Individuals with BDD are preoccupied with one or more aspects of their appearance and engage in repetitive behaviors in attempts to check, fix, or hide the appearance features (American Psychiatric Association, 2013). Although concerns about facial features are common in those with BDD, misperception of, and preoccupation with, appearance features related to the body are also common, including concerns about body weight and body shape (Phillips & Diaz, 1997). In one study (Phillips, 2005), of the 530 total appearance concerns, 222 (42%) were related to the body.

Eating disorders and BDD co-occur within individuals to a significant degree; up to 32% of BDD patients have a lifetime comorbid eating disorder (including binge-eating disorder) (Ruffolo et al., 2006) and 25% to 39% of those with AN are diagnosed with comorbid BDD during their lifetime (Grant et al., 2002; Rabe-Jablonska Jolanta & Sobow Tomasz, 2000). There is also overlap in specific areas of appearance concerns between those with AN and those with BDD (e.g., size of abdomen, hips, and thighs) (Grant & Phillips, 2004). Approximately 30% of individuals with BDD also report significant weight concerns, a phenomenon linked to significantly greater symptom severity and morbidity (Kittler et al., 2007). In the majority of individuals with comorbid eating disorders and BDD, the onset of BDD preceded the onset of eating disorder pathology (Grant et al., 2001), suggesting that body dysmorphic concerns may be a risk factor for the development of eating disorders in some.

AN and BDD demonstrate similarities in terms of comorbidities, ages of onset, illness trajectories, and clinical and personality characteristics (Hartmann et al., 2013), contributing to conceptualizations of BDD and eating disorders as being on a spectrum of body image disorders (Phillipou et al., 2017). This conceptualization fits as well with muscle dysmorphia, which demonstrates overlapping phenomenological features with AN such as restricted or ritualistic eating habits and excessive exercise (Murray et al., 2012; Pope Jr et al., 1993); further, in a small twin study, a high proportion of male co-twins of proband males with anorexia nervosa showed muscle dysmorphic symptoms (Raevuori et al., 2009). Similar functional neural abnormalities have been found in direct comparisons of adults with AN to those with BDD (Li, Lai, Bohon, et al., 2015; Moody et al., 2021; Vaughn et al., 2019), supporting the concept of a transdiagnostic neural phenotype related to perceptual disturbances.

Given the body image disturbance features in BDD, similar to that in some eating disorders, yet considering the overlap as well of BDD phenomenology with obsessive-compulsive disorder, somatoform disorders, and affective disorders, one study tested several empirical models of BDD symptoms classification using structural equation modeling (Hartmann et al., 2020). The strongest evidence was for a body image model of BDD, which showed gender invariance, demonstrating evidence of symptoms of BDD as on a body image disorders spectrum.

These data support the concept of body image disturbance, and potentially its underlying neural contributors, as a transdiagnostic phenomenon. Such a conceptualization may improve our nosological understandings of disorders involving body image from a dimensional perspective. This could have implications for determining if conditions that do not fit cleanly into diagnostic categories (e.g., "atypical AN") or those otherwise meeting criteria for BDD who specifically have body size/shape concerns but subclinical disturbances in eating or exercise and without low weight who may be best characterized by shared neural/behavioral phenotypes. This could help efforts in discovering transdiagnostic targets for the rational development and testing of new treatments.

Treatments may be effective for body image dissatisfaction in some with eating disorders but the field currently lacks robustly effective means to correct body image distortion

Body dissatisfaction might be improved in some individuals with eating disorders through cognitive behavioral therapy that includes mirror exposures, or with mirror exposures alone (reviewed in Butler & Heimberg, 2020). However, a meta-analysis of five studies, three of which were of cognitive behavioral therapy, found only small, nonsignificant effects on improving body dissatisfaction in those with AN (Gan et al., 2022). A meta-analysis of stand-alone treatments for improving body image (not limited to those with eating disorders) suggested small-magnitude effects (Alleva et al., 2015).

Body image distortions, distinct from body dissatisfaction, may reflect aberrancies in how the brain is creating one's internalized mental body image and may have contributions from intrinsic neural connectivity, behaviors, and emotions. Yet, the field currently has incomplete knowledge of neurobiological and behavioral contributors to an accurate body image. This likely accounts for evidence-based treatments being sparse, although there are early investigations in AN using VR with embodiment (Keizer et al., 2014; Keizer et al., 2016; Serino et al., 2019) and VR with eye-tracking (Meschberger-Annweiler et al., 2023). A deeper understanding of how one's body image is formed in healthy individuals and in psychiatric disorders will inform transdiagnostic treatment targets for body image disorders.

Conclusions

In conclusion, body image disturbances in individuals with eating disorders, particularly AN and BN, likely arise from a complex interplay of cognitive, affective, and sensory-perceptual factors. The neurobiological basis of body perception involves the integration of sensory inputs from multiple modalities, including visual perception, somatosensation, proprioception, and equilibrioception, within dynamic body-centered neural representations in the brain. The research to date has predominantly focused on AN, uncovering evidence of differences in visual perception, tactile somatosensation, proprioception, and multisensory integration as potential contributors to body image disturbances in this population. These perceptual factors, combined with heightened body dissatisfaction, may play pivotal roles in the development and maintenance of AN and potentially other eating disorders.

The significance of body image disturbance in eating disorders cannot be underestimated, as it has strong prognostic implications for their clinical course. Distorted perceptions of body size and shape are evident in AN and BN, potentially other eating disorders (Grilo et al., 2010), and body dysmorphic disorder. Given the high crude mortality rate associated with AN and the prevalence of relapse, effective treatment strategies are essential. Addressing body size distortions and body dissatisfaction could be crucial in improving clinical outcomes. Of additional clinical importance, body image disturbances may serve as risk factors for the development of certain eating disorders and could be considered a transdiagnostic phenomenon with implications for understanding and treating various conditions involving body image disturbances, such as body dysmorphic disorder.

The current understanding of the neurobiological and behavioral contributors to accurate body image is still incomplete, both in healthy individuals and across psychiatric disorders. A deeper knowledge of the formation of body image in both healthy and psychiatric populations can inform the development of transdiagnostic treatment targets for body image disorders. By adopting a dimensional perspective and identifying shared neural and behavioral phenotypes, researchers may be better equipped to discover transdiagnostic treatment approaches and improve interventions. Ultimately, advancing our understanding of the neurobiological underpinnings of body image disturbances can offer new hope for individuals struggling with eating disorders and related body image disorders.

References

Aleong, R., & Paus, T. (2010). Neural correlates of human body perception. *Journal of Cognitive Neuroscience, 22*(3), 482–495.

Ali, A. M., Hendawy, A. O., Abd Elhay, E. S., Ali, E. M., Alkhamees, A. A., Kunugi, H., & Hassan, N. I. (2022). The Bergen Facebook addiction scale: Its psychometric properties and invariance among women with eating disorders. *BMC Women's Health, 22*(1), 99. https://doi.org/10.1186/s12905-022-01677-2

Alleva, J. M., Sheeran, P., Webb, T. L., Martijn, C., & Miles, E. (2015). A meta-analytic review of stand-alone interventions to improve body image. *PLOS ONE, 10*(9), e0139177.

American Psychiatric Association. (2013). *Diagnostic and statistical manual of mental disorders: DSM-5* (Vol. 5). American Psychiatric Association.

Ango, F., & Dos Reis, R. (2019). Sensing how to balance. *Elife, 8*, e46973.

Arzy, S., Overney, L. S., Landis, T., & Blanke, O. (2006). Neural mechanisms of embodiment: Asomatognosia due to premotor cortex damage. *Archives of Neurology, 63*(7), 1022–1025. https://doi.org/10.1001/archneur.63.7.1022

Baker, C., & Wertheim, E. H. (2003). Review of *Body image: A handbook of theory, research, and clinical practice. Eating Disorders, 11*(3), 247–248. https://doi.org/10.1080/10640260390218738

Beato-Fernández, L., Rodríguez-Cano, T., Belmonte-Llario, A., & Martínez-Delgado, C. (2004). Risk factors for eating disorders in adolescents: A Spanish community-based longitudinal study. *European Child & Adolescent Psychiatry, 13*, 287–294.

Bellard, A., Trotter, P., McGlone, F., & Cazzato, V. (2022). Vicarious ratings of self vs. other-directed social touch in women with and recovered from anorexia nervosa. *Scientific Reports, 12*(1), 13429. https://doi.org/10.1038/s41598-022-17523-2

Berlucchi, G., & Aglioti, S. M. (2010). The body in the brain revisited. *Experimental Brain Research, 200*, 25–35.

Bischoff-Grethe, A., Wierenga, C. E., Berner, L. A., Simmons, A. N., Bailer, U., Paulus, M. P., & Kaye, W. H. (2018). Neural hypersensitivity to pleasant touch in women remitted from anorexia nervosa. *Translational Psychiatry, 8*(1), 161. https://doi.org/10.1038/s41398-018-0218-3

Blanke, O. (2012). Multisensory brain mechanisms of bodily self-consciousness. *Nature Reviews Neuroscience, 13*(8), 556–571. https://doi.org/10.1038/nrn3292

Blanke, O., Ionta, S., Fornari, E., Mohr, C., & Maeder, P. (2010). Mental imagery for full and upper human bodies: Common right hemisphere activations and distinct extrastriate activations. *Brain Topography, 23*(3), 321–332. https://doi.org/10.1007/s10548-010-0138-x

Blanke, O., Slater, M., & Serino, A. (2015). Behavioral, neural, and computational principles of bodily self-consciousness. *Neuron, 88*(1), 145–166.

Boepple, L., Choquette, E., & Thompson, J. (2015). Body distortion: Perceptual measurement of body image disturbance. In T. Wade (Ed.), *Encyclopedia of feeding and eating disorders* (pp. 978–981). Springer.

Bohon, C., Hembacher, E., Moller, H., Moody, T. D., & Feusner, J. D. (2012). Nonlinear relationships between anxiety and visual processing of own and others' faces in body dysmorphic disorder. *Psychiatry Research, 204*(2–3), 132–139. https://doi.org/10.1016/j.pscychresns.2012.09.003

Bolognini, N., Olgiati, E., Maravita, A., Ferraro, F., & Fregni, F. (2013). Motor and parietal cortex stimulation for phantom limb pain and sensations. *Pain, 154*(8), 1274–1280.

Botvinick, M. (2004). Probing the neural basis of body ownership. *Science, 305*(5685), 782–783.

Botvinick, M., & Cohen, J. (1998). Rubber hands "feel" touch that eyes see. *Nature, 391*(6669), 756–756. https://doi.org/10.1038/35784

Brown, T. A., Shott, M. E., & Frank, G. K. (2021). Body size overestimation in anorexia nervosa: Contributions of cognitive, affective, tactile and visual information. *Psychiatry Research, 297*, 113705.

Bruch, H. (1962). Perceptual and conceptual disturbances in anorexia nervosa. *Psychosomatic Medicine, 24*, 187–194. https://doi.org/10.1097/00006842-196203000-00009

Burr, D. C., Morrone, M. C., & Ross, J. (1994). Selective suppression of the magnocellular visual pathway during saccadic eye movements. *Nature, 371*(6497), 511–513. https://doi.org/10.1038/371511a0

Butler, R. M., & Heimberg, R. G. (2020). Exposure therapy for eating disorders: A systematic review. *Clinical Psychology Review, 78*, 101851.

Buzsáki, G. (2019). *The brain from inside out.* Oxford University Press. https://doi.org/10.1093/oso/9780190905385.001.0001

Buzsáki, G., & Tingley, D. (2023). Cognition from the body–brain partnership: Exaptation of memory. Annual Review of Neuroscience, 46, 191–210. https://doi.org/10.1146/annurev-neuro-101222-110632

Calvo-Merino, B., Urgesi, C., Orgs, G., Aglioti, S. M., & Haggard, P. (2010). Extrastriate body area underlies aesthetic evaluation of body stimuli. *Experimental Brain Research, 204*, 447–456.

Carey, M., Knight, R., & Preston, C. (2019). Distinct neural response to visual perspective and body size in the extrastriate body area. *Behavioural Brain Research, 372*, 112063.

Cash, T. F., & Brown, T. A. (1987). Body image in anorexia nervosa and bulimia nervosa. A review of the literature. *Behavior Modification, 11*(4), 487–521. https://doi.org/10.1177/01454455870114005

Cash, T. F., & Deagle III, E. A. (1997). The nature and extent of body-image disturbances in anorexia nervosa and bulimia nervosa: A meta-analysis. *International Journal of Eating Disorders, 22*(2), 107–126.

Cash, T. F., & Pruzinsky, T., eds. (2002). *Body image: A handbook of theory, research, and clinical practice.* Guilford Press.

Cazzato, V., Mele, S., & Urgesi, C. (2014). Gender differences in the neural underpinning of perceiving and appreciating the beauty of the body. *Behavioural Brain Research, 264*, 188–196.

Cazzato, V., Mele, S., & Urgesi, C. (2016). Different contributions of visual and motor brain areas during liking judgments of same-and different-gender bodies. *Brain Research, 1646*, 98–108.

Cazzato, V., Mian, E., Serino, A., Mele, S., & Urgesi, C. (2015). Distinct contributions of extrastriate body area and temporoparietal junction in perceiving one's own and others' body. *Cognitive, Affective, & Behavioral Neuroscience, 15*, 211–228.

Cornelissen, P. L., Hancock, P. J., Kiviniemi, V., George, H. R., & Tovée, M. J. (2009). Patterns of eye movements when male and female observers judge female attractiveness, body fat and waist-to-hip ratio. *Evolution and Human Behavior, 30*(6), 417–428.

Craig, A. D. (2003). Interoception: The sense of the physiological condition of the body. *Current Opinion in Neurobiology, 13*(4), 500–505.

Crucianelli, L., Cardi, V., Treasure, J., Jenkinson, P. M., & Fotopoulou, A. (2016). The perception of affective touch in anorexia nervosa. *Psychiatry Research, 239*, 72–78. https://doi.org/10.1016/j.psychres.2016.01.078

Crucianelli, L., Demartini, B., Goeta, D., Nisticò, V., Saramandi, A., Bertelli, S., Todisco, P., Gambini, O., & Fotopoulou, A. (2021). The anticipation and perception of affective touch in women with and recovered from anorexia nervosa. *Neuroscience, 464*, 143–155. https://doi.org/10.1016/j.neuroscience.2020.09.013

Davidovic, M., Karjalainen, L., Starck, G., Wentz, E., Björnsdotter, M., & Olausson, H. (2018). Abnormal brain processing of gentle touch in anorexia nervosa. *Psychiatry Research: Neuroimaging, 281*, 53–60. https://doi.org10.1016/j.pscychresns.2018.08.007

de Haan, E. H., & Dijkerman, H. C. (2020). Somatosensation in the brain: A theoretical re-evaluation and a new model. *Trends in Cognitive Sciences, 24*(7), 529–541.

Delle Monache, S., Indovina, I., Zago, M., Daprati, E., Lacquaniti, F., & Bosco, G. (2021). Watching the effects of gravity: Vestibular cortex and the neural representation of "visual" gravity. *Frontiers in Integrative Neuroscience, 15*, 793634.

Ehrsson, H. H. (2012). The concept of body ownership and its relation to multisensory integration. In B. E. Stein (Ed.), *The new handbook of multisensory processing* (pp. 775–792). MIT Press. https://doi.org/10.7551/mitpress/8466.003.0067

Ehrsson, H. H., Holmes, N. P., & Passingham, R. E. (2005). Touching a rubber hand: Feeling of body ownership is associated with activity in multisensory brain areas. *Journal of Neuroscience, 25*(45), 10564–10573.

Epstein, J., Wiseman, C. V., Sunday, S. R., Klapper, F., Alkalay, L., & Halmi, K. A. (2001). Neurocognitive evidence favors "top down" over "bottom up" mechanisms in the pathogenesis of body size distortions in anorexia nervosa. *Eating and Weight Disorders, 6*(3), 140–147. https://doi.org/10.1007/BF03339763

Ernst, M. O., & Bülthoff, H. H. (2004). Merging the senses into a robust percept. *Trends in Cognitive Sciences, 8*(4), 162–169.

Eshkevari, E., Rieger, E., Longo, M. R., Haggard, P., & Treasure, J. (2012). Increased plasticity of the bodily self in eating disorders. *Psychological Medicine, 42*(4), 819–828. https://doi.org/10.1017/S0033291711002091

Eshkevari, E., Rieger, E., Musiat, P., & Treasure, J. (2014). An investigation of interoceptive sensitivity in eating disorders using a heartbeat detection task and a self-report measure. *European Eating Disorders Review, 22*(5), 383–388. https://doi.org/10.1002/erv.2305

Evans, L., & Wertheim, E. (1998). Intimacy patterns and relationship satisfaction of women with eating problems and the mediating effects of depression, trait anxiety and social anxiety. *Journal of Psychosomatic Research, 44*(3–4), 355–365.

Fabello, M. (2020). *Appetite: Sex, touch, and desire in women with anorexia.* Routledge.

Farrell, C., Lee, M., & Shafran, R. (2005). Assessment of body size estimation: A review. *European Eating Disorders Review, 13*(2), 75–88. https://doi.org/10.1002/erv.622

Fassino, S., & Marzola, E. (2018). Diagnostic classification of body image disturbances. In M. Cuzzolaro and S. Fassino (Eds.), *Body image, eating, and weight: A guide to assessment, treatment, and prevention* (pp. 25–37). Springer.

Fetsch, C. R., DeAngelis, G. C., & Angelaki, D. E. (2013). Bridging the gap between theories of sensory cue integration and the physiology of multisensory neurons. *Nature Reviews Neuroscience, 14*(6), 429–442.

Feusner, J., Deshpande, R., & Strober, M. (2017). A translational neuroscience approach to body image disturbance and its remediation in anorexia nervosa. *International Journal of Eating Disorders, 50*(9), 1014–1017.

Fox, J. R. E., & Power, M. J. (2009). Eating disorders and multi-level models of emotion: An integrated model. *Clinical Psychology & Psychotherapy, 16*(4), 240–267. https://doi.org/10.1002/cpp.626

Frank, G. K., & Treasure, J. (2016). Authors' reply: Cognitive and emotional factors are involved in body-image distortion. *Nature Reviews Disease Primers, 2*(1), 16027. https://doi.org/10.1038/nrdp.2016.27

Frassinetti, F., Bolognini, N., & Làdavas, E. (2002). Enhancement of visual perception by crossmodal visuo-auditory interaction. *Experimental Brain Research, 147*, 332–343.

Fuchs, D. (2018). Dancing with gravity—Why the sense of balance is (the) fundamental. *Behavioral Sciences, 8*(1), 7.

Gallace, A., & Spence, C. (2014). *In touch with the future: The sense of touch from cognitive neuroscience to virtual reality*. Oxford University Press.

Gan, J. K. E., Wu, V. X., Chow, G., Chan, J. K. Y., & Klainin-Yobas, P. (2022). Effectiveness of non-pharmacological interventions on individuals with anorexia nervosa: A systematic review and meta-analysis. *Patient Education and Counseling, 105*(1), 44–55.

Gardner, R. M., & Brown, D. L. (2010). Body image assessment: A review of figural drawing scales. *Personality and Individual Differences, 48*(2), 107–111.

Gardner, R. M., & Brown, D. L. (2014). Body size estimation in anorexia nervosa: A brief review of findings from 2003 through 2013. *Psychiatry Research, 219*(3), 407–410. https://doi.org/10.1016/j.psychres.2014.06.029

Gardner, R. M., & Moncrieff, C. (1988). Body image distortion in anorexics as a non-sensory phenomenon: A signal detection approach. *Journal of Clinical Psychology, 44*(2), 101–107. https://doi.org/10.1002/1097-4679(198803)44:2<101::aid-jclp2270440203>3.0.co;2-u

Garfinkel, P. E., Moldofsky, H., Garner, D. M., Stancer, H. C., & Coscina, D. V. (1978). Body awareness in anorexia nervosa: disturbances in "body image" and "satiety." *Psychosomatic Medicine, 40*(6), 487–498.

Garner, D. M., & Garfinkel, P. E. (1981). Body image in anorexia nervosa: Measurement, theory and clinical implications. *International Journal of Psychiatry Medicine, 11*(3), 263–284. https://doi.org/10.2190/r55q-2u6t-lam7-rqr7

Goldzak-Kunik, G., Friedman, R., Spitz, M., Sandler, L., & Leshem, M. (2012). Intact sensory function in anorexia nervosa. *American Journal of Clinical Nutrition, 95*(2), 272–282.

Grant, J. E., Kim, S. W., & Crow, S. J. (2001). Prevalence and clinical features of body dysmorphic disorder in adolescent and adult psychiatric inpatients. *Journal of Clinical Psychiatry, 62*(7), 517–522.

Grant, J. E., Kim, S. W., & Eckert, E. D. (2002). Body dysmorphic disorder in patients with anorexia nervosa: Prevalence, clinical features, and delusionality of body image. *International Journal of Eating Disorders, 32*(3), 291–300. https://doi.org/10.1002/eat.10091

Grant, J. E., & Phillips, K. A. (2004). Is anorexia nervosa a subtype of body dysmorphic disorder? Probably not, but read on. *Harvard Review of Psychiatry, 12*(2), 123–126. https://doi.org/10.1080/10673220490447236

Grilo, C. M., Masheb, R. M., & White, M. A. (2010). Significance of overvaluation of shape/weight in binge-eating disorder: Comparative study with overweight and bulimia nervosa. *Obesity, 18*(3), 499–504.

Grogan, S. (2021). *Body image: Understanding body dissatisfaction in men, women and children*. Routledge.

Groves, K., Kennett, S., & Gillmeister, H. (2020). Evidence for altered configural body processing in women at risk of disorders characterized by body image disturbance. *British Journal of Psychology, 111*(3), 508–535.

Guardia, D., Carey, A., Cottencin, O., Thomas, P., & Luyat, M. (2013). Disruption of spatial task performance in anorexia nervosa. *PLOS ONE, 8*(1), e54928. https://doi.org/10.1371/journal.pone.0054928

Guardia, D., Cottencin, O., Thomas, P., Dodin, V., & Luyat, M. (2012). Spatial orientation constancy is impaired in anorexia nervosa. *Psychiatry Research, 195*(1), 56–59. https://doi.org/https://doi.org/10.1016/j.psychres.2011.08.003

Guldin, W., & Grüsser, O. (1998). Is there a vestibular cortex? *Trends in Neurosciences, 21*(6), 254–259.

Hagman, J., Gardner, R. M., Brown, D. L., Gralla, J., Fier, J. M., & Frank, G. K. W. (2015). Body size overestimation and its association with body mass index, body dissatisfaction, and drive for thinness in anorexia nervosa. *Eating and Weight Disorders, 20*(4), 449–455. https://doi.org/10.1007/s40519-015-0193-0

Hartmann, A. S., Greenberg, J. L., & Wilhelm, S. (2013). The relationship between anorexia nervosa and body dysmorphic disorder. *Clinical Psychology Review, 33*(5), 675–685.

Hartmann, A. S., Staufenbiel, T., Bielefeld, L., Buhlmann, U., Heinrichs, N., Martin, A., Ritter, V., Kollei, I., & Grocholewski, A. (2020). An empirically derived recommendation for the classification of body dysmorphic disorder: Findings from structural equation modeling. *PLOS ONE, 15*(6), e0233153.

Hennighausen, K., Enkelmann, D., Wewetzer, C., & Remschmidt, H. (1999). Body image distortion in anorexia nervosa—Is there really a perceptual deficit? *European Child & Adolescent Psychiatry, 8*, 200–206.

Hoek, H. W. (2006). Incidence, prevalence and mortality of anorexia nervosa and other eating disorders. *Current Opinions in Psychiatry, 19*(4), 389–394. https://doi.org/10.1097/01.yco.0000228759.95237.78

Jacobi, C., Hayward, C., de Zwaan, M., Kraemer, H. C., & Agras, W. S. (2004). Coming to terms with risk factors for eating disorders: Application of risk terminology and suggestions for a general taxonomy. *Psychological Bulletin, 130*(1), 19.

Jansen, A., Nederkoorn, C., & Mulkens, S. (2005). Selective visual attention for ugly and beautiful body parts in eating disorders. *Behaviour Research and Therapy, 43*(2), 183–196. https://doi.org/https://doi.org/10.1016/j.brat.2004.01.003

Jiotsa, B., Naccache, B., Duval, M., Rocher, B., & Grall-Bronnec, M. (2021). Social media use and body image disorders: Association between frequency of comparing one's own physical appearance to that of people being followed on social media and body dissatisfaction and drive for thinness. *International Journal of Environmental Research and Public Health, 18*(6), 2880. https://www.mdpi.com/1660-4601/18/6/2880

Johansson, R. S., & Flanagan, J. R. (2009). Coding and use of tactile signals from the fingertips in object manipulation tasks. *Nature Reviews Neuroscience, 10*(5), 345–359.

Keegan, E., Tchanturia, K., & Wade, T. D. (2021). Central coherence and set-shifting between nonunderweight eating disorders and anorexia nervosa: A systematic review and meta-analysis. *International Journal of Eating Disorders, 54*(3), 229–243.

Keizer, A., Engel, M. M., Bonekamp, J., & Van Elburg, A. (2019). Hoop training: A pilot study assessing the effectiveness of a multisensory approach to treatment of body image disturbance in anorexia nervosa. *Eating and Weight Disorders, 24*(5), 953–958. https://doi.org/10.1007/s40519-018-0585-z

Keizer, A., Smeets, M. A. M., Dijkerman, H. C., van den Hout, M., Klugkist, I., van Elburg, A., & Postma, A. (2011). Tactile body image disturbance in anorexia nervosa. *Psychiatry Research, 190*(1), 115–120. https://doi.org/10.1016/j.psychres.2011.04.031

Keizer, A., Smeets, M. A. M., Dijkerman, H. C., van Elburg, A., & Postma, A. (2012). Aberrant somatosensory perception in anorexia nervosa. *Psychiatry Research, 200*(2), 530–537. https://doi.org/10.1016/j.psychres.2012.05.001

Keizer, A., Smeets, M. A. M., Postma, A., van Elburg, A., & Dijkerman, H. C. (2014). Does the experience of ownership over a rubber hand change body size perception in anorexia nervosa patients? *Neuropsychologia, 62*, 26–37. https://doi.org/10.1016/j.neuropsychologia.2014.07.003

Keizer, A., van Elburg, A., Helms, R., & Dijkerman, H. C. (2016). A virtual reality full body illusion improves body image disturbance in anorexia nervosa. *PLOS ONE, 11*(10), e0163921. https://doi.org/10.1371/journal.pone.0163921

Kerr-Gaffney, J., Harrison, A., & Tchanturia, K. (2018). Eye-tracking research in eating disorders: A systematic review. *International Journal of Eating Disorders, 52*(1), 3–27. https://doi.org/10.1002/eat.22998

Kittler, J. E., Menard, W., & Phillips, K. A. (2007). Weight concerns in individuals with body dysmorphic disorder. *Eating Behaviors, 8*(1), 115–120. https://doi.org/10.1016/j.eatbeh.2006.02.006

Kosslyn, S. M. (1980). *Image and mind*. Harvard University Press.

Laeng, B., Bloem, I. M., D'Ascenzo, S., & Tommasi, L. (2014). Scrutinizing visual images: The role of gaze in mental imagery and memory. *Cognition, 131*(2), 263–283. https://doi.org/10.1016/j.cognition.2014.01.003

Lang, K., Lopez, C., Stahl, D., Tchanturia, K., & Treasure, J. (2014). Central coherence in eating disorders: An updated systematic review and meta-analysis. *World Journal of Biological Psychiatry, 15*(8), 586–598. https://doi.org/10.3109/15622975.2014.909606

Lang, P. J., Bradley, M. M., Fitzsimmons, J. R., Cuthbert, B. N., Scott, J. D., Moulder, B., & Nangia, V. (1998). Emotional arousal and activation of the visual cortex: An fMRI analysis. *Psychophysiology, 35*(2), 199–210.

Li, W., Lai, T. M., Bohon, C., Loo, S. K., McCurdy, D., Strober, M., Bookheimer, S., & Feusner, J. (2015). Anorexia nervosa and body dysmorphic disorder are associated with abnormalities in processing visual information. *Psychological Medicine, 45*(10), 2111–2122. https://doi.org/10.1017/s0033291715000045

Li, W., Lai, T. M., Loo, S. K., Strober, M., Mohammad-Rezazadeh, I., Khalsa, S., & Feusner, J. (2015). Aberrant early visual neural activity and brain-behavior relationships in anorexia nervosa and body dysmorphic disorder. *Frontiers in Human Neuroscience, 9*, 301. https://doi.org/10.3389/fnhum.2015.00301

Lopez, C., & Blanke, O. (2011). The thalamocortical vestibular system in animals and humans. *Brain Research Reviews, 67*(1–2), 119–146.

Mackrous, I., Carriot, J., Jamali, M., & Cullen, K. E. (2019). Cerebellar prediction of the dynamic sensory consequences of gravity. *Current Biology, 29*(16), 2698–2710.e2694.

Madsen, S. K., Bohon, C., & Feusner, J. D. (2013). Visual processing in anorexia nervosa and body dysmorphic disorder: Similarities, differences, and future research directions. *Journal of Psychiatric Research, 47*(10), 1483–1491. https://doi.org/https://doi.org/10.1016/j.jpsychires.2013.06.003

McGlone, F., Wessberg, J., & Olausson, H. (2014). Discriminative and affective touch: Sensing and feeling. *Neuron, 82*(4), 737–755. https://doi.org/10.1016/j.neuron.2014.05.001

Meredith, M. A., & Stein, B. E. (1986). Visual, auditory, and somatosensory convergence on cells in superior colliculus results in multisensory integration. *Journal of Neurophysiology, 56*(3), 640–662.

Meschberger-Annweiler, F.-A., Ascione, M., Porras-Garcia, B., Ferrer-Garcia, M., Moreno-Sanchez, M., Miquel-Nabau, H., Serrano-Troncoso, E., Carulla-Roig, M., & Gutiérrez-Maldonado, J. (2023). An attentional bias modification task, through virtual reality and eye-tracking technologies, to enhance the treatment of anorexia nervosa. *Journal of Clinical Medicine, 12*(6), 2185.

Mohr, C., Porter, G., & Benton, C. P. (2007). Psychophysics reveals a right hemispheric contribution to body image distortions in women but not men. *Neuropsychologia, 45*(13), 2942–2950.

Mohr, H. M., Röder, C., Zimmermann, J., Hummel, D., Negele, A., & Grabhorn, R. (2011). Body image distortions in bulimia nervosa: Investigating body size overestimation and body size satisfaction by fMRI. *Neuroimage, 56*(3), 1822–1831. https://doi.org/10.1016/j.neuroimage.2011.02.069

Mölbert, S. C., Klein, L., Thaler, A., Mohler, B. J., Brozzo, C., Martus, P., Karnath, H. O., Zipfel, S., & Giel, K. E. (2017). Depictive and metric body size estimation in anorexia nervosa and bulimia nervosa: A systematic review and meta-analysis. *Clinical Psychology Review, 57*, 21–31. https://doi.org/10.1016/j.cpr.2017.08.005

Mölbert, S. C., Thaler, A., Mohler, B. J., Streuber, S., Romero, J., Black, M. J., Zipfel, S., Karnath, H. O., & Giel, K. E. (2018). Assessing body image in anorexia nervosa using biometric self-avatars in virtual reality: Attitudinal components rather than visual body size estimation are distorted. *Psychological Medicine, 48*(4), 642–653. https://doi.org/10.1017/S0033291717002008

Molinari, E. (1995). Body-size estimation in anorexia nervosa. *Perceptual and Motor Skills, 81*(1), 23–31. https://doi.org/10.2466/pms.1995.81.1.23

Møller, P. (2014). Orosensory Perception. In D. Bar-Shalom & K. Rose (Eds.), *Pediatric formulations: A roadmap* (pp. 105–121). Springer New York. https://doi.org/10.1007/978-1-4899-8011-3_8

Moody, T. D., Morfini, F., Cheng, G., Sheen, C. L., Kerr, W. T., Strober, M., & Feusner, J. D. (2021). Brain activation and connectivity in anorexia nervosa and body dysmorphic disorder when viewing bodies: Relationships to clinical symptoms and perception of appearance. *Brain Imaging and Behavior, 15*(3), 1235–1252. https://doi.org/10.1007/s11682-020-00323-5

Moro, V., Urgesi, C., Pernigo, S., Lanteri, P., Pazzaglia, M., & Aglioti, S. M. (2008). The neural basis of body form and body action agnosia. *Neuron, 60*(2), 235–246.

Moseley, G. L., Gallace, A., & Spence, C. (2012). Bodily illusions in health and disease: Physiological and clinical perspectives and the concept of a cortical "body matrix." *Neuroscience & Biobehavioral Reviews, 36*(1), 34–46.

Murray, S. B., Rieger, E., Hildebrandt, T., Karlov, L., Russell, J., Boon, E., Dawson, R. T., & Touyz, S. W. (2012). A comparison of eating, exercise, shape, and weight related symptomatology in males with muscle dysmorphia and anorexia nervosa. *Body Image, 9*(2), 193–200.

Olausson, H., Lamarre, Y., Backlund, H., Morin, C., Wallin, B., Starck, G., Ekholm, S., Strigo, I., Worsley, K., & Vallbo, Å. (2002). Unmyelinated tactile afferents signal touch and project to insular cortex. *Nature Neuroscience, 5*(9), 900–904.

Olausson, H., Lamarre, Y., Backlund, H., Morin, C., Wallin, B. G., Starck, G., Ekholm, S., Strigo, I., Worsley, K., Vallbo, A. B., & Bushnell, M. C. (2002). Unmyelinated tactile afferents signal touch and project to insular cortex. *Nature Neuroscience, 5*(9), 900–904. https://doi.org/10.1038/nn896

Peelen, M. V., & Downing, P. E. (2007). The neural basis of visual body perception. *Nature Reviews Neuroscience, 8*(8), 636–648.

Perruchoud, D., Michels, L., Piccirelli, M., Gassert, R., & Ionta, S. (2016). Differential neural encoding of sensorimotor and visual body representations. *Scientific Reports, 6*, 37259. https://doi.org/10.1038/srep37259

Phillipou, A., Abel, L. A., Castle, D. J., Hughes, M. E., Gurvich, C., Nibbs, R. G., & Rossell, S. L. (2015). Self perception and facial emotion perception of others in anorexia nervosa. *Frontiers in Psychology, 6*, 1181. https://doi.org/10.3389/fpsyg.2015.01181

Phillipou, A., Mountjoy, R. L., & Rossell, S. L. (2017). Overvalued ideas or delusions in anorexia nervosa? *Australian & New Zealand Journal of Psychiatry, 51*(6), 563–564.

Phillipou, A., Rossell, S. L., Gurvich, C., Castle, D. J., Troje, N. F., & Abel, L. A. (2016). Body image in anorexia nervosa: Body size estimation utilising a biological motion task and eyetracking. *European Eating Disorders Review, 24*(2), 131–138. https://doi.org/10.1002/erv.2423

Phillips, K. A. (2005). *The broken mirror: Understanding and treating body dysmorphic disorder.* Oxford University Press.

Phillips, K. A., & Diaz, S. F. (1997). Gender differences in body dysmorphic disorder. *Journal of Nervous and Mental Disease, 185*(9), 570–577.

Pizzagalli, D. A., Lehmann, D., Hendrick, A. M., Regard, M., Pascual-Marqui, R. D., & Davidson, R. J. (2002). Affective judgments of faces modulate early activity (approximately 160 ms) within the fusiform gyri. *Neuroimage, 16*(3 Pt 1), 663–677. https://doi.org/10.1006/nimg.2002.1126

Pope Jr, H. G., Katz, D. L., & Hudson, J. I. (1993). Anorexia nervosa and "reverse anorexia" among 108 male bodybuilders. *Comprehensive Psychiatry, 34*(6), 406–409.

Preston, C., & Ehrsson, H. H. (2014). Illusory changes in body size modulate body satisfaction in a way that is related to non-clinical eating disorder psychopathology. *PLOS ONE, 9*(1), e85773. https://doi.org/10.1371/journal.pone.0085773

Proske, U., & Gandevia, S. C. (2012). The proprioceptive senses: Their roles in signaling body shape, body position and movement, and muscle force. *Physiological Reviews*, 92(4), 1651–1697. https://doi.org/10.1152/physrev.00048.2011

Provenzano, L., Porciello, G., Ciccarone, S., Lenggenhager, B., Tieri, G., Marucci, M., Dazzi, F., Loriedo, C., & Bufalari, I. (2019). Characterizing body image distortion and bodily self-plasticity in anorexia nervosa via visuo-tactile stimulation in virtual reality. *Journal of Clinical Medicine, 9*(1), 98. https://doi.org/10.3390/jcm9010098

Pruitt, N. A., Kappius, R. E., & Oorman, P. W. (1992). Bulimia and fear of intimacy. *Journal of Clinical Psychology, 48*(4), 472–476.

Rabe-Jablonska Jolanta, J., & Sobow Tomasz, M. (2000). The links between body dysmorphic disorder and eating disorders. *European Psychiatry, 15*(5), 302–305. https://doi.org/S0924-9338(00)00398-9

Raevuori, A., Hoek, H. W., Susser, E., Kaprio, J., Rissanen, A., & Keski-Rahkonen, A. (2009). Epidemiology of anorexia nervosa in men: A nationwide study of Finnish twins. *PLOS ONE, 4*(2), e4402.

Rodgers, R. F., Melioli, T., Laconi, S., Bui, E., & Chabrol, H. (2013). Internet addiction symptoms, disordered eating, and body image avoidance. *Cyberpsychology, Behavior, and Social Networking, 16*(1), 56–60. https://doi.org/10.1089/cyber.2012.1570

Ruffolo, J., Phillips, K., Menard, W., Fay, C., & Weisberg, R. (2006). Comorbidity of body dysmorphic disorder and eating disorders: Severity of psychopathology and body image disturbance. *International Journal of Eating Disorders, 39*(1), 11–19.

Sattler, F. A., Eickmeyer, S., & Eisenkolb, J. (2020). Body image disturbance in children and adolescents with anorexia nervosa and bulimia nervosa: a systematic review. *Eating and Weight Disorders, 25*, 857–865.

Sereno, M. I., & Huang, R.-S. (2014). Multisensory maps in parietal cortex. *Current Opinion in Neurobiology, 24*, 39–46.

Serino, S., Polli, N., & Riva, G. (2019). From avatars to body swapping: The use of virtual reality for assessing and treating body-size distortion in individuals with anorexia. *Journal of Clinical Psychology, 75*(2), 313–322.

Smeets, M. A., & Kosslyn, S. M. (2001). Hemispheric differences in body image in anorexia nervosa. *International Journal of Eating Disorders, 29*(4), 409–416.

Sperry, R. W. (1950). Neural basis of the spontaneous optokinetic response produced by visual inversion. *Journal of Comparative and Physiological Psychology, 43*(6), 482.

Spitoni, G. F., Serino, A., Cotugno, A., Mancini, F., Antonucci, G., & Pizzamiglio, L. (2015). The two dimensions of the body representation in women suffering from anorexia nervosa. *Psychiatry Research, 230*(2), 181–188. https://doi.org/https://doi.org/10.1016/j.psychres.2015.08.036

Stein, B. E., Meredith, M. A., Huneycutt, W. S., & McDade, L. (1989). Behavioral indices of multisensory integration: Orientation to visual cues is affected by auditory stimuli. *Journal of Cognitive Neuroscience, 1*(1), 12–24.

Stein, B. E., & Stanford, T. R. (2008). Multisensory integration: Current issues from the perspective of the single neuron. *Nature Reviews Neuroscience, 9*(4), 255–266. https://doi.org/10.1038/nrn2331

Stice, E., & Shaw, H. E. (2002). Role of body dissatisfaction in the onset and maintenance of eating pathology: A synthesis of research findings. *Journal of Psychosomatic Research, 53*(5), 985–993. https://doi.org/10.1016/S0022-3999(02)00488-9

Stott, N., Fox, J. R., & Williams, M. O. (2021). Attentional bias in eating disorders: A meta-review. *International Journal of Eating Disorders, 54*(8), 1377–1399.

Suchan, B., Busch, M., Schulte, D., Grönemeyer, D., Herpertz, S., & Vocks, S. (2010). Reduction of gray matter density in the extrastriate body area in women with anorexia nervosa. *Behavioural Brain Research, 206*(1), 63–67. https://doi.org/10.1016/j.bbr.2009.08.035

Tagini, S., Bastoni, I., Villa, V., Mendolicchio, L., Castelnuovo, G., Mauro, A., & Scarpina, F. (2023). Affective touch in anorexia nervosa: Exploring the role of social anhedonia and lifespan experiences. *Journal of Affective Disorders, 324*, 607–615. https://doi.org/https://doi.org/10.1016/j.jad.2022.12.137

Tan, T., Kuek, A., Goh, S. E., Lee, E. L., & Kwok, V. (2016). Internet and smartphone application usage in eating disorders: A descriptive study in Singapore. *Asian Journal of Psychiatry, 19*, 50–55. https://doi.org/10.1016/j.ajp.2015.11.007

Taylor, J. L. (2009). Proprioception. Larry R. Squire (eds), *Encyclopedia of Neuroscience*, Academic Press, 1143–1149, ISBN 9780080450469, https://doi.org/10.1016/B978-008045046-9.01907-0.

Thompson, J. K., Coovert, M. D., & Stormer, S. M. (1999). Body image, social comparison, and eating disturbance: A covariance structure modeling investigation. *International Journal of Eating Disorders, 26*(1), 43–51.

Thompson, J. K., & Stice, E. (2001). Thin-ideal internalization: Mounting evidence for a new risk factor for body-image disturbance and eating pathology. *Current Directions in Psychological Science, 10*(5), 181–183.

Tsakiris, M., Costantini, M., & Haggard, P. (2008). The role of the right temporo-parietal junction in maintaining a coherent sense of one's body. *Neuropsychologia, 46*(12), 3014–3018.

Uddin, L. Q., Molnar-Szakacs, I., Zaidel, E., & Iacoboni, M. (2006). rTMS to the right inferior parietal lobule disrupts self–other discrimination. *Social Cognitive and Affective Neuroscience, 1*(1), 65–71.

Urgesi, C., Berlucchi, G., & Aglioti, S. M. (2004). Magnetic stimulation of extrastriate body area impairs visual processing of nonfacial body parts. *Current Biology, 14*(23), 2130–2134.

Urgesi, C., Fornasari, L., Canalaz, F., Perini, L., Cremaschi, S., Faleschini, L., Thyrion, E. Z., Zuliani, M., Balestrieri, M., & Fabbro, F. (2014). Impaired configural body processing in anorexia nervosa: Evidence from the body inversion effect. *British Journal of Psychology, 105*(4), 486–508.

Vaughn, D. A., Kerr, W. T., Moody, T. D., Cheng, G. K., Morfini, F., Zhang, A., Leow, A. D., Strober, M. A., Cohen, M. S., & Feusner, J. D. (2019). Differentiating weight-restored anorexia nervosa and body dysmorphic disorder using neuroimaging and psychometric markers. *PLOS ONE, 14*(5), e0213974.

Via, E., Goldberg, X., Sánchez, I., Forcano, L., Harrison, B. J., Davey, C. G., Pujol, J., Martínez-Zalacaín, I., Fernández-Aranda, F., Soriano-Mas, C., Cardoner, N., & Menchón, J. M. (2018). Self and other body perception in anorexia nervosa: The role of posterior DMN nodes. *World Journal of Biological Psychiatry, 19*(3), 210–224. https://doi.org/10.1080/15622975.2016.1249951

Vitousek, K. B., & Hollon, S. D. (1990). The investigation of schematic content and processing in eating disorders. *Cognitive Therapy and Research, 14*(2), 191–214. https://doi.org/10.1007/BF01176209

Vocks, S., Busch, M., Grönemeyer, D., Schulte, D., Herpertz, S., & Suchan, B. (2010). Differential neuronal responses to the self and others in the extrastriate body area and the fusiform body area. *Cognitive, Affective, & Behavioral Neuroscience*, *10*(3), 422–429. https://doi.org/10.3758/cabn.10.3.422

Von Holst, E., & Mittelstaedt, H. (1950). Das reafferenzprinzip: Wechselwirkungen zwischen zentralnervensystem und peripherie. *Naturwissenschaften*, *37*(20), 464–476.

Vuilleumier, P., Richardson, M. P., Armony, J. L., Driver, J., & Dolan, R. J. (2004). Distant influences of amygdala lesion on visual cortical activation during emotional face processing. *Nature Neuroscience*, *7*(11), 1271–1278. https://doi.org/10.1038/nn1341

Waldman, A., Loomes, R., Mountford, V. A., & Tchanturia, K. (2013). Attitudinal and perceptual factors in body image distortion: an exploratory study in patients with anorexia nervosa. *Journal of Eating Disorders*, *1*, 1–9.

Wierenga, C. E., Bischoff-Grethe, A., Berner, L. A., Simmons, A. N., Bailer, U., Paulus, M. P., & Kaye, W. H. (2020). Increased anticipatory brain response to pleasant touch in women remitted from bulimia nervosa. *Translational Psychiatry*, *10*(1), 236.

Winlove, C. I. P., Milton, F., Ranson, J., Fulford, J., MacKisack, M., Macpherson, F., & Zeman, A. (2018). The neural correlates of visual imagery: A co-ordinate-based meta-analysis. *Cortex*, *105*, 4–25. https://doi.org/10.1016/j.cortex.2017.12.014

Woolf, C. J., & Ma, Q. (2007). Nociceptors—Noxious stimulus detectors. *Neuron*, *55*(3), 353–364.

World Health Organization. (2004). *International statistical classification of diseases and related health problems: Alphabetical index* (Vol. 3). World Health Organization.

Yong, E. (2022). *An immense world: How animal senses reveal the hidden realms around us.* Knopf Canada.

Zanetti, T., Santonastaso, P., Sgaravatti, E., Degortes, D., & Favaro, A. (2013). Clinical and temperamental correlates of body image disturbance in eating disorders. *European Eating Disorders Review*, *21*(1), 32–37.

PART IV

EMERGING NEUROBIOLOGICALLY INFORMED TREATMENTS

18

Habit-Centered Treatment for Anorexia Nervosa

Joanna E. Steinglass and Deborah R. Glasofer

Brief Definitional Overview

Habit: Behavior that is learned, is not innate, develops over time, and with repetition becomes relatively insensitive to the outcome. Habits are repeated because of an antecedent cue—regardless of whether there is a rewarding outcome or not.

Cue: Variable that precedes the initiation of an automatic behavior (or sequence of behaviors). Cues can be internal or external.

Reward: Consequence following an action that functions to strengthen behavior.

Goal-directed: Actions or decisions that are purposeful (i.e., driven explicitly by a desired outcome or reward).

Habit system: The neural substrate of overtrained, cue-dependent behavior shown (mostly in basic science research) to be localized to the dorsal striatum.

Introduction

A perplexing feature of anorexia nervosa (AN) is the rigidity of maladaptive restrictive eating: the tendency to eat low-calorie, low-energy dense foods. Individuals with AN consume 50% to 80% less food than their healthy peers. This has been measured using daily diaries/food records that patients fill out themselves over the course of a day, and in objective, laboratory-based meals where amounts can be standardized and measured (Fernstrom et al., 1994; Mayer et al., 2012). The behavior is so entrenched that the eating patterns are seen even among individuals who are voluntarily seeking treatment, when restrictive eating is in obvious conflict with the individual's goal of healthy eating and healthy weight. Moreover, even after full weight restoration, when patients are considered "in remission" and psychological symptoms have significantly improved, patients with AN often continue to make restrictive food choices (Mayer et al., 2012; Steinglass et al., 2023). The clear and sizeable disconnect between goals and behavior presents a clinical challenge and raises questions for research.

Joanna E. Steinglass and Deborah R. Glasofer, *Habit-Centered Treatment for Anorexia Nervosa*. In: *The Handbook of the Neurobiology of Eating Disorders*. Edited by: Christina E. Wierenga and Joanna E. Steinglass, Oxford University Press.
 DOI: 10.1093/9780197675212.003.0019

The habit-centered hypothesis of AN proposes that the maladaptive routines that perpetuate illness are stuck because they have acquired the behavioral and neural characteristics of a habit (Steinglass & Walsh, 2006; Walsh, 2013). That is, the behavior has become cue-dependent and outcome (i.e., reward) insensitive and the associated neural substrates that guide behavior have changed. It follows from the habit hypothesis that to achieve meaningful and lasting change, treatment needs to address habits specifically. Targeting habitual behavior with a psychological intervention is therefore a compelling mechanism-based approach to improve longer-term outcomes in the treatment of AN.

Biological Framework

Behavior is shaped, initially, through encountering rewards in the environment that reinforce actions. Purposeful activities that link behavior with a reward are termed action-outcome (A-O) behaviors (e.g., a mouse presses a lever to receive a pellet of food) (Yin & Knowlton, 2006). When an action or decision is paired with receipt of some type of reward, the behavior is more likely to be repeated when the context (or cue) occurs again. Even if the reward doesn't happen every time the behavior occurs, if it happens more often than not, it tends to reinforce that behavior in association with that cue. This is goal-directed behavior.

With sufficient repetition, the nature of an A-O behavior changes such that the behavior continues irrespective of the outcome (e.g., a mouse continues pressing the lever even when sated on the food). These over-learned behaviors are termed stimulus-response (S-R) behaviors, or habits. Animal studies indicate that acquiring A-O behaviors requires engagement of the ventral striatum, whereas S-R behaviors are mediated by dorsal striatal function (Graybiel, 2008). Moreover, when behavior transitions from goal-directed to habitual, there is a shift from ventral to dorsal frontostriatal neural circuits. Across species, inhibiting the ventral striatum interferes with reinforcement learning, while inhibiting the dorsal striatum interferes with the performance of learned behaviors (Atallah et al., 2007; Miyachi et al., 1997; Robbins et al., 2012).

Habits have their advantages. With goal-directed behavior, the brain is computing the value of outcomes and selecting choices/decisions—an effortful process. With sufficient repetition, the brain does not need to monitor for rewards and compute the value of behavior sequences. Rather, behavior proceeds on relative "autopilot" and the brain's cognitive resources can be devoted to other behaviors, choices, or processes. The classic example of this is the experience of driving to work: while each turn is initially attended to, over time one proceeds relatively automatically, allowing the driver to think about other things.

Once a behavior is a habit, even if it is specifically *not* desired, the behavior that has been learned will continue. Habitual behaviors are therefore defined as relatively insensitive to the desirability of an outcome—something a person keeps doing, even if their interest in the outcome has changed (Balleine & O'Doherty, 2010). Humans—in contrast to mice in experimental studies—develop habits in a complex environment. Consequently, behavioral routines are made up of a series of cues and actions. The brain links one thing with another for efficiency, by chunking behavior into highly elaborate sequences and creating habit chains. If the efficient, somewhat reflexive behavioral routine—the habit—is disadvantageous to overall health and well-being, it is no less entrenched; the behavior can persist, even when the outcome of the behavior is no longer desired.

The habit-centered hypothesis of anorexia nervosa

The habit model of AN proposes that, once established, specific patterns around eating (and specific eating choices) are made because they are tightly linked patterns of behavior set in motion by specific cues. Goals that may have been guiding behavior initially are less relevant over time (Walsh, 2013).

While restrictive eating is not the only problematic behavior characteristic of AN, it is the most stereotyped behavior seen in patients with this disorder and it is a *major* contributor to the need for hospitalization (Walsh, 2011). The central role of this behavior in illness—as well as the consistency of the pattern of reduced fat intake across individuals—led to a focus on this specific category of disordered behavior in efforts to test the role of habit systems in AN.

The habit model purports that when restrictive eating begins, it likely is a goal-directed behavior, in pursuit of a goal such as weight loss or some other individualized reward. This initial dieting behavior is presumed to be mediated by the ventral neural systems that reinforce and guide new behavior. Studies of the neural circuits underlying food choice in adolescents with AN indicate that there are no differences between patients and healthy peers in the engagement of these reward circuits. That is, both groups of adolescents show similar engagement of the ventral striatum while making decisions about what to eat (Lloyd et al., 2025).

With repetition over time and severity of illness, the maladaptive routines that perpetuate AN are thought to shift to become less related to the initial goal. Two separate studies have shown that among individuals with AN, but not healthy peers, neural activity in the dorsal striatum was significantly associated with decisions made about what to eat (see Chapter 14; Foerde et al., 2015; Foerde et al., 2022). Furthermore, individuals with the largest decrease in dorsal striatal engagement after inpatient weight restoration had the largest increase in selection of high-fat foods (Foerde et al., 2021). Together, these studies highlight the dorsal striatum as a substrate of restrictive eating. While one cannot infer motivation based on neuroimaging findings, the role of the dorsal striatum in guiding restrictive eating among patients with AN is at least consistent with the habit hypothesis and the behavioral findings and serves as the foundation of the habit focused behavioral intervention.

State of the Science in Eating Disorders

Habits in anorexia nervosa

The degree to which a behavior is governed by habit is commonly measured via the Self Report Habit Index (SRHI), quantified as "habit strength" (Verplanken & Orbell, 2003). The SRHI has been used to study habit strength in many health-related behaviors, including cigarette smoking, teeth brushing, and exercising (Gardner et al., 2011; Kremers & Brug, 2008; Ray et al., 2020). Habit strength has been shown reliably to predict the frequency and persistence of a behavior, and its emergence independent of explicit intention.

Individuals with AN and healthy controls alike can identify routines meeting the criteria for eating-related habits (Davis et al., 2020). Oftentimes, the behavior is the same (e.g., exercise, use of low-fat salad dressing). For individuals with AN, these routines have greater habit strength than similar routines in healthy controls (e.g., scores for exercise after eating and scores for delaying eating when hungry were greater among AN than healthy controls). Of course, there are also differences in the routines between groups such that individuals with AN describe habits that are clearly maladaptive (e.g., drinking an excess of water, fasting, purging) and healthy individuals' habits are generally not. For those with AN, habit strength increased with duration of illness (Coniglio et al., 2017; Davis et al., 2020). Relative to healthy controls, individuals with AN also have a greater frequency of behaviors that are considered "habits," both in the domain of personal hygiene and food (Seidel et al., 2022). In sum, evidence supports that restrictive eating behavior in AN has behavioral features of habit: it is learned, is not innate, occurs repeatedly, and, once learned, is elicited by specific stimuli.

The first support for a habit-focused intervention came from a pilot study of an adjunctive treatment for inpatients with AN (Steinglass et al., 2018). In this study, 22 hospitalized patients with AN received 12 adjunctive sessions of either a habit-focused intervention or supportive psychotherapy intervention (randomly assigned). The patients who received the habit-focused intervention demonstrated improvement in three key areas. One, they reported greater improvement in the habit strength of their maladaptive behaviors; that is, a decrease in the extent to which the behaviors were automatic, frequent, and interwoven with identity. This was the proximal target of the intervention and the most expected outcome. Two, the patients who received the habit-focused intervention also showed greater improvement in eating disorder severity as measured by the Eating Disorder Examination Questionnaire (Fairburn, 2008). Three, these individuals also showed greater improvement (although not statistically significant) in actual food intake in a laboratory meal.

Relapse Prevention and Changing Habits

Relapse Prevention and Changing Habits (REACH+) is the next iteration of a habit-focused intervention for AN. REACH+ aims to change routines in the outpatient, post-acute setting—a time when patients with AN are most vulnerable to relapse (Walsh et al., 2021). The rate of weight loss in the first month following hospital discharge predicts the outcome at one year (Kaplan et al., 2009). Cues for maladaptive routines likely contribute to the very high rehospitalization rates. REACH+ underscores the importance of developing adaptive behavior—and specifically, adaptive *eating* behavior—in the period immediately following discharge from intensive, structured treatment (Steinglass et al., 2022) and in an environment rich with cues for maladaptive behavior (i.e., home rather than the hospital).

REACH+ relies upon the habit hypothesis of AN and its neural basis. This psychological intervention builds from habit reversal therapy, known to be effective in changing semi-automatic behaviors in other illnesses (Mansueto, 2020). The critical elements of behavior change are identification of cues (external and internal), creation of new behavioral routines, and interruption of maladaptive routines.

Introducing Relapse Prevention and Changing Habits: Education, assessment, and motivation

REACH+ makes the habit framework explicit and conveys the importance of behaviorally—focused work to patients beginning in the first session. After reviewing basic principles of habits and the state of the research on the neural basis for habits in AN, there is a frank discussion about relapse risk in returning to an environment ripe with the contextual cues in which the eating disorder thrived.

The next early goal of REACH+ is to engage patients in learning more about the intricacies of their own habitual routines. Although individuals may be aware of their eating disorder habits, they may be less clear on the earliest antecedents for their actions. These antecedents precede the initiation of the automatic behavior (or sequence of behaviors). Through assessment and discussion of individualized examples, the concept of cues is elaborated upon, and their importance underscored.

Similar to other behavioral treatments, in REACH+ patients learn to identify cues. External cues for eating disorder-related habits can include settings where the behavior takes place (e.g., mirror, dining table); visual, tactile, or olfactory sensations (e.g., portion of food observed on plate, feeling of waistband against stomach, aroma of food); postural cues (e.g., thighs touching while seated, calorie labels on packaged meal items facing the patient); or the time of day. Internal cues can include affective states, such as anxiety, anger, or sadness, or thoughts (e.g., "I will never stop gaining weight if I eat three meals each day.").

REACH+ focuses on a habit sequence, a cue—or series of cues—preceding an action or series of actions in response to the particular stimulus. Often in AN, the actions involve "inaction" or avoidance. For example, an individual may skip breakfast (avoidant action). The cues preceding this behavior might include the alarm clock ringing (external cue) or thinking about a life stressor (internal cue). These cues set the stage for the fairly automatic, eating-disordered action of skipping a meal. Habit sequences—or chains—in AN are as elaborate as those in other human habit research, involving a series of cues and actions (or inactions) that get chunked together into routines.

In REACH+, the assessment of habits is codified in the creation of a personalized inventory of the kinds of behaviors/routines that the patient identifies as part of the eating disorder. Any discussion of habitual behavior in AN with a patient quickly illustrates the complexity of cues and actions. While restrictive eating is a core component of AN and its reduction is central to relapse prevention, it is not the only salient problematic routine for individuals with AN. Habitual routines are as complex as the environments in which they developed; therefore, they cannot exist in siloes. For example, some habits, such as body checking or calorie counting, may interface directly with restrictive eating. If walking past a mirror cues an individual to start scrutinizing, pinching, or measuring a part of their body, this checking behavior may subsequently cue the individual to select a small breakfast bowl, thus cuing under-portioning cereal.

Efficient, maladaptive habit chains, in which the brain links one behavior to the next, results in complex sequences that together contribute to inadequate intake. REACH+ posits that as "one thing leads to another," the behavior becomes increasingly charged and difficult to change. Treatment aims to find early antecedent cues where small behavior changes may meet with less resistance for the individual. Other behaviors, such as excessive exercise, purging, and eating or cooking rituals, may also share the features of habits for an individual and contribute to their risk of relapse over time. From the start of REACH+, the therapist uses habit reversal theory to motivate the patient by explaining that using cue awareness to make a small change in behavior may have big downstream effects on what comes next. Enhanced cue awareness in tandem with behavior change techniques introduced in REACH+ lead to alternate action and the ultimate goal; that is, to break a habit and take a different path.

Relapse Prevention and Changing Habits in Action: Interrupting habits and enacting change

Throughout the treatment, the therapist helps the patient to enhance cue awareness in a number of ways. First, as the therapist listens to the patient describe the fairly automatic routines that serve the eating disorder, they reflect the cues and categorize these elements as external or internal cues. This builds insight into cues and instructs the patient on general categories of cues to help them identify other examples. Second, personalized habit chains or timelines are created. When creating a behavior timeline or chain, the habit is placed toward the end of the sequence, encouraging reflection upon the complex sequence of cues that give rise to the behavior (see Figure 18.1). This serves as a visual illustration of cues and their temporal relationship to habitual behaviors, and it encourages collaborative brainstorming about cues ripe for intervention. In building the behavior timeline or chain, the expectation is that the patient will identify early cues that feel like an easy juncture to change course. Third, throughout REACH+, the patient tracks cues and their sequalae. Ultimately, the patient uses this monitoring to experiment with different options for behavior change in the setting of the cue, and to identify the points of least resistance or options for behavior change which might circumvent the cue entirely.

Eating-related behavioral experiments are central to REACH+. This reflects the stance that normalizing eating and adequacy of intake (e.g., diet variety and energy density) is critical to preventing relapse. It is therefore important that patients learn to implement REACH+ skills on eating- or intake-related habits before branching out to other kinds of routines of illness. Eating-related experiments—and subsequent recovery-related behavioral experiments—rely on principles from well-studied, behavioral principles (Albano & DiBartolo, 2007; Woods et al., 2008) including (1) habit reversal and competing responses, (2) stimulus control, and (3) exposure (see Table 18.1). Described briefly below, each strategy has

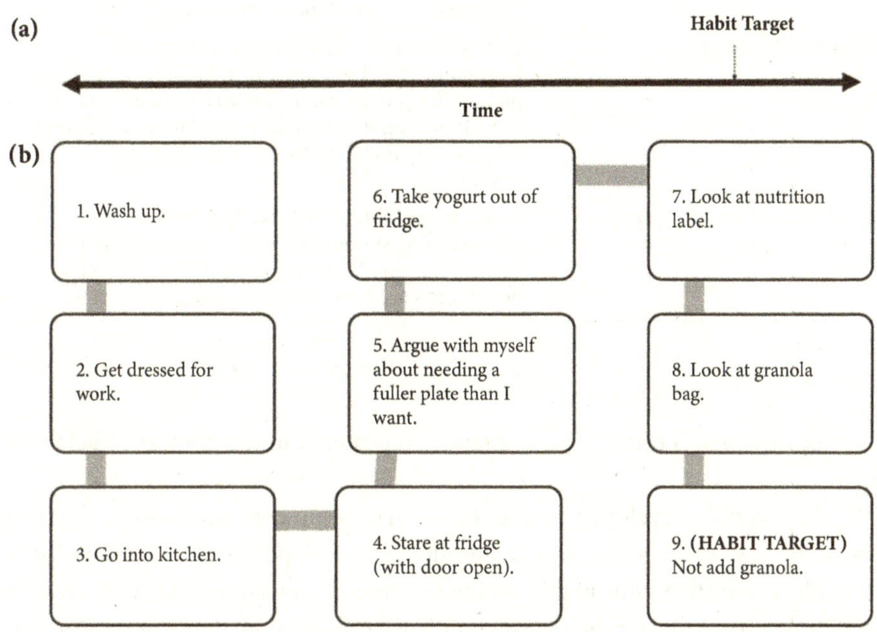

Figure 18.1 Habit worksheet. (a) Habit timeline. (b) Habit chain. Habit change experiment generated: Go to kitchen and eat breakfast in pajamas. *Hypothesis:* This may interrupt arguing with self by reducing amount of available time to eat and increase pressure to move onto the next activity (i.e., getting dressed).

Table 18.1 Behavior change principles

Habit	Competing Response
Rumination of food	Tongue on roof of mouth, talking
Pacing/fidgeting	Sitting on hands
Checking wrist size	Put hands in pocket
Sucking in stomach	Change posture; fully exhale
Eat food items separately	Add "unifying" seasoning (e.g., pepper) to multiple foods
Habit	**Stimulus Control**
Reading food/calorie labels	Reposition foods
Logging meals	Move notebook to difficult-to-access location
Delay eating through the use of meal "preparation" rituals	Use non-dominant hand, take bite of some food item before cutting anything
Use spoon to eat all items	Hide spoon, move spoon out of reach
Eat foods "separately"	Select "mixed" food items, alternate bites between items
Purge in the shower	Shower in the morning, when urge to purge is low
Habit	**Exposure**
Avoiding certain foods	Eating energy-dense snacks ranging from a bagel to dessert; caloric liquids of varying energy density; different food textures; high fat foods as part of meal (i.e., dessert); fearful main course (i.e., pizza)
Eating small portions	Eating from a buffet; having patient portion with a large empty bowl or plate and a "family size" serving plate of the chosen main course (e.g., pasta with sauce); putting similar quantities of food in different shaped containers; finished plate; eating one bite beyond planned
Eating "known" foods or amounts	Eating while blindfolded; eating from bowl behind a barrier; using spoons of different sizes; eating homemade food for which several different recipe possibilities are provided; eating unknown brand

its place in REACH+ and these are taught repeatedly in the context of behavior chains.

Habit reversal, developed in the 1970s, has been used successfully to treat tics, stuttering, excoriation, and trichotillomania (Woods et al., 2008), and it is particularly effective with highly automatic, simple behaviors. Habit reversal in REACH+ starts with cue awareness and identification in the moment, during eating experiments and in self-monitoring homework assignments. Experiments may occur in session or between sessions. The next critical step is the development of a competing response, a behavior that the patient will try to engage in every time they experience an urge to act out of habit. Commonly, competing responses are simple, motoric counteractions that can be done often or as long as needed (i.e., until the urge subsides), and must be incompatible with the target habit.

Stimulus control interventions involve using strategies that sufficiently alter the environment to encourage an alternate behavior (or absence of the problem behavior). These strategies may be particularly effective when a cue has been identified that precedes the individual's experience of strong affect or entrenched cognitions, when the cue reflects a confluence of factors, involves an aspect of the environment that is seemingly outside of the patient's control, or if habit reversal has been ineffective.

Exposure involves planned introduction of a stimulus that will provoke habitually avoided internal cues (e.g., emotions such as anxiety, disgust, anger, etc.) for the purpose of reducing avoidance (in all its forms), promoting new learning, and disconfirming the imagined consequence. Some stimulus control experiments—for example, alternating bites between items or tasting food without cutting it—could theoretically be conducted as part of an exposure eating experiment, if the intention is to activate an emotion. Experiments done in the "spirit" of exposure may not confirm to "normal" eating patterns or behaviors because the goal is to activate the affect and related cognitions and coach the patient to stick with it. For example, if an individual is alternating bites between items as part of an exposure exercise, the patient might intersperse bites of dessert and bites of salad to stay engaged with feared consequences and discomfort. The exposure experiment goal is to experience and tolerate a range of internal cues (i.e., affect and cognitions).

The role of rewards in Relapse Prevention and Changing Habits

Neither cue awareness nor brief behavioral experiments will be sufficient for the kind of sustained change that would prevent relapse. It is essential for new or alternate paths to be clearly linked with rewards to facilitate reinforcement and repetition of new behaviors. REACH+ involves intentionally building new routines using goal-directed systems, where action is driven by a desired (or, appreciated) reward or outcome.

Put another way, if habits are by definition insensitive to rewards, actions that are inconsistent with a habit can be meaningfully tied to rewards. Behavior change is hard, especially when it comes to habitual processes associated with the persistence of AN. When patients are discharged from intensive treatment, they leave an environment explicitly structured to support and reward health. Completing meals within the confines of a treatment setting, for example, may allow a patient to select their own menus or go on desired outings. The home environment is likely more variable in this regard.

Identifying meaningful rewards requires creativity. In REACH+, rewards are conceptualized as any reinforcement for behavior change that the individual interprets as intrinsically positive and desirable. These may be mild, especially compared with rewards that reinforced the eating disorder before it became habitual, and it may take some time for them to be identified and amplified. Rewards can be emotional (e.g., pride, relief, hopefulness, freedom), social (e.g., ability to participate in a group conversation or activity), cognitive (e.g., enhanced focus on something unrelated to food/eating/appearance), or eating-related (e.g., being less rushed to eat, having food be hot when it is eaten). See Box 18.1 for examples, as expressed by patients in session.

Box 18.1 Examples of rewards identified by patients in REACH+

Example #1

THERAPIST: Okay, great. Go ahead and talk me through these cue monitoring reward examples.

PATIENT: The first one was eating out twice. And usually I would not allow it and would prepare food at home like this would make me feel safe. But here I was able to eat at a diner for breakfast and eat pizza at dinner. And the reward was feeling normal.

THERAPIST: When you say feeling normal, can you tell me what that means for you?

PATIENT: I think like for a really long time, I was just stuck in this place where I didn't really feel like I fit in with my family. They would eat fast food or enjoy things and couldn't participate. But I did it and just feeling normal, feeling like I am able to do something with them, was really good.

THERAPIST: Yeah, you weren't separating yourself from your family. I think going to the diner is also an event, that's a social interaction. And it's not only just about like the food part of feeling normal but also feeling social involved, right?

PATIENT: Yes, definitely.

THERAPIST: I would add that in there too then because I think that those are two separate rewards. And then you wrote "no arguments." What do you mean by that?

PATIENT: Usually, because I will prepare my own food or when I don't want to eat what my family is eating, it would just cause a lot of arguments like between me and my parents. Looking back, / felt like they didn't understand me. but I think they were worried. And so this time, just being able to do something without us like yelling at each other or them forcing me to eat it, it was kind of nice.

Example #2

PATIENT: I've done a couple more like spontaneous things, too. Yesterday I grabbed lattes like after class in the morning with friends, and on the weekend/got together with another friend and we went and got hot drinks in the morning as well, which is harder for me for some reason, having something like that between breakfast and lunch has always been more challenging. But that was nice and spontaneous and then Friday, me and one of my roommates saw on Instagram that there was an event [at school] and they were giving out free muffins, so we went together and grabbed them, um which I don't know, was fine, I guess. Because I've been having muffins more, by the time I came it was not as big deal, which was kind of nice. And I could feel myself almost being able to look forward to that and enjoy it.

THERAPIST: How would you sort of summarize that [the benefits] for yourself?

PATIENT: Um, I'm more flexible, I think with things like that. And like, things aren't as big, as much of a big deal I think. Like before, like doing one of those things would be like, like the pinnacle of the week kind of thing, and now it's like just like a thing that 1 do.

It is common for an individual to experience anxiety around new behaviors. As the patient engages in behavioral experiments, the therapist helps the patient to identify and amplify focus on the experience of rewards. While treatment may include learning to tolerate anxiety, REACH+ sessions spend greater time focused on amplification of rewards.

Alternative Perspectives

The most straightforward "alternate perspective" on REACH+—and habit focus in general—is that this is not a new target at all. Cognitive behavior therapy (CBT) for eating disorders is one of the most empirically supported approaches, and it includes interventions to address maladaptive behavior. Indeed, many of the interventions in REACH+ rely heavily on the foundation of CBT for eating disorders (Fairburn, 2008). As such, a skeptic would be wise to wonder whether this approach is truly different from existing therapies. REACH+ differs in the way in which it focuses on cues and moving backward in time from the maladaptive behavior rather than thinking ahead to the outcome. And it differs somewhat in the fine-grained approach, although this of course borrows heavily from behavioral analysis approaches. The existing data are quite limited, and while they suggest that focus on habit may be able to target the deeply entrenched restrictive eating that perpetuates AN, clinical trial data are needed to determine whether this constitutes a valuable approach.

At the neural systems level, it is also important to wonder whether the distinction between habits and goal-directed behavior is warranted in the setting of complex maladaptive behavior that constitutes illness. While it may be true that cue-dependent behavior persists independent of the outcome, it may also be true that patients with AN are pursuing a goal. There are elements of the Western cultural environment that will reward pursuit of thinness, regardless of the individual's goal. Habitual and goal-directed behavior can be aligned, and this may require a different treatment approach. It may be that even those engaged in treatment continue to value, in some way, the outcome of restrictive eating. If so, changing habits may have limited benefit, and there may be a need to simultaneously assure that goals are open to re-evaluation in the pursuit of health.

Another key consideration is whether mechanisms of illness and health may differ. That is, even if habits underlie the maladaptive behavior that perpetuates AN, this may be unrelated to mechanisms of health. It may still be the case that focusing on goal-directed behavior is critical for interrupting maladaptive behavior. The REACH+ approach integrates this likely scenario through the skills that allow for goal directed pursuit of alternative behaviors that are more consistent with health maintenance.

Additional criticisms of the habit-centered approach come from consideration of other elements that are central to illness in AN. The cues that maintain habitual behaviors central to AN, such as restrictive eating, include unhelpful, often-erroneous, beliefs about food, eating, weight, and body shape/appearance. The idea that behavior change can support the reappraisal of certain eating disorder ideas is central to cognitive behavioral therapy for eating disorders (Fairburn, 2008); the idea that behavior change may be possible regardless of cognitive change via acceptance of the inevitable presence of eating disordered thoughts is a tenet of third wave behavioral therapies (Pisetsky et al., 2019). In REACH+, thoughts are acknowledged as an unavoidable contextual cue for certain behavioral routines and patients are taught different strategies to manage these thoughts.

Implications

The habit-centered hypothesis of AN led directly to the development of interventions that aim to change maladaptive habits to maintain health. A neuroscience-informed treatment approach for habits centers on understanding that if the behavior is relatively insensitive to the outcome, then interventions that focus on the outcome will be of limited benefit. Rather, to change habits, the intervention needs to address the cues for behavior, and the ways that behaviors get linked together. REACH+ heavily emphasizes fine-grained focus on sequences of behavior to raise an individual's attention to the moments in a day when small changes might lead to alternative paths. Raising attentiveness to cues and developing skills to maintain awareness allow the individual to make more adaptive choices and develop new routines. This approach may have particular utility in the post-acute setting when individuals with AN are renourished and goals are most aligned with health. It may provide a new set of tools for a time when patients are most vulnerable to relapse.

The neurobiological framework of the habit-centered hypothesis has additional implications for treatment. There may be neuromodulatory approaches that can access the dorsal striatum to influence restrictive eating choices. In one study, repetitive transcranial magnetic stimulation (TMS) applied to the dorsolateral prefrontal cortex changed food choices (to increase high-fat choices) acutely (Muratore et al., 2021). In another study, a full course of TMS was associated with changes in use of self-control when making food choices (Dalton et al., 2020). As TMS and other neuromodulatory approaches develop, it may be possible to directly target the dorsal frontostriatal circuits and change habits. As the neurobiological understanding of habits evolves, pharmacological interventions may also become plausible (Favier et al., 2020).

Aspects of this approach have implications for treatment research more broadly. The ability to create mechanism-based treatment interventions builds directly from the explosion of research in the past decade that has identified the neural bases of eating disorders. As an understanding of the biological basis of behavior increases, the potential to identify treatment targets increases. Furthermore, it will be increasingly possible to personalize interventions. For example, mechanistic studies will inform whether habit systems are relevant for long-term persistence versus remission of illness, and it will identify whether some individuals are more likely to benefit from an emphasis on habit change.

References

Albano, A. M., & DiBartolo, P. M. (2007). *Cognitive-behavioral therapy for social phobia in adolescents: Stand up, speak out.* Oxford University Press.

Atallah, H. E., Lopez-Paniagua, D., Rudy, J. W., & O'Reilly, R. C. (2007). Separate neural substrates for skill learning and performance in the ventral and dorsal striatum. *Nature Neuroscience, 10*(1), 126–131. https://doi.org/10.1038/nn1817

Balleine, B. W., & O'Doherty, J. P. (2010). Human and rodent homologies in action control: Corticostriatal determinants of goal-directed and habitual action. *Neuropsychopharmacology, 35*(1), 48–69. https://doi.org/npp2009131

Coniglio, K. A., Becker, K. R., Franko, D. L., Zayas, L. V., Plessow, F., Eddy, K. T., & Thomas, J. J. (2017). Won't stop or can't stop? Food restriction as a habitual behavior among individuals with anorexia nervosa or atypical anorexia nervosa. *Eating Behaviors, 26*, 144–147. https://doi.org/10.1016/j.eatbeh.2017.03.005

Dalton, B., Foerde, K., Bartholdy, S., McClelland, J., Kekic, M., Grycuk, L., Campbell, I. C., Schmidt, U., & Steinglass, J. E. (2020). The effect of repetitive transcranial magnetic stimulation on food choice-related self-control in patients with severe, enduring anorexia nervosa. *International Journal of Eating Disorders*, 53(8), 1326–1336. https://doi.org/10.1002/eat.23267

Davis, L., Walsh, B. T., Schebendach, J., Glasofer, D. R., & Steinglass, J. E. (2020). Habits are stronger with longer duration of illness and greater severity in anorexia nervosa. *International Journal of Eating Disorders, 53*(5), 413–419. https://doi.org/10.1002/eat.23265

Fairburn, C. G. (2008). *Cognitive behavior therapy and eating disorders.* Guilford Press.

Favier, M., Janickova, H., Justo, D., Kljakic, O., Runtz, L., Natsheh, J. Y., Pascoal, T. A., Germann, J., Gallino, D., Kang, J. I., Meng, X. Q., Antinora, C., Raulic, S., Jacobsen, J. P., Moquin, L., Vigneault, E., Gratton, A., Caron, M. G., Duriez, P., . . . El Mestikawy, S. (2020). Cholinergic dysfunction in the dorsal striatum promotes habit formation and maladaptive eating. *Journal of Clinical Investigation, 130*(12), 6616–6630. https://doi.org/10.1172/JCI138532

Fernstrom, M. H., Weltzin, T. E., Neuberger, S., Srinivasagam, N., & Kaye, W. H. (1994). Twenty-four-hour food intake in patients with anorexia nervosa and in healthy control subjects. *Biological Psychiatry, 36*(10), 696–702. https://doi.org/10.1016/0006-3223(94)91179-7

Foerde, K., Schebendach, J. E., Davis, L., Daw, N., Walsh, B. T., Shohamy, D., & Steinglass, J. E. (2022). Restrictive eating across a spectrum from healthy to unhealthy: Behavioral and neural mechanisms. *Psychological Medicine, 52*(9), 1755–1764. https://doi.org/10.1017/S0033291720003542

Foerde, K., Steinglass, J. E., Shohamy, D., & Walsh, B. T. (2015). Neural mechanisms supporting maladaptive food choices in anorexia nervosa. *Nature Neuroscience*, *18*(11), 1571–1573. https://doi.org/10.1038/nn.4136

Foerde, K., Walsh, B. T., Dalack, M., Daw, N., Shohamy, D., & Steinglass, J. E. (2021). Changes in brain and behavior during food-based decision-making following treatment of anorexia nervosa. *Journal of Eating Disorders*, *9*(1), 48. https://doi.org/10.1186/s40337-021-00402-y

Gardner, B., de Bruijn, G.-J., & Lally, P. (2011). A systematic review and meta-analysis of applications of the self-report habit index to nutrition and physical activity behaviours. *Annals of Behavioral Medicine*, *42*(2), 174–187.

Graybiel, A. M. (2008). Habits, rituals, and the evaluative brain. *Annual Review of Neuroscience*, *31*, 359–387. https://doi.org/10.1146/annurev.neuro.29.051605.112851

Kaplan, A. S., Walsh, B. T., Olmsted, M., Attia, E., Carter, J. C., Devlin, M. J., Pike, K. M., Woodside, B., Rockert, W., Roberto, C. A., & Parides, M. (2009). The slippery slope: Prediction of successful weight maintenance in anorexia nervosa. *Psychological Medicine*, *39*(6), 1037–1045. https://doi.org/S003329170800442X

Kremers, S. P., & Brug, J. (2008). Habit strength of physical activity and sedentary behavior among children and adolescents. *Pediatric Exercise Science*, *20*(1), 5–17.

Lloyd, E. C., Posner, J., Schebendach, J., Muratore, A. F., Hong, S., Ojeda, J., Rafanello, E., Steinglass, J. E., & Foerde, K. (2025). Food choice and neural reward systems in adolescents with anorexia nervosa and atypical anorexia nervosa. *Journal of Child Psychology and Psychiatry*, *66*(3), 378–389. https://doi.org/10.1111/jcpp.14066

Mansueto, C. S., Vavrichek, S. M., & Golomb, R. G. (2020). *Overcoming body-focused repetitive behaviors: A comprehensive behavioral treatment for hair pulling and skin picking*. New Harbinger Publications.

Mayer, L. E., Schebendach, J., Bodell, L. P., Shingleton, R. M., & Walsh, B. T. (2012). Eating behavior in anorexia nervosa: Before and after treatment. *International Journal of Eating Disorders*, *45*(2), 290–293. https://doi.org/10.1002/eat.20924

Miyachi, S., Hikosaka, O., Miyashita, K., Karadi, Z., & Rand, M. K. (1997). Differential roles of monkey striatum in learning of sequential hand movement. *Experimental Brain Research*, *115*(1), 1–5. https://doi.org/10.1007/pl00005669

Muratore, A. F., Bershad, M., Steinglass, J. E., Foerde, K. E., Gianini, L., Broft, A., & Attia, E. (2021). Use of high-frequency repetitive transcranial magnetic stimulation to probe the neural circuitry of food choice in anorexia nervosa: A proof-of-concept study. *International Journal of Eating Disorders*, *54*(11), 2031–2036. https://doi.org/10.1002/eat.23597

Pisetsky, E. M., Schaefer, L. M., Wonderlich, S. A., & Peterson, C. B. (2019). Emerging psychological treatments in eating disorders. *Psychiatric Clinics of North America*, *42*(2), 219–229. https://doi.org/10.1016/j.psc.2019.01.005

Ray, L. A., Du, H., Grodin, E., Bujarski, S., Meredith, L., Ho, D., Nieto, S., & Wassum, K. (2020). Capturing habitualness of drinking and smoking behavior in humans. *Drug and Alcohol Dependence*, *207*, 107738.

Robbins, T. W., Gillan, C. M., Smith, D. G., de Wit, S., & Ersche, K. D. (2012). Neurocognitive endophenotypes of impulsivity and compulsivity: Towards dimensional psychiatry. *Trends in Cognitive Science*, *16*(1), 81–91. https://doi.org/S1364-6613(11)00242-7

Seidel, M., King, J. A., Furtjes, S., Labitzke, N., Wronski, M. L., Boehm, I., Hennig, J., Gramatke, K., Roessner, V., & Ehrlich, S. (2022). Increased habit frequency in the daily lives of patients with acute anorexia nervosa. *Nutrients*, *14*(19), 3905. https://doi.org/10.3390/nu14193905

Steinglass, J., & Walsh, B. T. (2006). Habit learning and anorexia nervosa: A cognitive neuroscience hypothesis. *International Journal of Eating Disorders*, *39*(4), 267–275. https://doi.org/10.1002/eat.20244

Steinglass, J. E., Attia, E., Glasofer, D. R., Wang, Y., Ruggiero, J., Walsh, B. T., & Thomas, J. G. (2022). Optimizing relapse prevention and changing habits (REACH+) in anorexia nervosa. *International Journal of Eating Disorders*, *55*(6), 851–857. https://doi.org/10.1002/eat.23724

Steinglass, J. E., Fei, W., Foerde, K., Touzeau, C., Ruggiero, J., Lloyd, C., Attia, E., Wang, Y., & Walsh, B. T. (2023). Change in food choice during acute treatment and the effect on longer-term outcome in patients with anorexia nervosa. *Psychological Medicine*, *54*(6), 1133–1141. https://doi.org/10.1017/S0033291723002933

Steinglass, J. E., Glasofer, D. R., Walsh, E., Guzman, G., Peterson, C. B., Walsh, B. T., Attia, E., & Wonderlich, S. A. (2018). Targeting habits in anorexia nervosa: A proof-of-concept randomized trial. *Psychological Medicine*, *48*(15), 2584–2591. https://doi.org/10.1017/S003329171800020X

Verplanken, B., & Orbell, S. (2003). Reflections on past behavior: A self-report index of habit strength. *Journal of Applied Social Psychology*, *33*(6), 1313–1330.

Walsh, B. T. (2011). The importance of eating behavior in eating disorders. *Physiology & Behavior*, *104*(4), 525–529. https://doi.org/10.1016/j.physbeh.2011.05.007

Walsh, B. T. (2013). The enigmatic persistence of anorexia nervosa. *American Journal of Psychiatry*, *170*(5), 477–484. https://doi.org/10.1176/appi.ajp.2012.12081074

Walsh, B. T., Xu, T., Wang, Y., Attia, E., & Kaplan, A. S. (2021). Time course of relapse following acute treatment for anorexia nervosa. *American Journal of Psychiatry*, *178*(9), 848–853. https://doi.org/10.1176/appi.ajp.2021.21010026

Woods, D. W., Piacentini, J., Chang, S., Deckersbach, T., Ginsburg, G., Peterson, A., Scahill, L., Walkup, J., & Wilhelm, S. (2008). *Managing tourette syndrome: A behavioral intervention for children and adults*. Oxford University Press.

Yin, H. H., & Knowlton, B. J. (2006). The role of the basal ganglia in habit formation. *Nature Reviews Neuroscience*, *7*(6), 464–476. https://doi.org/10.1038/nrn1919

19

Temperament-Informed Treatment for Anorexia Nervosa

Christina E. Wierenga, Stephanie Knatz Peck, and Laura Hill

Brief Definitional Overview

Temperament: Temperament is the biological basis of personality, and includes endogenous basic tendencies of behavior, cognition, and emotion that contribute to individual differences (Cloninger, 1994; Rothbart, 2012). Temperament is genetically influenced, and this heritability is thought to contribute risk for the development of mental health problems in adolescence and adulthood (Whittle et al., 2006).

Introduction

Advances in the ability to characterize a range of psychopathology on the basis of underlying neurobiology have driven new etiological models and targets of intervention. There is growing enthusiasm for applying neuroscience-informed interventions to eating disorders (Schmidt & Campbell, 2013; Touyz et al., 2023). This chapter explores the biological framework underlying the temperament model of anorexia nervosa (AN), which proposes that certain biologically based and heritable traits confer risk for the development and persistence of AN and may also facilitate recovery. Temperament Based Therapy with Support (TBT-S) is introduced as an emerging treatment approach informed by this model. TBT-S applies contemporary neuroscience research findings to inform treatment targets, and it addresses AN from a framework of temperament and altered brain function affecting the regulation of emotion and eating. Rather than aiming to change traits, TBT-S focuses on the development of compensatory strategies to manage maladaptive expression of these traits to reduce eating disorder symptoms, and uses multiple strategies, including neurobiological psychoeducation, experiential exercises, massed practice skills training, meal coaching, and behavioral contracting, within a developmentally tailored model of social support.

Christina E. Wierenga, Stephanie Knatz Peck, and Laura Hill, *Temperament-Informed Treatment for Anorexia Nervosa*. In: *The Handbook of the Neurobiology of Eating Disorders*. Edited by: Christina E. Wierenga and Joanna E. Steinglass, Oxford University Press. © Oxford University Press (2025). DOI: 10.1093/9780197675212.003.0020

Biological Framework

The role of temperament in psychopathology

In its broadest sense, the term temperament refers to endogenous, basic tendencies of behavior, cognitions, and emotions (Mitchell, 2018; Whittle et al., 2006). Core temperament dimensions are observable in infancy and remain relatively stable across the lifespan (Cole, 2020). While there is some disagreement about the relationship between temperament and personality, prominent models view temperament as the biological basis of personality (Cloninger, 1994; Rothbart, 2012). Temperament is both heritable and shaped by environmental influences, which may alter trait expression across the lifespan (Steiger & Booij, 2020). Supporting this notion, a recent meta-analysis of behavior genetic studies (studies that use genetic methods to examine the basis of individual differences in behavior) found that 40% of individual differences in personality are due to genetic influences while 60% are due to environmental influences (Vukasovic & Bratko, 2015). Longitudinal work suggests that environment may have a stronger influence on trait expression in youth whereas genetics confer greater influence in adolescence and adulthood (Klump et al., 2007; Mervilde & De Pauw, 2012). The heritability of temperament is thought to contribute to the risk for behavioral and mental health problems, particularly during adolescence when the onset of such problems is particularly pronounced (Cloninger, 2000; Ormel et al., 2005; Steinberg, 2005; Whittle et al., 2006).

Three higher-order trait dimensions tend to be shared across models of temperament: negative affectivity (characterized by inhibition, avoidance, and punishment sensitivity), positive affectivity (characterized by high approach and reward sensitivity), and constraint or inhibition (characterized by degree of control over impulses and emotions, ability to direct attention and delay gratification) (Bijttebier et al., 2009; Clark & Watson, 1999; Cloninger et al., 1993; Eysenck, 1967). Notably, psychopathology is thought to reflect extreme expressions of these trait dimensions, supporting the widely held view that temperament is strongly related to most mental health conditions (Clark, 2005; Whittle et al., 2006). For instance, elevated positive affectivity characterized by externalizing behaviors and extreme approach motivation is thought to contribute to substance use disorders, whereas elevated negative affectivity characterized by internalizing behaviors and extreme avoidance is thought to contribute to anxiety and depression (Bijttebier et al., 2009). Accumulating evidence from animal neurophysiology and human brain imaging studies suggests that these trait dimensions have roots in separate neurobiological systems including subcortical-limbic and prefrontal circuits (Cloninger, 2000), which overlap with systems that have been associated with psychiatric disorders (Whittle et al., 2006). Models linking temperament and psychopathology have posited both a causal role for temperament, by increasing vulnerability and likelihood of developing mental health problems, and a complicating role, whereby psychopathology and temperament interact to maintain illness.

The role of temperament in treatment

While an individual's traits are relatively stable across the lifespan, trait expression can vary and be disadvantageous in one situation and advantageous in others. Collectively, the notion that traits can be both vulnerability factors and assets has led to the idea that interventions managing trait expression may improve psychological functioning (Duckworth et al., 2005; Hower et al., 2021). Early compensatory management interventions were derived from a deficit model, stemming from their focus on neurological and cognitive rehabilitation (Carney et al., 1999; Sitzer et al., 2006). More recent compensatory interventions have taken a strength-based, capitalization approach, teaching new strategies for working around or improving cognitive or behavioral difficulties. These capitalization approaches focus on leveraging existing endogenous strengths or external support and adapting environments that represent challenges for given temperament profiles (McClowry et al., 2008). Often the goal is to form new habits or routines in thinking, learning, and problem-solving to circumvent deficits and improve functioning (Cheavens et al., 2012; McClowry et al., 2008). Studies conducted in depression, psychosis, and autism spectrum disorder support tailoring interventions to an individual's strengths, demonstrating enhanced treatment effects and better clinical outcome (Allott et al., 2020; Brookman-Frazee et al., 2019; Cheavens et al., 2012; McGurk et al., 2007; Twamley et al., 2012; Zhang & Perivoliotis, 2022).

State of the Science in Eating Disorders

The role of temperament in anorexia nervosa

Accumulating behavioral and neuroimaging evidence suggests that individuals with AN tend to have common traits and altered neural circuit function that may contribute to the development and maintenance of the disorder (for a review of behavioral expression and neurobiological mechanisms, see Kaye et al., 2015). Many of these traits predate the illness, and they often persist in a mild to modest degree after recovery (Anderluh et al., 2003; Cassin & von Ranson, 2005; Wagner et al., 2006). For example, AN is frequently associated with increased anxiety, characterized by elevated trait anxiety (Lilenfeld et al., 2006); increased state anxiety, especially related to food and eating (Steinglass et al., 2010); elevated intolerance of uncertainty (Frank et al., 2012); and exaggerated harm avoidance, which is a multifaceted trait (Cloninger et al., 1994) characterized by anxiety, inhibition, and inflexibility (Cassin & von Ranson, 2005; Fassino, Amianto, et al., 2004; Klump et al., 2004; Wagner et al., 2006). Individuals with AN also have a high incidence of co-morbid anxiety disorders (Kaye et al., 2004). Anxiety in AN has been associated with lower body mass index, increased dietary restriction (avoiding food often serves to reduce anxiety), poorer clinical outcome, and may have a genetic basis as genes linked to anxiety are also associated with AN (Bloss et al., 2011; Dellava et al., 2010; Steinglass et al., 2010). Anxiety in AN has been associated with altered function of executive dorsal caudate and limbic regions, including altered dopamine and serotonin function (Bailer et al., 2013; Frank & Kaye 2005; Kaye, Wierenga, Bailer, Simmons, & Bischoff-Grethe, 2013). For instance, a small positron emission tomography that assessed [11C]raclopride binding following amphetamine administration to measure endogenous dopamine production found that dopamine release in the dorsal caudate was associated with increased anxiety in women recovered from AN (Bailer et al., 2012), in contrast to the normative experience of euphoria in response to limbic dopamine release (Brauer & de Wit, 1996; Gabbay, 2003). This suggests that dopamine release associated with usually pleasurable events (e.g., eating) may be experienced as anxiogenic in AN. Animal studies (Eagle et al., 2011; Simon et al., 2011) confirm that risk avoidance and inhibition correlate with dopamine function in the dorsal caudate and related regions, suggesting that such neural processes may contribute to anxiety and avoidant behaviors in AN. Imaging studies have also demonstrated altered anticipatory dorsal caudate and insula response to cues for food and interoceptive experience in AN that is associated with elevated harm avoidance (Berner et al., 2018; Kaye et al., 2020; Oberndorfer et al., 2013; Strigo et al., 2013). Collectively, these studies suggest a biological basis for anxiety in AN.

In addition to anxiety, the AN temperament is characterized by perfectionism (Bardone-Cone et al., 2007), cognitive inflexibility (see Chapter 11), inhibition (see Chapter 10), altered sensitivity to reward and punishment (see Chapter 7), and altered interoceptive function (see Chapter 8) (Kaye, Wierenga, Bailer, Simmons, Wagner, et al., 2013; Wierenga, 2023; Wierenga et al., 2014). Recent theories have begun to take an integrative approach by considering the relationships of these traits to each other and their association with eating disorder symptoms. For instance, AN has been proposed to reflect dysregulation of approach/avoidance motivational systems, characterized by decreased approach motivation to rewarding outcomes and increased avoidance of aversive outcomes (Harrison et al., 2011; Kaye, Wierenga, Bailer, Simmons, Wagner, et al., 2013; Wierenga et al., 2014). Studies assessing individual differences in the strength of the Behavior Activation System (BAS; a tendency to experience strong positive affect or behavioral approach in response to specific goal-oriented outcomes) and Behavior Inhibition System (BIS; a tendency to experience strong negative affect or behavioral inhibition in response to perceived threats) generally find increased BIS and decreased BAS in AN samples (Harrison et al., 2010; Harrison et al., 2011; Jonker et al., 2020; Turner et al., 2014), with a greater motivational bias toward BIS versus

BAS (Abber et al., 2024). Similarly, others have shown that trait-based phenotypes based on BIS, BAS, and effortful control can identify clinically meaningful groups that may better reflect core dimensions of eating disorders than traditional diagnostic classification (Claes et al., 2006; Turner et al., 2014). For instance, clustering approaches have identified eating disorder groups characterized by over-control (high inhibition, anxiety, and motivation to avoid aversive stimuli) and under-control (high impulsivity, approach motivation, and reward responsivity) that cross eating disorder diagnostic boundaries, with the under-control group experiencing more severe bulimic symptoms and emotion dysregulation (Turner et al., 2014).

Temperament and neurobiological model of anorexia nervosa

Figure 19.1 depicts the updated temperament and neurobiological model of AN (Kaye et al., 2009). The model incorporates the findings that AN is a heritable illness with a strong genetic component (see Chapter 4) (Bulik, Blake, et al., 2019; Bulik et al., 2006; Hinney et al., 2017) with trait findings in AN. Accordingly, heritable risk is thought to be conferred through traits that increase susceptibility to developing AN, and also serve to maintain the illness. Traits are viewed as being expressed on a continuum ranging from destructive expression contributing to illness to productive expression contributing to health and recovery. As such, traits are conceptualized as stable but that can be modified by channeling their expression to eliminate symptoms without eliminating one's personality in the process

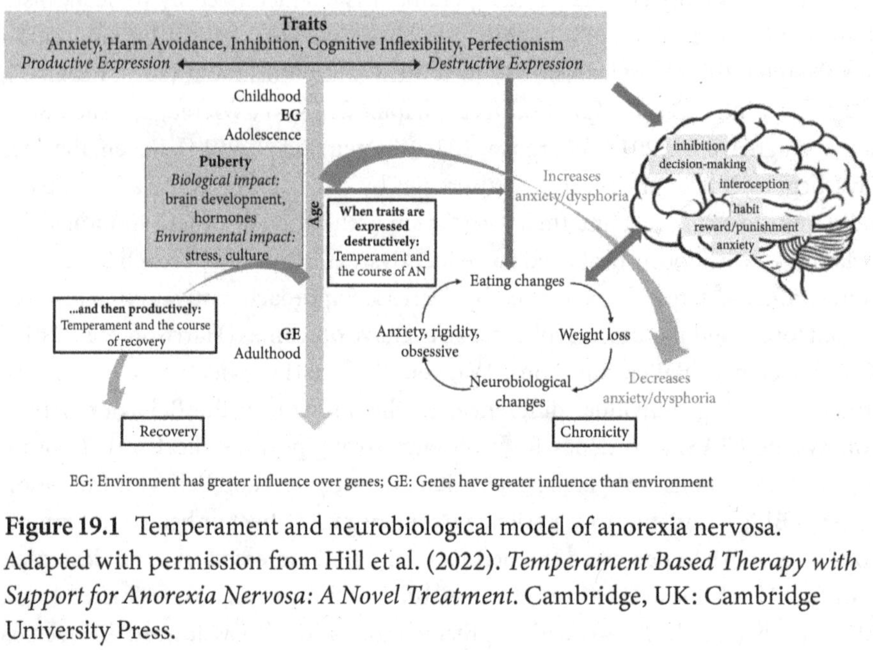

Figure 19.1 Temperament and neurobiological model of anorexia nervosa. Adapted with permission from Hill et al. (2022). *Temperament Based Therapy with Support for Anorexia Nervosa: A Novel Treatment.* Cambridge, UK: Cambridge University Press.

(e.g., instead of rigidly and perfectly adhering to a diet, the focus shifts to leveraging perfectionism to adhere to prescribed meal and recovery plan).

The model acknowledges the role of developmental, pubertal, environmental, and epigenetic factors in the development of AN (Bang et al., 2023; Bulik, 2005; Bulik, Blake, et al., 2019; Bulik, Flatt, et al., 2019; Klump, 2013; Watson et al., 2019) and the reinforcing cycle of dietary restriction and weight loss on emotion regulation (Lavender et al., 2015). In addition to the traditional traits implicated in AN, the model also integrates neuroscience research that has elucidated altered function in brain systems regulating food intake in AN (see Chapter 2 and Chapter 6). This includes altered anxiety (i.e., high harm avoidance, intolerance of uncertainty, worry about future consequences, obsessiveness), interoception (i.e., disturbed hunger and satiety signaling, altered body-state experience; see Chapter 6 and Chapter 8), reward and punishment sensitivity (which impacts motivation and learning; see Chapter 5), and decision-making and inhibitory control (i.e., cognitive inflexibility, ability to suppress impulses; see Chapter 10) (Cassin & von Ranson, 2005; Fassino, Piero, et al., 2004; Harrison et al., 2010; Kaye et al., 2004; Lilenfeld, 2011; Wagner et al., 2006). The model suggests that individuals with AN recover, in part, by developing constructive, rather than destructive, ways to use their temperament.

Temperament Based Therapy with Support

TBT-S is an emerging treatment for adults with AN that is designed to augment existing treatments. It is based on the premise that a mechanistic understanding of eating disorder behavior grounded in neurobiological and cognitive neuroscience research can inform treatment targets and interventions to improve outcome (Hill et al., 2016; Hill et al., 2022; Kaye et al., 2015). Approaching AN from a temperament-based neurobiological perspective provides a biological foundation and conceptual framework from which to view symptoms and the underlying mechanisms that drive behavior. Temperament informs targeted interventions directed at the cause of the behavior, rather than the behavior itself. By adopting a temperament-based neurobiological model of AN, the treatment emphasis shifts away from attempts to understand how behaviors developed and toward a focus on their functional impact to guide strategies to redirect trait expressions to achieve a reduction in eating disorder symptoms.

TBT-S treatment targets include common AN traits (e.g., anxiety, uncertainty intolerance, harm avoidance, cognitive inflexibility) and related cognitive functions such as altered reward and punishment sensitivity, interoception, inhibitory control, and decision-making. The focus of TBT-S is to work with adults who have AN and their support person(s) to acknowledge, understand, and use their own temperament as a primary source for strength and change. Support persons can include members of one's family of origin (e.g., parents, siblings, grandparents, adult children) and of one's "family" of choice (e.g., spouses, partners, friends, housemates, or colleagues). The TBT-S approach was developed and refined over a 10-year period, integrating AN research with ongoing patient and support person feedback to assure the intervention strategies accurately reflect patient experiences and traits.

Key principles of Temperament Based Therapy with Support

Treat to the trait. The TBT-S interventional approach focuses on development of compensatory strategies to manage common traits and associated cognitive-emotional processes to reduce eating disorder symptoms. It involves in vivo practice of new compensatory skills to facilitate learning and behavior change. In this way, TBT-S "treats to the trait," which means that treatment is personalized to align with the traits endorsed by each patient as the most instrumental in driving their maladaptive behavior and eating disorder symptoms. Treatment modules and activities are specifically designed to target destructive trait expressions and help patients realize how to leverage these traits in productive ways to achieve recovery goals. Table 19.1 provides an example of re-conceptualizing traits as strengths and corresponding treatment strategies that are used when treating to the trait.

Table 19.1 Traits as strengths and TBT-S treatment strategies

Trait	Trait as Strength (Productive expression)	TBT-S Treatment Strategy
Intolerance of uncertainty	Thrives with structure	• Increase predictability • Structure treatment • Structure meal plan • Establish explicit and consistent rules and response-sets
Anticipatory anxiety	Ability to plan and prepare	• Distraction techniques • Pre- & post-meal routine • Redirect attention
Harm avoidant	Cautious	• Implement negative contingencies to motivate their avoidance
Obsessiveness	Attention to detail	• Detail-oriented recovery plan

Trait	Trait as Strength (Productive expression)	TBT-S Treatment Strategy
Cognitive inflexibility, perseverations, set-shifting difficulties	Rule bound	• Re-direction • Prompting • Establish consistent rule-set for treatment and recovery
Perfectionism	Strives for excellence High error detection	• Set explicit, specific and concrete rules and recovery goals
Achievement-oriented	Driven for success	• Leverage treatment rules
Altered sensitivity to reward/punishment; altered intrinsic motivation (to recover)	Motivated by avoiding consequences, ability to focus on long-term goals	• Identify external reinforcers and consequences • Contingency management tailored to individual reward/punishment sensitivity
Poor interoceptive awareness (altered hunger/satiety)	Altered body-state experience	• Highly structured meal/snack schedule
Difficulty trusting decisions	Rely on external feedback	• Establish external structure and protocols
Inhibited	Ability to resist impulses and delay gratification	• Use long-term rewards and consequences via contingency management
Difficulty making decisions	Conscientious, striving for excellence	• Plan ahead • Provide two- or three-choice options (avoid open-ended choices)

Although not all the strategies used in TBT-S are novel, the rationale for their use is based on a neurobiological understanding of AN, which is taught to patients and support people to enhance buy-in to treatment. Examples of compensatory management strategies include developing (1) strategies to compensate for altered physiological signaling/interoception (e.g., structured and planned meals rather than relying on hunger/fullness signaling to guide eating); (2) techniques to enhance motivation given known alterations in motivation circuitry (e.g., psychoeducation framing AN as a biological illness to destigmatize and instill hope that change is possible, contingency management based on one's sensitivity to reward/punishment to individually tailor external incentives and compensate for lack of intrinsic motivation); and (3) methods to help reduce anxiety/inhibition and initiate eating (e.g., distraction, pre-meal routines). Support people are taught to modify the environment and establish predictable rules to reduce uncertainty, shifting reliance from internal to external cues to guide behavior, and helping patients practice new skills and routines.

Support persons are a necessary part of treatment for all ages. TBT-S adopts a developmentally tailored model of support to leverage parent/support person involvement in the management of AN. There is growing evidence that family involvement aids in recovery in adult AN (Bulik et al., 2012; Chen et al., 2016; Dimitropoulos et al., 2018; Tozzi et al., 2003). Parents and/or other support people play a critical role in the treatment of adults with AN by providing accountability, leverage, and emotional and instrumental assistance to manage AN. TBT-S is delivered in a multi-family format, where multiple patients and their families are treated simultaneously in a group format. The multi-family format is used to capitalize on lived experience expertise and create a support community, and to facilitate in vivo experiential activities and skill practice to enhance learning and recovery (Hill et al., 2022; Kaye et al., 2015; Knatz Peck et al., 2021; Knatz et al., 2015; Wierenga et al., 2018). Traditional multi-family therapy techniques and principles are used to increase engagement by fostering group affiliation and support networks, and later, inter-family communication and peer-to-peer consultation. This facilitates learning from one another via sharing, feedback, modeling, observation, and comradery, and it improves understanding of the illness as participants hear multiple perspectives that broaden viewpoints on effective ways to manage recovery.

An intensive format may improve learning through in vivo *massed practice.* TBT-S was initially developed and tested as a short-term, intensive treatment to be delivered in a five-day, 40-hour, multi-family format. The intensive format leverages aspects of traditional long-term intensive treatment programs that may contribute to behavior change, such as structure and monitored meal practice while allowing for in vivo massed practice and corrective feedback to maximize learning and improve and facilitate behavior change. This is in line with tenets of neuroplasticity based on Hebbian learning and the principle that "neurons that fire together wire together," or in other words, that repetition of behavior and skill acquisition builds stronger neural circuit pathways to rewire the brain (Kolb, 1995; Santucci et al., 2009; Storch et al., 2007; Whiteside & Jacobsen, 2010). Participants receive therapist-assisted practice of skills and strategies throughout the day. This intensive format is in keeping with evidence showing that early aggressive interventions can have beneficial effect on the course of AN (Eisler et al., 1997), that early weight gain is associated with better outcome (Doyle et al., 2010), and that a short-term, family-based treatment was as effective as a longer-term treatment (Lock & le Grange, 2005).

Temperament Based Therapy with Support intervention strategies

TBT-S uses five primary intervention strategies designed to reduce AN symptoms by "treating to the trait" (e.g., teaching compensatory management skills from a framework of neurobiology and aligned with temperament). A brief description of the TBT-S interventions follows. (For in-depth descriptions of these interventions and activities, see Hill et al., 2022).

Neurobiological psychoeducation. Didactic sessions educate patients and support people on relevant neurobiological constructs (anxiety, interoception, sensitivity to reward/punishment, altered inhibitory control, cognitive flexibility, and decision-making), traits (perfectionism, obsessionality, intolerance of uncertainty, harm avoidance), and associated symptom expression (dietary restriction, purging), and provide a framework and rationale for TBT-S intervention strategies. TBT-S psychoeducation frames AN as a malleable biological illness, which serves as an interventional strategy to increase hope, motivation to change and willingness to engage in treatment, to validate and reduce blame, and to increase insight and awareness to inform skill use and drive behavior change.

Experiential learning via activities addressing (1) AN neurobiology and traits, (2) problem solving and role of support person, and (3) multi-family therapy activities to improve family function. TBT-S is a treatment of doing, based on the notion that active behavior and practice enhance learning (Hebb, 1949). TBT-S addresses traits and neurobiology via simple games/activities that serve as metaphors of the AN experience to improve support person understanding of biological contributions to symptoms. The therapeutic aim is to reduce blame, mobilize appropriate support, and provide a rationale for TBT-S skills and management strategies. Activities also target communication and collaboration amongst families to support effective parent–patient working relationships (e.g., increase perceived support; decrease expressed emotion, enabling and accommodating). As mentioned, a stakeholder-engaged, iterative, systematic approach was used to collaboratively develop many of the experiential exercises and skills taught in TBT-S.

Skills training. Patients and support people receive training in effective management of AN symptoms individualized to traits self-identified as the most extreme or problematic. Patient coping skills focus on temperament-congruent management (vs. change) strategies targeting symptom reduction. Support people receive training on effective tools to assist the patient. In the version of TBT-S tailored to young adults, this includes parenting skills to achieve a balance between providing emotional support and accountability and reducing accommodation and expressed emotion.

Nutritional rehabilitation and meal support. Patients and support people are prescribed and learn a meal plan tailored to the patient's needs. TBT-S builds structure and routine around meals to compensate for altered interoception (e.g., altered hunger and/or satiety signaling that promotes food restriction or binge eating, altered trust in body-related signals), decision-making (e.g., difficulty deciding what foods to eat, tendency to choose lower calorie option), and reward sensitivity (e.g., reduced brain response for pleasure to motivate eating). TBT-S involves in-vivo meal practice with patients, support people, and therapists, who provide feedback and coaching as necessary to navigate barriers to dietary success and build mastery.

Behavioral agreement. Patients and their support people collaboratively develop a written Behavioral Agreement that establishes a mutually agreed upon framework for necessary action and contingencies that the patient has identified to achieve recovery. The behavioral agreement is a treatment strategy that facilitates consistency, clarity, and continuation of effective structure and behaviors practiced during treatment to the patient's home environment and outpatient treatment team. It is intended to appeal to the rule-bound, highly structured, and achievement-oriented nature of many individuals with AN and enhances engagement and motivation by using the oversight of the support people and response via contingency management tailored to the patient's sensitivity to rewards and consequences.

State of the evidence for Temperament Based Therapy with Support

Preliminary feasibility, acceptability, and efficacy have been examined in several open trials of TBT-S delivered in a five-day multi-family intensive format, including a multi-site trial for adults with longstanding AN (Wierenga et al., 2018), a single-site trial for young adults aged 18 to 27 (Knatz Peck et al., 2021), and a single-site trial for adults receiving outpatient treatment in Oslo, Norway (Stedal et al., 2023). Patients attended with at least one support person, and completed symptom assessments at pre-treatment, post-treatment, and variable follow-up lengths. Attrition was low across these trials (0–5.3%). Significant decreases in eating disorder psychopathology (global score on the Eating Disorder Examination Questionnaire) were observed in adults with longstanding AN atpost-treatment and six-month follow-up, in young adults with AN over 12 months, and in Norwegian adults with AN immediately after treatment. Decreases in psychosocial impairment at follow-up were also observed in young adults and in the Norwegian sample. Of the adult patients with longstanding AN who completed follow-up assessment, 62% met criteria for full or partial remission at six-month follow-up (Bardone-Cone et al., 2010). Similarly, 56% of the young adult participants were in full or partial remission at 12-month follow-up. Young adult patient adherence ratings of skill-use at 12-month follow-up ranged from 50% to 75% and parents of the young adults reported improved parental self-efficacy post-treatment (Peck et al., 2024).

Across these trials, patients and parents/support people rated TBT-S as highly acceptable with high ratings on items assessing increased motivation for recovery, understanding of the eating disorder through neurobiology exercises, feeling better equipped with tools to manage the eating disorder, confidence in ability to change, and commitment to using TBT-S skills. These early trials suggest TBT-S is a promising new treatment for AN with high acceptability. Open trials suggest a reduction in eating disorder symptoms and an increase in motivation.

Randomized controlled trials are needed to further assess treatment efficacy as well as to evaluate treatment delivery in different formats.

Alternative Perspectives

An interesting alternative perspective to consider is whether management versus change strategies are best indicated in effective treatment of AN. The National Institute for Mental Health focus on experimental therapeutics has prioritized target engagement, or the demonstration of sufficient change in an identified mechanism that is ultimately associated with change in clinical outcome. An advantage of this approach is that it places greater emphasis not only on identifying mechanisms of action of treatment to elucidate how effective treatments actually work, but it also appreciates the value of intervening on underlying mechanisms (e.g., reduced reward sensitivity) rather than observable behavior (e.g., dietary restriction). Among the target mechanisms that have gained recent attention in AN are those pertaining to the positive valence or reward system, the habit system, and cognitive flexibility, with growing evidence for the efficacy of behavioral interventions, such as positive affect treatment (Haynos et al., 2023), habit-reversal treatment approach (e.g., Relapse Prevention and Changing Habits for anorexia nervosa; see Chapter 18), and cognitive remediation therapy (Tchanturia et al., 2010). It is somewhat challenging to couch TBT-S within the experimental therapeutics framework; although its focus is on applying knowledge of underlying mechanisms driving maladaptive behavior to develop personalized skills, the goal is to compensate for these biologically based alterations rather than to change them (e.g., rather than increasing the neural reward response to food, instead establish external rewards and structure to facilitate meal completion). Teaching management skills does not preclude change; instead, management skills may foster behavior change that is necessary to elicit cognitive and neural circuit change. Qualitative data suggest TBT-S increases motivation to recover, but the change in motivational systems has not yet been evaluated. Precision medicine and idiographic treatment approaches are gaining attention in psychiatry, yet it remains to be determined which treatments may be most effective for which patients and at what timepoint during their course of illness (Insel, 2014). It is our opinion that given the heterogeneity of clinical expression, frequent chronicity of symptoms, and high relapse rates in AN, it is beneficial to develop a broad arsenal of effective treatments that work to both alter neurocognitive processes that maintain persistence of disordered eating that are potentially malleable and compensate for those processes that are not.

Another alternative perspective is that there are other important temperament features relevant to AN that are not targeted by TBT-S. TBT-S is not the definitive temperament-based treatment for AN. There are other promising temperament-informed treatments for AN. For instance, Radically

Open Dialectical Behavior Therapy (RO DBT) is a transdiagnostic treatment that aims to treat maladaptive over-control, defined as deficits in receptivity and openness, flexible-responding, emotional expression and awareness, and social connectedness and intimacy (Lynch et al., 2018). There is growing interest in the application of RO DBT to AN (Baudinet et al., 2020; Baudinet et al., 2021; Chen et al., 2015) because AN is often considered a prototypical disorder of maladaptive over-control. RO DBT posits social signaling deficits stemming from maladaptive over-control is the core issue in AN; restrictive and ritualized eating are conceptualized as symptoms or consequences stemming from rigid, maladaptive over-controlled coping. RO DBT prioritizes social signaling as the primary mechanism of change. RO DBT balances acceptance and change strategies to increase openness, flexibility, connectedness, and help clients obtain valued goals. While both TBT-S and RO DBT adhere to the notion that temperament contributes to symptom expression and illness maintenance, TBT-S addresses a wide range of traits to reduce eating disorder symptoms whereas RO-DBT is developed for "over-controlled" individuals and aims to improve social signaling.

Finally, as is the case with any treatment with multiple components, it can be challenging to identify the mechanism(s) of action. This concern applies to TBT-S when administered in the five-day, multi-family format, raising the possibility that although it is a neurobiologically informed approach, the neurobiological content and intervention strategies may not be the active component(s) of the treatment. Future work is needed to dismantle whether the intensive format, multi-family approach and/or the TBT-S content and intervention strategies are the active component(s). It is also possible that the conceptual framework of TBT-S is the agent of change. As mentioned, many of the strategies used in TBT-S were adopted from other evidence-based practices (e.g., dialectical behavior therapy, cognitive behavior therapy, exposure response prevention, parent management training) and it is their strategic combination and neurobiological rationale that distinguishes TBT-S from other approaches. Many existing treatments focus on changing observable behavior or cognitions—TBT-S targets the underlying neurobiologically mediated mechanisms driving the maladaptive behavior.

Implications

TBT-S includes a collection of interventional approaches designed to augment existing treatments for adults with AN. However, it is also a philosophy and conceptual framework that can be integrated into clinical practice at all levels of care. Viewing eating disorders from a neurobiological perspective can inform case conceptualization to identify key constructs and underlying mechanisms driving symptom expression and guide individually tailored and targeted treatment interventions. While TBT-S currently addresses temperament (e.g., anxiety, harm avoidance, intolerance of uncertainty, cognitive inflexibility) and altered cognitive function (e.g., sensitivity to reward and punishment, interoception, decision-making), both implicated in the maintenance of AN due to their involvement in the regulation of eating and emotion (Berner et al., 2018; Bischoff-Grethe et al., 2013; Bischoff-Grethe et al., 2018; DeGuzman et al., 2017; Foerde et al., 2015; Frank et al., 2018; Holsen et al., 2012; Kaye et al., 2020; Kerr et al., 2016; Oberndorfer et al., 2013; Strigo et al., 2013; Wagner et al., 2007; Wierenga et al., 2015), these targets will likely expand as the neurobiological understanding of AN continues to advance. Moreover, adopting the principle that family members and support people are integral in the recovery process can inform clinical decisions regarding the involvement of these individuals in treatment. Recognizing the value of innovative treatment formats, such as the multi-family format and intense delivery of treatment can inform efforts to optimize current treatments.

References

Abber, S. R., Murray, S. M., Brown, C. S., & Wierenga, C. E. (2024). Change in motivational bias during treatment predicts outcome in anorexia nervosa. *International Journal of Eating Disorders, 57*(3), 671–681. https://doi.org/10.1002/eat.24156

Allott, K., Van-der-El, K., Bryce, S., Parrish, E. M., McGurk, S. R., Hetrick, S., Bowie, C. R., Kidd, S., Hamilton, M., Killackey, E., & Velligan, D. (2020). Compensatory interventions for cognitive impairments in psychosis: A systematic review and meta-analysis. *Schizophrenia Bulletin, 46*(4), 869–883. https://doi.org/10.1093/schbul/sbz134

Anderluh, M. B., Tchanturia, K., Rabe-Hesketh, S., & Treasure, J. (2003). Childhood obsessive-compulsive personality traits in adult women with eating disorders: Defining a broader eating disorder phenotype. *American Journal of Psychiatry, 160*(2), 242–247. https://doi.org/10.1176/appi.ajp.160.2.242

Bailer, U., Frank, G., Price, J., Meltzer, C., Becker, C., Mathis, C., Wagner, A., Barbarich-Marsteller, N., Bloss, C., Putnam, K., Schork, N., Gamst, A., & Kaye, W. (2013). Interaction between serotonin transporter and dopamine D2/D3 receptor radioligand measures is associated with harm avoidant symptoms in anorexia and bulimia nervosa. *Psychiatry Research: Neuroimaging, 211*(2), 160–168. https://doi.org/10.1016/j.pscychresns.2012.06.010

Bailer, U., Narendran, R., Frankle, W., Himes, M., Duvvuri, V., Mathis, C., & Kaye, W. (2012). Amphetamine induced dopamine release increases anxiety in individuals recovered from anorexia nervosa. *International Journal of Eating Disorders, 45*(2), 263–271. https://doi.org/10.1002/eat.20937

Bang, L., Bahrami, S., Hindley, G., Smeland, O. B., Rodevand, L., Jaholkowski, P. P., Shadrin, A., Connell, K. S. O., Frei, O., Lin, A., Rahman, Z., Cheng, W., Parker, N., Fan, C. C., Dale, A. M., Djurovic, S., Bulik, C. M., & Andreassen, O. A. (2023). Genome-wide analysis of anorexia nervosa and major psychiatric disorders and related traits reveals genetic overlap and identifies novel risk loci for anorexia nervosa. *Translational Psychiatry, 13*(1), 291. https://doi.org/10.1038/s41398-023-02585-1

Bardone-Cone, A., Harney, M., Maldonado, C., Lawson, M., Robinson, D., Smith, R., & Tosh, A. (2010). Defining recovery from an eating disorder: Conceptualization, validation, and examination of psychosocial functioning and psychiatric comorbidity. *Behaviour Research and Therapy, 48*(3), 194–202. https://doi.org/10.1016/j.brat.2009.11.001

Bardone-Cone, A., Wonderlich, S., Frost, R., Bulik, C., Mitchell, J., Uppala, S., & Simonich, H. (2007). Perfectionism and eating disorders: Current status and future directions. *Clinical Psychology Review, 27*(3), 384–405.

Baudinet, J., Simic, M., Griffiths, H., Donnelly, C., Stewart, C., & Goddard, E. (2020). Targeting maladaptive overcontrol with radically open dialectical behaviour therapy in a day programme for adolescents with restrictive eating disorders: An uncontrolled case series. *Journal of Eating Disorders, 8*(1), 68. https://doi.org/10.1186/s40337-020-00338-9

Baudinet, J., Stewart, C., Bennett, E., Konstantellou, A., Parham, R., Smith, K., Hunt, K., Eisler, I., & Simic, M. (2021). Radically open dialectical behaviour therapy adapted for adolescents: A case series. *BMC Psychiatry, 21*(1), 462. https://doi.org/10.1186/s12888-021-03460-3

Berner, L., Simmons, A., Wierenga, C., Bischoff-Grethe, A., Paulus, M., Bailer, U., Ely, A., & Kaye, W. (2018). Altered interoceptive activation before, during, and after aversive breathing load in women remitted from anorexia nervosa. *Psychological Medicine, 48*(1), 142–154. https://doi.org/10.1017/S0033291717001635

Bijttebier, P., Beck, I., Claes, L., & Vandereycken, W. (2009). Gray's reinforcement sensitivity theory as a framework for research on personality-psychopathology associations. *Clinical Psychology Review, 29*(5), 421–430.

Bischoff-Grethe, A., McCurdy, D., Grenesko-Stevens, E., Irvine, L., Wagner, A., Yau, W.-Y., Fennema-Notestine, C., Fudge, J., Delgado, M., & Kaye, W. (2013). Altered brain response to reward and punishment in adolescents with anorexia nervosa. *Psychiatry Research, 214*(3), 331–340. https://doi.org/10.1016/j.pscychresns.2013.07.004

Bischoff-Grethe, A., Wierenga, C., Berner, L., Simmons, A., Bailer, U., Paulus, M., & Kaye, W. (2018). Neural hypersensitivity to pleasant touch in women remitted from anorexia nervosa. *Translational Psychiatry, 8*(1), 161. https://doi.org/10.1038/s41398-018-0218-3

Bloss, C., Berrettini, W., Bergen, A., Magistretti, P., Duvvuri, V., Strober, M., Brandt, H., Crawford, S., Crow, S., Fichter, M., Halmi, K., Johnson, C., Kaplan, A., Keel, P., Klump, K., Mitchell, J., Treasure, J., Woodside, D., Marzola, E., . . . Kaye, W. (2011). Genetic association of recovery from eating disorders: The role of GABA receptor SNPs. *Neuropsychopharmocology, 36*(11), 2222–2232. https://doi.org/10.1038/npp.2011.108

Brauer, L., & de Wit, H. (1996). Subjective responses to D-amphetamine alone and after pimozide pretreatment in normal, healthy volunteers. *Biological Psychiatry, 39*, 26–31.

Brookman-Frazee, L., Roesch, S., Chlebowski, C., Baker-Ericzen, M., & Ganger, W. (2019). Effectiveness of training therapists to deliver an individualized mental health intervention for children with ASD in publicly funded mental health services: A cluster randomized clinical trial. *JAMA Psychiatry, 76*(6), 574–583. https://doi.org/10.1001/jamapsychiatry.2019.0011

Bulik, C. (2005). Exploring the gene-environment nexus in eating disorders. *Journal of Psychiatry and Neuroscience, 30*(5), 335–339.

Bulik, C., Baucom, D., & Kirby, J. (2012). Treating anorexia nervosa in the couple context. *Journal of Cognitive Psychotherapy, 26*(1), 19–33. https://doi.org/10.1891%2F0889-8391.26.1.19

Bulik, C., Blake, L., & Austin, J. (2019). Genetics of eating disorders: What the clinician needs to know. *Psychiatric Clinics of North America, 42*(1), 59–73. https://doi.org/10.1016/j.psc.2018.10.007

Bulik, C., Flatt, R., Abbaspour, A., & Carroll, I. (2019). Reconceptualizing anorexia nervosa. *Psychiatry and Clinical Neurosciences, 73*(9), 518–525. https://doi.org/10.1111/pcn.12857

Bulik, C., Sullivan, P. F., Tozzi, F., Furberg, H., Lichtenstein, P., & Pedersen, N. L. (2006). Prevalence, heritability and prospective risk factors for anorexia nervosa. *Archives of General Psychiatry, 63*(3), 305–312. https://doi.org/10.1001/archpsyc.63.3.305

Carney, N., Chesnut, R. M., Maynard, H., Mann, N. C., Patterson, P., & Helfand, M. (1999). Effect of cognitive rehabilitation on outcomes for persons with traumatic brain injury: A systematic review. *Journal of Head Trauma Rehabilitation, 14*(3), 277–307. https://doi.org/10.1097/00001199-199906000-00008

Cassin, S., & von Ranson, K. (2005). Personality and eating disorders: A decade in review. *Clinical Psychology Review, 25*(7), 895–916. https://doi.org/10.1016/j.cpr.2005.04.012

Cheavens, J. S., Strunk, D. R., Lazarus, S. A., & Goldstein, L. A. (2012). The compensation and capitalization models: A test of two approaches to individualizing the treatment of depression. *Behaviour Research and Therapy, 50*(11), 699–706. https://doi.org/10.1016/j.brat.2012.08.002

Chen, E., Segal, K., Weissman, J., Zeffiro, T., Gallop, R., Linehan, M., Bohus, M., & Lynch, T. (2015). Adapting dialectical behavior therapy for outpatient adult anorexia nervosa—A pilot study. *International Journal of Eating Disorders, 48*(1), 23–132. https://doi.org/10.1002/eat.22360

Chen, E., Weissman, J., Zeffiro, G., Yiu, A., Eneva, K., Arlt, J., & Swantek, M. (2016). Family-based therapy for young adults with anorexia nervosa restores weight. *International Journal of Eating Disorders, 49*(7), 701–707. https://doi.org/10.1002/eat.22513

Claes, L., Nederkoorn, C., Vandereycken, W., Guerrieri, R., & Vertommen, H. (2006). Impulsiveness and lack of inhibitory control in eating disorders. *Eating Behaviors, 7*(3), 196–203. https://doi.org/10.1016/j.eatbeh.2006.05.001

Clark, L., & Watson, D. (1999). *Temperament: A new paradigm for trait psychology.* Guilford Press.

Clark, L. A. (2005). Temperament as a unifying basis for personality and psychopathology. *Journal of Abnormal Psychology, 114*(4), 505–521. https://doi.org/10.1037/0021-843X.114.4.505

Cloninger, C. R. (1994). Temperament and personality. *Current Opinion in Neurobiology, 4*(2), 266–273.

Cloninger, C. R. (2000). Biology of personality dimensions. *Current Opinion in Psychiatry, 13*(6), 611–616. https://doi.org/10.1097/00001504-200011000-00024

Cloninger, C. R., Przybeck, T. R., Svrakic, D. M., & Wetzel, R. D. (1994). *The temperament and character inventory (TCI): A guide to its development and use.* Center for Psychobiology of Personality, Washington University.

Cloninger, C. R., Svrakic, D. M., & Przybeck, T. R. (1993). A psychobiological model of temperament and character. *Archives of General Psychiatry, 50*(12), 975–990.

Cole, C. (2020). Infant temperament predicts personality more than 20 years later. NIH Record, May 15.

DeGuzman, M., Shott, M., Yang, T., Riederer, J., & Frank, G. (2017). Association of elevated reward prediction error response with weight gain in adolescent anorexia nervosa. *American Journal of Psychiatry, 174*(6), 557–565. https://doi.org/10.1176/appi.ajp.2016.16060671

Dellava, J., Thornton, L., Hamer, R., Strober, M., Plotnicov, K., Klump, K., Brandt, H., Crawford, S., Fichter, M., Halmi, K., Jones, I., Johnson, C., Kaplan, A., La Via, M., Mitchell, J., Rotondo, A., Treasure, J., Woodside, D., Berrettini, W., . . . Bulik, C. (2010). Childhood anxiety associated with low BMI in women with anorexia nervosa. *Behaviour Research and Therapy, 48*(1), 60–67. https://doi.org/10.1016/j.brat.2009.09.009

Dimitropoulos, G., Landers, A., Freeman, V., Novick, J., Garger, A., & Le Grange, D. (2018). Open trial of family-based treatment of anorexia nervosa for transition age youth. *Journal of the Canadian Academy of Child and Adolescent Psychiatry, 27*(1), 50–61.

Doyle, P., Le Grange, D., Loeb, K., Doyle, A., & Crosby, R. (2010). Early response to family-based treatment for adolescent anorexia nervosa. *International Journal of Eating Disorders, 43*(7), 659–662. https://doi.org/10.1002/eat.20764

Duckworth, A. L., Steen, T. A., & Seligman, M. E. (2005). Positive psychology in clinical practice. *Annual Review of Clinical Psychology, 1*, 629–651. https://doi.org/10.1146/annurev.clinpsy.1.102803.144154

Eagle, D., Wong, J., Allan, M., Mar, A., Theobald, D., & Robbins, T. (2011). Contrasting roles for dopamine D1 and D2 receptor subtypes in the dorsomedial striatum but not the nucleus accumbens core during behavioral inhibition in the stop-signal task in rats. *Journal of Neuroscience, 31*(20), 7349–7356. https://doi.org/10.1523/JNEUROSCI.6182-10.2011

Eisler, I., Dare, C., Russell, G. F., Szmukler, G., Le Grange, D., & Dodge, E. (1997). Family and individual therapy in anorexia nervosa. A 5-year follow-up. *Archives of Genernal Psychiatry, 54*, 1025–1030. https://doi.org/10.1001/archpsyc.1997.01830230063008

Eysenck, H. (1967). *The biological basis of personality.* Charles C. Thomas Pub.

Fassino, S., Amianto, F., Gramaglia, C., Facchini, F., & Abbate Daga, G. (2004). Temperament and character in eating disorders: ten years of studies. *Eating and Weight Disorders, 9*(2), 81–90. https://doi.org/10.1007/BF03325050

Fassino, S., Piero, A., Gramaglia, C., & Abbate-Daga, G. (2004). Clinical, psychopathological and personality correlates of interoceptive awareness in anorexia nervosa, bulimia nervosa and obesity. *Psychopathology, 37*(4), 168–174. https://doi.org/10.1159/000079420

Foerde, K., Steinglass, J., Shohamy, D., & Walsh, B. (2015). Neural mechanisms supporting maladaptive food choices in anorexia nervosa. *Nature Neuroscience, 18*(11), 1571–1573. https://doi.org/10.1038/nn.4136

Frank, G., DeGuzman, M., Shott, M., Laudenslager, M., Rossi, B., & Pryor, T. (2018). Association of brain reward learning response with harm avoidance, weight gain, and hypothalamic effective connectivity in adolescent anorexia nervosa. *JAMA Psychiatry, 75*(10), 1071–1080. https://doi.org/10.1001/jamapsychiatry.2018.2151

Frank, G., & Kaye, W. H. (2005). Positron emission tomography studies in eating disorders: Multireceptor brain imaging, correlates with behavior and implications for pharmacotherapy. *Nuclear Medicine and Biology, 32*(7), 755–761.

Frank, G., Roblek, T., Shott, M., Jappe, L., Rollin, M., Hagman, J., & Pryor, T. (2012). Heightened fear of uncertainty in anorexia and bulimia nervosa. *International Journal of Eating Disorders, 45*(2), 227–232. https://doi.org/10.1002/eat.20929

Gabbay, F. (2003). Variations in affect following amphetamine and placebo: Markers of stimulant drug preference. *Experimental and Clinical Psychopharmacology, 11*, 91–101.

Harrison, A., O'Brien, N., Lopez, C., & Treasure, J. (2010). Sensitivity to reward and punishment in eating disorders. *Psychiatry Research, 177*(1–2), 1–11. https://doi.org/10.1016/j.psychres.2009.06.010

Harrison, A., Treasure, J., & Smillie, L. (2011). Approach and avoidance motivation in eating disorders. *Psychiatry Research, 188*(3), 396–401. https://doi.org/10.1016/j.psychres.2011.04.022

Haynos, A. F., Anderson, L. M., Askew, A. J., Liu, C., Venables, K., Craske, M. G., & Peterson, C. B. (2023). A randomized, controlled pilot study of positive affect treatment adapted for anorexia nervosa. *International Journal of Eating Disorders*, 57(5), 1253–1259. https://doi.org/10.1002/eat.24071

Hebb, D. (1949). *The organization of behavior*. McGraw-Hill.

Hill, L., Peck, S., Wierenga, C., & Kaye, W. (2016). Applying neurobiology to the treatment of adults with anorexia nervosa. *Journal of Eating Disorders, 4*, 31. https://doi.org/10.1186/s40337-016-0119-x

Hill, L. L., Knatz Peck, S., & Wierenga, C. E. (2022). *Temperament based therapy with support for anorexia nervosa: A novel treatment*. Cambridge University Press.

Hinney, A., Kesselmeier, M., Jall, S., Volckmar, A., Focker, M., Antel, J., CGAN, WTCC3, Heid, I., Winkler, T., GIANT, Grant, S., Egger, H., Guo, Y., Bergen, A., Kaye, W., Berrettini, W., Hakonarson, H., Price Foundation Collaborative Group, . . . Hebebrand, J. (2017). Evidence for three genetic loci involved in both anorexia nervosa risk and variation of body mass index. *Molecular Psychiatry, 22*(2), 321–322. https://doi.org/10.1038/mp.2016.126

Holsen, L., Lawson, E., Blum, K., Ko, E., Makris, N., Fazeli, P., Klibanski, A., & Goldstein, J. (2012). Food motivation circuitry hypoactivation related to hedonic and nonhedonic aspects of hunger and satiety in women with active anorexia nervosa and weight-restored women with anorexia nervosa. *Journal of Psychiatry & Neuroscience, 37*(5), 322–332. https://doi.org/10.1503/jpn.110156

Hower, H., Reilly, E. E., Wierenga, C. E., & Kaye, W. H. (2021). Last word: A call to view temperamental traits as dual vulnerabilities and strengths in anorexia nervosa. *Eating Disorders, 29*(2), 151–160. https://doi.org/10.1080/10640266.2021.1883882

Insel, T. (2014). The NIMH research domain criteria (RDoC) project: Precision medicine for psychiatry. *American Journal of Psychiatry, 171*(4), 395–397. https://doi.org/10.1176/appi.ajp.2014.14020138

Jonker, N. C., Glashouwer, K. A., Hoekzema, A., Ostafin, B. D., & de Jong, P. J. (2020). Heightened self-reported punishment sensitivity, but no differential attention to cues signaling punishment or reward in anorexia nervosa. *PLOS ONE, 15*(3), e0229742.

Kaye, W., Bulik, C., Thornton, L., Barbarich, N., Masters, K., Fichter, M., Halmi, K., Kaplan, A., Strober, M., Woodside, D. B., Bergen, A., Crow, S., Mitchell, J., Rotondo, A., Mauri, M., Cassano, G., Keel, P. K., Plotnicov, K., Pollice, C., . . . Berrettini, W. H. (2004). Comorbidity of anxiety disorders with anorexia and bulimia nervosa. *American Journal of Psychiatry, 161*(12), 2215–2221. https://doi.org/10.1176/appi.ajp.161.12.2215

Kaye, W., Fudge, J., & Paulus, M. (2009). New insights into symptoms and neurocircuit function of anorexia nervosa. *Nature Reviews Neuroscience, 10*(8), 573–584. https://doi.org/10.1038/nrn2682

Kaye, W., Wierenga, C., Bailer, U., Simmons, A., & Bischoff-Grethe, A. (2013). Nothing tastes as good as skinny feels: The neurobiology of anorexia nervosa. *Trends in Neuroscience: Special Issue on Neural Control of Appetite, 36*(2), 110–120. https://doi.org/10.1016/j.tins.2013.01.003

Kaye, W., Wierenga, C., Bailer, U., Simmons, A., Wagner, A., & Bischoff-Grethe, A. (2013). Does a shared neurobiology for foods and drugs of abuse contribute to extremes of food ingestion in anorexia and bulimia nervosa? *Biological Psychiatry, 73*(9), 836–842. https://doi.org/10.1016/j.biopsych.2013.01.002

Kaye, W., Wierenga, C., Bischoff-Grethe, A., Berner, L., Ely, A., Bailer, U., Paulus, M., & Fudge, J. (2020). Neural insensitivity to the effects of hunger in women remitted from anorexia nervosa. *American Journal of Psychiatry, 177*(7), 601–610. https://doi.org/10.1176/appi.ajp.2019.19030261

Kaye, W., Wierenga, C., Knatz, S., Liang, J., Boutelle, K., Hill, L., & Eisler, I. (2015). Temperament-based treatment for anorexia nervosa. *European Eating Disorders Review, 23*(1), 12–18. https://doi.org/10.1002/erv.2330

Kerr, K., Moseman, S., Avery, J., Bodurka, J., Zucker, N., & Kyle Simmons, W. (2016). Altered insula activity during visceral interoception in weight-restored patients with anorexia nervosa *Neuropsychopharmacology*, *41*(2), 521–528. https://doi.org/10.1038/npp.2015.174

Klump, K. (2013). Puberty as a critical risk period for eating disorders: a review of human and animal studies. *Hormones and Behavior*, *64*(2), 399–410. https://doi.org/10.1016/j.yhbeh.2013.02.019

Klump, K., Burt, S., McGue, M., & Iacono, W. (2007). Changes in genetic and environmental influences on disordered eating across adolescence. A longitudinal twin study. *Archives of General Psychiatry*, *64*(12), 1409–1415.

Klump, K., Strober, M., Johnson, C., Thornton, L., Bulik, C., Devlin, B., Fichter, M., Halmi, K., Kaplan, A., Woodside, D. B., Crow, S., Mitchell, J., Rotondo, A., Keel, P., Berrettini, W. H., Plotnicov, K., Pollice, C., Lilenfeld, L. R., & Kaye, W. (2004). Personality characteristics of women before and after recovery from an eating disorder. *Psychological Medicine*, *34*(8), 1407–1418. https://doi.org/10.1017/s0033291704002442

Knatz Peck, S., Towne, T., Wierenga, C., Hill, L., Eisler, I., Brown, T., E, H., Miller, M., Perry, T., & Kaye, W. (2021). Temperament-based treatment for young adults with eating disorders: Acceptability and initial efficacy of an intensive, multi-family, parent-involved treatment. *Journal of Eating Disorders*, *9*(1), 110. https://doi.org/10.21203/rs.3.rs-529512/v1

Knatz, S., Wierenga, C., Murray, S., Hill, L., & Kaye, W. (2015). Neurobiologically-informed treatment for adults with anorexia nervosa: A novel approach to a chronic disorder. *Dialogues in Clinical Neuroscience*, *17*(2), 229–236. https://doi.org/10.31887/DCNS.2015.17.2/sknatz

Kolb, B. (1995). *Brain plasticity and recovery of function in adulthood.* Lawrence Erlbaum Associates.

Lavender, J., S, W., Engel, S., Gordon, K., Kaye, W., & Mitchell, J. (2015). Dimensions of emotion dysregulation in anorexia nervosa and bulimia nervosa: A conceptual review of the empirical literature. *Clinical Psychology Review 40*, 111–122. https://doi.org/10.1016/j.cpr.2015.05.010

Lilenfeld, L. (2011). Personality and temperament. *Current Topics in Behavioral Neurosciences*, *6*, 3–9. https://doi.org/10.1007/7854_2010_86

Lilenfeld, L., Wonderlich, S., Riso, L. P., Crosby, R., & Mitchell, J. (2006). Eating disorders and personality: A methodological and empirical review. *Clinical Psychology Review*, *26*(3), 299–320. https://doi.org/10.1016/j.cpr.2005.10.003

Lock, J., & le Grange, D. (2005). Family-based treatment of eating disorders. *International Journal of Eating Disorders*, *37*, S64–S67. https://doi.org/10.1002/eat.20122

Lynch, T. R., Hempel, R. J., Whalley, B., Byford, S., Chamba, R., Clarke, P., Clarke, S., Kingdon, D., O'Mahen, H., Remington, B., Rushbrook, S. C., Shearer, J., Stanton, M., Swales, M., Watkins, A., & Russell, I. T. (2018). Radically open dialectical behaviour therapy for refractory depression: the RefraMED RCT. *NIHR Journals Library*. https://doi.org/10.3310/eme05070

McClowry, S. G., Rodriguez, E. T., & Koslowitz, R. (2008). Temperament-based intervention: Re-examining goodness of fit. *European Journal of Developmental Science*, *2*(1–2), 120–135. https://www.ncbi.nlm.nih.gov/pubmed/20354571

McGurk, S., Twamley, E., Sitzer, D., McHugo, G., & Mueser, K. (2007). A meta-analysis of cognitive remediation in schizophrenia. *American Journal of Psychiatry*, *164*(12), 1791–1802. https://doi.org/10.1176/appi.ajp.2007.07060906

Mervilde, I., & De Pauw, S. (2012). Models of child temperament. In M. Zentner and R. Shiner (Eds.), *Handbook of temperament.* 21–40. New York: Guilford Press.

Mitchell, K. (2018). *Innate.* Princeton University Press.

Oberndorfer, T., Frank, G., Fudge, J., Simmons, A., Paulus, M., Wagner, A., Yang, T., & Kaye, W. (2013). Altered insula response to sweet taste processing after recovery from anorexia and bulimia nervosa. *American Journal of Psychiatry*, *214*(2), 132–141. https://doi.org/10.1176/appi.ajp.2013.11111745

Oberndorfer, T., Simmons, A., McCurdy, D., Strigo, I., Matthews, S., Yang, T., Irvine, Z., & Kaye, W. (2013). Greater anterior insula activation during anticipation of food images in women recovered from anorexia nervosa versus controls. *Psychiatry Research*, *214*(2), 132–141. https://doi.org/10.1016/j.pscychresns.2013.06.010

Ormel, J., Oldehinkel, A. J., Ferdinand, R. F., Hartman, C. A., De Winter, A. F., Veenstra, R., Vollebergh, W., Minderaa, R. B., Buitelaar, J. K., & Verhulst, F. C. (2005). Internalizing and externalizing problems in adolescence: General and dimension-specific effects of familial loadings and preadolescent temperament traits. *Psychological Medicine*, *35*(12), 1825–1835. https://doi.org/10.1017/S0033291705005829

Peck, S. K., Towne, T., Wierenga, C., Perry, T., Miller, M., Kim, J., & Kaye, W. (2024). Parental perceptions of participation in young adult-focused eating disorder treatment. *European Eating Disorders Review*. Advance online publication. https://doi.org/10.1002/erv.3084

Rothbart, M. (2012). Advances in temperament, history, concepts and measures. In M. Zentner and R. Shiner (Eds.), *Handbook of temperament* (p. 3). Guilford Publications.

Santucci, L., Ehrenreich, J., Trosper, S., Bennett, S., & Pincus, D. (2009). Development and preliminary evaluation of a one-week summer treatment program for separation anxiety disorder. *Cognitive and Behavioral Practice, 16*, 317–331. https://doi.org/10.1016/j.cbpra.2008.12.005

Schmidt, U., & Campbell, I. (2013). Treatment of eating disorders can not remain "brainless": The case for brain-directed treatments *European Eating Disorders Review, 21*(6), 425–427. https://doi.org/10.1002/erv.2257

Simon, N., Montgomery, K., Beas, B., Mitchell, M., LaSarge, C., Mendez, I., Banuelos, C., Vokes, C., Taylor, A., Haberman, R., Bizon, J., & Setlow, B. (2011). Dopaminergic modulation of risky decision-making. *Journal of Neuroscience, 31*(48), 17460–17470. https://doi.org/10.1523/JNEUROSCI.3772-11.2011

Sitzer, D. I., Twamley, E. W., & Jeste, D. V. (2006). Cognitive training in Alzheimer's disease: A meta-analysis of the literature. Acta Psychiatrica Scandinavica, *114*(2), 75–90. https://doi.org/10.1111/j.1600-0447.2006.00789.x

Stedal, K., Funderud, I., Wierenga, C. E., Knatz-Peck, S., & Hill, L. (2023). Acceptability, feasibility and short-term outcomes of temperament based therapy with support (TBT-S): A novel 5-day treatment for eating disorders. *Journal of Eating Disorders, 11*(1), 156. https://doi.org/10.1186/s40337-023-00878-w

Steiger, H., & Booij, L. (2020). Eating disorders, heredity and environmental activation: Getting epigenetic concepts into practice. *Journal of Clinical Medicine, 9*(5), E1332. https://doi.org/10.3390/jcm9051332

Steinberg, L. (2005). Cognitive and affective development in adolescence. *Trends in Cognitive Sciences, 9*(2), 69–74. https://doi.org/10.1016/j.tics.2004.12.005

Steinglass, J., Sysko, R., Mayer, L., Berner, L., Schebendach, J., Wang, Y., Chen, H., Albano, A., Simpson, H., & Walsh, B. (2010). Pre-meal anxiety and food intake in anorexia nervosa. *Appetite, 55*(2), 214–218. https://doi.org/10.1016/j.appet.2010.05.090

Storch, E., Geffken, G., Merlo, L., Mann, G., Duke, D., Munson, M., Adkins, J., Grabill, K., Murphy, T., & Goodman, W. (2007). Family-based cognitive-behavioral therapy for pediatric obsessive-compulsive disorder: Comparison of intensive and weekly appraoches. *Journal of the American Academy of Child and Adolescent Psychiatry, 26*, 469–478. https://doi.org/10.1097/chi.0b013e31803062e7

Strigo, I., Matthews, S., Simmons, A., Oberndorfer, T., Reinhardt, L., Klabunde, M., & Kaye, W. (2013). Altered insula activation during pain anticipation in individuals recovered from anorexia nervosa: evidence of interocetive dysregulation. *International Journal of Eating Disorders, 46*, 23–33. https://doi.org/10.1002/eat.22045

Tchanturia, K., Davies, H., Reeder, C., & Wykes, T. (2010). Cognitive remediation therapy for anorexia nervosa. https://img3.reoveme.com/m/243251c42ccb2de4.pdf

Touyz, S., Bryant, E., Dann, K. M., Polivy, J., Le Grange, D., Hay, P., Lacey, H., Aouad, P., Barakat, S., Miskovic-Wheatley, J., Griffiths, K., Carroll, B., Calvert, S., & Maguire, S. (2023). What kind of illness is anorexia nervosa? Revisited: Some preliminary thoughts to finding a cure. *Journal of Eating Disorders, 11*(1), 221. https://doi.org/10.1186/s40337-023-00944-3

Tozzi, F., Sullivan, P., Fear, J., McKenzie, J., & Bulik, C. (2003). Causes and recovery in anorexia nervosa: The patient's perspective. *International Journal of Eating Disorders, 33*(2), 143–154. https://doi.org/10.1002/eat.10120

Turner, B., Claes, L., Wilderjans, T., Pauwels, E., Dierckx, E., Chapman, A., & Schoevaerts, K. (2014). Personality profiles in eating disorders: Further evidence of the clinical utility of examining subtypes based on temperament *Psychiatry Research, 219*(1), 157–165. https://doi.org/10.1016/j.psychres.2014.04.036

Twamley, E. W., Vella, L., Burton, C. Z., Heaton, R. K., & Jeste, D. V. (2012). Compensatory cognitive training for psychosis: Effects in a randomized controlled trial. *Journal of Clinical Psychiatry, 73*(9), 1212–1219. https://doi.org/10.4088/JCP.12m07686

Vukasovic, T., & Bratko, D. (2015). Heritability of personality: A meta-analysis of behavior genetic studies. *Psychological Bulletin, 141*(4), 769–785. https://doi.org/10.1037/bul0000017

Wagner, A., Aizenstein, H., Venkatraman, M., Fudge, J., May, J., Mazurkewicz, L., Frank, G., Bailer, U. F., Fischer, L., Nguyen, V., Carter, C., Putnam, K., & Kaye, W. H. (2007). Altered reward processing in women recovered from anorexia nervosa. *American Journal of Psychiatry, 164*(12), 1842–1849. https://doi.org/10.1176/appi.ajp.2007.07040575

Wagner, A., Barbarich, N., Frank, G., Bailer, U., Weissfeld, L., Henry, S., Achenbach, S., Vogel, V., Plotnicov, K., McConaha, C., Kaye, W., & Wonderlich, S. (2006). Personality traits after recovery from eating disorders: Do subtypes differ? *International Journal of Eating Disorders, 39*(4), 276–284. https://doi.org/10.1002/eat.20251

Watson, H. J., Yilmaz, Z., Thornton, L. M., Hubel, C., Coleman, J. R. I., Gaspar, H. A., Bryois, J., Hinney, A., Leppa, V. M., Mattheisen, M., Medland, S. E., Ripke, S., Yao, S., Giusti-Rodriguez, P., Anorexia Nervosa Genetics, I., Hanscombe, K. B., Purves, K. L., Eating Disorders Working Group of the Psychiatric Genomics, C., Adan, R. A. H., . . . Bulik, C. M. (2019). Genome-wide association study identifies eight risk loci and implicates metabo-psychiatric origins for anorexia nervosa. *Nature Genetics, 51*(8), 1207–1214. https://doi.org/10.1038/s41588-019-0439-2

Whiteside, S., & Jacobsen, A. (2010). An uncontrolled examination of a 5-day intensive treatment for pediatric OCD. *Behavior Therapy, 41*, 414–422. https://doi.org/10.1016/j.beth.2009.11.003

Whittle, S., Allen, N., Lubman, D., & Yucel, M. (2006). The neurobiological basis of temperament: Towards a better understanding of psychopathology. *Neuroscience & Biobehavioral Reviews, 30*(4), 511–525. https://doi.org/10.1016/j.neubiorev.2005.09.003

Wierenga, C. (2023). Eating disorders. In G. G. Brown, T. Z. King, K. Y. Haaland, & B. Crosson (Eds.), *APA handbook of neuropsychology*. American Psychological Association.

Wierenga, C., Bischoff-Grethe, A., Melrose, A., Irvine, Z., Torres, L., Bailer, U., Simmons, A., Fudge, J., McClure, S., Ely, A., & Kaye, W. (2015). Hunger does not motivate reward in women remitted from anorexia nervosa. *Biological Psychiatry, 77*(7), 642–652. https://doi.org/10.1016/j.biopsych.2014.09.024

Wierenga, C., Ely, A., Bischoff-Grethe, A., Bailer, U., Simmons, A., & Kaye, W. (2014). Are extremes of consumption in eating disorders related to an altered balance between reward and inhibition? *Frontiers in Behavioral Neuroscience, 9*(8), 410. https://doi.org/10.3389/fnbeh.2014.00410

Wierenga, C., L, H., Knatz Peck, S., McCray, J., Greathouse, L., Peterson, D., Scott, A., Eisler, I., & WH, K. (2018). The acceptability, feasibility, and possible benefits of a neurobiologically-informed 5-day multifamily treatment for adults with anorexia nervosa. *International Journal of Eating Disorders, 51*(8), 863–869. https://doi.org/10.1002/eat.22876

Zhang, W., & Perivoliotis, D. (2022). Promoting recovery among persons with schizophrenia using recovery-oriented cognitive therapy (CT-R). *Schizophrenia Research, 250*, 125–126. https://doi.org/10.1016/j.schres.2022.11.014

20

Interoceptive Exposure

Developing Capacities to Discriminate and Adaptively Respond to Visceral Signals

Nancy Zucker

Brief Definitional Overview

Interoception: A fundamental process whereby an individual learns to map the moment-to-moment state of their body.

Interoceptive responsivity: Refers to how an individual responds to interoceptive signals, which can be adaptive or maladaptive.

Visceral hypersensitivity: An individual difference whereby a person has a lower threshold for noticing changes in their body.

Interoceptive exposure: A therapeutic technique designed to augment prior learning histories such that an individual's response to their body not only does not impair functioning but also helps them to flourish.

Fear generalization: A learning process whereby one's fear of a given stimulus, given prior direct or indirect experience, extends to stimuli that are similar to, associated with, or predictive of, the initial feared stimulus.

Introduction

> "The conditions favorable to proper digestion are wholly abolished when unpleasant feelings such as vexation and worry and anxiety, or great emotions such as anger and fear, are allowed to prevail."
>
> —Walter Cannon (1925), *Bodily Changes in Pain, Hunger, Fear, and Rage*

Consider this scenario. A new parent is faced with a distressed infant. (We use the term "parent" as a blanket term to encompass any individual who is responsible for the care of a child.) The parent engages in a back-and-forth exchange with the infant—a sequence of trial and error learning as the parent tries to decipher what the infant is communicating, attempts to respond to that perceived need, and

Nancy Zucker, *Interoceptive Exposure*. In: *The Handbook of the Neurobiology of Eating Disorders*. Edited by: Christina E. Wierenga and Joanna E. Steinglass, Oxford University Press. © Oxford University Press (2025).
DOI: 10.1093/9780197675212.003.0021

then evaluates whether that response was effective in satisfying the child's need and/or ameliorating the child's distress. With practice, the parent–infant interaction system becomes increasingly precise and efficient: the parent can decipher what the child is communicating and responds adeptly to those signals. The parent learns to discriminate signals of hunger from signals of fatigue and from the need to snuggle. As a result, several important experiences presumably happen for the infant. According to tenets of attachment theory (Ainsworth et al., 2015), when an infant's needs are reliably responded to by a given parent, the infant comes to trust that parent and to develop a secure attachment—an experience of interpersonal safety that provides a secure base from which the child can turn to get their needs met. The infant also learns that they exist: that they exert influence on their environment. The environment responds when they communicate a need. This felt sense of safety, in turn, gives the child the courage to explore new things and engage in adventures as they trust they will be cared for if something unwanted or unexpected happens. The child is set up to have the courage to explore their world.

As children age, they must master these tasks themselves. They need to learn to tune into their bodies, notice different visceral sensations, discriminate what those sensations might be communicating—fear, hunger, fatigue, and so on—and learn how to adaptively respond to those signals. This process of tuning in to internal organs of the body and perceiving the signals that the body is communicating is referred to as interoception. Interoception refers to the "process by which the nervous system senses, interprets, and integrates signals originating from within the body, providing a moment-by-moment mapping of the body's internal landscape across conscious and unconscious levels" (Khalsa et al., 2018). Interoceptive responsivity refers to the process of adaptively responding to interoceptive signals (Oswald et al., 2017). Just like the parent–child scenario, over time the child would get better at deciphering their body signals and responding adeptly to these signals. As a result, several important outcomes may occur. Children and adolescents would learn to know themselves (e.g., what they like or dislike, how much sleep they need) and trust themselves—they learn to "self-parent." And because they know they can take care of themselves even if unwanted or uncertain things occur, they develop the courage to explore the world—to take reasonable risks and to try new things.

Capacities to sense, discriminate, and/or respond to the body have been shown to be disrupted across eating disorder diagnoses (Datta et al., 2021; Khalsa et al., 2015), and one could argue that such disruptions are pivotal to understanding the phenomenology of disorders such as anorexia nervosa (AN), avoidant/restrictive food intake disorder (ARFID), bulimia nervosa (BN), and binge-eating disorder (BED). This chapter does not attempt to explain how interoception or interoceptive responsivity became disrupted in those with eating disorders (see Chapter 8). Rather, the main thrust of this chapter is on considerations when treating disruptions in interoception and interoceptive responsivity with the ultimate goal of helping individuals with eating disorders to learn to trust their bodies. This chapter focuses on the techniques and principles underlying the use of interoceptive exposure, a behavioral intervention that is intended to reduce anxiety and distress regarding physical sensations (Boettcher et al., 2016).

Biological Framework

Discriminating and responding to interoceptive signals

How does fear of the body emerge? An individual's learning history may offer clues as to how fear and distrust of internal bodily sensations may develop. Consider this example. An infant has frequent and severe gastroesophageal reflux disease (GERD) that is misdiagnosed and misconstrued as the "typical" spitting up of babies. Eventually, the infant is properly diagnosed and treated. Yet, the infant continues to have problems with feeding and is very resistant around mealtimes. This may be an example of classic Pavlovian conditioning (Pavlov, 1957): food, eating, and mealtimes become conditioned aversive stimuli due to their frequent past associations with pain (the unconditioned stimulus). Eating occasions become triggers for fear-based avoidance.

This example is apropos because gastrointestinal issues are highly prevalent in individuals with eating disorders (Hetterich et al., 2019; Salvioli et al., 2013). Gastrointestinal symptoms and disorders are proposed to be both a vulnerability for eating disorder emergence (Stein et al., 2021; van Tilburg et al., 2014) and may be exacerbated by disordered eating behaviors (Hetterich et al., 2019). The visceral sensations of eating and digesting foods, sensations that may resemble the aversive symptoms of disorders of gut–brain interaction, may become cues for fear-based avoidance of food quantity and variety. However, not every individual with an eating disorder will develop a disorder of gut–brain interaction and vice versa.

One individual difference that may be important in understanding vulnerable somatic experiences of those with eating disorders is that of visceral hypersensitivity (Simren et al., 2017). This is an individual difference whereby a person has a lower threshold for noticing changes in their viscera. Visceral hypersensitivity has been associated with and predictive of more intense pain experiences (Simren et al., 2017). If individuals are more sensitive to changes in their bodies, they may allocate more attention to these changes. Amplified attention toward the body that occurs through a fear-based lens (e.g., fearful of future gastrointestinal discomfort or pain) may interact to create setting conditions whereby individuals are hypervigilant to sensations of their body and interpret even innocuous sensations as predictive of future threat (Figure 20.1). Thus, early gastrointestinal distress and visceral hypersensitivity may interact resulting in fear-based hypervigilance to

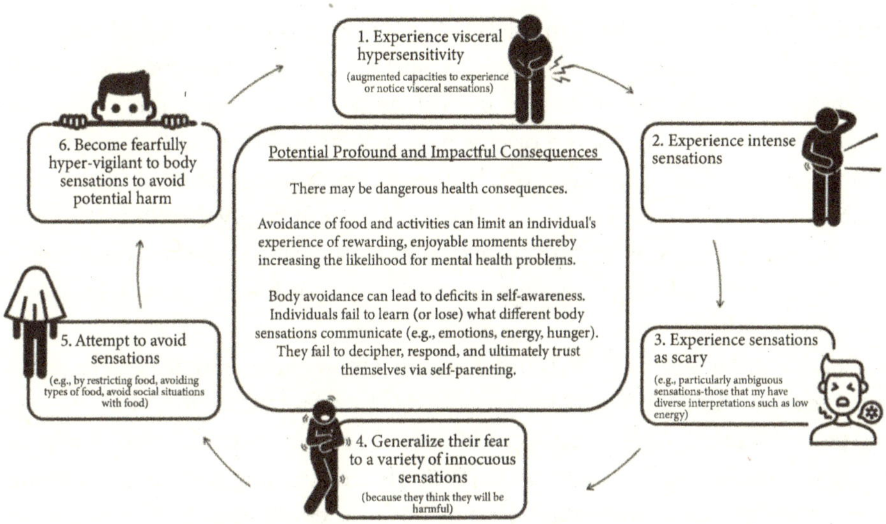

Figure 20.1 A model of the emergence of somatic fear in the presence of visceral hypersensitivity. Given that visceral sensations communicate needs that often require behavioral responses, attempts to avoid or suppress visceral sensations may disrupt the emergence of adaptive self-awareness or "self-parenting."

potential somatic threat which may intensify the experience of visceral sensations as aversive.

Fear generalizes (LaBar & Phelps, 2005). It is adaptive that fear experienced in response to a threatening object or circumstance generalizes to similar objects or circumstances. An individual should not have to directly experience that a novel stimulus is threatening if it shares the threatening properties of a scary object. As an example, if an individual has an allergic reaction to peanut butter served in a peanut butter and jelly sandwich at their school, they should also be cautious around peanut butter in whatever context it appears, however it is prepared, and whatever brand it is. The individual does not have to taste each different brand of peanut butter to determine that they will have an allergic reaction. They might also be cautious around other nuts until they determine the boundaries of their allergy. This is an example of adaptive fear generalization.

Fear generalization becomes maladaptive when situations or objects are avoided that have a very low probability of threat. Continuing with the example, if that individual subsequently avoids all carbohydrates and all jellies because their peanut butter was served on bread with jelly that would be an example of maladaptive fear generalization. This fear generalization may be compounded by our brain's prioritization of threatening information relative to safety signaling. LeDoux describes a fast (low road) and slow (high road) of processing potentially threatening or salient stimuli by different brain regions (LeDoux, 1996). The fast road (or subcortical route) is proposed to process crude features (think shadows and contours—not the detailed features of the high road) (Méndez-Bértolo et al., 2016). This system alerts you that something potentially important or dangerous may be unfolding before you can correctly identify just quite what is going on. This is an adaptive system that alerts and orients us to potential threats so that responsive actions are mobilized quickly, even before we are aware of what is happening. Problems can arise however, when individuals have difficulty discriminating safe stimuli from dangerous stimuli. Consider the application of this reasoning to another disorder in which individuals have a fear of bodily sensations—panic disorder.

Panic disorder is an anxiety disorder in which individuals exhibit a fear response to a variety of innocuous somatic sensations as they fear these sensations may signal potential harm. A panic attack is an acute fear reaction constituted of intense visceral sensations such as tachycardia, that, while distressing, are physically harmless. Notwithstanding, individuals with panic disorder may fear the potential harm of a panic attack and thus become hypervigilant to visceral sensations that they think may predict the onset of an emerging attack. In other words, they may exhibit startle or related fear responses to innocuous body sensations for fear these sensations predict harm. A maladaptive cycle emerges: a fear response to innocuous sensations is itself constituted of intensified visceral sensations—such as sweating or a pounding heart—which brings on many of the sensations the person was trying to avoid, though they are also harmless. In an attempt to avoid a future panic attack, individuals with panic disorder are often on the alert for various body sensations that they think are warning signals for a future attack (such as their heart beating faster). They also start avoiding activities (e.g., like exercise) that provoke the sensations that they think may cause a potential attack. The end result is that this generalized fear response to safe somatic signals contributes to impairment in functioning: a greatly restricted repertoire of life activities as a way to manage this increasingly pervasive fear of the body.

The theoretical basis for interoceptive exposures

Applying this model and logic to individuals with eating disorders reveals a broad array of interoceptive sensations that may provoke negative emotions such as guilt, fear, self-disgust, or despair in individuals with eating disorders. These interoceptive sensations may also serve as conditioned stimuli that provoke disordered eating behaviors (Figure 20.2). The acts of eating and digesting food are interoceptive experiences. For example, an individual with an eating disorder may sense fullness in their gut while eating and the initial stretch of mechanoreceptors as their gut fills. Such cues may adaptively trigger meal termination. However, someone struggling with an eating disorder may interpret these cues as threatening—a sign that they have overeaten—which may trigger a binge eating episode (an example of an abstinence violation effect because according to their own rigid dietary rules,

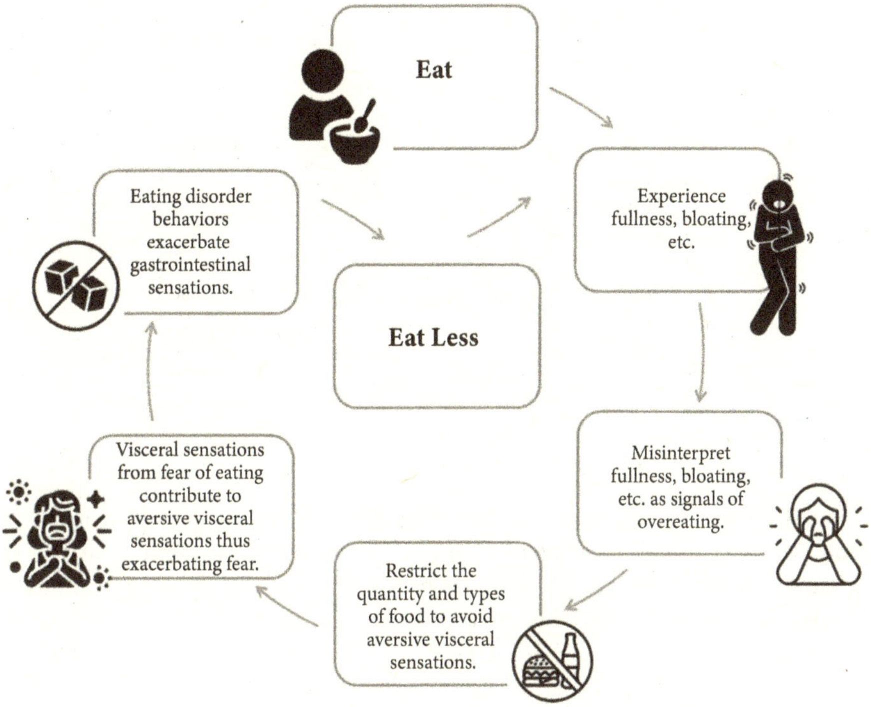

Figure 20.2 Interoceptively conditioned food restriction and avoidance.

feeling full cues guilty feelings and subsequent additional eating) (Grilo & Shiffman, 1994). Now the sensation of fullness is a threatening stimulus because it has been a trigger for a binge eating episode (Figure 20.2). Consequently, the individual tries to restrict the quantity of food at an eating episode to avoid the sensation of fullness. Imagine that they succeed in doing this over time, resulting in severe weight loss. Such disordered eating behaviors, weight loss, and the physical health consequences of these behaviors can paradoxically exacerbate the intensity of interoceptive signaling. Extreme food restriction and weight loss can disrupt digestive functioning such as delayed gastric emptying and bloating—making the act of eating and digesting food an increasingly aversive task. Disordered eating behaviors can exacerbate gastrointestinal symptoms, such as constipation, heartburn, and bloating (Zucker & Bulik, 2020). Feelings of fullness are more easily experienced and trigger further restriction (Figure 20.2).

Strong emotions can further impede digestion, which strengthens this vicious cycle: individuals who have a fear of food, eating, or the consequences of eating may experience physiological changes related to fear (e.g., decreased salivary output, decreased gastric secretions, reduced gastric motility) that can contribute to make the visceral sensations that accompany eating more aversive, further impeding abilities to approach and consume optimal food volume and variety (Cannon, 1925). Focusing on minimizing the harm of interoceptive sensations

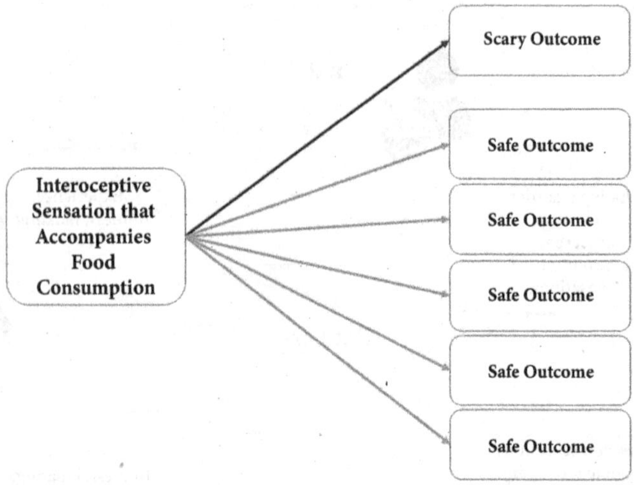

Figure 20.3 A symbolic depiction of inhibitory learning. An interoceptive sensation becomes feared because it may predict a future aversive consequence. Repeated experiences of that stimulus with safe outcomes provide competing interpretations of that sensation as threatening.

as depicted in this diagram may provide a very powerful intervention strategy (Figure 20.2).

Interoceptive exposure as an intervention strategy

Interoceptive exposure exercises are therapeutic strategies designed to break this cycle of behavioral avoidance and ultimately to reduce negative emotional reactions to somatic sensations. Interoceptive exposure activities are designed to intentionally evoke sensations that are feared and to create new associations with that sensation and a new outcome—one different from the feared outcome. The result is that a given stimulus (a previously feared interoceptive sensation) now has multiple associations—the interceptive sensation is associated with multiple outcomes, not just the one that is feared (Figure 20.3).

One mechanism proposed to underlie the effects of interoceptive exposure, and exposure as a therapeutic strategy for pathological fear-based reactions more broadly, is inhibitory learning (Craske et al., 2014). Inhibitory learning refers to competing associations with a feared stimulus that provide alternative interpretations of the potential danger of a previously feared object, sensation, and so on. Imagine an individual developed food poisoning eating a peanut butter and strawberry jam sandwich with tainted jam. The sight of jam provokes a fear response, and the individual avoids all forms of strawberry jam. The individual engages with a therapist who will conduct interoceptive exposure exercises with them to help them overcome their fear of jam. The individual consumes their first peanut butter and strawberry jam sandwich since the incident and feel butterflies in gut, mild queasiness, a tightening of their throat, difficulty swallowing,—but they do not throw up. They subsequently eat peanut butter and strawberry jam for 50 days in a row with no aversive consequences. Via the process of extinction, the conditioned stimulus (strawberry jam) is no longer associated with the unconditioned response (vomiting). However, according to the model of inhibitory learning, the feared memory is not erased, it is inhibited. Spontaneous recovery is one form of support for the inhibitory learning model: a fear-based reaction can be rapidly ignited after extinction learning; for example, upon seeing a dented container of jam in the grocery store.

There have been suggestions on ways to improve the potency of exposure therapy and thus inhibitory learning (Craske et al., 2014). One strategy is maximizing the creation of a prediction error: designing exposure activities so that new learning experiences violate previously formed expectancies. A prediction error is a difference between one's expectancies about a situation and the outcome (Pine et al., 2018). Accumulating evidence demonstrates prediction errors contribute to the brain's updating of previously held models, beliefs, assumptions, or expectations to improve future predictions and minimize future prediction errors. In other words, prediction errors contribute to new learning and some evidence indicates that the larger the prediction error, the greater learning that will occur (Pine et al., 2018). According to Craske and colleagues (2014), exposures should be developed around the new learning that needs to occur and so that expectancy violations are maximized.

This differs from exposure exercises designed to help an individual to habituate to fear or another negative affect. For example, imagine that an individual with AN did not want to eat until fullness when eating out with friends. They were afraid that if they ate to fullness, they would become preoccupied during the remainder of the meal, not be able to enjoy the time with their friends, and that their friends would evaluate them negatively because they were not fun to be around. An exposure designed to create an expectancy violation might have the individual with AN eat to fullness in the therapist's office and then demonstrate that they can continue to have an engaged conversation about some timely topic. In contrast, an interoceptive exposure activity designed to maximize habituation would try to demonstrate that the intensity of an individual's fear or guilt following eating to fullness dissipates over time—or, with repeated practices, does not occur as strongly. Mechanisms of inhibitory learning do not require reductions in negative affect—the new learned outcome can occur even in the presence of guilt or fear (e.g., the patient can continue to have meaningful conversations with the therapist even though she is feeling a bit guilty about eating to fullness). In this way, inhibitory learning models can be construed as acceptance-based—they help individuals approach avoided, feared circumstances while accepting the negative thoughts and feelings that may accompany that approach.

There are other ways to potentiate exposure. Deepened exposure occurs when multiple feared cues or contexts are integrated into an exposure activity. Sticking with the previous example, an example of deepened extinction would be if the individual with AN ate to fullness while at a birthday dinner with her friends and while consuming feared and previously avoided foods such as birthday cake. Removal of safety signals can also potentiate interoceptive exposures. Again with the previous example, if the individual ate to fullness but then went on a walk after the meal with her friend this may weaken inhibitory learning because the individual has not learned that they can be socially adept in the presence of fullness—they have attempted to reduce that sensation. While such safety signals may first be necessary to increase an individual's capacity and willingness to approach feared contexts, ultimately these signals need to fade for potent inhibitory learning to occur. Otherwise, a situation may be created where the individual is dependent on the safety signal to approach a challenging circumstance (e.g., an individual with AN panics when not able to walk after a meal).

Occasional reinforced exposure may further strengthen inhibitory learning. In this case, the unconditioned stimulus and conditioned stimulus occasionally do co-occur (e.g., the feeling of fullness is associated with socially debilitating distraction). The adaptive learning that may occur from such reinforced exposures are that the individual can tolerate uncertainty and master an aversive circumstance, potentially decreasing the potency of the feared outcome and furthering inhibitory learning. In our extended example, the individual who was distracted while feeling full might learn "So what. Everyone is boring sometimes."

State of the Science in Eating Disorders

Family-based interoceptive exposure for low-weight adolescents

The application of interoceptive exposure exercises into the treatment of adolescent low-weight eating disorders, ARFID in children, and disorders of gut–brain interaction in children are next considered. Hildebrandt and colleagues (2021) describe an elegant model of family-based interoceptive exposure for adolescent low-weight eating disorders. The researchers developed a six-session module that was designed as an adjunct to family-based treatment for low-weight eating disorders. A core emphasis of this protocol is to give the adolescent and family tools to manage the aversive visceral sensations often provoked by food cues or the ingestion of food by engaging in counter-conditioning of visceral sensations with positively valenced experiences or stimuli. Further, interoceptive exposure activities were embedded in an acceptance framework where one goal of the activity was to demonstrate to both the adolescent and parents that they could tolerate discomfort (e.g., feeling uncomfortably full) in the service of moving toward valued goals (e.g., having the freedom to eat out with friends). An emphasis is on the experience of disgust, an emotional experience designed to protect an organism from contamination or infection from pathogens, such as pathogens that exert their influence by crossing some form of body barrier (i.e., as happens with food ingestion).

The use of interoceptive exposure in the context of disgust warrants consideration. Disgust has been shown to be more resistant to extinction using exposure-based methods that adhere to principles of Pavlovian conditioning (Mason & Richardson, 2010; Olatunji et al., 2007). Although it is unclear why this is the case, there are several hypotheses that attempt to explain this relative resistance to extinction. First, disgust is considered to be a form of evaluative conditioning, learned associations that alter a person's preference or liking of a stimulus (De Houwer et al., 2005). In classical Pavlovian conditioning, the conditioned stimulus signals the future onset of a feared stimulus. When this predictive signaling is weakened via non-reinforced experiences of the conditioned stimulus without the feared outcome, fear of the conditioned stimulus may weaken. In contrast, evaluative conditioning concerns whether one likes or dislikes something. A conditioned stimulus in a disgust-conditioning paradigm is associated with the disgusting properties of the unconditioned stimulus (i.e., it has acquired the negative valence properties of the unconditioned stimulus) and may come to elicit these negative evaluations irrespective of the predictive function of the conditioned stimulus. For example, a person learns that cleaning up vomit does not make them sick. After cleaning up vomit repeatedly with no harm befalling them, the person no longer fears contamination from vomit, but they still find vomit disgusting; that is, the person's evaluation of vomit has not changed (Mason & Richardson, 2010). Alternatively, the function of disgust may help to explain this resistance to extinction. If disgust signals the potential contamination from pathogens, there may be an uncertain time course from exposure to later infection as when an incubation period occurs with a pathogen or as in the delayed time course of vomiting or malaise resulting from ingestion of contaminated food. A related hypothesis is that a potential agent of contamination maintains its harmful qualities and thus it would not be adaptive to extinguish a disgust response. Despite this, people approach disgusting things every day. They change diapers, wipe their children's noses, and so on. Thus, it may be that the context or meaning of the associations between approaching a disgusting stimulus and the outcome of that approach needs to change. For example, one could facilitate an approach to something disgusting by making the behavior of approach a valued action (e.g., a person values helping people) with a valued outcome (e.g., sick individuals are helped when someone cares for them) (Harris et al., 2019). This does not alter the evaluation of the stimulus but that of approaching the stimulus. Understanding the conditions under which one's evaluations change will provide critical information for intervention design in eating disorders in which the experience of disgust is central.

Rather than trying to terminate or reduce feelings of disgust, Hildebrandt and colleagues (2021) taught families methods of counter-conditioning. Adolescents were taught to mindfully observe and describe visceral sensations associated with food or eating. Mindful observations and descriptions are those that are present, focused, non-judgmental, and deliberate as one directs one's attention to ongoing experience. Counter-conditioning was designed to help adolescents integrate and associate aversive visceral experiences with positive images or experiences, as in thinking of the stomach pulsations of food ingestions as synchronizing with the beat of their favorite song. The empathy of parents was accentuated by having parents engage in an activity they found to be disgusting (e.g., eating a despised food). Acceptance-based metaphors and demonstrations were used to demonstrate the paradoxical nature of control. For example, the adolescent might be guided to compare the experience of natural breathing versus paced breathing. All didactic exercises were integrated with an interoceptive exposure activity designed to increase uncertainty—the consumption of a shake of unknown nutritional properties. This six-session module was designed to potentiate family-based treatment for low-weight eating disorders by providing the family with tools to manage the aversive visceral sensations associated with food and food ingestion.

Aspects of this intervention are consistent with principles of inhibitory learning. The intervention is designed such that new, potentially pleasant experiences are created in association with prior aversive post-meal digestive sensations. There are competing associations created with a given gut visceral sensation. While this sensation may have been interpreted by someone with an eating disorder as a signal of the threat of weight gain, instead this sensation is immediately associated with support, community, and enjoyable experience via counter-conditioning, while also being linked to future value-based goals or aspirations (e.g., being a good friend). The therapists communicate that they are not expecting habituation of negative affect, particularly disgust, to post-ingestive sensations. Rather, the interoceptive exposure activities are framed so that they are similar to other hard things the adolescent and parents have done that are important to them. The therapists try to eliminate distraction as a potential safety signal while the acceptance-based framework establishes the expectation of occasional reinforced exposures. (For more details regarding the protocol, see Hildebrandt et al., 2021.)

Interoceptive exposures for young children with food avoidance or disorders of gut–brain interaction

Zucker and colleagues (2017, 2019) designed and tested an acceptance-based interoceptive exposure intervention for young children with disorders of gut–brain interaction, such as functional abdominal pain and a modified version for

ARFID. The term acceptance indicated that exposure activities were designed such that individuals embraced, tolerated, enjoyed, and so on, strong visceral sensations and the affective responses to these sensations rather than trying to terminate the sensations or their reactions to these sensations. Instead, exposure activities were designed to maximize expectancy violations. Parents and children were given a mindset that guided the intervention. Rather than viewing the body and body sensations as threatening, as may happen in the presence of chronic functional abdominal pain or the fears of aversive outcomes of ARFID, children and parents learned that bodies are amazingly strong and smart. While everyone's body is smart, children with visceral hypersensitivity (called "sensory superpowers") had bodies that were particularly strong and smart. Children were given data about their somatic or sensory sensitivities to further support these superpowers. This superpower was framed as a gift "that enables them to see things that others cannot see and feel things more deeply . . . feelings that help make the world a more beautiful and joyful place." Children were given stories about how such superpowers would be adaptive (e.g., as in enhanced capacities to detect poisonous or spoiled foods) and they were encouraged to think through all the occupations and tasks they would be experts at given their superpowers.

In line with this formulation, children were also given several tools. When children fear their bodies, they may experience an initial startle when they experience a somatic sensation (Figure 20.1). To alter their initial perception of threat toward a visceral sensation, they were taught to associate body sensations with cute and playful cartoon characters (e.g., Georgia the Gut Growler). Characters were used to provide psychoeducation about the wise messages communicated by different visceral sensations. Coloring pages and character buttons served as further memory cues of these sensations. A goal was to alter the initial perception of a visceral sensation from that of harm to that of curiosity, a task particularly suited for elite Feeling and Body Investigators (FBI agent; Figure 20.4), individuals with sensory superpowers.

Another tool to increase curiosity toward the body was a set of interoceptive exposure exercises that were designed to create expectancy violations that demonstrate that the body is even smarter than the children may have thought. The body is constantly learning and thus is getting stronger, wiser, faster, and so on. Armed with these concepts, interoceptive exposures are designed to demonstrate this wisdom of the body and, to the extent possible, to demonstrate expectancy violations regarding the body's ability to adapt and learn. For example, each session began with a Henry Heartbeat activity in which the child chose some activities to raise and lower the heartrate. Therapists, parents, and children all made predictions about how much the heart will change while supporting various activities or regarding how long it will take the heart to return to baseline after performing certain skills. The discrepancy between the prediction and the actual heartbeat is one example of a lesson learned about the body: *My heart is so smart, it knows how*

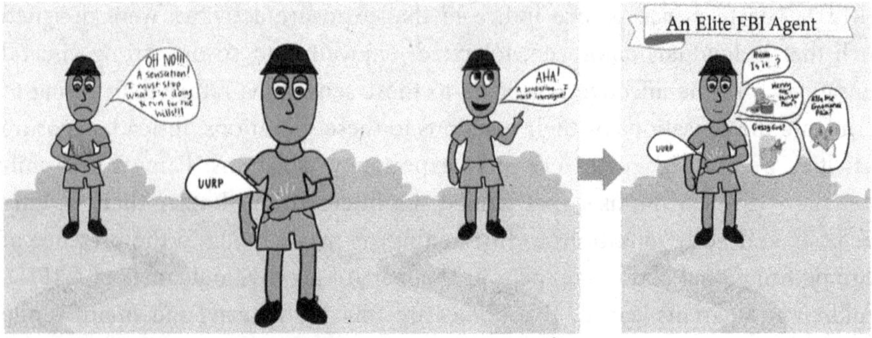

Figure 20.4 The framework of an elite FBI Agent in Feeling and Body Investigators. Children and parents are guided to use a mindset of investigative curiosity and humor to the initial perception of visceral sensations.

much it needs to beat to support me in certain situations. Or, if the child guessed correctly: *I can really learn to listen to my body with practice*. With each investigation, there was a lesson learned about the body. To consolidate the memory about the wisdom of the body, children created a Body Map. This was a life-size tracing of their body on butcher paper to which they added, via drawings and captions, the wise things they have learned their body can do. For example, they wrote "My stomach growls to let me know I need more energy." Interoceptive exposures were designed to help children learn how smart their body is, sometimes in the form of expectancy violations that demonstrate that the body knows what to do more than the person making the predictions.

Children and self-parenting

Children in FBI learned to decode and respond to body messages, in other words, to "self-parent." While Body Investigations (i.e., interoceptive exposures) helped children learn about the wisdom of the body, Body Clues Worksheets helped children learn that visceral and other somatic sensations communicate needs and that they can do investigations to figure out how to respond to those body messages (Figure 20.5). For example, when they notice Harold the Hunger Pain, they may learn that they have let themselves get too hungry and that they have a tough time making a decision about what to eat when they are that hungry. If they have a menu of snacks available when they feel Harold the Hunger Pain, that may help them decide and their hunger pains go away more quickly. Children may work this out by going through the steps of the worksheet (Figure 20.5). Parents and children were instructed to use a Body Clues Worksheet in many ways. They might go through a worksheet after a moment of strong feelings to figure out what happened and what to do next time. They might review a worksheet as a summary of the most intense sensations they felt that day. They might use it to

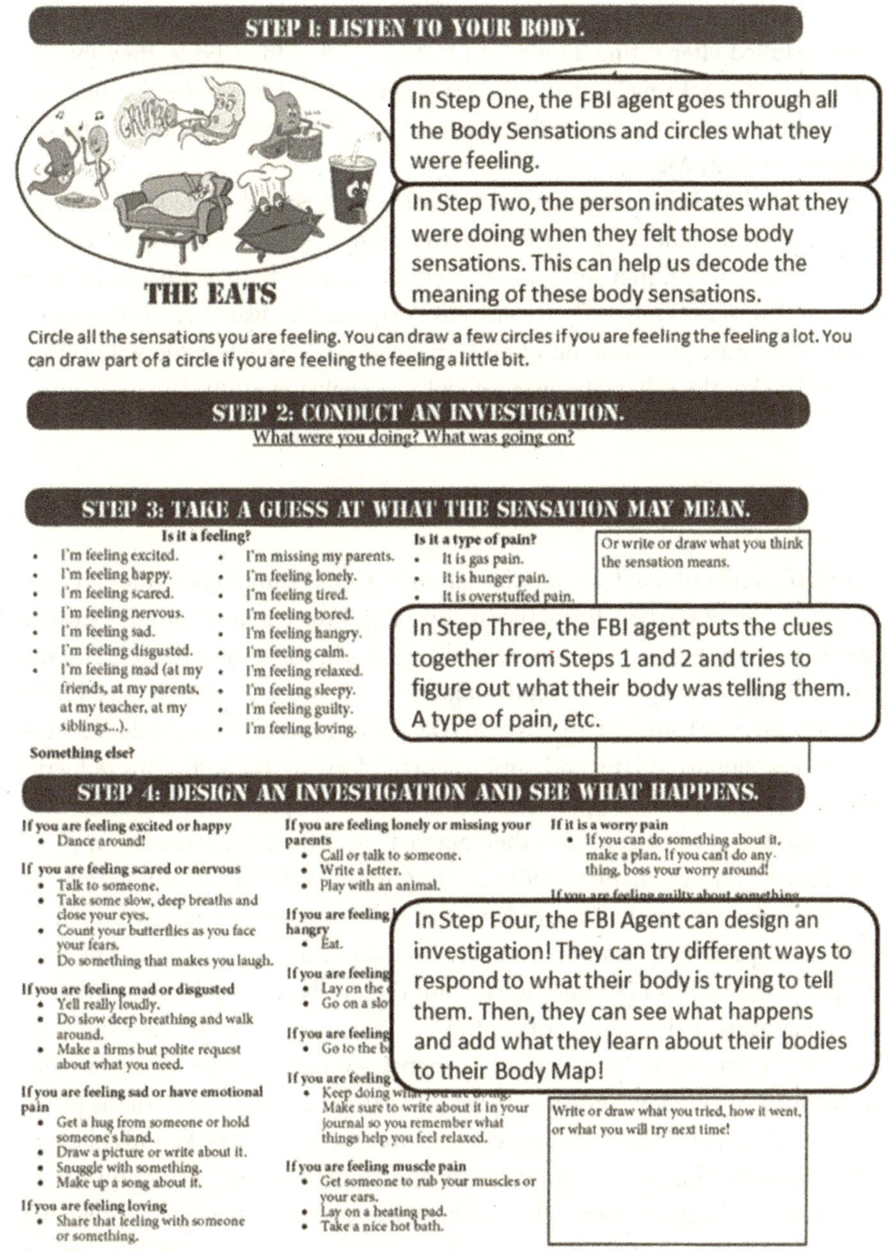

Figure 20.5 A sample body clues worksheet.

plan an upcoming investigation. All these uses were intended to facilitate interoceptive responsivity, responsiveness to the needs the body is communicating, or "self-parenting."

Body Clues Worksheets also served as a guide to help parents and children learn to design "on-the-spot investigations" when they feel strong visceral sensations. In other words, they learned to design their own interoceptive exposure activities in response to actual visceral sensations as they occur in daily life. If a child feels Sabrina Stuffed after eating an amount of food to fuel their body, they may see what happens to Sabrina Stuffed if she reads her favorite book or lies on the couch with a heating pad. The wisdom that she learns from this investigation will then be added to her Body Map.

Feeling and Body Investigators is an intervention that is designed to go beyond decreasing a fear of the body. Rather, the over-arching intention is to build trusting self-awareness in children so that they feel safe in their bodies broadly. As such, it is intended to not only improve current symptoms of disordered eating but to prevent the future exacerbation of body mistrust during such vulnerable periods as puberty. (For the full treatment protocol, see Zucker et al. 2023.)

Alternative Perspectives

Historically, reduction of fear via habituation to a scary stimulus was thought to be a central driver of the benefits of therapeutic exposure activities for the treatment of anxiety (Foa & Kozak, 1986). A patient's report of initial fear or distress and subsequent changes in negative affect throughout the exposure (often reported in the form of Subjective Units of Distress or SUDS ratings) would guide the design of the session: a session would not end until a patient's fear was reduced. This reduction or habituation of a feared response in the presence of the previously feared stimulus was hypothesized to be central to therapeutic benefit from exposure therapy.

In contrast, accumulating evidence supports a different interpretation: in-session change in fear is not predictive of later post-session negative affect in response to previously feared stimuli (Kircanski et al., 2012; Prenoveau et al., 2013). These findings raise questions about the mechanisms of therapeutic benefit for exposure activities. In contrast, exposures designed to create expectancy violations, according to the tenets of inhibitory learning, do not require a reduction in anxiety in session. Sessions are designed around changes in what the patient expects will happen when these expectancies are challenged. Craske and colleagues (2014) describe this as overlapping with the strategy of belief disconfirmation (Salkovskis et al., 2007), although inhibitory learning activities do not have to be designed around a belief. Work by Pine and colleagues (2018) found that semantic knowledge (knowledge of facts) and episodic memory (events) are also updated by prediction errors, as one's brain tries to update previously held knowledge or memories with new information. Strikingly, the larger the prediction error, the greater the updating of previously held models. By corollary, if a patient had a strongly held expectancy about the impact of an interoceptive experience, and this expectancy was violated (i.e., a large prediction error), that may lead to strong updating of previously held assumptions. For example, if an individual with an eating disorder believed there was "absolutely no way" they could concentrate on studying if they felt full and then preceded to be extremely efficient with their studying when full, even better than was typical, this may lead to potent updating of prior expectancies. It is exciting to think of the design of interoceptive exposure exercises in light of these findings.

Summary

Interoception is a fundamental process whereby an individual learns to map the moment-to-moment state of their body, while interoceptive responsivity is when an individual learns to respond adaptively to these signals. Fear of the body can disrupt the emergence of such adaptive self-awareness and attunement. Interoceptive exposure is a therapeutic technique designed to augment prior learning histories so that an individual's response to their body not only does not impair functioning, but also helps them to flourish.

References

Ainsworth, M. D. S., Blehar, M. C., Waters, E., & Wall, S. N. (2015). Theoretical background. In *Patterns of attachment: A psychological study of the strange situation* (pp. 1–22). Taylor & Francis.

Boettcher, H., Brake, C. A., & Barlow, D. H. (2016). Origins and outlook of interoceptive exposure. *Journal of Behavior Therapy and Experimental Psychiatry, 53*, 41–51. https://doi.org/10.1016/j.jbtep.2015.10.009

Cannon, W. B. (1925). The effect of the emotions on digestion. In *Bodily changes in pain, hunger, fear, and rage* (pp. 1–21). Martino Fine Books.

Craske, M. G., Treanor, M., Conway, C. C., Zbozinek, T., & Vervliet, B. (2014). Maximizing exposure therapy: An inhibitory learning approach. *Behaviour Research and Therapy, 58*, 10–23. https://doi.org/10.1016/j.brat.2014.04.006

Datta, N., Bidopia, T., Datta, S., Mittal, G., Alphin, F., Herbert, B. M., Marsh, E. J., Fitzsimons, G. J., Strauman, T. J., & Zucker, N. L. (2021). Internal states and interoception along a spectrum of eating disorder symptomology. *Physiology & Behaviour, 230*, 113307. https://doi.org/10.1016/j.physbeh.2020.113307

De Houwer, J. D., Baeyens, F., & Field, A. P. (2005). Associative learning of likes and dislikes: Some current controversies and possible ways forward. *Cognition and Emotion, 19*(2), 161–174. https://doi.org/10.1080/02699930441000265

Foa, E. B., & Kozak, M. J. (1986). Emotional processing of fear: Exposure to corrective information. *Psychological Bulletin, 99*(1), 20–35. https://doi.org/10.1037/0033-2909.99.1.20

Grilo, C. M., & Shiffman, S. (1994). Longitudinal investigation of the abstinence violation effect in binge eaters. *Journal of Consulting and Clinical Psychology, 62*(3), 611–619. https://doi.org/10.1037//0022-006x.62.3.611

Harris, A. A., Romer, A. L., Hanna, E. K., Keeling, L. A., LaBar, K. S., Sinnott-Armstrong, W., Strauman, T. J., Wagner, H. R., Marcus, M. D., & Zucker, N. L. (2019). The central role of disgust in disorders of food avoidance. *International Journal of Eating Disorders, 52*(5), 543–553. https://doi.org/10.1002/eat.23047

Hetterich, L., Mack, I., Giel, K. E., Zipfel, S., & Stengel, A. (2019). An update on gastrointestinal disturbances in eating disorders. *Molecular and Cellular Endocrinology, 497*, 110318. https://doi.org/10.1016/j.mce.2018.10.016

Hildebrandt, T., Peyser, D., & Sysko, R. (2021). Lessons learned developing and testing family-based interoceptive exposure for adolescents with low-weight eating disorders. *International Journal of Eating Disorders, 54*(11), 2037–2045. https://doi.org/10.1002/eat.23605

Khalsa, S. S., Adolphs, R., Cameron, O. G., Critchley, H. D., Davenport, P. W., Feinstein, J. S., Feusner, J. D., Garfinkel, S. N., Lane, R. D., Mehling, W. E., Meuret, A. E., Nemeroff, C. B., Oppenheimer, S., Petzschner, F. H., Pollatos, O., Rhudy, J. L., Schramm, L. P., Simmons, W. K., Stein,

M. B., . . . Paulus, M. P. (2018). Interoception and mental health: A roadmap. *Biological Psychiatry: Cognitive Neuroscience and Neuroimaging, 3*(6), 501–513. https://doi.org/10.1016/j.bpsc.2017.12.004

Khalsa, S. S., Craske, M. G., Li, W., Vangala, S., Strober, M., & Feusner, J. D. (2015). Altered interoceptive awareness in anorexia nervosa: Effects of meal anticipation, consumption and bodily arousal. *International Journal of Eating Disorders, 48*(7), 889–897. https://doi.org/10.1002/eat.22387

Kircanski, K., Mortazavi, A., Castriotta, N., Baker, A. S., Mystkowski, J. L., Yi, R., & Craske, M. G. (2012). Challenges to the traditional exposure paradigm: Variability in exposure therapy for contamination fears. *Journal of Behavior Therapy and Experimental Psychiatry, 43*(2), 745–751. https://doi.org/10.1016/j.jbtep.2011.10.010

LaBar, K. S., & Phelps, E. A. (2005). Reinstatement of conditioned fear in humans is context dependent and impaired in amnesia. *Behavioral Neuroscience, 119*(3), 677–686. https://doi.org/10.1037/0735-7044.119.3.677

LeDoux, J. (1996). *The emotional brain: The mysterious underpinnings of emotional life.* Simon & Schuster.

Mason, E. C., & Richardson, R. (2010). Looking beyond fear: The extinction of other emotions implicated in anxiety disorders. *Journal of Anxiety Disorders, 24*(1), 63–70. https://doi.org/10.1016/j.janxdis.2009.08.007

Méndez-Bértolo, C., Moratti, S., Toledano, R., Lopez-Sosa, F., Martínez-Alvarez, R., Mah, Y. H., Vuilleumier, P., Gil-Nagel, A., & Strange, B. A. (2016). A fast pathway for fear in human amygdala. *Nature Neuroscience, 19*(8), 1041–1049. https://doi.org/10.1038/nn.4324

Olatunji, B. O., Forsyth, J. P., & Cherian, A. (2007). Evaluative differential conditioning of disgust: a sticky form of relational learning that is resistant to extinction. *Journal of Anxiety Disorders, 21*(6), 820–834. https://doi.org/10.1016/j.janxdis.2006.11.004

Oswald, A., Chapman, J., & Wilson, C. (2017). Do interoceptive awareness and interoceptive responsiveness mediate the relationship between body appreciation and intuitive eating in young women? *Appetite, 109*, 66–72. https://doi.org/10.1016/j.appet.2016.11.019

Pavlov, I. P. (1957). Physiological facts, human instinct, and medical empiricism. In *Experimental psychology.* Philosophical Library.

Pine, A., Sadeh, N., Ben-Yakov, A., Dudai, Y., & Mendelsohn, A. (2018). Knowledge acquisition is governed by striatal prediction errors. *Nature Communications, 9*(1), 1673. https://doi.org/10.1038/s41467-018-03992-5

Prenoveau, J. M., Craske, M. G., Liao, B., & Ornitz, E. M. (2013). Human fear conditioning and extinction: timing is everythingor is it? *Biological Psychology, 92*(1), 59–68. https://doi.org/10.1016/j.biopsycho.2012.02.005

Salkovskis, P. M., Hackmann, A., Wells, A., Gelder, M. G., & Clark, D. M. (2007). Belief disconfirmation versus habituation approaches to situational exposure in panic disorder with agoraphobia: a pilot study. *Behaviour Research and Therapy, 45*(5), 877–885. https://doi.org/10.1016/j.brat.2006.02.008

Salvioli, B., Pellicciari, A., Iero, L., Di Pietro, E., Moscano, F., Gualandi, S., Stanghellini, V., De Giorgio, R., Ruggeri, E., & Franzoni, E. (2013). Audit of digestive complaints and psychopathological traits in patients with eating disorders: A prospective study. *Digestive and Liver Disease, 45*(8), 639–644. https://doi.org/10.1016/j.dld.2013.02.022

Simren, M., Tornblom, H., Palsson, O. S., van Tilburg, M. A., Van Oudenhove, L., Tack, J., & Whitehead, W. E. (2017). Visceral hypersensitivity is associated with GI symptom severity in functional GI disorders: Consistent findings from five different patient cohorts. *Gut.* https://doi.org/10.1136/gutjnl-2016-312361

Stein, K., Warne, N., Heron, J., Zucker, N., & Bould, H. (2021). Do children with recurrent abdominal pain grow up to become adolescents who control their weight by fasting? Results from a UK population-based cohort. *International Journal of Eating Disorders, 54*(6), 915–924. https://doi.org/10.1002/eat.23513

van Tilburg, M. A. L., Fortunato, J. E., Squires, M., Drossman, D. A., Dalton, C., Lichtman, S., & Whitehead, W. E. (2014). Impact of eating restriction on gastrointestinal motility in adolescents with IBS. *Journal of Pediatric Gastroenterology and Nutrition, 58*(4), 491–494. https://doi.org/10.1097/mpg.0000000000000228

Zucker, N., & Bulik, C. M. (2020). On bells, saliva, and abdominal pain or discomfort: Early aversive visceral conditioning and vulnerability for anorexia nervosa. *International Journal of Eating Disorders, 53*(4), 508–512. https://doi.org/10.1002/eat.23255

Zucker, N., Mauro, C., Craske, M., Wagner, H. R., Datta, N., Hopkins, H., Caldwell, K., Kiridly, A., Marsan, S., Maslow, G., Mayer, E., & Egger, H. (2017). Acceptance-based interoceptive exposure for young children with functional abdominal pain. *Behaviour Research and Therapy*, *97*, 200–212. https://doi.org/10.1016/j.brat.2017.07.009

Zucker, N. L., LaVia, M. C., Craske, M. G., Foukal, M., Harris, A. A., Datta, N., Savereide, E., & Maslow, G. R. (2019). Feeling and body investigators (FBI): ARFID division—An acceptance-based interoceptive exposure treatment for children with ARFID. *International Journal of Eating Disorders*, *52*(4), 466–472. https://doi.org/10.1002/eat.22996

Zucker, N. L., Loeb, K. L., & Gagliano, M. E. (2023). *Treating functional abdominal pain in children: A clinical guide using feeling and body investigators*. Cambridge University Press

21

Neurosurgery and Neuromodulation for Eating Disorders

Philippe De Vloo, Elske Vrieze, Nir Lipsman, D. Blake Woodside, and Andres Lozano

Brief Definitional Overview

Neuromodulation: Neuromodulation refers to the alteration of neural activity through targeted delivery of a stimulus, such as electrical or magnetic stimulation to specific neurological sites. These stimuli can be delivered invasively (i.e., after a skin incision) or non-invasively (i.e. from outside the body).

Deep brain stimulation (DBS): DBS is an invasive neurosurgical technique in which electrodes (typically one or two) are implanted with high precision in the brain (targeting deep grey nuclei or white matter tracts) to allow electrical stimulation by means of an implantable neurostimulator. DBS is an established technique for several movement disorders (including Parkinson's Disease, tremor, and dystonia) and obsessive-compulsive disorder (OCD). All other indications, including eating disorders, are considered experimental at this stage.

Repetitive transcranial magnetic stimulation (rTMS): rTMS is a non-invasive neuromodulation technique where energy is transmitted through the intact skin and skull by means of differentially oriented electromagnets positioned over a specific brain area, where the excitability of the cortex and subcortical white matter can be modulated. The US Food and Drug Administration has approved rTMS for major depression, migraine with aura, OCD, and combined anxiety and major depressive disorder (MDD). rTMS can be delivered with different frequencies: high-frequency rTMS (5–20 Hz) is thought to increase cortical excitability (potentially through long-term potentiation).

Transcranial direct current stimulation (tDCS): tDCS is a non-invasive neuromodulation technique in which scalp electrodes are applied through which a weak direct current is delivered, either cathodal or anodal.

Electroconvulsive therapy (ECT): ECT is an old, non-invasive neuromodulation technique which has been mainly applied in major depression (often with suicidality), bipolar disorder, and schizophrenia. It uses an electrical current to induce a brief generalized tonic-clonic seizure under general anesthesia.

Philippe De Vloo et al., *Neurosurgery and Neuromodulation for Eating Disorders*. In: *The Handbook of the Neurobiology of Eating Disorders*. Edited by: Christina E. Wierenga and Joanna E. Steinglass, Oxford University Press.
 DOI: 10.1093/9780197675212.003.0022

Introduction

Neurosurgical treatment for anorexia nervosa (AN) dates back to the 1940s. Initially, mainly leucotomies (also known as lobotomies) were applied, based on (1) observed disinhibition of appetitive behaviors after local brain damage, (2) alleviation of chronic anxiety associated with the perceived threat of weight gain, and (3) the now-obsolete concept that AN was a subtype of obsessive compulsive disorder (OCD) (Lipsman, Woodside, Giacobbe, & Lozano, 2013; Wu et al., 2013). Lesioning procedures, including limbic leucotomy and thalamotomy (lesioning of the thalamus), were also applied but clinical outcome was inconclusive due to the heterogeneity in diagnostic standards, surgical procedures, and outcome parameters (Carmody & Vibber, 1952; Crisp & Kalucy, 1973; D'Andrea et al., 1974; Drury, 1950; Glazebrook & Prosen, 1956; Heath et al., 1979; Morgan & Crisp, 2000; Sargant, 1951; Sifneos, 1952). In the following decades, neurosurgery for psychiatric disorders, including AN, was almost abandoned when the scientific community and the public opinion reacted heavily to psychosurgery in general, and frontal lobotomies in particular, although some centers continued until the 1990s (Zamboni et al., 1993). Although many authors refer to a better understanding of the neurobiology and dysfunctional neurocircuitry as the main trigger to pursue neuromodulation treatments for eating disorders in modern times, as with many treatments in medicine in general, and in neuromodulation in particular, the truth is that serendipity and re-use of historic targets have played a big role. This chapter provides a comprehensive overview of the outcome and safety of neuromodulation and lesioning techniques applied in eating disorders to date, and recommendations for future studies.

Biological Framework

Attention to neurosurgical treatment for eating disorders re-emerged from 2007 to 2011, following several case reports describing beneficial effects on comorbid AN among patients who underwent deep brain stimulation (DBS) for major depressive disorder (MDD) (Israël et al., 2010) or OCD (Barbier et al., 2011). In 2007, a patient underwent successful DBS for AN as the primary illness, but this case is rarely mentioned because it was presented as a poster at a neurosurgical meeting and was not otherwise published (Wu et al., 2007). Since the early ages of stereotactic surgery, lesioning of specific brain areas has been used to alter diseased neurocircuitry. In the pre-DBS era, radiofrequency lesioning was the standard technique, although brain lesions can also be created through stereotactic radiotherapy. All stereotactic brain lesions induce necrosis of brain tissue resulting in a brain cavity. Although with the advent of DBS in the early 1990s, stereotactic brain lesioning had been largely replaced, the optimization of focused ultrasound

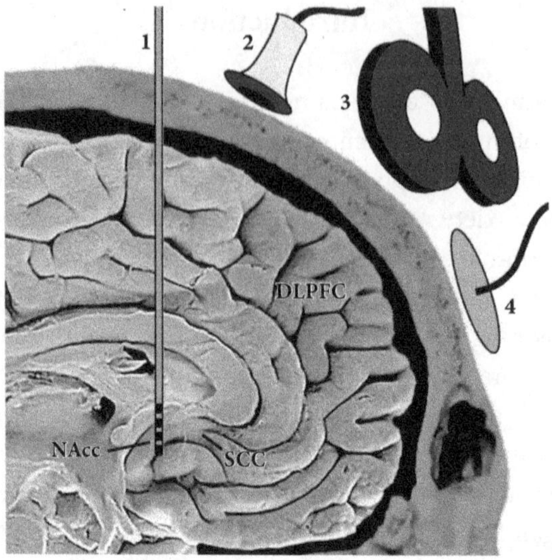

Figure 21.1 A diagram depicting neuromodulatory techniques applied to the brain, including deep brain stimulation targeting the nucleus accumbens (NAcc) and nearby subcollosal cingulate (SCC) (1), electroconvulsive therapy (2), and repetitive transcranial magnetic stimulation (3) and transcranial direct current stimulation (4) targeting the dorsolateral prefrontal cortex (DLPFC).

lesioning in the mid-2010s through MRI guidance has created a new surge in brain lesioning procedures. The novel technology of MRI-guided focused ultrasound has opened the possibility of non-invasive brain lesioning. MRI-guided focused ultrasound anterior capsulotomy for treatment of AN was described in a large series from China (Liu et al., 2018).

In addition to these neurosurgical interventions, studies have investigated non-invasive neuromodulation, including repetitive transcranial magnetic stimulation (rTMS), transcranial direct current stimulation (tDCS), and electroconvulsive therapy (ECT). Nevertheless, for many of these techniques, the role in the management of eating disorders remains unclear (Figure 21.1).

State of the Science in Eating Disorders

Deep brain stimulation

The modern era of DBS for eating disorders started in the late 2000s to the early 2010s, when two case reports were published of DBS for MDD (targeting the subcallosal cingulate [SCC]) (Israël et al., 2010) and capsulotomy for OCD (targeting the bed nucleus of the stria terminalis [BNST]) (Barbier et al., 2011) in patients with comorbid AN. Both patients experienced beneficial effects not only on their MDD/OCD but also on measures of AN severity. A few years prior, a successful case of nucleus accumbens deep brain stimulation (NAcc-DBS) to specifically treat AN had been presented at a neurosurgical meeting (H. Wu et al., 2007).

Both SCC and NAcc—and neighboring BNST, ventral striatum/ventral caudate (VC/VS), and anterior limb of the internal capsule (ALIC)—were considered theoretically promising DBS targets in eating disorders given their (1) prominent afferent and efferent connection with the anterior insula, (2) involvement in reward-processing through corticostriatothalamic loops, (3) involvement in AN-related provocation and imaging studies, and (4) involvement in anxiety and dysphoric mood (Karaszewska et al., 2022; Lipsman, Woodside, Giacobbe, & Lozano, 2013; Steinglass & Walsh, 2006). These two targets have been further explored in a series of mainly open-label feasibility studies and one small randomized double-blind ON/OFF crossover trial. In neuromodulation for OCD, the BNST, NAcc, VC/VS, and ALIC are often considered as one target, because (1) they are spatially very close to each other; (2) often very high stimulation energy is applied, resulting in large volumes of tissue activated covering more than just the targeted brain area; (3) these targets share connectivity and functionality; and (4) although DBS surgeons target NAcc, often the stimulating cathode is anatomically in ALIC. BNST, NAcc, VC/VS, and ALIC are considered as one target in this chapter.

Interestingly, whilst only 83 reported patients have undergone DBS for AN over the course of more than 15 years globally, this topic has been extensively discussed in the literature, with 111 articles found on PubMed from a search in April 2024 with "anorexia" AND "deep brain stimulation" as search terms. This reflects the particular interest of the neurosurgical community, despite the very limited experience in a disease with a prevalence similar to Parkinson's Disease, for which more than 200,000 patients have undergone DBS worldwide.

Eligibility criteria

Given the invasiveness and associated risks of DBS, this intervention has typically been offered after other treatments have been unsuccessful. However, there is no consensus on who should be eligible for this technique and each study has used its own inclusion criteria. Mostly, eligibility is based on (1) illness duration, (2) history of unsuccessful treatments, and (3) AN severity. The latter is often expressed as body mass index (BMI), although an extremely low BMI (e.g., $<10 kg/m^2$) is often also an exclusion criterion, for which in-hospital refeeding is administered to lower the anesthesiologic risk prior to surgery. An overview of eligibility criteria for the published trials (not case reports) is provided in Table 21.1.

Deep brain stimulation studies targeting NAcc, BNST, ALIC, or VC/VS

A total of 56 patients who underwent DBS for (comorbid) AN targeting NAcc, BNST, ALIC, or VC/VS have been reported across a total of 13 publications originating from China, the United Kingdom (UK), Spain, the United States (US), the

Table 21.1 Eligibility criteria for studies (not case reports) of deep brain stimulation (DBS) for anorexia nervosa (AN)

Study	Illness duration (years)	Patient age (years)	Pharmacotherapy history	Other treatment history requirements	BMI (kg/m^2)	Additional criteria
Liu 2020 (Shanghai, China) (Liu et al., 2020)	≥3	≥18	≥2 SSRIs or anti-psychotics	≥3 months of psychotherapy	n.s.	Life-threatening AN, physiologically or mentally (e.g. past suicide attempts); functionally impaired
Wang 2013 (Xi'an, China) (Wang et al., 2013)	≥2	≥18	n.s.	n.s.	n.s.	Life-threatening as declared by doctor
Scaife 2022 (Oxford, UK) (Scaife et al., 2022)	≥7	21–60	n.s.	≥2 psychotherapy trials; ≥3 voluntary partial or full hospitalizations	13–16	Restricting subtype
Oudijn 2021 (Amsterdam, the Netherlands) (Oudijn et al., 2021)	≥10	n.s.	n.s.	Lack of response to ≥2 typical treatment modes, including 1 hospital admission or inpatient treatment in ED specialized clinic	<15	Functional impairment (GAF ≤45 for ≥2 years, DSM-IV criteria)
Wu 2013 (Shanghai, China) (H. Wu et al., 2013)	n.s.	n.s.	Lack of response to anti-depressant medication	Lack of response to standard psychiatric treatment program of at least 12 months	n.s.	Substantial suffering, significant reduction of psychosocial function, hormonal disturbance due to malnutrition
Vilalba-Martinez 2020 (Barcelona, Spain) (Villalba Martínez et al., 2020)	≥10	18–60	n.s.	Lack of response to ≥3 voluntary intensive treatments (full or partial hospitalization) or clinical worsening and unwillingness to receive any further treatment, including ≥2 hospital admissions for involuntary feeding	13–16	

AN: anorexia nervosa; BMI: body mass index; GAF: global assessment of functioning; n.s.: not specified; SSRI: selective serotonin reuptake inhibitor

Netherlands, Luxemburg, Italy, and Sweden—largely in case reports. All but one were female, with a mean age at surgery of 29 years (range of 16 to 60 years) and a median disease duration of 11 years (range of 1 to 42 years). Follow-up ranged from six months to five years (Table 21.2).

Case series. The Shanghai group described bilateral NAcc-DBS in four adolescents (mean age 15 years) with acute AN (duration of illness 13 to 28 months) and reported a mean BMI increase from 11.9 to 19.6 kg/m^2 and normalization of obsessive-compulsive symptoms, anxiety, and menstruation after nine to 50 months (Wu et al., 2013). The Xi'an group described bilateral NAcc-DBS in two patients with AN (duration of illness from 24 to 36 months) and reported normalization of BMI (from 13.1 to 20.0 kg/m^2) and menstruation, with improvement in depression, anxiety, obsessions, and compulsions following one year of stimulation at the DBS site (Wang et al., 2013). In a study from Barcelona, eight patients received either SCC-DBS or NAcc-DBS, and there was no significant change in BMI at six months post-operatively, although five of the eight patients experienced a BMI increase of more than 10%, with no difference between the surgical targets (Villalba Martínez et al., 2020). A larger study from Shanghai with 28 patients with AN (mean duration of illness 5.1 years; mean pre-operative BMI 13 kg/m^2) provided NAcc-DBS and reported a mean two-year post-operative BMI of 17.7 kg/m^2 and improvement in obsessions/compulsions, anxiety, depression, social functioning, and cognitive functioning (Liu et al., 2020). In a study from Amsterdam that had four patients with AN (Oudijn et al., 2021), BMI increased from 12.5 to 17.8kg/m^2 at one-year post ALIC-DBS, and eating disorder severity, anxiety, depression, and quality of life also improved. A phase 1 double-blind cross-over trial from Oxford investigating the value of NAcc-DBS among seven patients with AN (mean illness duration 21 years, mean pre-operative BMI 12.6 kg/m^2) showed no change in BMI but a greater than 35% reduction in eating disorder severity score at 12 months in three of the patients (Scaife et al., 2022).

Single case reports. A 52-year-old woman with childhood-onset OCD and comorbid mild AN (lowest BMI 17.4 kg/m^2) who underwent VC/VS-DBS in the United States demonstrated an increase in her BMI from 18.5 to 18.9–19.6 kg/m^2 during follow-up. When the contact with ventral caudate was turned on, anxiety, mood, and OCD symptoms worsened, and she lost weight. When turned off, she gained four pounds and her symptoms improved (McLaughlin et al., 2013). A 56-year-old woman with a childhood onset of anxiety and AN, who later also developed MDD, underwent bilateral medial forebrain bundle DBS in Sweden to treat MDD, and had initially a good effect on depression and anxiety symptoms. However, because of stimulation induced blurred-vision, DBS amplitude had to be lowered to levels where her symptoms recurred, after which she underwent BNST-DBS, with again good effect on depression and anxiety, and on eating behavior and obsession with food (Blomstedt et al., 2017). A 37-year-old woman underwent BNST-DBS to treat AN in Italy, and her BMI increased from 16.3 to 18.1 kg/m^2 at

Table 21.2 Deep brain stimulation (DBS) targeting nucleus accumbens (NAcc), bed nucleus of the stria terminalis (BNST), ventral anterior limb of the internal capsule (vALIC), or ventral caudate/ventral striatum (VC/VS)

Study	Number of patients	Sex, age	AN subtype	Illness duration (years)	BMI historic low/preop* (kg/m^2)	Psychiatric comorbidity	Surgical target	Reported complications (excluding post-operative pain and fever <1 week post-op)
Wu 2013 (Shanghai, China) (H. Wu et al., 2013)	4	F, 16	n.s.	2	12.2*	OCD	NAcc	None
		F, 17	n.s.	1	13.3*	OCD	NAcc	none
		F, 17	n.s.	1	12.0*	GAD	NAcc	None
		F, 16	n.s.	1	10.0*	OCD	NAcc	none
Wang 2013 (Xi'an, China) (Wang et al., 2013)	2	F, 28	n.s.	2	13.3*		NAcc	none
		F, 18	n.s.	3	12.9*		NAcc	
McLaughlin 2013 (Providence, US) (McLaughlin et al., 2013)	1	F, 48	R	ns	17.4/18.5*	OCD, MDD, GAD, ADHD	VC/VS	none
Blomstedt 2017 (Umea, Sweden) (Blomstedt et al., 2017)	1	F, 60	R-P	>42	16.6*	MDD	MFB*/ BNST	Blurred vision
Manuelli 2020 (Italy) (Manuelli et al., 2020; Vismara M et al., 2020)	1	F, 37	R-P	18	15.48	OCD	BNST	none
Lin 2020 (Shanghai, China) (Lin et al., 2020)	1	ns	ns	ns	Ns	ns	BNST	none

Villalba-Martinez 2020 (Barcelona, Spain) (Villalba Martínez et al., 2020)	4	M, 45	R	32	13.44/13.44*	GAD, OCD, MDD	NAcc	Skin necrosis requiring flap surgery
		F, 39	P	25	11.47/11.83*	GAD	NAcc	none
		F, 57	R	41	11.92/12.33*	GAD, MDD, OCD	NAcc	none
		F, 34	B-P	19	11.61/11.98*	GAD, MDD, OCD	NAcc	none
Fernandes Arroteia 2020 (Luxemburg) (Fernandes Arroteia et al., 2020)	1	F, 42	B-P	26	12.8*	MDD	NAcc	Erosion leading to infection over burr hole cap
Liu 2020 (Shanghai, China) (Liu et al., 2020)	28*	F, 22.8±4	13 R15 B-P	5 (3–10)	13.01(+-1.86)*	12 MDD 9 OCD 7 anxiety	NAcc	1/28 infection
Oudijn 2021 (Amsterdam, the Netherlands) (Oudijn et al., 2021)	4	F, 32	P	18	9.5/12.4*	MDD, GAD, PDnos	vALIC	(hypo)manic symptoms in 2 patients
		F, 39	P	24	10.2/11.2*	SUD, PDnos	vALIC	
		F, 33	P	19	10.6/13.4*	MDD, OCD, BPD	vALIC	
		F, 53	P	24	9.7/13.1*	PDnos	vALIC	
Lin 2021 (China) (Lin et al., 2021)	1	F, 18	R	4	13.28	OCD, MDD, GAD	NAcc	None+

continued

Table 21.2 *continued*

Study	Number of patients	Sex, age	AN subtype	Illness duration (years)	BMI historic low/preop* (kg/m^2)	Psychiatric comorbidity	Surgical target	Reported complications (excluding post-operative pain and fever <1 week post-op)
		F, 54	R	40	13.0	OCD	NAcc	None
		F, 26	R	13	12.0	OCD, MDD	NAcc	None
Scaife 2022 (Oxford, UK) (Scaife et al., 2022)	7	F, 28	R	14	13.0	OCD, MDD, GAD	NAcc	Facial tingling (stimulation dependent)
		M, 38	R	12	12.0	OCPD, MDD	NAcc	None
		F, 58	R	38	14.0	MDD	NAcc	none
		F, 25	R	15	13.0	OCD	NAcc	Nausea (stimulation dependent)
		F, 30	R	17	11.0	MDD	vALIC	
Lara-Almunia 2023 (Madrid, Spain) (Lara-Almunia et al., 2023)	1	F, 46	R	21	12.7	OCD, MDD, anxiety	NAcc	none

[+]went on to undergo capsulotomy given absence of effect of DBS;
*Individual data not available; AN subtype: B: binging; P: purging; B-P: binging-purging; R: restricting; BPD: borderline personality disorder; F: female; M: male; MDD: major depressive disorder; ns: not specified; OCD: obsessive compulsive disorder; OCPD: obsessive compulsive personality disorder; PDnos: personality disorder not otherwise specified; SUD: substance use disorder

one-year post-operatively, and obsessive/compulsive symptoms, anxiety, depression, and eating attitude improved (Manuelli et al., 2020; Vismara M et al., 2020). A 42-year-old patient from Luxemburg with AN underwent NAcc-DBS, and her BMI increased from 12.8 to 16.8 kg/m^2 one-year post-operatively, with no improvement in comorbid depression (Fernandes Arroteia et al., 2020). An 18-year-old woman underwent NAcc-DBS in China, with no associated improvement six-months post-operatively. A rescue anterior capsulotomy was conducted, after which her BMI normalized and her symptoms of AN improved (Lin et al., 2021). A 46-year-old woman with AN underwent NAcc-DBS in Spain, and her BMI increased from 13.2 to 17.3kg/m^2 and remained stable 50 months post-operatively, with improvements in anxiety, depression, obsessions/compulsions, and quality of life (Lara-Almunia et al., 2023).

Deep brain stimulation studies targeting SCC

A total of 27 patients who underwent SCC-DBS for (comorbid) AN have been reported in the literature; 23 from Canada and four from Spain (Table 21.3). All patients were female, with a median age of 35 years (range of 20 to 57 years), and a median disease duration of 20 years (range of seven to 35 years).

Case series and single case reports. The first report on SCC-DBS, from Montreal, Canada, was of a 52-year-old female with AN and it demonstrated that DBS was associated with remission of AN, and maintenance of normal BMI and improvement in eating disorder symptoms at a three-year follow-up (Israël et al., 2010). The Toronto group treated 22 patients with AN with longstanding and treatment refractory illness using SCC-DBS. They have described nine-months outcomes of the first six patients (Lipsman, Woodside, Giacobbe, Hamani, et al., 2013), one-year outcomes of 16 patients (Lipsman et al., 2017), and longer-term outcomes of 22 patients (of whom 15 had at least three years of follow-up data available, with a maximum of 6.8 years) (De Vloo et al., 2021). Mean BMI increased significantly from 14.0 kg/m^2 at baseline to 17.5 kg/m^2 and 16.3 kg/m^2 at one- and three-year follow-ups, respectively. Following three years of SCC-DBS, BMI had increased by more than 25% in four patients (27%) and more than 10% in nine patients (60%). BMI had decreased, by 4% at most, in two (13%) patients. At last follow-up, three (20%) patients had obtained and maintained a normal BMI (≥18.5 kg/m^2) for at least one year. Further, there was a significant improvement in obsessions and compulsions, depression, and anxiety after one year of SCC-DBS. However, none of these were sustained at long-term follow-up. Mean quality of life did not improve after one or three years post-SCC-DBS (De Vloo et al., 2021). In a study from Barcelona of four SCC-DBS patients, three were considered responders (≥10% increase in BMI), and had improved depression, although overall there was no significant improvement in BMI and the follow-up was limited to six months (Villalba Martínez et al., 2020).

Table 21.3 Overview of patients with anorexia nervosa (AN) who underwent subcallosal cingulate deep brain stimulation (SCC-DBS)

	Number of patients	Sex, age	AN subtype	Illness duration (years)	BMI historic low/preop* (kg/m²)	Psychiatric comorbidity	Reported Complications
Israel 2010 (Montreal, Canada) (Israël et al., 2010)	1	F, 52	P	35	14.4	MDD	None
Lipsman 2013 (Lipsman, Woodside, Giacobbe, Hamani, et al., 2013)/Lipsman 2017 (Lipsman et al., 2017)/De Vloo 2021 (De Vloo et al., 2021) (Toronto, Canada)	22	F, 24	BP	10	11.0	MDD, GAD	Medication overdose, pain, nausea
		F, 39	R	21	11.9	MDD, PTSD, SUD, OCD	Pancreatitis, hypo-K, pain, intraoperative panic attack, death (alcoholic ketoacidosis)
		F, 35	R	15	12.4	MDD, PTSD	Refeeding delirium, hypophosphatemia, battery depletion, increased lead impedance
		F, 40	R	10	13.1	MDD, PTSD	Worsening mood, pain, scalp sebaceous cyst
		F, 35	R	19	13.5	MDD, PTSD, GAD	QT prolongation, seizure, hypo-Na
		F, 57	R	27	13.0	None	Air embolism
		F, 20	R	8	11.2	MDD, GAD, OCD, BPD	None
		F, 32	BP	19	12.9	MDD, PTSD	Hypo-K, surgical site infection x2, battery depletion

		F, 26	BP	14	14.8	PTSD	Hypo-K, surgical site infection
		F, 30	R	19	10.6	OCD, MDD	Seizures, medication overdose, battery depletion
		F, 39	BP	24	10.3	PTSD, OCD, MDD	Surgical site infection
		F, 39	BP	29	7.2	GAD, PTSD	None
		F, 32	R	20	11.4	OCD, MDD, PTSD	Seizure, extension wire fracture, recharging difficulties
		F, 42	R	27	15.1	PTSD, MDD, GAD	Seizure, fracture
		F, 33	BP	20	10.0	MDD, OCD, BPD	Medication overdose, pain
		F, 31	R	8	13.7	None	Pain
		F, 29	BP	15	12.8	PTSD, OCD, MDD	Hypo-K, death (heart failure during purging?)
		F, 30	BP	15	14.5	MDD	None
		F, 35	R	21	10.1	MDD, PTSD	Battery depletion, hypo-K
		F, 33	BP	20	9.3	MDD, PTSD	None
		F, 38	R	23	11.7	None	None
		F, 23	R	7	12.6	MDD, BPD	None
Villalba Martinez 2020 (Barcelona, Spain) (Villalba Martínez et al., 2020)	4	F, 37	R	26	14.64/ 16.22*	MDD	None
		F, 45	R	16	10.06/ 10.94*	MDD	None
		F, 36	R	22	13.07/ 13.07*	MDD	Skin dehiscence (fiducial site)
		F, 33	R	21	9.64/ 11.57*	MDD	Skin infection (fiducial site)

AN subtype: B: binge eating; P: purging; B-P: binge eating/purging; R: restricting; BPD: borderline personality disorder: F: female; GAD: generalized anxiety disorder; MDD: major depressive disorder; OCD: obsessive compulsive disorder; PTSD: posttraumatic stress disorder; SUD: substance use disorder

Safety of deep brain stimulation for anorexia nervosa

The main surgical concern of performing DBS in this population is the risk of infection and skin erosion. With a published rate of eight out of 83 (10%), skin dehiscence and infection indeed seem more prevalent in DBS for AN than in DBS for movement disorders or OCD, where 5% is a commonly reported rate. No published patients died in the perioperative period. The Toronto group reported two deaths: one from presumed heart failure while purging 5.5 years post-operatively, and one from alcoholic ketoacidosis 2.5 years post-operatively. Unfortunately, the mortality rate in AN is high and these deaths may be consistent with illness progression. Data are insufficient to determine whether the mortality rate is higher with DBS.

Predictors of deep brain stimulation response

Several studies have examined possible factors which may predict a response to DBS. In the Oxford series, childhood OCD preceding AN appeared to be predictive of response to NAcc-DBS: all responders had OCD preceding the onset of AN, while this was only the case in one non-responder (Scaife et al., 2022). In the Shanghai series, the restricting subtype of AN appeared to be associated with a worse response to NAcc-DBS compared to the binge eating/purging subtype (Liu et al., 2020).

Which deep brain stimulation target is the best?

Due to differences in population (e.g., age, illness duration, AN subtype), comorbidities (mainly OCD, MDD, GAD, and PTSD), setting (quality of and access to conservative psychiatric care), study design, outcome scales, and length of follow-up, it is not possible to make a head-to-head comparison between the aforementioned studies. Some have suggested that SCC and BNST had the most favorable BMI outcomes (Hsu et al., 2022; McClelland, Bozhilova, Campbell, et al., 2013; Shaffer et al., 2023). One Spanish study was set up in such a way that NAcc or SCC were chosen individually based on the predominant psychiatric comorbidity (anxiety: NAcc; affective: SCC), or if inconclusive the subtype of AN (binge/purge: NAcc; restrictive: SCC). However, given the very small sample size (n=8), it is difficult to draw conclusions (Villalba Martínez et al., 2020).

Brain lesioning

Brain lesioning is the oldest neurosurgical treatment for AN, with reports dating back to the 1940s. In these historic case reports, mainly leucotomy, limbic leucotomy, and dorsomedial thalamotomy were applied, but due to inconsistencies in diagnostic standards, surgical procedures and outcome parameters, the clinical utility of these procedures remains inconclusive (Carmody & Vibber, 1952; Crisp & Kalucy, 1973; D'Andrea et al., 1974; Drury, 1950; Glazebrook & Prosen, 1956;

Heath et al., 1979; Morgan & Crisp, 2000; Sargant, 1951; Sifneos, 1952). Herein, we will focus on the modern era of brain lesioning for eating disorders, in which mainly anterior capsulotomy has been applied (Table 21.4).

Case series and single case reports

In 2011, the Leuven group published a single case in which lesioning of the BNST and anterior capsule was performed to treat OCD, after which not only OCD but also comorbid AN symptoms improved, including long-term normalization of BMI (Barbier et al., 2011). Wang and colleagues (2013) performed a lesioning procedure of the NAcc in six patients with AN, with normalization of BMI at one-year post-operatively, alongside improvement in OCD symptoms, anxiety, and depressive symptoms. In a single case report from Shanghai, a patient with AN who showed no response to NAcc-DBS was successfully treated by a "rescue" bilateral anterior capsulotomy (Lin et al., 2021). In the largest series on anterior capsulotomy in AN published so far, originating from Shanghai, 74 patients (a mean age of 25 years; a mean illness duration of five years) underwent bilateral radiofrequency capsulotomy. Post-operatively, the mean BMI increased from 13.6 kg/m^2 to 18.2 kg/m^2 at one year and 19.3 kg/m^2 after three years, with associated improvement in measures of depression, obsessions/compulsions, and anxiety (Liu et al., 2018). Although this study has shortcomings (Zanello et al., 2018) and cannot be easily generalized, it is by far the largest case series and the results are encouraging.

Safety of brain lesioning for anorexia nervosa

Overall, the complication rate in AN seems to be in line with the complications observed after capsulotomy for OCD, with mainly urinary incontinence, sleep disorders, and fatigue, which are usually transient, and disinhibition, lethargy, and memory disturbances, which may be long-lasting. It is noteworthy that there were no surgical infections over 82 published cases. In summary, capsulotomy represents a promising treatment option in AN, with remission in a large subset of patients in several studies from China, although the illness duration was often less than five years.

Possible mechanisms of DBS and brain lesioning

To examine possible mechanisms of NAcc-DBS, a group in China performed fluorodeoxyglucose-positron emission tomography (FDG-PET) scans preoperatively and at three-to-six months post NAcc-DBS. They noted a reduction of resting brain (hyper)metabolism in the lentiform nucleus, hippocampus, and frontal lobe (Zhang et al., 2013). In the Oxford cohort, a magnetoencephalogram study was performed pre-DBS, post-DBS, and following each phase of a randomized on/off comparison. An increase in alpha power and evoked power at latencies typically associated with visual processing, working memory, and contextual integration

Table 21.4 Brain lesioning studies in patients with anorexia nervosa (AN)

	N	Sex, age	AN subtype	Illness duration (years)	BMI historic low/baseline*	Psychiatric comorbidity	Surgical target	Reported Complications
Barbier 2011 (Belgium)	1	F, 38	R	24	9.1/13.1*	OCD	BNST/Anterior capsule	None
Wang 2013 (China)	6	F, 20 (19–25)	n.s.	3 (2–4)	13.4 (12.8–14.4)*	OCD (n=4), MDD (n=6), Anxiety (n=1)	NAcc	None (headaches and central fever in first post-op days)
Liu 2018 (China)	74	F, 25±7.9	n.s.	5.0 (3.7–6.0)	13.6±1.6*	OCD (n=19), MDD (n=32), Anxiety (n=15)	Anterior capsule	*Short term (<1 month)* Headache (all) Urinary incontinence (n=7) Sleep disorders (n=8) Fatigue (n=6) *Long term (>1 month)* Disinhibition (n=6) Memory loss (n=3) Lethargy (n=4).
Lin 2021 (China)	1	F, 18	R	4	13.3	OCD, MDD, GAD	Anterior capsule	Transient disinhibition

AN: anorexia nervosa; BNST: bed nucleus of the stria terminalis; F: female; GAD: generalized anxiety disorder; MDD: major depressive disorder; NAcc: nucleus accumbens; n.s.: not specified; OCD: obsessive compulsive disorder; R: restricting subtype was observed in ON compared to OFF sessions across all seven patients. In a reward and loss anticipation task-based functional MRI study among patients who underwent ventral ALIC DBS, the Amsterdam group observed a difference in the response of reward-related brain areas post-DBS, with a decrease in the right precuneus, right putamen, and right ventral striatum activation, and an increase in medial orbitofrontal cortex activation following DBS (Oudijn et al., 2023).

To examine mechanisms of SCC-DBS, the Toronto group performed FDG-PET scans preoperatively and six-months post-operatively. Following six months of SCC-DBS, voxel-wise analysis showed decreased brain metabolism in the anterior cingulate (Brodmann area [BA] right 24, 25), medial frontal gyrus (left BA 6, right BA 9), bilateral insula (BA13), left caudate, left claustrum, and left cerebellum (culmen, vermis, and declive). Metabolism was increased in posterior cortical regions, the right middle and right inferior temporal gyrus (BA 21, 20), left postcentral gyrus (BA 1), right precuneus (BA 7), right supramarginal gyrus (BA 40), right inferior parietal lobule (BA 40), and left cuneus (BA 19) (Lipsman, Woodside, Giacobbe, Hamani, et al., 2013). In another Toronto publication, multi-tensor tractography was used to compare patients with AN and controls, and the correlation between imaging and SCC-DBS response. Preoperative left fornix fractional anisotropy, a measure of white matter integrity, was related to post SCC-DBS improvement in quality of life, and right ALIC fractional anisotropy was related to post-operative improvement in depressive symptoms (Hayes et al., 2015).

To explore mechanisms of brain lesioning, the Belgian group reported FDG-PET scans acquired in a single case preoperatively and three-months post-operatively. When comparing the post-operative to preoperative tracer uptake, there was a strong metabolic decrease in the caudate nucleus and medial thalamus (Barbier et al., 2011). In summary, little is known about the mechanisms by which DBS and brain lesioning lead to symptom improvement.

Repetitive transcranial magnetic stimulation

rTMS for anorexia nervosa

Two studies suggest a beneficial effect of rTMS on mood and, to a lesser extent, on BMI in patients with AN (Table 21.5) (Choudhary et al., 2017; Kamolz et al., 2008; McClelland et al., 2016; Van den Eynde et al., 2013). In 2018, the TIARA trial, the first randomized controlled trial (RCT) of high-frequency rTMS applied to the left dorsolateral prefrontal cortex (DLPFC) was published (Dalton et al., 2018). In this trial, 34 patients with longstanding AN (more than three years) were randomized to either active (n=22) or sham (n=12) DLPFC-rTMS. At four months post-randomization, quality of life, mood, BMI, and eating disorder symptoms were significantly better in the active versus sham rTMS group. These improvements in the active rTMS group were largely maintained in an 18-month open label extension of the study, and in the sham rTMS group, improvements were

Table 21.5 Repetitive transcranial magnetic stimulation (rTMS) studies in patients with anorexia nervosa (AN)

Study	Number of patients	Number of sessions	TMS pulses per session	TMS target	Follow-up duration (mo)	Outcome
Kamolz 2008 (Germany) (Kamolz et al., 2008)	1	26	2000	DLPFC	5	BMI: from 12.4 to 16.0 kg/m^2 HAMD: from 28 to 11
Van den Eynde 2013 (UK) (Van den Eynde et al., 2013)	10	1	1000	Left DLPFC	0	Reduced feelings of anxiety. Improvement in "urge to exercise," "feeling fat" and "feeling full"
McClelland 2013 (UK) (McClelland, Bozhilova, Nestler, et al., 2013)	2	20	1000	Left DLPFC	1	BMI: from 15.7 to 14.7; and from 16.4 to 16.0 EDE: from 4.3 to 2.7; and from 4.1 to 3.4 DASS: from 23 to 18; and from 40 to 21
Dunlop 2015 (Canada) (Dunlop et al., 2015)	28	20–30	3000	Bilateral DMPFC	4	EDE: from 4.1 to 3.2 HAMD from 19.3 to 12.1 BDI: from 35.8 to 25.3
McClelland 2016 (UK) (McClelland et al., 2016)	49	1	1000	Left DLPFC	0	Improvement in "urge to restrict," "feeling fat" and "feeling full"
Choudhary 2017 (India) (Choudhary et al., 2017)	1	21	1000	Left DLPFC	2	BMI: from 10.9 to 18.6kg/m^2
Jaššová 2018 (Czech Republic) (Jaššová et al., 2018)	1	10	1500	Left DLPFC	24	BMI: from 13.2 to 22.9kg/m^2 Zung self-rating scale: from 70 to 70
Dalton 2018 (UK) (Dalton et al., 2018; Dalton, Lewis, et al., 2020)	34	20	1000	Left DLPFC	18	BMI: no significant increase weight recovery in 46% (TMS) vs. 9% (sham) DASS: improvement in TMS>sham EDE-Q: no significant change
Knyahnytska 2019 (Canada) (Knyahnytska et al., 2019)	8	42	2880	Insula	6	YBC-EDS, HDRS, MADRS, BDI, BAI: improved up to 6 months post rTMS
Woodside 2021 (Canada) (Woodside et al., 2021)	19	20–30	1000	Bilateral DMFPC	1.5	BMI: from 16.4 to 16.3kg/m^2 EDE weight and shape concerns: improvement BAI and BDI: improvement
Muratore 2021 (USA) (Muratore et al., 2021)	10	1	3000	Right DLPFC	0	Food Choice Task: reduction of fat avoidance after rTMS vs sham

BAI: Beck Anxiety Inventory; BDI: Beck Depression Inventory; BMI: Body Mass Index; DASS: Depression Anxiety Stress scale; DLPFC: dorsolateral prefrontal cortex; DMPFC: dorsomedial prefrontal cortex; EDE: Eating Disorder Examination; HAMD: Hamilton Depression Rating Scale also observed, likely due to the fact that 10 of the 12 patients decided to undergo active rTMS during this stage. Weight recovery (BMI >18.5kg/m^2) at 18 months post-randomization was achieved in 46% of the active rTMS group and 9% of the sham group, suggesting that substantial weight changes may take more time to occur than mood effects (Dalton, Lewis, et al., 2020). Subjectively, study participants reported an improvement in flexibility and relaxation around eating and food choices and this was confirmed in a Food Choice Task (Dalton, Foerde, et al., 2020). There were no significant changes in the cerebral blood flow in DLPFC, and there was a reduction in amygdala cerebral blood flow, which was associated with long term weight gain (Dalton et al., 2021).

In 2021, the Toronto group published a series of 19 patients with AN who received rTMS to the dorsomedial prefrontal cortex (DMPFC). They reported significant improvements in eating disorder symptoms, anxiety, and depressive mood versus baseline. Resting-state MRI functional connectivity data suggested that weak pre-rTMS functional connectivity between DMPFC and the right frontal pole and the left angular gyrus correlated with eating disorder symptom improvement post-rTMS (Woodside et al., 2021). All studies were conducted with an rTMS frequency of 10Hz.

rTMS for bulimia nervosa and binge-eating disorder

rTMS has also been used with patients with bulimia nervosa (BN) (Table 21.6), almost always targeting the left DLPFC. Despite encouraging results on binge eating and purging derived from case reports and small case series (Downar et al., 2012; Dunlop et al., 2015), two RCTs have not found group differences in binge eating and purging symptoms between active and sham DLPFC-rTMS (Gay et al., 2016; Walpoth et al., 2008). Although eating disorder symptoms did not improve, there may be an effect on inhibitory control and impulsivity (Guillaume et al., 2018). In the largest RCT on rTMS in BN conducted so far (n=38), self-reported food cravings and frequency of binge-eating episodes were significantly decreased with active versus sham rTMS, but all other measures did not differ between the active and sham rTMS group (Van den Eynde et al., 2010). Importantly, the follow-up terms were extremely short. Overall, rTMS for BN does not appear very promising. Evidence for rTMS for binge-eating disorder (BED) is limited to uncontrolled case reports in patients with BED and comorbid bipolar disorder (Sciortino et al., 2021).

Additional neuromodulatory approaches

Several additional non-invasive techniques have been studied in patients with eating disorders. In transcranial direct current stimulation (tDCS), scalp electrodes are applied and a weak direct current is delivered, either cathodal or anodal. In ECT, electrical current is used to induce a brief generalized tonic-clonic seizure

Table 21.6 Repetitive transcranial magnetic stimulation (rTMS) studies in patients with bulimia nervosa (BN)

Study	Number of patients	Number of sessions	TMS pulses per session	TMS target	Follow-up duration (mo)	Outcome
Hausmann 2004 (Austria) (Hausmann et al., 2004)	1	10	2000	Left DLPFC	0.5	Normalization of binge-purge behavior HAMD: −50%
Walpoth 2008 (Austria) (Walpoth et al., 2008)	14	15	2000	Left DLPFC	1	BDI, YBOCS, binge and vomiting frequency per day: no difference between TMS and sham group
Van den Eynde 2010 (UK) (Van den Eynde et al., 2010)	38	1	1000	Left DLPFC	0	Urge-to-eat VAS: significant decrease in TMS group Hunger, urge to binge, mood, tension, FCQ-S: no changes
Downar 2012 (Canada) (Downar et al., 2012)	1	20	3000	Bilateral DMPFC	2	HAMD: from 26 to 0 BDI: from 28 to 7 Binge-purge behavior: from 5 to 0 hours/d
Gay 2016 (France) (Gay et al., 2016)	47	10	1000	Left DLPFC	0.5	Binging, purging, craving, MADRS, duration of binging: no significant changes

BDI: Beck Depression Inventory; DASS: Depression Anxiety Stress scale; EDE: Eating Disorder Examination; FCQ-S: Food Craving Questionnaire-State; HAMD: Hamilton Depression Rating Scale; MADRS: Montgomery–Asberg Depression Rating Scale; VAS: Visual Analogue Scale; YBOCS: Yale-Brown Obsessive-Compulsive Scale under general anesthesia. ECT is an established treatment for MDD, bipolar disorder, and schizophrenia.

Transcranial direct current stimulation

A summary of published studies of tDCS in eating disorders is provided in Table 21.7. An Italian study of 23 adolescents with AN compared treatment-as-usual combined with 18 sessions of DLPFC tDCS (n=12) to treatment-as-usual combined with family therapy (n=11). Six weeks later, a single-blinded assessment revealed a BMI increase in the tDCS group (persisting one month later). Both groups showed improvement in mood, anxiety, and eating disorder severity, with no significant differences (Costanzo et al., 2018). In the 2019 French STAR study of 10 patients with AN who underwent 20 sessions of tDCS, similar improvements in AN psychopathology post-tDCS versus pre-tDCS were noted alongside a decrease in depression symptoms, but no change in functioning or physical activity (Strumila et al., 2019). In a Czech double-blind controlled trial, 43 female inpatients with moderate to severe AN were randomized to receive either 10 sessions of anodal tDCS treatment over the left DLPFC or sham tDCS. There were no between-group differences in BMI, EDE-Q, or depression scores (Baumann et al., 2021). In a study from London, UK, on BN, three sessions of DLPFC tDCS led to a decrease in self-reported urge to binge eat and an increase in self-regulatory control. In BED, an American 2016 sham-controlled RCT with a single session of tDCS demonstrated decreased craving for sweets, savory proteins, and an all-foods category in tDCS versus sham tDCS also decreased total and preferred food intake. In a sham-controlled RCT conducted in Tübingen, comparing 1 milliampere (mA) of current (n=16) and 2 mA (n=15) right DLPFC-tDCS versus sham tDCS, focusing on a food-modified antisaccade task, only the 2 mA group noted a significant decrease in self-reported binge-eating episodes (Max et al., 2021).

In a 2019 transdiagnostic study in 21 patients with AN, 13 patients with BN and two patients with an eating disorder not otherwise specified, tDCS to the medial prefrontal cortex modulated preferences for food and body images (Mattavelli et al., 2019).

Electroconvulsive therapy

Publications reporting ECT in eating disorders are limited (Table 21.8). There is one large retrospective case series from Israel of 30 adolescent female patients with AN (14 restricting type and 16 binge eating/purging type). BMI increased from 17.3±1.9 to 20.1±1.2 kg/m^2 following several months of ECT, alongside a subjective improvement in eating disorder and depression severity as rated by two independent psychiatrists (Shilton et al., 2020).

Noteworthy, only a small proportion of the published cases classify patients as having extreme AN. In 2023, Andersson and colleagues (2023) published a systematic review on neuromodulation for AN, including ECT, which was applied

Table 21.7 Transcranial direct current stimulation (tDCS) studies in patients with eating disorders

Study	Number of patients	Number of sessions	tDCS parameters	tDCS target	Groups	Outcome
AN						
Khedr 2014 (Egypt) (Khedr et al., 2014)	7	10	2 mA 25 min	+ left DLPFC - ?	1/tDCS 2/FBT	EDI Body dissatisfaction, interpersonal distrust, interoceptive awareness, ineffectiveness: significant decrease BDI: significant increase from 22.4 to 13.3
Costanzo 2018 (Italy) (Costanzo et al., 2018)	23	18	1 mA	+ left DLPFC - right DLPFC	1/tDCS 2/FBT	BMI, EDI-3, EAT-26, BUT, MASC, CDI: no difference between tDCS and FBT
Strumila 2019 (France) (Strumila et al., 2019)	10	20	2 mA	+ left DLPFC - right DLPFC	Single group (post vs. pre)	EDI: from 95 to 79 EDE-Q: from 3.7 to 3.1 BSQ: from 114 to 102 BDI: from 17 to 14 BMI, YMRS, MOCI, C-SSRS, WSAS, GAF, EDS-R: no difference
Baumann 2021 (Czech Republic) (Baumann et al., 2021)	43	1	2mA 30 min	+ left DLPFC - right orbitofrontal cortex	1/tDCS 2/sham	BMI, ZUNG, EDE-Q: no between-group differences

BN						
Kekic 2017 (UK) (Kekic et al., 2017)	39	3	2mA 20 min	1/+ left DLPFC - right DLFPC 2/+ right DLPFC - left DLPFC		Self-reported urge to binge eat: decrease Self-regulatory control: increase MEDCQ-R: reduction in group 1 vs. others
BED						
Burgess 2016 (USA) (Burgess et al., 2016)	30	1	2mA 20 min	+ right DLPFC - left DLPFC	tDCS vs sham in all patients	Total calories consumed: 75kcals fewer in tDCS vs. sham Consumption of preferred foods: 70kcals fewer in tDCS vs. sham Cravings for desserts: less in tDCS vs. sham Binge frequency: no effect
Max 2021 (Germany) (Max et al., 2021)	31	1	1–2 mA 20 min	+ right DLPFC - left deltoid muscle	1/1mA tDCS 2/2mA tDCS	Binge episodes: significantly fewer in 2 mA, no change in 1 mA group. Food inhibition in UPPS: improved in 2 mA
Giel 2023 (Giel et al., 2023) (Germany)	41	6	2 mA 15 min	+ right DLPFC - left deltoid muscle	1/tDCS+FRIC 2/sham+FRIC	EDE-Q and QoL scales: improved in both groups Binge eating frequency: greater reduction in tDCS + FRIC vs. sham + FRIC group

BDI: Beck Depression Inventory; BSQ: The Body Shape Questionnaire; DLPFC: dorsolateral prefrontal cortex; EDI: Eating Disorders Inventory; EDE-Q: Eating Disorder Examination Questionnaire; FBT: family-based therapy; FRIC: food-related inhibitory control training; mA: milliampere; MEDCQ-R: Mizes Eating Disorder Cognition Questionnaire-Revised; UPPS: Impulsive Behavior Scale in 46 patients, but only three of the 46 patients were classified as extreme AN. A minimal average increase in BMI of 0.4kg/m^2 and consistent reduction in depression were reported (Andersson et al., 2023). There is only one published case of BED who underwent ECT, with long-lasting beneficial effects (Rapinesi et al., 2013). Overall, the results in terms of eating disorder symptoms and BMI have been poorly described and appear to be highly variable and not very promising.

Alternative Perspectives

Fierce ethical debates have always been part of neurosurgery for psychiatric disorders. Currently, there is general agreement that it is ethically justifiable to perform neurosurgery for psychiatric disorders if clinicians agree that there is a diseased state which is refractory to less invasive treatment modalities, and in the context of a clinical study until evidence has been obtained from randomized trials (i.e., Level 1 evidence). This has been discussed extensively in the context of the neurosurgical treatment for OCD (Grant et al., 2014). For neurosurgical treatment of AN, some have questioned whether individuals with AN can provide informed consent for neurosurgery. In part, this stems from the experimental nature of DBS, with unknown risks and benefits, both with respect to the invasive procedure and with respect to changes to mood or behavior. Additionally, some have proposed that individuals with AN may prefer DBS or lesioning over alternative renourishment options (such as tube feeding, and, in some cases, involuntary tube feeding). In this case, the consent for surgical treatment is complicated by the possibility that the illness drives the patient to avoid of a treatment with known benefit (Maslen et al., 2015; Park et al., 2017; Wu et al., 2024). One group suggested these risks can be mitigated through the inclusion of an independent qualified clinical ethicist and/or clinician to assess the patient's capacity and independently advocate for the patient (Park et al., 2017).

Questions have also arisen about the optimal study design for DBS and other neurosurgical treatments for AN. A RCT design with a sham stimulation control group may be considered unethical when AN is severe and possibly life-threatening (which is sometimes an inclusion criterion) (Karaszewska et al., 2022). Most studies have used within-subject comparisons rather than parallel group designs to assess the effect of DBS on an outcome. Another possibility for DBS is a blinded ON/OFF crossover design. With careful follow-up, this design can be used even among severely ill patients (Scaife et al., 2022). A challenge for before/after design is the reliance on preoperative assessments, which may vary substantially over time due to the waxing and waning illness course and treatments. Challenges for crossover design are that the stimulation settings must be optimized first, the trial duration needs to be sufficiently long to detect slow changes, and there needs to be a clear indicator to turn the stimulation back on (e.g., the explicit wish of the patient) to be ethically sound. One group has questioned whether DBS and

Table 21.8 Electroconvulsive therapy (ECT) studies in patients with eating disorders

Study	Number of patients	Patient characteristics (sex, age)	AN subtype	Psychiatric comorbidities	Number of sessions	Outcome
Davis 1961 (Davis, 1961)	1	F, 12	R	MDD	12	Weight: from 26.3 to 32.0kg
Bernstein 1964 (Bernstein, 1964)	1	F, 19	n.s.	MDD, SZ	21	Weight: from 34.0 to 41.3kg
Bernstein 1972 (Bernstein, 1972)	1	F, 94	R	SZ	5	Weight: +2.3kg
Ferguson 1993 (Ferguson, 1993)	3	F, 23 F, 35 F, 42	n.s.	None MDD MDD	16 8 11	Weight: no change Weight: +20 lbs Weight: +18 lbs
Ben 1996 (Bek & Hotujak, 1996)	2	F,16–22	n.s.	n.s.	n.s.	Unclear (total study 8 patients, of whom 2 had ECT)
Hill 2001 (Hill et al., 2001)	1	F, 77	R	MDD	9	Weight: from 40 to 42 kg
Poutanen 2009 (Poutanen et al., 2009)	1	F, 21	BP	MDD	45	BMI: from 15.0 to 16.4 kg/m^2 BDI: from 52 to 43
Andrews 2014 (Andrews et al., 2014)	1	F, 17	BP	MDD, NSSI	31	Weight stabilization
Andersen 2017 (Andersen et al., 2017)	1	F, 14	R	MDD, GAD	22	Weight: from 50.1 to 63.7 kg CDRS-R: from 43 to 17
Sağlam 2018 (Sağlam et al., 2018)	1	M, 24	BP	MDD, OCD	12	BMI: from 16.5 to 20.5 kg/m^2 HMDRS: from 23 to 10

continued

Table 21.8 *continued*

Study	Number of patients	Patient characteristics (sex, age)	AN subtype	Psychiatric comorbidities	Number of sessions	Outcome
Pacillo 2019 (Pacilio et al., 2019)	1	F, 30	n.s.	MDD	11	BMI: from 15.2 to 15.7 kg/m^2 MADRS: from 33 to 10
Naguy 2019 (Naguy et al., 2019)	1	F, 16	n.s.	PDnos	6	Weight: +4 kg
Duriez 2020 (Duriez et al., 2020)	1	F, 21	n.s.	none	10	HADS: from 10 to 9
Shilton 2020 (Shilton et al., 2020)	30	F, 16.1±1.6	14R 16BP	MDD (n=30), OCD (n=11), GAD (n=7), PTSD (n=6), NSSI (n=28)	16.7±6.8	BMI: from 17.3±1.9 to 20.1±1.2 kg/m^2 CGI-S: from 6.0±0.5 to 3.7±1.0

BDI: Beck Depression Inventory; CDRS-R: Children's Depression Rating Scale-Revised; CGI-S: Clinical Global Impression Scale; F: female; GAD: generalized anxiety disorder; HADS: Hospital Anxiety and Depression Score; HMDRS: Hamilton Depression Rating Scale; M: male; MADRS: Montgomery Asberg Depression Rating Scale; MDD: major depressive disorder; n.s.: not specified; NSSI: non-suicidal self-injury; OCD: obsessive compulsive disorder; PDnos: personality disorder not otherwise specified; PTSD: posttraumatic stress disorder; SZ: schizophrenia lesioning procedures can both be offered at this stage (Pugh et al., 2018). Whilst lesioning carries the negative stigma of psychosurgery from the 1950s to the 1970s, DBS has a more positive connotation, mainly due to its relative reversibility and adjustability. DBS also offers the option to carry out blinded ON/OFF comparisons which is a scientifically valid method to gather high-class evidence without exposing patients to sham surgeries. However, DBS increases the risk of hardware-related complications. Further, it is possible that DBS and lesioning procedures have different safety and efficacy profiles, as illustrated by a case report of a patient who was successfully treated with capsulotomy after not responding to NAcc-DBS (Lin et al., 2021).

Criticism of DBS also comes from the variability of critical study design elements across studies. Participant inclusion criteria have varied by site. All recent European and North American studies of neuromodulation for eating disorders have focused exclusively on adult patients with longstanding AN (for more than five years and often more than 10 years). Several Chinese studies have described neuromodulation with adolescent patients, often with a disease duration of one or two years (Liu et al., 2018, 2020; Wu et al., 2013). This group may have a higher likelihood of remission without neuromodulation. Further, there is no consensus on the severity or refractoriness of AN required for inclusion (Oudijn et al., 2021), as illustrated in Table 21.1. Consequently, it is impossible to perform a meta-analysis of outcomes in a scientifically sound fashion. It is difficult to determine whether DBS should be considered as a last resort; that is, is DBS only for patients for whom every other possible treatment option has been tried, or can it be tried earlier in the treatment pathway (Park et al., 2017)? An international consensus on severity grading and definition of refractoriness could align patient characteristics in future studies.

Challenges in the interpretation of findings also come from variability in definition of outcome and in assessment tools used. In modern neuromodulation techniques, the programming space is almost indefinite. In the absence of symptoms that respond immediately and reliably to stimulation, such as in movement disorders, neuromodulation programming in eating disorders is often based on predefined arbitrary programming paradigms and/or trial-and-error adjustments with very regular follow-up visits. This complicates the interpretation of findings, and studies should be as clear as possible on the choices made during programming. A wide range of outcome scales have been used across the published studies. Most studies have assessed BMI, obsessive/compulsive symptoms, and depression. It is unclear which measures are the best choices. Optimal scales for measurement of depressive symptoms in the context of AN is not clear. This is particularly important given the effect of DBS on depression (Ali et al., 2021; Andersson et al., 2023; Dêbska et al., 2011). Self-report questionnaires are, for example, susceptible to recall bias and the volatile and time-dependent nature of some eating disorder symptoms are not taken into account with these scales. BMI in the context of neurosurgery has several complexities. One is that the pre-treatment BMI may need to be considered as the BMI outside of a structured/medical setting (in some cases medical hospitalization is used to increase BMI pre-operatively; Scaife et al., 2022). In addition, the post-treatment effect evolves over time. Furthermore, BMI has limitations as an outcome measure for this severely ill group because it may not reflect some important quality of life changes. No international consensus has been reached on the definition of response to treatment or remission in AN in general, and of response to DBS in AN in particular. This limits research into predictors for optimal response, counselling of patients, and benchmarking between treatment options (Karaszewska et al., 2022). Clarification of a core outcome set, with input from specialists and patient partners, would be of great value for future studies, not only to ascertain relevant outcome measures, but also to allow the creation of multi-center registries and meta-analyses of publications (Andersson et al., 2023).

One perspective on the use of DBS, neurosurgery, and neuromodulation is that it is part of a treatment in which the adjuvant psychotherapy may be important. Yet studies of DBS have not standardized or evaluated the post-surgical treatments. It remains to be elucidated whether a potentially beneficial effect of neuromodulation may be (partially) due to improved response to psychotherapeutic interventions. Hence, a clear description of the psychotherapeutic treatment offered along with neuromodulation is an important feature of future studies on neuromodulation for eating disorders (Karaszewska et al., 2022).

Implications

In patients with eating disorders who are resistant to conventional psychotherapy, various neuromodulation techniques (especially rTMS, tDCS, and capsulotomy, with DBS providing more variable results) appear to be effective not only in increasing BMI but also in improving the associated psychiatric symptoms (mainly anxiety, depression, and obsessive-compulsive symptoms). Nevertheless, it seems that none of these neuromodulation treatments are currently considered as standard of care. To ultimately determine the role of neurosurgical neuromodulation treatments in eating disorders, close collaboration between psychiatrists and neurosurgeons will be crucial, alongside several improvements in study design. For now, we suggest that all these neurosurgical treatments take place in the context of a clinical study or, at least, a prospective registry under strong ethical supervision.

References

Ali, A. M., Alkhamees, A. A., Hori, H., Kim, Y., & Kunugi, H. (2021). The depression anxiety stress scale 21: Development and validation of the depression anxiety stress scale 8-item in psychiatric patients and the general public for easier mental health measurement in a post COVID-19 world. *International Journal of Environmental Research and Public Health, 18*(19), 10142. https://doi.org/10.3390/ijerph181910142

Andersen, L., LaRosa, C., & Gih, D. E. (2017). Reexamining the role of electroconvulsive therapy in anorexia nervosa in adolescents. *Journal of ECT*, *33*(4), 294–296. https://doi.org/10.1097/YCT.0000000000000418

Andersson, P., Jamshidi, E., Ekman, C.-J., Tedroff, K., Björkander, J., Sjögren, M., Lundberg, J., Jokinen, J., & Desai Boström, A. E. (2023). Anorexia nervosa with comorbid severe depression: A systematic scoping review of brain stimulation treatments. *Journal of ECT*, *39*(4), 227–234. https://doi.org/10.1097/YCT.0000000000000922

Andrews, J. T., Seide, M., Guarda, A. S., Redgrave, G. W., & Coffey, D. B. J. (2014). Electroconvulsive therapy in an adolescent with severe major depression and anorexia nervosa. *Journal of Child and Adolescent Psychopharmacology*, *24*(2), 94–98. https://doi.org/10.1089/cap.2014.2422

Barbier, J., Gabriëls, L., van Laere, K., & Nuttin, B. (2011). Successful anterior capsulotomy in comorbid anorexia nervosa and obsessive-compulsive disorder: Case report. *Neurosurgery*, *69*(3), E745-751; discussion E751. https://doi.org/10.1227/NEU.0b013e31821964d2

Baumann, S., Mareš, T., Albrecht, J., Anders, M., Vochosková, K., Hill, M., Bulant, J., Yamamotová, A., Štastný, O., Novák, T., Holanová, P., Lambertová, A., & Papežová, H. (2021). Effects of transcranial direct current stimulation treatment for anorexia nervosa. *Frontiers in Psychiatry*, 12. https://doi.org/10.3389/fpsyt.2021.717255

Bek, R., & Hotujak, L. (1996). Clinical characteristics of female patients suffering from anorexia nervosa. *Soc. Psihijat.*, 24, 159–161.

Bernstein, I. C. (1964). Anorexia nervosa treated successfully with electroshock therapy and subsequently followed by pregnancy. *American Journal of Psychiatry*, *120*, 1023–1024. https://doi.org/10.1176/ajp.120.10.1023

Bernstein, I. C. (1972). Anorexia nervosa, 94-year-old woman treated with electroshock. *Minnesota Medicine*, *55*(6), 552–553.

Blomstedt, P., Naesström, M., & Bodlund, O. (2017). Deep brain stimulation in the bed nucleus of the stria terminalis and medial forebrain bundle in a patient with major depressive disorder and anorexia nervosa. *Clinical Case Reports*, *5*(5), 679–684. https://doi.org/10.1002/ccr3.856

Burgess, E. E., Sylvester, M. D., Morse, K. E., Amthor, F. R., Mrug, S., Lokken, K. L., Osborn, M. K., Soleymani, T., & Boggiano, M. M. (2016). Effects of transcranial direct current stimulation (tDCS) on binge-eating disorder. *International Journal of Eating Disorders*, *49*(10), 930–936. https://doi.org/10.1002/eat.22554

Carmody, J. T. B., & Vibber, F. L. (1952). Anorexia nervosa treated by prefrontal lobotomy. *Annals of Internal Medicine*, *36*(2:2), 647–652. https://doi.org/10.7326/0003-4819-36-2-647

Choudhary, P., Roy, P., & Kumar Kar, S. (2017). Improvement of weight and attitude towards eating behaviour with high frequency rTMS augmentation in anorexia nervosa. *Asian Journal of Psychiatry*, *28*, 160. https://doi.org/10.1016/j.ajp.2017.05.010

Costanzo, F., Menghini, D., Maritato, A., Castiglioni, M. C., Mereu, A., Varuzza, C., Zanna, V., & Vicari, S. (2018). New treatment perspectives in adolescents with anorexia nervosa: The efficacy of non-invasive brain-directed treatment. *Frontiers in Behavioral Neuroscience*, 12. https://doi.org/10.3389/fnbeh.2018.00133

Crisp, A. H., & Kalucy, R. S. (1973). The effect of leucotomy in intractable adolescent weight phobia (primary anorexia nervosa). *Postgraduate Medical Journal*, *49*(578), 883–893. https://doi.org/10.1136/pgmj.49.578.883

Dalton, B., Bartholdy, S., McClelland, J., Kekic, M., Rennalls, S. J., Werthmann, J., Carter, B., O'Daly, O. G., Campbell, I. C., David, A. S., Glennon, D., Kern, N., & Schmidt, U. (2018). Randomised controlled feasibility trial of real versus sham repetitive transcranial magnetic stimulation treatment in adults with severe and enduring anorexia nervosa: The TIARA study. *BMJ Open*, *8*(7), e021531. https://doi.org/10.1136/bmjopen-2018-021531

Dalton, B., Foerde, K., Bartholdy, S., McClelland, J., Kekic, M., Grycuk, L., Campbell, I. C., Schmidt, U., & Steinglass, J. E. (2020). The effect of repetitive transcranial magnetic stimulation on food choice-related self-control in patients with severe, enduring anorexia nervosa. *International Journal of Eating Disorders*, *53*(8), 1326–1336. https://doi.org/10.1002/eat.23267

Dalton, B., Lewis, Y. D., Bartholdy, S., Kekic, M., McClelland, J., Campbell, I. C., & Schmidt, U. (2020). Repetitive transcranial magnetic stimulation treatment in severe, enduring anorexia nervosa: An open longer-term follow-up. *European Eating Disorders Review*, *28*(6), 773–781. https://doi.org/10.1002/erv.2766

Dalton, B., Maloney, E., Rennalls, S. J., Bartholdy, S., Kekic, M., McClelland, J., Campbell, I. C., Schmidt, U., & O'Daly, O. G. (2021). A pilot study exploring the effect of repetitive transcranial magnetic stimulation (rTMS) treatment on cerebral blood flow and its relation to clinical outcomes in severe enduring anorexia nervosa. *Journal of Eating Disorders, 9*(1). https://doi.org/10.1186/s40337-021-00420-w

D'Andrea, F., De Divitiis, E., Megna, G., De Giacomo, P., & Pierri, G. (1974). [Remission of "mental anorexia" following stereotaxic thalamolysis (previously resistant to other therapies) (author's transl)]. *Rivista Di Patologia Nervosa E Mentale, 95*(5), 579–590.

Davis, H. K. (1961). Anorexia nervosa: Treatment with hypnosis and ECT. *Diseases of the Nervous System, 22*, 627–631.

De Vloo, P., Lam, E., Elias, G. J., Boutet, A., Sutandar, K., Giacobbe, P., Woodside, D. B., Lipsman, N., & Lozano, A. (2021). Long-term follow-up of deep brain stimulation for anorexia nervosa. *Journal of Neurology, Neurosurgery, and Psychiatry, 92*(10), 1135–1136. https://doi.org/10.1136/jnnp-2020-325711

Dêbska, E., Janas, A., Bañczyk, W., & Janas-Kozik, M. (2011). Depression or depressiveness in patients diagnosed with anorexia nervosa and bulimia nervosa—Pilot research. *Psychiatria Danubina, 23*(Suppl 1), S87–90.

Downar, J., Sankar, A., Giacobbe, P., Woodside, B., & Colton, P. (2012). Unanticipated rapid remission of refractory bulimia nervosa, during high-dose repetitive transcranial magnetic stimulation of the dorsomedial prefrontal cortex: A case report. *Frontiers in Psychiatry*, 3. https://doi.org/10.3389/fpsyt.2012.00030

Drury, M. O. (1950). An emergency leucotomy. *British Medical Journal, 2*(4679), 609. https://doi.org/10.1136/bmj.2.4679.609

Dunlop, K., Woodside, B., Lam, E., Olmsted, M., Colton, P., Giacobbe, P., & Downar, J. (2015). Increases in frontostriatal connectivity are associated with response to dorsomedial repetitive transcranial magnetic stimulation in refractory binge/purge behaviors. *NeuroImage: Clinical, 8*, 611–618. https://doi.org/10.1016/j.nicl.2015.06.008

Duriez, P., Maatoug, R., & Verbe, J. (2020). Failure of electroconvulsive therapy to improve anorexia nervosa in the absence of other psychiatric comorbidities: A case report. *Journal of ECT, 36*(4), e44–e45. https://doi.org/10.1097/YCT.0000000000000678

Ferguson, J. M. (1993). The use of electroconvulsive therapy in patients with intractable anorexia nervosa. *International Journal of Eating Disorders, 13*(2), 195–201. https://doi.org/10.1002/1098-108x(199303)13:2<195::aid-eat2260130207>3.0.co;2-5

Fernandes Arroteia, I., Husch, A., Baniasadi, M., & Hertel, F. (2020). Impressive weight gain after deep brain stimulation of nucleus accumbens in treatment-resistant bulimic anorexia nervosa. *BMJ Case Reports, 13*(11), e239316. 10.1136/bcr-2020-239316

Gay, A., Jaussent, I., Sigaud, T., Billard, S., Attal, J., Seneque, M., Galusca, B., Van Den Eynde, F., Massoubre, C., Courtet, P., & Guillaume, S. (2016). A lack of clinical effect of high-frequency rTMS to dorsolateral prefrontal cortex on bulimic symptoms: A randomised, double-blind trial. *European Eating Disorders Review, 24*(6), 474–481. https://doi.org/10.1002/erv.2475

Giel, K. E., Schag, K., Max, S. M., Martus, P., Zipfel, S., Fallgatter, A. J., & Plewnia, C. (2023). Inhibitory control training enhanced by transcranial direct current stimulation to reduce binge eating episodes: Findings from the randomized phase II ACCElect trial. *Psychotherapy and Psychosomatics, 92*(2), 101–112. https://doi.org/10.1159/000529117

Glazebrook, A. J., & Prosen, H. (1956). Compulsive neurosis with cachexia. *Canadian Medical Association Journal, 75*(1), 40–42.

Grant, R. A., Halpern, C. H., Baltuch, G. H., O'Reardon, J. P., & Caplan, A. (2014). Ethical considerations in deep brain stimulation for psychiatric illness. *Journal of Clinical Neuroscience, 21*(1), 1–5. https://doi.org/10.1016/j.jocn.2013.04.004

Guillaume, S., Gay, A., Jaussent, I., Sigaud, T., Billard, S., Attal, J., Seneque, M., Galusca, B., Thiebaut, S., Massoubre, C., & Courtet, P. (2018). Improving decision-making and cognitive impulse control in bulimia nervosa by rTMS: An ancillary randomized controlled study. *International Journal of Eating Disorders, 51*(9), 1103–1106. https://doi.org/10.1002/eat.22942

Hausmann, A., Mangweth, B., Walpoth, M., Hoertnagel, C., Kramer-Reinstadler, K., Rupp, C. I., & Hinterhuber, H. (2004). Repetitive transcranial magnetic stimulation (rTMS) in the double-blind treatment of a depressed patient suffering from bulimia nervosa: A case report. *International Journal of Neuropsychopharmacology, 7*(3), 371–373. https://doi.org/10.1017/S1461145704004420

Hayes, D. J., Lipsman, N., Chen, D. Q., Woodside, D. B., Davis, K. D., Lozano, A. M., & Hodaie, M. (2015). Subcallosal cingulate connectivity in anorexia nervosa patients differs from healthy controls: A multi-tensor tractography study. *Brain Stimulation, 8*(4), 758–768. https://doi.org/10.1016/j.brs.2015.03.005

Heath, R., Llewellyn, R., & Rouchell, A. (1979). Brain mechanisms in psychiatric illness: Rationale for and results of treatment with cerebellar stimulation. In E. R. Hitchcock, H. Ballantine, & B. A. Meyerson (Eds.), *Modern concepts in psychiatric surgery* (pp. 85–93). Elsevier.

Hemphill, R. E. (1944). Return of virility after prefrontal leucotomy: With enlargement of gonads. *Lancet, 244*(6315), 345–346. https://doi.org/10.1016/S0140-6736(00)42682-6

Hill, R., Haslett, C., & Kumar, S. (2001). Anorexia nervosa in an elderly woman. *Australian and New Zealand Journal of Psychiatry, 35*(2), 246–248. https://doi.org/10.1046/j.1440-1614.2001.00871.x

Hsu, T. I., Nguyen, A., Gupta, N., Godbole, N., Perisetla, N., Hatter, M. J., Beyer, R. S., Bui, N. E., Jagan, J., Yang, C., Gendreau, J., Brown, N. J., & Oh, M. (2022). Effectiveness of deep brain stimulation in treatment of anorexia nervosa and obesity: A systematic review. *World Neurosurgery, 168*, 179–189. https://doi.org/10.1016/j.wneu.2022.09.114

Israël, M., Steiger, H., Kolivakis, T., McGregor, L., & Sadikot, A. F. (2010). Deep brain stimulation in the subgenual cingulate cortex for an intractable eating disorder. *Biological Psychiatry, 67*(9), e53–54. https://doi.org/10.1016/j.biopsych.2009.11.016

Jaššová, K., Albrecht, J., Papežová, H., & Anders, M. (2018). Repetitive transcranial magnetic stimulation (rTMS) treatment of depression and anxiety in a patient with anorexia nervosa. *Medical Science Monitor, 24*, 5279–5281. https://doi.org/10.12659/MSM.908250

Kamolz, S., Richter, M. M., Schmidtke, A., & Fallgatter, A. J. (2008). [Transcranial magnetic stimulation for comorbid depression in anorexia]. *Der Nervenarzt, 79*(9), 1071–1073. https://doi.org/10.1007/s00115-008-2537-8

Karaszewska, D., Cleintuar, P., Oudijn, M., Lok, A., van Elburg, A., Denys, D., & Mocking, R. (2022). Efficacy and safety of deep brain stimulation for treatment-refractory anorexia nervosa: A systematic review and meta-analysis. *Translational Psychiatry, 12*(1), 333. https://doi.org/10.1038/s41398-022-02102-w

Kekic, M., McClelland, J., Bartholdy, S., Boysen, E., Musiat, P., Dalton, B., Tiza, M., David, A. S., Campbell, I. C., & Schmidt, U. (2017). Single-session transcranial direct current stimulation temporarily improves symptoms, mood, and self-regulatory control in bulimia nervosa: A randomised controlled trial. *PLOS ONE, 12*(1), e0167606. https://doi.org/10.1371/journal.pone.0167606

Khedr, E. M., Elfetoh, N. A., Ali, A. M., & Noamany, M. (2014). Anodal transcranial direct current stimulation over the dorsolateral prefrontal cortex improves anorexia nervosa: A pilot study. *Restorative Neurology and Neuroscience, 32*(6), 789–797. https://doi.org/10.3233/RNN-140392

Knyahnytska, Y. O., Blumberger, D. M., Daskalakis, Z. J., Zomorrodi, R., & Kaplan, A. S. (2019). Insula H-coil deep transcranial magnetic stimulation in severe and enduring anorexia nervosa (SE-AN): A pilot study. *Neuropsychiatric Disease and Treatment, 15*, 2247–2256. https://doi.org/10.2147/NDT.S207630

Lara-Almunia, M., Aguirre-Orue, I., Roset-Ferrer, C., Bermudez-Andion, C., Alvarez, A. S., Mas-Bonet, A., Miguel-Pueyo, J., & Hernandez-Vicente, J. (2023). Refractory anorexia nervosa in adulthood and nucleus accumbens deep brain stimulation. *Surgical Neurology International, 14*, 14. https://doi.org/10.25259/SNI_1112_2022

Lin, Z., Dai, L., Zhang, C., Li, D., & Sun, B. (2021). Rescue anterior capsulotomy after failure of nucleus accumbens deep brain stimulation in anorexia nervosa: A case report. *Stereotactic and Functional Neurosurgery, 99*(6), 491–495. https://doi.org/10.1159/000517105

Lin, Z., Zhang, C., Zhang, Y., Dai, L., Voon, V., Li, D., & Sun, B. (2020). Deep brain stimulation telemedicine programming during the COVID-19 pandemic: Treatment of patients with psychiatric disorders. *Neurosurgical Focus, 49*(6), E11. https://doi.org/10.3171/2020.9.FOCUS20666

Lipsman, N., Lam, E., Volpini, M., Sutandar, K., Twose, R., Giacobbe, P., Sodums, D. J., Smith, G. S., Woodside, D. B., & Lozano, A. M. (2017). Deep brain stimulation of the subcallosal cingulate for treatment-refractory anorexia nervosa: 1 year follow-up of an open-label trial. *Lancet. Psychiatry, 4*(4), 285–294. https://doi.org/10.1016/S2215-0366(17)30076-7

Lipsman, N., Woodside, D. B., Giacobbe, P., Hamani, C., Carter, J. C., Norwood, S. J., Sutandar, K., Staab, R., Elias, G., Lyman, C. H., Smith, G. S., & Lozano, A. M. (2013). Subcallosal cingulate deep brain stimulation for treatment-refractory anorexia nervosa: A phase 1 pilot trial. *Lancet, 381*(9875), 1361–1370. https://doi.org/10.1016/S0140-6736(12)62188-6

Lipsman, N., Woodside, D. B., Giacobbe, P., & Lozano, A. M. (2013). Neurosurgical treatment of anorexia nervosa: Review of the literature from leucotomy to deep brain stimulation. *European Eating Disorders Review, 21*(6), 428–435. https://doi.org/10.1002/erv.2246

Liu, W., Li, D., Sun, F., Zhang, X., Wang, T., Zhan, S., Pan, Y., Huang, P., Jin, H., Li, Y., & Sun, B. (2018). Long-term follow-up study of mri-guided bilateral anterior capsulotomy in patients with refractory anorexia nervosa. *Neurosurgery, 83*(1), 86–92. https://doi.org/10.1093/neuros/nyx366

Liu, W., Zhan, S., Li, D., Lin, Z., Zhang, C., Wang, T., Pan, S., Zhang, J., Cao, C., Jin, H., Li, Y., & Sun, B. (2020). Deep brain stimulation of the nucleus accumbens for treatment-refractory anorexia nervosa: A long-term follow-up study. *Brain Stimulation, 13*(3), 643–649. https://doi.org/10.1016/j.brs.2020.02.004

Manuelli, M., Franzini, A., Galentino, R., Bidone, R., Dell'Osso, B., Porta, M., Servello, D., & Cena, H. (2020). Changes in eating behavior after deep brain stimulation for anorexia nervosa. A case study. *Eating and Weight Disorders, 25*(5), 1481–1486. https://doi.org/10.1007/s40519-019-00742-4

Maslen, H., Pugh, J., & Savulescu, J. (2015). The ethics of deep brain stimulation for the treatment of anorexia nervosa. *Neuroethics, 8*(3), 215–230. https://doi.org/10.1007/s12152-015-9240-9

Mattavelli, G., Gallucci, A., Schiena, G., D'Agostino, A., Sassetti, T., Bonora, S., Bertelli, S., Benetti, A., Tugnoli, E., Ruggiero, G. M., Sassaroli, S., Romero Lauro, L., Gambini, O., & Papagno, C. (2019). Transcranial direct current stimulation modulates implicit attitudes towards food in eating disorders. *International Journal of Eating Disorders, 52*(5), 576–581. https://doi.org/10.1002/eat.23046

Max, S. M., Plewnia, C., Zipfel, S., Giel, K. E., & Schag, K. (2021). Combined antisaccade task and transcranial direct current stimulation to increase response inhibition in binge eating disorder. *European Archives of Psychiatry and Clinical Neuroscience, 271*(1), 17–28. https://doi.org/10.1007/s00406-020-01164-5

McClelland, J., Bozhilova, N., Campbell, I., & Schmidt, U. (2013). A systematic review of the effects of neuromodulation on eating and body weight: Evidence from human and animal studies. *European Eating Disorders Review, 21*(6), 436–455. https://doi.org/10.1002/erv.2256

McClelland, J., Bozhilova, N., Nestler, S., Campbell, I. C., Jacob, S., Johnson-Sabine, E., & Schmidt, U. (2013). Improvements in symptoms following neuronavigated repetitive transcranial magnetic stimulation (rTMS) in severe and enduring anorexia nervosa: findings from two case studies. *European Eating Disorders Review, 21*(6), 500–506. https://doi.org/10.1002/erv.2266

McClelland, J., Kekic, M., Campbell, I. C., & Schmidt, U. (2016). Repetitive transcranial magnetic stimulation (rTMS) treatment in enduring anorexia nervosa: A case series. *European Eating Disorders Review, 24*(2), 157–163. https://doi.org/10.1002/erv.2414

McLaughlin, N. C. R., Didie, E. R., Machado, A. G., Haber, S. N., Eskandar, E. N., & Greenberg, B. D. (2013). Improvements in anorexia symptoms after deep brain stimulation for intractable obsessive-compulsive disorder. *Biological Psychiatry, 73*(9), e29-31. https://doi.org/10.1016/j.biopsych.2012.09.015

Morgan, J. F., & Crisp, A. H. (2000). Use of leucotomy for intractable anorexia nervosa: A long-term follow-up study. *International Journal of Eating Disorders, 27*(3), 249–258. https://doi.org/10.1002/(SICI)1098-108X(200004)27:3<249::AID-EAT1>3.0.CO;2-K

Muratore, A. F., Bershad, M., Steinglass, J. E., Foerde, K. E., Gianini, L., Broft, A., & Attia, E. (2021). Use of high-frequency repetitive transcranial magnetic stimulation to probe the neural circuitry of food choice in anorexia nervosa: A proof-of-concept study. *International Journal of Eating Disorders, 54*(11), 2031–2036. https://doi.org/10.1002/eat.23597

Naguy, A., Al-Tajali, A., & Alamiri, B. (2019). An adolescent case of treatment-refractory anorexia nervosa favorably responded to electroconvulsive therapy. *Journal of ECT, 35*(3), 217–218. https://doi.org/10.1097/YCT.0000000000000582

Oudijn, M. S., Linders, J. T. W., Lok, A., Schuurman, P. R., van den Munckhof, P., van Elburg, A. A., van Wingen, G. A., Mocking, R. J. T., & Denys, D. (2023). Neural effects of deep brain stimulation on reward and loss anticipation and food viewing in anorexia nervosa: A pilot study. *Journal of Eating Disorders, 11*(1), 140. https://doi.org/10.1186/s40337-023-00863-3

Oudijn, M. S., Mocking, R. J. T., Wijnker, R. R., Lok, A., Schuurman, P. R., van den Munckhof, P., van Elburg, A. A., & Denys, D. (2021). Deep brain stimulation of the ventral anterior limb of the capsula interna in patients with treatment-refractory anorexia nervosa. *Brain Stimulation, 14*(6), 1528–1530. https://doi.org/10.1016/j.brs.2021.10.387

Pacilio, R. M., Livingston, R. K., & Gordon, M. R. (2019). The use of electroconvulsive therapy in eating disorders: A systematic literature review and case report. *Journal of ECT, 35*(4), 272–278. https://doi.org/10.1097/YCT.0000000000000599

Park, R. J., Singh, I., Pike, A. C., & Tan, J. O. A. (2017). Deep brain stimulation in anorexia nervosa: Hope for the hopeless or exploitation of the vulnerable? The Oxford neuroethics gold standard framework. *Frontiers in Psychiatry, 8*, 44. https://doi.org/10.3389/fpsyt.2017.00044

Poutanen, O., Huuhka, K., & Perko, K. (2009). Severe anorexia nervosa, co-occurring major depressive disorder and electroconvulsive therapy as maintenance treatment: A case report. *Cases Journal, 2*, 9362. https://doi.org/10.1186/1757-1626-2-9362

Pugh, J., Tan, J., Aziz, T., & Park, R. J. (2018). The moral obligation to prioritize research into deep brain stimulation over brain lesioning procedures for severe enduring anorexia nervosa. *Frontiers in Psychiatry*, *9*, 523. https://doi.org/10.3389/fpsyt.2018.00523

Rapinesi, C., Del Casale, A., Serata, D., Caccia, F., Di Pietro, S., Scatena, P., Carbonetti, P., Fensore, C., Angeletti, G., Tatarelli, R., Kotzalidis, G. D., & Girardi, P. (2013). Electroconvulsive therapy in a man with comorbid severe obesity, binge eating disorder, and bipolar disorder. *Journal of ECT*, *29*(2), 142–144. https://doi.org/10.1097/YCT.0b013e31827a7f85

Sağlam, T., Aksoy Poyraz, C., Poyraz, B. Ç., & Tosun, M. (2018). Successful use of electroconvulsive therapy in a patient with anorexia nervosa and severe acute-onset obsessive-compulsive disorder. *International Journal of Eating Disorders*, *51*(8), 1026–1028. https://doi.org/10.1002/eat.22923

Sargant, W. (1951). Leucotomy in psychosomatic disorders. *Lancet*, *2*(6673), 87–91. https://doi.org/10.1016/s0140-6736(51)91351-7

Scaife, J. C., Eraifej, J., Green, A. L., Petric, B., Aziz, T. Z., & Park, R. J. (2022). Deep brain stimulation of the nucleus accumbens in severe enduring anorexia nervosa: A pilot study. *Frontiers in Behavioral Neuroscience*, *16*, 842184. https://doi.org/10.3389/fnbeh.2022.842184

Sciortino, D., Schiena, G., Cantù, F., Maggioni, E., & Brambilla, P. (2021). Case report: Repeated transcranial magnetic stimulation improves comorbid binge eating disorder in two female patients with treatment-resistant bipolar depression. *Frontiers in Psychiatry*, *12*, 732066. https://doi.org/10.3389/fpsyt.2021.732066

Shaffer, A., Naik, A., Bederson, M., Arnold, P. M., & Hassaneen, W. (2023). Efficacy of deep brain stimulation for the treatment of anorexia nervosa: A systematic review and network meta-analysis of patient-level data. *Neurosurgical Focus*, *54*(2), E5. https://doi.org/10.3171/2022.11.FOCUS22616

Shilton, T., Enoch-Levy, A., Giron, Y., Yaroslavsky, A., Amiaz, R., Gothelf, D., Weizman, A., & Stein, D. (2020). A retrospective case series of electroconvulsive therapy in the management of comorbid depression and anorexia nervosa. *International Journal of Eating Disorders*, *53*(2), 210–218. https://doi.org/10.1002/eat.23181

Sifneos, P. E. (1952). A case of anorexia nervosa treated successfully by leucotomy. *American Journal of Psychiatry*, *109*(5), 356–360. https://doi.org/10.1176/ajp.109.5.356

Steinglass, J., & Walsh, B. T. (2006). Habit learning and anorexia nervosa: A cognitive neuroscience hypothesis. *International Journal of Eating Disorders*, *39*(4), 267–275. https://doi.org/10.1002/eat.20244

Strumila, R., Thiebaut, S., Jaussent, I., Seneque, M., Attal, J., Courtet, P., & Guillaume, S. (2019). Safety and efficacy of transcranial direct current stimulation (tDCS) in the treatment of anorexia nervosa. The open-label STAR study. *Brain Stimulation*, *12*(5), 1325–1327. https://doi.org/10.1016/j.brs.2019.06.017

Van den Eynde, F., Claudino, A. M., Mogg, A., Horrell, L., Stahl, D., Ribeiro, W., Uher, R., Campbell, I., & Schmidt, U. (2010). Repetitive transcranial magnetic stimulation reduces cue-induced food craving in bulimic disorders. *Biological Psychiatry*, *67*(8), 793–795. https://doi.org/10.1016/j.biopsych.2009.11.023

Van den Eynde, F., Guillaume, S., Broadbent, H., Campbell, I. C., & Schmidt, U. (2013). Repetitive transcranial magnetic stimulation in anorexia nervosa: A pilot study. *European Psychiatry*, *28*(2), 98–101. https://doi.org/10.1016/j.eurpsy.2011.06.002

Villalba Martínez, G., Justicia, A., Salgado, P., Ginés, J. M., Guardiola, R., Cedrón, C., Polo, M., Delgado-Martínez, I., Medrano, S., Manero, R. M., Conesa, G., Faus, G., Grau, A., Elices, M., & Pérez, V. (2020). A randomized trial of deep brain stimulation to the subcallosal cingulate and nucleus accumbens in patients with treatment-refractory, chronic, and severe anorexia nervosa: Initial results at 6 months of follow up. *Journal of Clinical Medicine*, *9*(6), 1946. https://doi.org/10.3390/jcm9061946

Vismara M, Franzini, A., Manuelli, M., Galentino, R., Porta, M., Servello, D., Cena, H., & Dell'Osso, B. (2020). Deep brain stimulation in treating anorexia nervosa and comorbid obsessive compulsive disorder: A 12 months follow-up case study. *European Neuropsychopharmacology*, *40*, 232-S233.

Walpoth, M., Hoertnagl, C., Mangweth-Matzek, B., Kemmler, G., Hinterhölzl, J., Conca, A., & Hausmann, A. (2008). Repetitive transcranial magnetic stimulation in bulimia nervosa: Preliminary results of a single-centre, randomised, double-blind, sham-controlled trial in female outpatients. *Psychotherapy and Psychosomatics*, *77*(1), 57–60. https://doi.org/10.1159/000110061

Wang, J., Chang, C., Geng, N., Wang, X., & Gao, G. (2013). Treatment of intractable anorexia nervosa with inactivation of the nucleus accumbens using stereotactic surgery. *Stereotactic and Functional Neurosurgery*, *91*(6), 364–372. https://doi.org/10.1159/000348278

Woodside, D. B., Dunlop, K., Sathi, C., Lam, E., McDonald, B., & Downar, J. (2021). A pilot trial of repetitive transcranial magnetic stimulation of the dorsomedial prefrontal cortex in anorexia nervosa: Resting fMRI correlates of response. *Journal of Eating Disorders*, *9*(1). https://doi.org/10.1186/s40337-021-00411-x

Wu, H., Van Dyck-Lippens, P. J., Santegoeds, R., van Kuyck, K., Gabriëls, L., Lin, G., Pan, G., Li, Y., Li, D., Zhan, S., Sun, B., & Nuttin, B. (2013). Deep-brain stimulation for anorexia nervosa. *World Neurosurgery*, *80*(3–4), S29.e1–10. https://doi.org/10.1016/j.wneu.2012.06.039

Wu, H., Zhang, W., Chen, Y., Li, D., Zhan, S., Ma, R., & Sun, B. (2007). Anorexia nervosa: A functional stereotactic neurosurgery case report and correlations with obsessive-compulsive disorder. Proceeding of the 2nd Congress of International Society of Reconstructive Neurosurgery, Taipei, Taiwan, September 13–16.

Wu, K., Lo, Y. T., Cavaleri, J., Bergosh, M., Ipe, J., Briggs, R. G., Jann, K. B., Murray, S. B., Mason, X. L., Liu, C. Y., & Lee, D. J. (2024). Neuromodulation of eating disorders: A review of underlying neural network activity and neuromodulatory treatments. *Brain Sciences*, *14*(3), 200. https://doi.org/10.3390/brainsci14030200

Zamboni, R., Larach, V., Poblete, M., Mancini, R., Mancini, H., Charlin, V., Parr, F., Carvajal, C., & Gallardo, R. (1993). Dorsomedial thalamotomy as a treatment for terminal anorexia: a report of two cases. In B. A. Meyerson, G. Broggi, J. Martin-Rodriguez, C. Ostertag, & M. Sindou (Eds.), *Advances in stereotactic and functional neurosurgery* (pp. 34–35). Springer Vienna.

Zanello, M., Duriez, P., Pallud, J., Roux, A., Sharshar, T., Gorwood, P., & Devaux, B. (2018). Letter: Long-term follow-up study of MRI-guided bilateral anterior capsulotomy in patients with refractory anorexia nervosa. *Neurosurgery*, *83*(1), E39–E40. https://doi.org/10.1093/neuros/nyy123

Zhang, H.-W., Li, D.-Y., Zhao, J., Guan, Y.-H., Sun, B.-M., & Zuo, C.-T. (2013). Metabolic imaging of deep brain stimulation in anorexia nervosa: A 18F-FDG PET/CT study. *Clinical Nuclear Medicine*, *38*(12), 943–948. https://doi.org/10.1097/RLU.0000000000000261

PART V

EMERGING TOPICS

22

Advances in the Activity-Based Anorexia Paradigm

An Animal Model for Aspects of Anorexia Nervosa

Stephanie C. Dulawa

Brief Definitional Overview

Animal model: An animal model is an experimental preparation developed for the purpose of studying a condition in the same or different species.

Activity-based anorexia (ABA) paradigm: An experimental preparation in which rodents are singly housed with a running wheel and exposed to time-scheduled feeding, resulting in extreme weight loss, hypophagia, and hyperactivity.

Predictive validity: The degree to which an animal model makes accurate predictions about the condition being modelled.

Introduction

The activity-based anorexia (ABA) phenomenon, sometimes also referred to as food restriction-induced hyperactivity, was first reported in 1953 by Hall and Hanford (Hall et al., 1953). They found that rats housed with running wheels and subjected to restricted food access for the same one-hour period a day showed significant decreases in body weight and food intake, and a paradoxical increase in running wheel activity (Hall et al., 1953). On the other hand, rats provided with running wheels and ad libitum food access and food-restricted rats housed without running wheels were able to maintain a normal body weight (Hall et al., 1953). Virtually all strains of rats and mice exposed to ABA conditions consistently show rapid decreases in body weight, food intake, and hyperactivity. If allowed to continue in the ABA paradigm unchecked, animals will develop hypothermia, loss of estrus, increases in hypothalamic–pituitary–adrenal (HPA) axis activity, stomach ulceration, and death (Dixon et al., 2003; Fraga et al., 2021; Routtenberg & Kuznesof, 1967; Vincent & Pare, 1976). The ABA phenomenon has been observed in

Stephanie C. Dulawa Advances in the Activity-Based Anorexia Paradigm. In: *The Handbook of the Neurobiology of Eating Disorders*. Edited by: Christina E. Wierenga and Joanna E. Steinglass, Oxford University Press. © Oxford University Press (2025). DOI: 10.1093/9780197675212.003.0023 many other mammalian species, including the hamster, gerbil, guinea pig, chipmunk, pig, and mouse (Kyriakis et al., 1990; Treasure & Owen, 1997; Vincent & Pare, 1976; Vincent et al., 1977). Thus, the ABA phenomenon can be readily induced in normal animals, and it does not require the use of genetically manipulated rodents. The ABA phenomenon has been hypothesized to be an adaptive mechanism that facilitates migration in response to famine (Duclos et al., 2013), not only in animals but also in humans (Guisinger, 2003), who evolved as nomadic foragers (Lee & Daly, 1999). This intriguing hypothesis remains largely untestable and neither contributes to nor detracts from the predictive validity of the ABA model.

Biological Framework

The ABA paradigm is an experimental preparation that can be used to study specific aspects of anorexia nervosa (AN). When neuropsychopharmacology was an emerging field, animal models were expected to recapitulate nearly all aspects of a neuropsychiatric disorder; however, decades of work have revealed the weaknesses of this approach. A more current approach to the development and use of animal models relies on recapitulating only specific aspects of the neuropsychiatric disorder of interest (Geyer & Markou, 1995), allowing an investigator to obtain more definitive information about a more circumscribed domain of the disorder. By limiting the scope of the animal model, one can increase the confidence in the cross-species validity (Geyer & Markou, 1995).

Predictive validity of activity-based anorexia

The ABA paradigm makes accurate predictions about specific aspects of AN. Although no approved pharmacological treatments for AN exist, atypical antipsychotics are frequently used off label in individuals with AN with some limited success (Attia et al., 2019; Dold et al., 2015; Thorey et al., 2023). Likewise, chronic treatment with the atypical antipsychotic olanzapine was reported to reduce the rate of weight loss in mice in the ABA paradigm (Hillebrand, van Elburg, et al., 2005; Klenotich et al., 2012; Klenotich et al., 2015), in the absence of a sedative effect. However, the lack of approved pharmacological treatments for AN presents an obstacle for further validating the ABA model using pharmacological responses.

The ABA paradigm recapitulates important behavioral characteristics of AN. Both patients with AN and rodents in ABA exhibit voluntary reductions in food intake, and increases in physical activity, despite significantly decreased energy balance (Zhang & Dulawa, 2021). Specifically, in the ABA paradigm, the experimental conditions induce animals to reduce voluntary food intake, run compulsively on wheels, and show dramatic weight loss. Nearly all patients with AN exhibit weight-loss, voluntary hypophagia, and hyperactivity is observed in approximately 70% of patients. Hyperactivity in AN can consist of both compulsive exercise, and also general restlessness (Casper, 2022; Casper et al., 2020; Scheurink et al., 2010; Shroff et al., 2006). Animals in the ABA paradigm exhibit robust increases in wheel running, and additionally can also show increased locomotor activity in the home cage aside from wheel running (unpublished observations), although this "non-wheel" form of hyperactivity has received little attention. Furthermore, AN is a disorder with peak onset during adolescence (Neale & Hudson, 2020; Ranzenhofer et al., 2022), and adolescent mice and rats are more vulnerable to developing ABA than older rodents (Frintrop et al., 2018). Another feature of AN that might be recapitulated in the ABA paradigm is food anticipatory activity (FAA). Reduced food availability induces hyperactivity in humans and animals, and is thought to reflect foraging behavior (Illius et al., 2002; Sodersten et al., 2008). In animals, when food is only available for a limited time period each day during the ABA paradigm, food delivery is preceded by a pronounced increase in physical activity (Moran & Tamashiro, 2007), termed FAA. At least one report suggests that patients with AN also exhibit FAA (Bruch, 1962), although this finding requires further study. As will be discussed, many recent advances have further validated the ABA paradigm as a rodent model for aspects of AN.

Differences between activity-based anorexia and anorexia nervosa

The ABA model also differs from AN in many aspects. Because an animal model cannot recapitulate every aspect of a neuropsychiatric disorder, such differences between AN and ABA do not invalidate the model. For example, AN affects approximately 0.5% to 1.0% of females during their lifetime, and affects about one-tenth of as many males (Attia, 2010). Although our work and that of others suggests that the ABA phenotype develops more quickly in female than male rodents (Hancock & Grant, 2009; Klenotich & Dulawa, 2012; Martin et al., 2007), a number of additional reports suggest that male and female rodents show comparable sensitivity to developing ABA (Boakes et al., 1999; Lambert & Kinsley, 1993), and still others report that male rodents are more vulnerable to ABA (Achamrah et al., 2017; Doerries et al., 1991). Another manner in which AN and ABA diverge is that rodents only develop ABA if macronutrient-balanced chow is used in the paradigm. A study using rats showed that when sweet high-fat chow is provided during the restriction phase, weight loss is completely prevented. Additionally, presenting fat alone results in weight loss intermediate between that obtained when presenting normal chow and sweet high-fat chow (Brown et al., 2008). However, it is interesting to note that individuals with AN tend to strongly avoid high-fat foods (Dalton et al., 2020; Uniacke et al., 2020; Yanovski, 2003). Another limitation of the ABA model is that the experimenter must impose a time-scheduled feeding regimen and a running wheel onto rodents to induce ABA, and this phenotype resolves when ad libitum feeding is restored or when the running wheel is removed. On the other hand, individuals with AN self-initiate restricted feeding and compulsive exercise. The thoughts of the rodent regarding their body weight and shape, or their ruminations regarding food during ABA, remain unknowable. Nevertheless, the ABA model recapitulates the voluntary reduction of food intake, hyperactivity, and weight loss observed in AN, providing an experimental preparation for studying these core aspects.

Physiology, neuroanatomy, and genetics of activity-based anorexia

Research examining the neural substrates underlying ABA are thought to broadly overlap with those implicated in AN, although differences between the methods used to identify the neural substrates underlying AN and ABA limit the ability to make definitive comparisons. Human neuroimaging approaches have identified changes in the activity of specific brain regions, which may be a cause or a consequence of AN. This work has largely used positron emission tomography (PET), functional magnetic resonance imaging (fMRI), and biochemical studies of blood or cerebrospinal fluid (CSF) in patients with AN, in the ill or recovered state. Much preclinical work over the past decades has enumerated the changes in neurobiology and physiology induced by exposure to the ABA paradigm (Spadini et al., 2021). Many of these findings in rodents may be best conceptualized as corresponding to the ill state in AN, and as reflecting the consequences of starvation. Thus, many preclinical studies of ABA have identified consequences, rather than causes, of ABA. For example, in rodents exposed to ABA, the mean brain volumes and the number of astrocytes are reduced in the cerebral cortex and corpus callosum (Frintrop et al., 2019), mirroring volumetric brain changes found in human subjects with AN (Seitz et al., 2021). Rodents exposed to the ABA paradigm also exhibit increased brain-derived neurotrophic factor (BDNF) levels and increased GABA receptor expression in the hippocampus. Studies using Golgi staining found that adolescent female rats exposed to ABA showed less total dendritic length and fewer dendritic branches in stratum radiatum of the dorsal hippocampus, which preferentially mediates spatial learning and cognition, and more branching in stratum radiatum of the ventral hippocampus, which preferentially mediates anxiety. Although these results suggest that ABA elicits pathway-specific changes in the hippocampus that could contribute to the increased anxiety and reduced behavioral flexibility observed in AN, it remains unknown whether these brain changes exist in patients with AN. Studying the consequences of ABA in rodents might also provide clues to identifying novel treatments for AN, as some of these consequences may drive the chronicity of the disorder.

The effects of ABA on additional neurotransmitter systems and hormones have also been reported. For example, ABA is also well known to activate the HPA axis in rodents (de Rijke et al., 2005; Scharner et al., 2018). Two exposures to ABA during adolescence produce long-term effects on HPA axis activation (Lee & Kinzig, 2017). Likewise, in AN, a common finding is that of hypercortisolism, associated with increased central corticotropin-releasing hormone levels (Licinio et al., 1996; Seed et al., 2000). This sustained hypercortisolism is thought to contribute to impairments in learning, memory, and attention in AN (Seed et al., 2000). Furthermore, the ABA paradigm was also reported to increase endogenous opioid peptides levels such that naloxone treatment induced significant withdrawal symptoms (Kanarek et al., 2009). Inconsistent effects of ABA on leptin levels have been reported (Exner et al., 2000; Fraga et al., 2020; Gelegen et al., 2007), and administration of leptin to rats undergoing ABA reduced hyperactivity but also food intake, leading to increased ABA severity (Hillebrand, Koeners, et al., 2005). Currently, there is insufficient evidence regarding the effects of ABA on dopamine and serotonin levels and their release dynamics during ABA. For example, experiments using dopamine or serotonin biosensors to assess neurotransmitter release during the ABA paradigm are greatly needed (Kubitschke et al., 2022; Sun et al., 2020) because alterations of the dopaminergic and serotonergic systems have also been consistently found in AN. For example, in both ill and recovered individuals with AN, reduced cerebrospinal levels of dopamine metabolites have been found, suggesting reduced dopaminergic turnover (Kaye et al., 1984; Kaye et al., 1999; Kontis & Theochari, 2012). Furthermore, decreased cerebrospinal levels of 5-HIAA, a serotonin metabolite, have been found in people ill with AN (Haleem, 2009; Kaye et al., 1988), and increased levels of 5-HIAA are found following recovery (Kaye, 1997).

Current knowledge of the genetic basis of the ABA phenomenon in rodents remains very limited. Although genome-wide analysis (GWAS) has been applied to other behavioral traits in rodents (Gunturkun et al., 2022; Wang et al., 2018), GWAS of the ABA phenotype in rodents has never been conducted to identify genetic loci. On the other hand, major progress has been made during the past decade in elucidating the genetic basis of AN, which will ultimately enhance our understanding of the underlying biological mechanisms. Watson and colleagues (2019) performed the largest genome-wide association study to date for AN, with 16,992 cases and 55,525 controls, and identified eight risk loci. Their genetic findings also showed that the genetic architecture of AN shows significant genetic correlations with psychiatric disorders, but also physical activity, metabolic, and anthropometric traits, independent of the effects of common variants associated with body mass index (BMI). However, the genes driving the significance of each of these loci remain to be determined. Thus, it remains unknown whether these loci would overlap with potential loci for ABA in rodents. The current state of the genetics of ABA in rodents consists of evidence that ABA is strongly heritable.

Indeed, ABA progression varies substantially between different inbred mouse strains (Gelegen et al., 2007; Pjetri et al., 2012) and is altered by the knockout of various genes (Belmonte et al., 2016; Daimon & Hentges, 2021; Robinette et al., 2020; Verhagen et al., 2011). Once the genes underlying the significant hits in the GWAS of AN are identified, mouse genetic models can be generated to study how these genes contribute to the ABA phenotype.

State of the Science in Eating Disorders

Recent work during the past decade using mice has provided substantial conceptual advances in understanding ABA as a model for aspects of AN, and in dissecting the neural substrates that regulate ABA. These reports have shown that biomarkers of AN can be recapitulated by the ABA model. While a trait of a disorder can be a pattern of thinking, reacting, or behaving that is different from controls, a biomarker is an objective and measurable characteristic that marks either risk or manifestation of illness (Gottesman & Gould, 2003). One report by Milton and colleagues (2021) has shown that ABA also induces cognitive inflexibility (Milton et al., 2021), a major trait of AN (Dulawa, 2021). Another report by Welch and colleagues (2019) has shown that a biomarker observed in individuals recovered from AN, dopamine D2 receptor overexpression in the nucleus accumbens, may actually play a causal role in AN (Welch et al., 2019).

Relationship between activity-based anorexia and cognitive flexibility

AN is strongly associated with several cognitive traits that are observed before the onset of illness. Impaired cognitive flexibility, defined as the inability to modify cognitive strategies and behavior to adapt to changing environmental demands, is a major feature of AN (Berner et al., 2019; Foldi et al., 2021; Sternheim et al., 2022; Wierenga et al., 2022). For example, perseverative thinking and rigid behavior including preoccupation with food, body shape, and compulsive exercise are hallmarks of cognitive inflexibility in AN. Cognitive inflexibility has also been objectively measured in individuals with AN using experimental tests of attentional set shifting, response inhibition, and reversal learning (Steinglass et al., 2006). Reduced cognitive flexibility is likely an endophenotype of AN, which is a special type of biomarker with a genetic basis (Gottesman & Gould, 2003) because this trait is also observed in healthy siblings of individuals with AN, is independent of current body weight, and persists following recovery from AN (Holliday et al., 2005).

Milton and colleagues (2021) examined the role of the projection from the medial prefrontal cortex (mPFC) to the nucleus accumbens shell (AcbSh) in modulating both cognitive flexibility and ABA in mice (Milton et al., 2021). They selected this neural projection for study because top-down control of the mPFC over the AcbSh is important for modulating both reward-based feeding and cognitive flexibility. Specifically, altering mPFC activity has been reported to impair reversal learning and set-shifting, and activating the mPFC decreases AcbSh-evoked feeding behavior (Richard & Berridge, 2013). Milton and colleagues (2021) used a two-virus chemogenetic strategy to bidirectionally manipulate the activity of the mPFC to AcbSh projection. They found that chemogenetic inhibition of the mPFC to AcbSh projection robustly reduced the development of ABA. Additionally, chemogenetic activation of this pathway resulted in an increase of the ABA phenotype, with mice showing an increased "dropout rate," reflecting attainment of a weight-loss criterion, compared to mice receiving chemogenetic inhibition. Importantly, Milton and colleagues (2021) also revealed that chemogenetic activation of this neural projection increased the perseveration index in the reversal learning task, while chemogenetic inhibition of the mPFC to AcbSh projection increased accuracy in a reversal learning task. Thus, inhibiting the mPFC to AcbSh projection reduces vulnerability to ABA and increases reversal learning, while activating this pathway produces the opposite effects. Although this study does not determine whether changes in ABA cause alterations in reversal learning, or vice versa, an earlier report using rats suggested that the development of ABA induces impairments in reversal learning, which normalize following recovery from ABA (Allen et al., 2017). Together, these studies have shown that ABA can induce reversal learning deficits, and that a specific corticostriatal projection regulates both cognitive flexibility and ABA. The findings challenge the notion that the ABA paradigm cannot be used to study cognitive aspects of AN (Dulawa, 2021).

Effects of dopamine D2 receptor overexpression in the nucleus accumbens on activity-based anorexia

Another potential biomarker in AN is the finding that in a small sample of individuals recovered from AN, increased dopamine D2/D3 receptor binding in the anteroventral striatum, as measured by [11C] raclopride binding using PET, was found (Frank et al., 2005). This imaging finding suggests that in the anteroventral striatum of individuals recovered from AN, either D2/D3 receptors are upregulated, or extracellular dopamine levels are reduced, or both. Furthermore, upregulation of D2/D3 receptors in the anteroventral striatum might either predispose to the development of AN or be a consequence of illness. To explore both these questions, Welch and colleagues (2019) virally overexpressed D2Rs on nucleus accumbens core (D2R-OE_{Nac}) neurons that endogenously express D2Rs, and tested mice of both sexes in the ABA paradigm. Remarkably, only female D2R-OE_{Nac} mice rapidly lost 25% of their initial body weight, reduced food intake, and substantially increased wheel running in the paradigm. To assess the importance of running wheel access to the observed phenotype, an identical study was performed without wheel access. Surprisingly, only female D2R-OE_{Nac} mice rapidly lost 25% of their initial body weight during scheduled fasting without wheel access, and showed no changes in food intake. Interestingly, female D2R-OE_{Nac} mice also appeared more active in their home cages than ad libitum-fed controls (unpublished observations). This observation suggests that animals can exhibit an ABA-like phenotype, with rapid weight loss and increased activity, even without wheel access. It is also possible that this hyperactivity is similar to the restlessness observed in AN.

Furthermore, D2R-OE_{Nac} mice of both sexes showed glucose intolerance in the intraperitoneal glucose tolerance test (IGTT); glucose intolerance reflects a delay in the clearance of elevated blood glucose, such as following a meal (Michaelides et al., 2017). Individuals with AN have been shown to exhibit glucose intolerance (Drossman et al., 1979; Scheen et al., 1988; Warren & Vande Wiele, 1973; Yasuhara et al., 2005), which is associated with a poor refeeding outcome (Yasuhara et al., 2005). These findings suggest that metabolic mechanisms may contribute to the effect of D2R-OE_{Nac} on ABA, and they are consistent with the GWAS findings of significant genetic correlations with both psychiatric disorders and metabolic traits (Duncan et al., 2017; Watson et al., 2019). Lastly, these results suggest that D2R overexpression in the anteroventral striatum may predispose to AN, rather than being a consequence of starvation.

Circuit-dissecting techniques applied to activity-based anorexia

A number of recent studies using modern neuroscience circuit-dissecting approaches have provided novel insights into the mechanisms that modulate the ABA phenotype (Cai et al., 2022; Daimon & Hentges, 2022; Foldi et al., 2017; Miletta et al., 2020; Milton et al., 2021; Santiago et al., 2021; Sutton Hickey et al., 2023). Modern circuit-dissecting techniques, including optogenetics, chemogenetics, and fiber photometry, have been used in rodents to dissect the role of specific neuron subtypes and projections in ABA. For example, fiber photometry is a calcium imaging technique that measures bulk or population level calcium activity from neurons expressing a biosensor; calcium activity provides a proxy for neuronal activity which can then be correlated with the behavior of the animal. The biosensor is expressed in the desired neuronal populations using a viral platform with an appropriate serotype and promoter, and other elements (Hui et al., 2022). Fiber photometry-based studies therefore allow highly spatially and temporally precise measurements of neuronal activity in awake and behaving animals (Byron & Sakata, 2024; Simpson et al., 2024). While fiber photometry can reveal correlations between neural activity and behavior, optogenetic and chemogenetic techniques can directly manipulate neural activity to determine causal effects on behavior. Optogenetic techniques allow control over the activity of selected neurons using a combination of genetic engineering and light (Deisseroth, 2015; Emiliani et al., 2022). Either natural or engineered microbial photoreceptors are genetically introduced into the neurons of interest, typically using viral injections. Thus, neurons of interest are made photosensitive, and can be precisely excited or inhibited in time and space using illumination from a fiber optic implant. Chemogenetics uses designer receptors exclusively activated by designer drugs (DREADDs) to manipulate specific neuronal populations of interest in a time and region-specific manner (Michaelides & Hurd, 2016; Smith et al., 2016). Many DREADDs have been generated which allow for selective interrogation of G-protein coupled receptor (GPCR) signaling cascades activated by Gq, Gi, Gs, Golf, and β-arrestin (Michaelides & Hurd, 2016). The most popular DREADD to date, the hM3Dq, was generated two decades ago using mutagenesis of the Gq-coupled human M3 muscarinic acetylcholine receptor (Smith et al., 2016). The ligand clozapine-N-oxide (CNO) has substantially higher affinity for this mutated receptor than acetylcholine, and thus CNO can be administered to animals to activate the receptor and determine effects on behavior. However, other ligands have recently been identified that potently bind to hM3Dq and may have more desirable properties (Thompson et al., 2018). Chemogenetic approaches have the advantage of not requiring tethering of the animal during behavior, which is required to deliver light in optogenetic approaches. However, optogenetic approaches have the advantage of highly temporally precise control over neuronal activity, while neuronal activity is altered for hours after hM3Dq activation by CNO. Therefore, a suite of powerful circuit-dissecting techniques is available to dissect the neural circuits of ABA.

Dopaminergic circuits regulating activity-based anorexia

A role for midbrain ventral tegmental area (VTA) projection neurons has been identified in modulating ABA (Cai et al., 2022; Foldi et al., 2017; Frank et al., 2005). For example, in rats, excitation of predominantly dopaminergic neurons in the VTA to nucleus accumbens reward pathway using chemogenetics increased food intake and wheel running just prior to food delivery (i.e., FAA) and prevented drop out from the ABA paradigm (Foldi et al., 2017). This finding is consistent with reports from human studies that dopamine turnover may be reduced in AN (Johnston et al., 1984; Kaye et al., 1999) and that reward processing in the nucleus accumbens is altered (Frank et al., 2020; Frank et al., 2022; Tadayonnejad et al., 2022). Other work examined the role of dopaminergic VTA projections onto serotonergic neurons in the dorsal raphe nucleus (DRN) using optogenetics in mice (Cai et al., 2022). They reported that dopaminergic neurons in the VTA can bidirectionally regulate serotonin neuron activity in the DRN, with weaker stimulation inducing dopamine receptor D2 (DRD2)-dependent inhibition and overeating, and stronger stimulation causing DRD1-dependent activation. Furthermore, they observed a DRD2 to DRD1 shift of dopamine neurotransmission on DRN serotonergic neurons, which causes constant activation of these neurons and contributes to AN-like behaviors in the ABA paradigm (Cai et al., 2022). Using refined neural circuit dissection of ABA behavior, which is only possible in rodents, these findings define a more specific role for the serotonergic system in AN-related behavior.

Medial-prefrontal cortical projections regulating activity-based anorexia

Recent work has also begun elucidating the role of medial prefrontal cortical (mPFC) projections to the nucleus accumbens and to the raphe in the regulation of ABA. As previously detailed, Milton and colleagues (2021) showed that chemogenetic inhibition of the mPFC to AcbSh projection robustly reduced the development of ABA, while chemogenetic activation of this pathway resulted in an increase of the ABA phenotype. Other work by Du and colleagues (2022) found that chemogenetic activation of a mPFC to the DRN pathway did not alter ABA. Interestingly, chemogenetic activation of either the general mPFC pyramidal cell population, or the subpopulation projecting to the dorsal striatum, did not alter food intake or bodyweight during ABA, but drove wheel running specifically during hours preceding limited food availability (i.e., FAA), but not during ad libitum food availability (Santiago et al., 2021). Conversely, suppression of mPFC pyramidal cells generally, or targeting mPFC-to-DS cells, reduced wheel running specifically during the FAA period and not during ad libitum food access. Although modulation of this circuit did not alter ABA outcomes, results indicate that this circuit plays a specific and causal role in the decision to run during food scarcity (Santiago et al., 2021). These reports demonstrating a role for the rodent mPFC in ABA broadly align with the notion that in humans, a dorsal cognitive neurocircuit including the dorsolateral prefrontal cortex (DLPFC) (Kaye et al., 2009; Phillips et al., 2003a, 2003b), an analog of the rodent mPFC, plays a role in AN.

Hypothalamic circuits regulating activity-based anorexia

Recent experiments have also uncovered an essential role for various populations of hypothalamic neurons in ABA. Specifically, neurons expressing agouti-related peptide (AgRP) and neuropeptide Y (NPY), and another population of neurons expressing proopiomelanocortin (POMC) in the arcuate nucleus of the hypothalamus have been shown to affect vulnerability to developing ABA. AgRP neurons have been well characterized for their role in feeding, energy homeostasis, foraging, and even compulsive behaviors (Aponte et al., 2011; Betley et al., 2013; Dietrich et al., 2012; Krashes et al., 2011; Li et al., 2019). Moreover, AgRP plasma levels are elevated in ill individuals with AN reflecting undernutrition, suggesting that AgRP neurons or receptors might provide a target for treatment during the ill state

(Mequinion et al., 2019; Merle et al., 2011). One recent report using mice showed that early life ablation of AgRP neurons using a combined genetic and pharmacological strategy resulted in accelerated weight loss of five- to six-week-old female mice in the ABA paradigm. These animals with ablated AgRP neurons were unable to properly mobilize fuels during ABA conditions; however, when provided with elevated fat content through diet, dropout from the ABA paradigm was completely prevented (Dietrich et al., 2012). On the other hand, daily chemogenetic activation of AgRP neurons, by expressing transient receptor potential cation channel subfamily V member 1 (Trpv1) on AgRP neurons plus IP administration of capsaicin, caused an extension of days of voluntary running with no dropout under ABA conditions (Dietrich et al., 2012). These observations suggest that AgRP neurons interact with peripheral signals to regulate compulsive exercise and body weight. Using fiber photometry, Miletta and colleagues (2020) found rapid AgRP neuronal inhibition following voluntary cessation of running, as is normally observed following the sensory detection of food (Dietrich et al., 2012); these findings suggests that AgRP neurons also regulate activity. Yet another investigation further characterized the role of AgRP neuron activity in ABA modulation, using fiber photometry and chemogenetics during different times of the ABA paradigm, such as with or without food availability. Photometry recordings of AgRP neurons during ABA versus control conditions showed that mice under ABA conditions exhibit a reduction of AgRP neuronal inhibition following food intake (Sutton Hickey et al., 2023). This reduction persisted for up to four days, until ABA mice lost a significant amount of weight and this normal neural response returned. The investigators also demonstrated that ABA progression was mitigated by chemogenetic AgRP activation through the reprioritization of food intake over hyperactivity (Sutton Hickey et al., 2023). Importantly, chemogenetic activation reduced ABA once the ABA phenotype was already established for three days, rather than merely preventing ABA development. However, this effect of AgRP neuron activation was only observed when applied during periods of food availability (Sutton Hickey et al., 2023). Lastly, Daimon and Hentges (2022) reported that chemogenetic inhibition of POMC neurons during ABA reduces FAA in male and female mice, without changing body weight or food intake. They suggest that POMC neurons may contribute preferentially to excessive exercise habits in patients with AN (Daimon & Hentges, 2022).

Central–peripheral interactions regulate activity-based anorexia

Recent findings have furthered the mechanistic understanding of ABA by investigating brain and adipose tissue interactions (Yoon et al., 2024). Recent transcriptomic studies identified white adipose tissue (WAT) as a primary location of the "metabolic memory" of prior obesity, and implicated WAT-derived signals as drivers of recidivism to obesity following weight loss (Hernandez-Carretero et al., 2018; MacLean et al., 2015; Zapata et al., 2022). Yoon and colleagues (2024) therefore tested whether transplanting WAT from high fat diet (HFD)-fed obese mice into normal weight recipient mice would attenuate ABA. Female recipient mice received a small (~150 mg) WAT transplant harvested from either normal chow-fed, or HFD-fed obese female mice; four weeks later, obese WAT recipients and control WAT recipient mice were tested in the ABA paradigm (Yoon et al., 2024). It was found that obese WAT recipient mice survived longer in the paradigm than control fat recipient mice, defined as maintaining 75% of their baseline body weight (Yoon et al., 2024). However, no consistent group differences in food intake or wheel running were found, suggesting that obese WAT might have induced metabolic changes that altered survival (Yoon et al., 2024). The findings are consistent with the emerging hypothesis that AN is a metabo-psychiatric disorder (Watson et al., 2019). Much work will be required to identify the mechanisms by which the contents of obese WAT interact with the brain to modulate body weight during ABA. To begin addressing this question, Yoon and colleagues (2024) show that neonatal ablation of AgRP neurons in the hypothalamus prevents the ability of an obese WAT transplant to reduce weight loss in recipient mice during ABA. These studies suggest novel potential approaches to treating AN, including autologous WAT transfer following reprogramming.

Individual variability in activity-based anorexia

Beeler and colleagues (2021) have furthered our understanding of the ABA phenomenon, and emphasized the importance of considering individual variability in the use of the ABA model to study aspects of AN. Only some individuals succumb to AN, while the majority can be exposed to dieting and physical activity without developing the disorder. Thus, capturing and studying resilience and vulnerability to ABA may be valuable to research. Both adolescent and young adult female C57BL/6N mice were assessed in the ABA model. Mice that adapted to ABA conditions and maintained body weight past 10 days of ABA conditions were characterized as "resilient" (Beeler et al., 2021), while the rest were "vulnerable." While all adolescent mice were vulnerable under the parameters used (two hours of food availability), in adult mice, both vulnerable and resilient phenotypes emerged. Interestingly, vulnerable mice exhibited a marked increase in running during the light cycle as well as the dark cycle, the cycle when food was provided (Beeler et al., 2021). The increase in running activity exhibited by vulnerable mice peaked dramatically just prior to removal from the experiment due to reaching the dropout weight criterion (Beeler et al., 2021). Resilient mice, on the other hand, ran during the dark cycle and increased consumption, thereby achieving stable body weight. Thus, disruption of the normal circadian rhythm for activity may be a key feature underlying vulnerability to ABA, and perhaps aspects of AN. Furthermore, this work suggests that studies assessing ABA should consider whether experimental manipulations affect resilient and/or vulnerable mice; although, defining resilient/vulnerable groups across studies might not always be straightforward.

Alternative Perspectives

One major alternative perspective of the ABA paradigm is the basic criticism that the ABA phenomenon does not model AN. This criticism could be based on the false assumption that an animal model should recapitulate a neuropsychiatric disorder in its entirety (Geyer & Markou, 1995), which the ABA model does not. Alternatively, this perspective could result from the idea that the paradoxical response to negative energy balance in ABA (eating less and running more despite very low body weight) does not drive AN. Arguments could be put forward that disordered body image and obsession with thinness are more central to AN, are not captured by the ABA model. Additionally, intense anxiety is a feature of AN that is thought to interfere with eating (Kaye et al., 2013), and a role for anxiety in the ABA paradigm has not been suggested. This encourages the development of a model that incorporates anxiogenic conditions. Another critique of ABA is that the phenomenon only occurs with macronutrient-balanced food, and that sweet and fat foods prevent ABA development.

Another perspective is that AN is too complex to be approached using an animal model such as the ABA paradigm. Questions that have highlighted the complexity of AN include: Are there several forms of anorexia nervosa (Chavez & Insel, 2007)? Can prognosis be predicted? Can risk for AN be detected (Chavez & Insel, 2007)? Is AN a disorder of body image, self-esteem, obsessive thoughts, or compulsive behavior (Chavez & Insel, 2007)?

Another potential view regarding the utility of the ABA paradigm which is far more narrow, is using the paradigm as a weight-loss model. Specifically, intermittent fasting is a popular diet used for weight loss that uses both scheduled fasting and exercise, and it has similarity to the ABA paradigm. If the ABA paradigm were used with substantially longer food access periods so that animals did not lose as much body weight, and rather, reached a plateau, these experimental conditions may be useful for studying intermittent fasting in animals. In support of this idea, dieters often show a marked increase in eating after prolonged food restriction (Polivy & Herman, 1985), and this is also observed in rodents when ad lib feeding follows a period of ABA. Yet, some patients with AN develop binge eating behavior (Serra et al., 2022; Vervaet et al., 2004), which is also similar to rodent behavior during recovery from ABA.

Despite these criticisms, the ABA model is useful for addressing specific questions regarding AN because humans cannot be extensively and invasively manipulated like rodents to determine the precise role of various neurotransmitters, neural subtypes, and projections in specific features of AN. Using both translational research findings in patients with AN and investigations using the rodent ABA paradigm provides the greatest power to ultimately uncover mechanisms underlying AN.

Implications

Studies identifying the mechanisms underlying the ABA phenomenon are hoped to ultimately lead to the first approved pharmacological treatments for AN. The recent application of circuit-dissecting techniques, also used in combination with novel transcriptomic approaches that can identify gene expression changes within specific neuron subpopulations, could identify novel targets for drug development. Other experiments aimed at identifying the factors within the periphery, such as active substances released by obese WAT (Dulawa et al., 2022), could lead to novel treatment targets. For example, obese WAT releases extracellular vesicles containing many active substances, including microRNAs (Mori et al., 2023), which could communicate with the brain (Yerrapragada & Bihl, 2022; Zhou et al., 2023) to regulate ABA and could become treatment targets for AN.

As vulnerability genes for AN are identified within the loci identified by recent GWAS studies (Watson et al., 2019), mouse genetic models can be generated and assessed for ABA to determine their effects on behavior. For example, different genetic factors likely give rise to at least somewhat different behavioral phenotypes in AN, which may be responsive to different treatments and yield different outcomes. If a human genetic variant was found to strongly associate with anxiety in mice, then individuals with AN harboring that variant could be tested for response to anti-anxiety drugs, such as selective serotonin reuptake inhibitors (SSRIs), even though patients with AN as a whole do not respond to SSRIs with weight gain (Flament et al., 2012; Pittenger, 2023; Womperski & Wozniak, 2021). Genetic etiological rodent models of AN will provide a powerful resource for understanding subtypes and could ultimately influence treatment development.

The ABA model may provide some insights for behavioral management of AN. For example, Beeler and colleagues (2021) found that vulnerable animals develop hyperactivity during their sleep cycle, while resilient animals do not. Could preventing night-time activity in patients with AN improve outcomes? Could monitoring night-time activity in patients with AN provide a warning of relapse? As previously described, ABA studies in rodents have determined that a biomarker for AN, D2R overexpression in the anteroventral striatum (Frank et al., 2005), is likely a cause rather than a consequence of AN (Welch et al., 2019); these findings encourage the development of D2R antagonists or partial agonists in the treatment of AN.

In conclusion, the ABA rodent model cannot be used to better understand the psychological correlates of AN, such as body image disturbance. However, the

ABA paradigm is a powerful preparation for dissecting the biological mechanisms underlying the paradoxical response to negative energy balance and associated biomarkers of AN. Thus, the ABA model provides an important tool for identifying potential treatment targets for AN.

References

Achamrah, N., Nobis, S., Goichon, A., Breton, J., Legrand, R., do Rego, J. L., do Rego, J. C., Dechelotte, P., Fetissov, S. O., Belmonte, L., & Coeffier, M. (2017). Sex differences in response to activity-based anorexia model in C57Bl/6 mice. *Physiology & Behavior, 170*, 1–5. https://doi.org/10.1016/j.physbeh.2016.12.014

Allen, P. J., Jimerson, D. C., Kanarek, R. B., & Kocsis, B. (2017). Impaired reversal learning in an animal model of anorexia nervosa. *Physiology & Behavior, 179*, 313–318. https://doi.org/10.1016/j.physbeh.2017.06.013

Aponte, Y., Atasoy, D., & Sternson, S. M. (2011). AGRP neurons are sufficient to orchestrate feeding behavior rapidly and without training. *Nature Neuroscience, 14*(3), 351–355. https://doi.org/10.1038/nn.2739

Attia, E. (2010). Anorexia nervosa: Current status and future directions. *Annual Review of Medicine, 61*, 425–435. https://doi.org/10.1146/annurev.med.050208.200745

Attia, E., Steinglass, J. E., Walsh, B. T., Wang, Y., Wu, P., Schreyer, C., Wildes, J., Yilmaz, Z., Guarda, A. S., Kaplan, A. S., & Marcus, M. D. (2019). Olanzapine versus placebo in adult outpatients with anorexia nervosa: A randomized clinical trial. *American Journal of Psychiatry, 176*(6), 449–456. https://doi.org/10.1176/appi.ajp.2018.18101125

Beeler, J. A., Mourra, D., Zanca, R. M., Kalmbach, A., Gellman, C., Klein, B. Y., Ravenelle, R., Serrano, P., Moore, H., Rayport, S., Mingote, S., & Burghardt, N. S. (2021). Vulnerable and resilient phenotypes in a mouse model of anorexia nervosa. *Biological Psychiatry, 90*(12), 829–842. https://doi.org/10.1016/j.biopsych.2020.06.030

Belmonte, L., Achamrah, N., Nobis, S., Guerin, C., Riou, G., Bole-Feysot, C., Boyer, O., Richard, V., Rego, J. C., Dechelotte, P., Goichon, A., & Coeffier, M. (2016). A role for intestinal TLR4-driven inflammatory response during activity-based anorexia. *Scientific Reports, 6*, 35813. https://doi.org/10.1038/srep35813

Berner, L. A., Romero, E. M., Reilly, E. E., Lavender, J. M., Kaye, W. H., & Wierenga, C. E. (2019). Task-switching inefficiencies in currently ill, but not remitted anorexia nervosa. *International Journal of Eating Disorders, 52*(11), 1316–1321. https://doi.org/10.1002/eat.23175

Betley, J. N., Cao, Z. F., Ritola, K. D., & Sternson, S. M. (2013). Parallel, redundant circuit organization for homeostatic control of feeding behavior. *Cell, 155*(6), 1337–1350. https://doi.org/10.1016/j.cell.2013.11.002

Boakes, R. A., Mills, K. J., & Single, J. P. (1999). Sex differences in the relationship between activity and weight loss in the rat. *Behavioral Neuroscience, 113*(5), 1080–1089. https://doi.org/10.1037/0735-7044.113.5.1080

Brown, A. J., Avena, N. M., & Hoebel, B. G. (2008). A high-fat diet prevents and reverses the development of activity-based anorexia in rats. *International Journal of Eating Disorders, 41*(5), 383–389. https://doi.org/10.1002/eat.20510

Bruch, H. (1962). Perceptual and conceptual disturbances in anorexia nervosa. *Psychosomatic Medicine, 24*, 187–194. https://doi.org/10.1097/00006842-196203000-00009

Byron, N., & Sakata, S. (2024). Fiber photometry-based investigation of brain function and dysfunction. *Neurophotonics, 11*(Suppl 1), S11502. https://doi.org/10.1117/1.NPh.11.S1.S11502

Cai, X., Liu, H., Feng, B., Yu, M., He, Y., Liu, H., Liang, C., Yang, Y., Tu, L., Zhang, N., Wang, L., Yin, N., Han, J., Yan, Z., Wang, C., Xu, P., Wu, Q., Tong, Q., He, Y., & Xu, Y. (2022). A D2 to D1 shift in dopaminergic inputs to midbrain 5-HT neurons causes anorexia in mice. *Nature Neuroscience, 25*(5), 646–658. https://doi.org/10.1038/s41593-022-01062-0

Casper, R. C. (2022). Restlessness and an increased urge to move (drive for activity) in anorexia nervosa may strengthen personal motivation to maintain caloric restriction and may augment body awareness and proprioception: A lesson from leptin administration in anorexia nervosa. *Frontiers in Psychology, 13*, 885274. https://doi.org/10.3389/fpsyg.2022.885274

Casper, R. C., Voderholzer, U., Naab, S., & Schlegl, S. (2020). Increased urge for movement, physical and mental restlessness, fundamental symptoms of restricting anorexia nervosa? *Brain and Behavior, 10*(3), e01556. https://doi.org/10.1002/brb3.1556

Chavez, M., & Insel, T. R. (2007). Eating disorders—National Institute of Mental Health's perspective. *American Psychologist, 62*(3), 159–166. https://doi.org/10.1037/0003-066x.62.3.159

Daimon, C. M., & Hentges, S. T. (2021). Beta-endorphin differentially contributes to food anticipatory activity in male and female mice undergoing activity-based anorexia. *Physiological Reports, 9*(5), e14788. https://doi.org/10.14814/phy2.14788

Daimon, C. M., & Hentges, S. T. (2022). Inhibition of POMC neurons in mice undergoing activity-based anorexia selectively blunts food anticipatory activity without affecting body weight or food intake. *American Journal of Physiology-Regulatory, Integrative and Comparative Physiology, 322*(3), R219–R227. https://doi.org/10.1152/ajpregu.00313.2021

Dalton, B., Foerde, K., Bartholdy, S., McClelland, J., Kekic, M., Grycuk, L., Campbell, I. C., Schmidt, U., & Steinglass, J. E. (2020). The effect of repetitive transcranial magnetic stimulation on food choice-related self-control in patients with severe, enduring anorexia nervosa. *International Journal of Eating Disorders, 53*(8), 1326–1336. https://doi.org/10.1002/eat.23267

de Rijke, C. E., Hillebrand, J. J., Verhagen, L. A., Roeling, T. A., & Adan, R. A. (2005). Hypothalamic neuropeptide expression following chronic food restriction in sedentary and wheel-running rats. *Journal of Molecular Endocrinology, 35*(2), 381–390. https://doi.org/10.1677/jme.1.01808

Deisseroth, K. (2015). Optogenetics: 10 years of microbial opsins in neuroscience. *Nature Neuroscience, 18*(9), 1213–1225. https://doi.org/10.1038/nn.4091

Dietrich, M. O., Bober, J., Ferreira, J. G., Tellez, L. A., Mineur, Y. S., Souza, D. O., Gao, X. B., Picciotto, M. R., Araujo, I., Liu, Z. W., & Horvath, T. L. (2012). AgRP neurons regulate development of dopamine neuronal plasticity and nonfood-associated behaviors. *Nature Neuroscience, 15*(8), 1108–1110. https://doi.org/10.1038/nn.3147

Dixon, D. P., Ackert, A. M., & Eckel, L. A. (2003). Development of, and recovery from, activity-based anorexia in female rats. *Physiology & Behavior, 80*(2–3), 273–279. https://doi.org/10.1016/j.physbeh.2003.08.008

Doerries, L. E., Stanley, E. Z., & Aravich, P. F. (1991). Activity-based anorexia: Relationship to gender and activity-stress ulcers. *Physiology & Behavior, 50*(5), 945–949. https://doi.org/10.1016/0031-9384(91)90419-o

Dold, M., Aigner, M., Klabunde, M., Treasure, J., & Kasper, S. (2015). Second-generation antipsychotic drugs in anorexia nervosa: A meta-analysis of randomized controlled trials. *Psychotherapy and Psychosomatics, 84*(2), 110–116. https://doi.org/10.1159/000369978

Drossman, D. A., Ontjes, D. A., & Heizer, W. D. (1979). Clinical conference. Anorexia nervosa. *Gastroenterology, 77*(5), 1115–1131. https://www.ncbi.nlm.nih.gov/pubmed/488639

Du, M., Santiago, A., Akiz, C., & Aoki, C. (2022). GABAergic interneurons' feedback inhibition of dorsal raphe-projecting pyramidal neurons of the medial prefrontal cortex suppresses feeding of adolescent female mice undergoing activity-based anorexia. *Brain Structure and Function, 227*(6), 2127–2151. https://doi.org/10.1007/s00429-022-02507-9

Duclos, M., Ouerdani, A., Mormede, P., & Konsman, J. P. (2013). Food restriction-induced hyperactivity: Addiction or adaptation to famine? *Psychoneuroendocrinology, 38*(6), 884–897. https://doi.org/10.1016/j.psyneuen.2012.09.012

Dulawa, S. C. (2021). Overlapping neural circuitry links cognitive flexibility and activity-based anorexia. *Biological Psychiatry, 90*(12), 803–805. https://doi.org/10.1016/j.biopsych.2021.10.002

Dulawa, S. C. Z., J. Zapata, R., & Osborn, O. (2022). Attenuation of anorexia-related phenotype in recipients of obese adipose tissue transplant. *Neuropsychopharmacology, 47*(1), 171–172.

Duncan, L., Yilmaz, Z., Gaspar, H., Walters, R., Goldstein, J., Anttila, V., Bulik-Sullivan, B., Ripke, S., Eating Disorders Working Group of the Psychiatric Genomics Consortium, Thornton, L., Hinney, A., Daly, M., Sullivan, P. F., Zeggini, E., Breen, G., & Bulik, C. M. (2017). Significant locus and metabolic genetic correlations revealed in genome-wide association study of anorexia nervosa. *American Journal of Psychiatry, 174*(9), 850–858. https://doi.org/10.1176/appi.ajp.2017.16121402

Emiliani, V., Entcheva, E., Hedrich, R., Hegemann, P., Konrad, K. R., Luscher, C., Mahn, M., Pan, Z. H., Sims, R. R., Vierock, J., & Yizhar, O. (2022). Optogenetics for light control of biological systems. *Nature Reviews Methods Primers, 2*, 55. https://doi.org/10.1038/s43586-022-00136-4

Exner, C., Hebebrand, J., Remschmidt, H., Wewetzer, C., Ziegler, A., Herpertz, S., Schweiger, U., Blum, W. F., Preibisch, G., Heldmaier, G., & Klingenspor, M. (2000). Leptin suppresses semi-starvation induced hyperactivity in rats: implications for anorexia nervosa. *Molecular Psychiatry, 5*(5), 476–481. https://doi.org/10.1038/sj.mp.4000771

Flament, M. F., Bissada, H., & Spettigue, W. (2012). Evidence-based pharmacotherapy of eating disorders. *International Journal of Neuropsychopharmacology, 15*(2), 189–207. https://doi.org/10.1017/S1461145711000381

Foldi, C. J., Milton, L. K., & Oldfield, B. J. (2017). The role of mesolimbic reward neurocircuitry in prevention and rescue of the activity-based anorexia (ABA) phenotype in rats. *Neuropsychopharmacology, 42*(12), 2292–2300. https://doi.org/10.1038/npp.2017.63

Foldi, C. J., Morris, M. J., & Oldfield, B. J. (2021). Executive function in obesity and anorexia nervosa: Opposite ends of a spectrum of disordered feeding behaviour? *Progress in Neuro-Psychopharmacological & Biological Psychiatry, 111*, 110395. https://doi.org/10.1016/j.pnpbp.2021.110395

Fraga, A., Carreira, M. C., Gonzalez-Izquierdo, A., Dieguez, C., Lopez, M., & Gutierrez, E. (2020). Temperature but not leptin prevents semi-starvation induced hyperactivity in rats: Implications for anorexia nervosa treatment. *Science Reports, 10*(1), 5300. https://doi.org/10.1038/s41598-020-62147-z

Fraga, A., Rial-Pensado, E., Nogueiras, R., Ferno, J., Dieguez, C., Gutierrez, E., & Lopez, M. (2021). Activity-based anorexia induces browning of adipose tissue independent of hypothalamic AMPK. *Frontiers in Endocrinology, 12*, 669980. https://doi.org/10.3389/fendo.2021.669980

Frank, G. K., Bailer, U. F., Henry, S. E., Drevets, W., Meltzer, C. C., Price, J. C., Mathis, C. A., Wagner, A., Hoge, J., Ziolko, S., Barbarich-Marsteller, N., Weissfeld, L., & Kaye, W. H. (2005). Increased dopamine D2/D3 receptor binding after recovery from anorexia nervosa measured by positron emission tomography and [11c]raclopride. *Biological Psychiatry, 58*(11), 908–912. https://doi.org/10.1016/j.biopsych.2005.05.003

Frank, G. K. W., Kalina, C., DeGuzman, M. C., & Shott, M. E. (2020). Eye blink and reward prediction error response in anorexia nervosa. *International Journal of Eating Disorders, 53*(9), 1544–1549. https://doi.org/10.1002/eat.23332

Frank, G. K. W., Shott, M. E., Pryor, T., Swindle, S., & Stoddard, J. (2022). Brain reward response in adolescents and young adults with anorexia nervosa is moderated by changes in body weight and sweetness perception. *International Journal of Eating Disorders, 55*(12), 1799–1810. https://doi.org/10.1002/eat.23814

Frintrop, L., Trinh, S., Liesbrock, J., Leunissen, C., Kempermann, J., Etdoger, S., Kas, M. J., Tolba, R., Heussen, N., Neulen, J., Konrad, K., Pafgen, V., Kiessling, F., Herpertz-Dahlmann, B., Beyer, C., & Seitz, J. (2019). The reduction of astrocytes and brain volume loss in anorexia nervosa-the impact of starvation and refeeding in a rodent model. *Translational Psychiatry, 9*(1), 159. https://doi.org/10.1038/s41398-019-0493-7

Frintrop, L., Trinh, S., Liesbrock, J., Paulukat, L., Kas, M. J., Tolba, R., Konrad, K., Herpertz-Dahlmann, B., Beyer, C., & Seitz, J. (2018). Establishment of a chronic activity-based anorexia rat model. *Journal of Neuroscience Methods, 293*, 191–198. https://doi.org/10.1016/j.jneumeth.2017.09.018

Gelegen, C., Collier, D. A., Campbell, I. C., Oppelaar, H., van den Heuvel, J., Adan, R. A., & Kas, M. J. (2007). Difference in susceptibility to activity-based anorexia in two inbred strains of mice. *European Neuropsychopharmacology, 17*(3), 199–205. https://doi.org/10.1016/j.euroneuro.2006.04.007

Geyer, M. A. & Markou, A. (1995). Animal models of psychiatric disorders. In F. E. Bloom & D. Kupfer (Eds.), *Psychopharmacology: Fourth Generation of Progress* (pp. 787–798). Raven Press.

Gottesman, I. I., & Gould, T. D. (2003). The endophenotype concept in psychiatry: Etymology and strategic intentions. *American Journal of Psychiatry, 160*(4), 636–645. https://doi.org/10.1176/appi.ajp.160.4.636

Guisinger, S. (2003). Adapted to flee famine: Adding an evolutionary perspective on anorexia nervosa. *Psychological Review, 110*(4), 745–761. https://doi.org/10.1037/0033-295X.110.4.745

Gunturkun, M. H., Wang, T., Chitre, A. S., Garcia Martinez, A., Holl, K., St Pierre, C., Bimschleger, H., Gao, J., Cheng, R., Polesskaya, O., Solberg Woods, L. C., Palmer, A. A., & Chen, H. (2022). Genome-wide association study on three behaviors tested in an open field in heterogeneous stock rats identifies multiple loci implicated in psychiatric disorders. *Frontiers in Psychiatry, 13*, 790566. https://doi.org/10.3389/fpsyt.2022.790566

Haleem, D. J. (2009). Exaggerated feedback control decreases brain serotonin concentration and elicits hyperactivity in a rat model of diet-restriction-induced anorexia nervosa. *Appetite, 52*(1), 44–50. https://doi.org/10.1016/j.appet.2008.07.009

Hall, J. F., Smith, K., Schnitzer, S. B., & Hanford, P. V. (1953). Elevation of activity level in the rat following transition from ad libitum to restricted feeding. *Journal of Comparative and Physiological Psychology, 46*(6), 429–433. https://doi.org/10.1037/h0062565

Hancock, S., & Grant, V. (2009). Early maternal separation increases symptoms of activity-based anorexia in male and female rats. *Journal of Experimental Psychology: Animal Behavior Processes*, *35*(3), 394–406. https://doi.org/10.1037/a0014736

Hernandez-Carretero, A., Weber, N., La Frano, M. R., Ying, W., Lantero Rodriguez, J., Sears, D. D., Wallenius, V., Borgeson, E., Newman, J. W., & Osborn, O. (2018). Obesity-induced changes in lipid mediators persist after weight loss. *International Journal of Obesity*, *42*(4), 728–736. https://doi.org/10.1038/ijo.2017.266

Hillebrand, J. J., Koeners, M. P., de Rijke, C. E., Kas, M. J., & Adan, R. A. (2005). Leptin treatment in activity-based anorexia. *Biological Psychiatry*, *58*(2), 165–171. https://doi.org/10.1016/j.biopsych.2005.03.011

Hillebrand, J. J., van Elburg, A. A., Kas, M. J., van Engeland, H., & Adan, R. A. (2005). Olanzapine reduces physical activity in rats exposed to activity-based anorexia: possible implications for treatment of anorexia nervosa? *Biological Psychiatry*, *58*(8), 651–657. https://doi.org/10.1016/j.biopsych.2005.04.008

Holliday, J., Tchanturia, K., Landau, S., Collier, D., & Treasure, J. (2005). Is impaired set-shifting an endophenotype of anorexia nervosa? *American Journal of Psychiatry*, *162*(12), 2269–2275. https://doi.org/10.1176/appi.ajp.162.12.2269

Hui, Y. Q., Zheng, X. F., Zhang, H. J., Li, F., Yu, G. Y., Li, J., Zhang, J. F., Gong, X. B., & Guo, G. Q. (2022). Strategies for targeting neural circuits: how to manipulate neurons using virus vehicles. *Frontiers in Neural Circuits*, 16. https://doi.org/ARTN88236610.3389/fncir.2022.882366

Illius, A. W., Tolkamp, B. J., & Yearsley, J. (2002). The evolution of the control of food intake. *Proceedings of the Nutrition Society*, *61*(4), 465–472. https://doi.org/10.1079/pns2002179

Johnston, J. L., Leiter, L. A., Burrow, G. N., Garfinkel, P. E., & Anderson, G. H. (1984). Excretion of urinary catecholamine metabolites in anorexia nervosa: effect of body composition and energy intake. *American Journal of Clinical Nutrition*, *40*(5), 1001–1006. https://doi.org/10.1093/ajcn/40.5.1001

Kanarek, R. B., D'Anci, K. E., Jurdak, N., & Mathes, W. F. (2009). Running and addiction: Precipitated withdrawal in a rat model of activity-based anorexia. *Behavioral Neuroscience*, *123*(4), 905–912. https://doi.org/10.1037/a0015896

Kaye, W. H. (1997). Anorexia nervosa, obsessional behavior, and serotonin. *Psychopharmacology Bulletin*, *33*(3), 335–344. https://www.ncbi.nlm.nih.gov/pubmed/9550876

Kaye, W. H., Ebert, M. H., Raleigh, M., & Lake, R. (1984). Abnormalities in CNS monoamine metabolism in anorexia nervosa. *Archives of General Psychiatry*, *41*(4), 350–355. https://doi.org/10.1001/archpsyc.1984.01790150040007

Kaye, W. H., Frank, G. K., & McConaha, C. (1999). Altered dopamine activity after recovery from restricting-type anorexia nervosa. *Neuropsychopharmacology*, *21*(4), 503–506. https://doi.org/10.1016/S0893-133X(99)00053-6

Kaye, W. H., Fudge, J. L., & Paulus, M. (2009). New insights into symptoms and neurocircuit function of anorexia nervosa. *Nature Reviews Neuroscience*, *10*(8), 573–584. https://doi.org/10.1038/nrn2682

Kaye, W. H., Gwirtsman, H. E., George, D. T., Jimerson, D. C., & Ebert, M. H. (1988). CSF 5-HIAA concentrations in anorexia nervosa: reduced values in underweight subjects normalize after weight gain. *Biological Psychiatry*, *23*(1), 102–105. https://doi.org/10.1016/0006-3223(88)90113-8

Kaye, W. H., Wierenga, C. E., Bailer, U. F., Simmons, A. N., & Bischoff-Grethe, A. (2013). Nothing tastes as good as skinny feels: The neurobiology of anorexia nervosa. *Trends in Neuroscience*, *36*(2), 110–120. https://doi.org/10.1016/j.tins.2013.01.003

Klenotich, S. J., & Dulawa, S. C. (2012). The activity-based anorexia mouse model. *Methods in Molecular Biology*, *829*, 377–393. https://doi.org/10.1007/978-1-61779-458-2_25

Klenotich, S. J., Ho, E. V., McMurray, M. S., Server, C. H., & Dulawa, S. C. (2015). Dopamine D2/3 receptor antagonism reduces activity-based anorexia. *Translational Psychiatry*, *5*(8), e613. https://doi.org/10.1038/tp.2015.109

Klenotich, S. J., Seiglie, M. P., McMurray, M. S., Roitman, J. D., Le Grange, D., Dugad, P., & Dulawa, S. C. (2012). Olanzapine, but not fluoxetine, treatment increases survival in activity-based anorexia in mice. *Neuropsychopharmacology*, *37*(7), 1620–1631. https://doi.org/10.1038/npp.2012.7

Kontis, D., & Theochari, E. (2012). Dopamine in anorexia nervosa: A systematic review. *Behavioural Pharmacology*, *23*(5–6), 496–515. https://doi.org/10.1097/FBP.0b013e328357e115

Krashes, M. J., Koda, S., Ye, C., Rogan, S. C., Adams, A. C., Cusher, D. S., Maratos-Flier, E., Roth, B. L., & Lowell, B. B. (2011). Rapid, reversible activation of AgRP neurons drives feeding behavior in mice. *Journal of Clinical Investigations*, *121*(4), 1424–1428. https://doi.org/10.1172/JCI46229

Kubitschke, M., Muller, M., Wallhorn, L., Pulin, M., Mittag, M., Pollok, S., Ziebarth, T., Bremshey, S., Gerdey, J., Claussen, K. C., Renken, K., Gross, J., Gneisse, P., Meyer, N., Wiegert, J. S., Reiner, A., Fuhrmann, M., & Masseck, O. A. (2022). Next generation genetically encoded fluorescent sensors for serotonin. *Nature Communications, 13*(1), 7525. https://doi.org/10.1038/s41467-022-35200-w

Kyriakis, S. C., Martinsson, K., Olsson, N. G., & Bjork, A. (1990). Thin sow syndrome (TSS): The effect of amperozide. *British Veterinary Journal, 146*(5), 463–467. https://doi.org/10.1016/0007-1935(90)90036-3

Lambert, K. G., & Kinsley, C. H. (1993). Sex differences and gonadal hormones influence susceptibility to the activity-stress paradigm. *Physiology & Behavior, 53*(6), 1085–1090. https://doi.org/10.1016/0031-9384(93)90363-k

Lee, R. B., & Daly, R. (1999). Introduction: Foragers & others. In R. B. Lee & R. Daly (Eds.), *The Cambridge encyclopedia of hunters & gatherers* (pp. 1–20). Cambridge University Press.

Lee, T. J., & Kinzig, K. P. (2017). Repeated adolescent activity-based anorexia influences central estrogen signaling and adulthood anxiety-like behaviors in rats. *Physiology & Behavior, 171*, 199–206. https://doi.org/10.1016/j.physbeh.2016.12.039

Li, C., Hou, Y., Zhang, J., Sui, G., Du, X., Licinio, J., Wong, M. L., & Yang, Y. (2019). AGRP neurons modulate fasting-induced anxiolytic effects. *Translational Psychiatry, 9*(1), 111. https://doi.org/10.1038/s41398-019-0438-1

Licinio, J., Wong, M. L., & Gold, P. W. (1996). The hypothalamic-pituitary-adrenal axis in anorexia nervosa. *Psychiatry Research, 62*(1), 75–83. https://doi.org/10.1016/0165-1781(96)02991-5

MacLean, P. S., Higgins, J. A., Giles, E. D., Sherk, V. D., & Jackman, M. R. (2015). The role for adipose tissue in weight regain after weight loss. *Obesity Review, 16*(Suppl 1), 45–54. https://doi.org/10.1111/obr.12255

Martin, B., Pearson, M., Kebejian, L., Golden, E., Keselman, A., Bender, M., Carlson, O., Egan, J., Ladenheim, B., Cadet, J. L., Becker, K. G., Wood, W., Duffy, K., Vinayakumar, P., Maudsley, S., & Mattson, M. P. (2007). Sex-dependent metabolic, neuroendocrine, and cognitive responses to dietary energy restriction and excess. *Endocrinology, 148*(9), 4318–4333. https://doi.org/10.1210/en.2007-0161

Mequinion, M., Foldi, C. J., & Andrews, Z. B. (2019). The ghrelin-AgRP neuron nexus in anorexia nervosa: Implications for metabolic and behavioral adaptations. *Frontiers in Nutrition, 6*, 190. https://doi.org/10.3389/fnut.2019.00190

Merle, J. V., Haas, V., Burghardt, R., Dohler, N., Schneider, N., Lehmkuhl, U., & Ehrlich, S. (2011). Agouti-related protein in patients with acute and weight-restored anorexia nervosa. *Psychological Medicine, 41*(10), 2183–2192. https://doi.org/10.1017/S0033291711000365

Michaelides, M., & Hurd, Y. L. (2016). Chemogenetics: DREADDs. In D. W. Pfaff, N. D. Volkow, & J. L. Rubenstein (Eds.), *Neuroscience in the 21st century: From basic to clinical* (2nd ed.) (pp. 2847–2856). Springer. https://doi.org/10.1007/978-1-4939-3474-4_147

Michaelides, M., Miller, M. L., DiNieri, J. A., Gomez, J. L., Schwartz, E., Egervari, G., Wang, G. J., Mobbs, C. V., Volkow, N. D., & Hurd, Y. L. (2017). Dopamine D2 receptor signaling in the nucleus accumbens comprises a metabolic-cognitive brain interface regulating metabolic components of glucose reinforcement. *Neuropsychopharmacology, 42*(12), 2365–2376. https://doi.org/10.1038/npp.2017.112

Miletta, M. C., Iyilikci, O., Shanabrough, M., Sestan-Pesa, M., Cammisa, A., Zeiss, C. J., Dietrich, M. O., & Horvath, T. L. (2020). AgRP neurons control compulsive exercise and survival in an activity-based anorexia model. *Nature Metabolism, 2*(11), 1204–1211. https://doi.org/10.1038/s42255-020-00300-8

Milton, L. K., Mirabella, P. N., Greaves, E., Spanswick, D. C., van den Buuse, M., Oldfield, B. J., & Foldi, C. J. (2021). Suppression of corticostriatal circuit activity improves cognitive flexibility and prevents body weight loss in activity-based anorexia in rats. *Biological Psychiatry, 90*(12), 819–828. https://doi.org/10.1016/j.biopsych.2020.06.022

Moran, T. H., & Tamashiro, K. L. K. (2007). Curt Richter: Spontaneous activity and food intake. *Appetite, 49*(2), 368–375. https://doi.org/10.1016/j.appet.2006.09.016

Mori, T., Giovannelli, L., Bilia, A. R., & Margheri, F. (2023). Exosomes: Potential next-generation nanocarriers for the therapy of inflammatory diseases. *Pharmaceutics, 15*(9). https://doi.org/10.3390/pharmaceutics15092276

Neale, J., & Hudson, L. D. (2020). Anorexia nervosa in adolescents. *British Journal of Hospital Medicine, 81*(6), 1–8. https://doi.org/10.12968/hmed.2020.0099

Phillips, M. L., Drevets, W. C., Rauch, S. L., & Lane, R. (2003a). Neurobiology of emotion perception I: The neural basis of normal emotion perception. *Biological Psychiatry, 54*(5), 504–514. https://doi.org/10.1016/s0006-3223(03)00168-9

Phillips, M. L., Drevets, W. C., Rauch, S. L., & Lane, R. (2003b). Neurobiology of emotion perception II: Implications for major psychiatric disorders. *Biological Psychiatry, 54*(5), 515–528. https://doi.org/10.1016/s0006-3223(03)00171-9

Pittenger, C. (2023). The pharmacological treatment of obsessive-compulsive disorder. *Psychiatric Clinics of North America, 46*(1), 107–119. https://doi.org/10.1016/j.psc.2022.11.005

Pjetri, E., de Haas, R., de Jong, S., Gelegen, C., Oppelaar, H., Verhagen, L. A., Eijkemans, M. J., Adan, R. A., Olivier, B., & Kas, M. J. (2012). Identifying predictors of activity based anorexia susceptibility in diverse genetic rodent populations. *PLOS ONE, 7*(11), e50453. https://doi.org/10.1371/journal.pone.0050453

Polivy, J., & Herman, C. P. (1985). Dieting and binging. A causal analysis. *American Psychologist, 40*(2), 193–201. https://doi.org/10.1037//0003-066x.40.2.193

Ranzenhofer, L. M., Jablonski, M., Davis, L., Posner, J., Walsh, B. T., & Steinglass, J. E. (2022). Early course of symptom development in anorexia nervosa. *Journal of Adolescent Health, 71*(5), 587–593. https://doi.org/10.1016/j.jadohealth.2022.06.010

Richard, J. M., & Berridge, K. C. (2013). Prefrontal cortex modulates desire and dread generated by nucleus accumbens glutamate disruption. *Biological Psychiatry, 73*(4), 360–370. https://doi.org/10.1016/j.biopsych.2012.08.009

Robinette, T. M., Nicholatos, J. W., Francisco, A. B., Brooks, K. E., Diao, R. Y., Sorbi, S., Ricca, V., Nacmias, B., Brieno-Enriquez, M. A., & Libert, S. (2020). SIRT1 accelerates the progression of activity-based anorexia. *Nature Communications, 11*(1), 2814. https://doi.org/10.1038/s41467-020-16348-9

Routtenberg, A., & Kuznesof, A. W. (1967). Self-starvation of rats living in activity wheels on a restricted feeding schedule. *Journal of Comparative Physiological Psychology, 64*(3), 414–421. https://doi.org/10.1037/h0025205

Santiago, A. N., Makowicz, E. A., Du, M., & Aoki, C. (2021). Food restriction engages prefrontal corticostriatal cells and local microcircuitry to drive the decision to run versus conserve energy. *Cerebral Cortex, 31*(6), 2868–2885. https://doi.org/10.1093/cercor/bhaa394

Scharner, S., Friedrich, T., Goebel-Stengel, M., Kobelt, P., Rose, M., & Stengel, A. (2018). Activity-based anorexia activates CRF immunoreactive neurons in female rats. *Neuroscience Letters, 674*, 142–147. https://doi.org/10.1016/j.neulet.2018.03.049

Scheen, A. J., Castillo, M., & Lefebvre, P. J. (1988). Insulin sensitivity in anorexia nervosa: A mirror image of obesity? *Diabetes/Metabolism Reviews, 4*(7), 681–690. https://doi.org/10.1002/dmr.5610040705

Scheurink, A. J., Boersma, G. J., Nergardh, R., & Sodersten, P. (2010). Neurobiology of hyperactivity and reward: Agreeable restlessness in anorexia nervosa. *Physiology & Behavior, 100*(5), 490–495. https://doi.org/10.1016/j.physbeh.2010.03.016

Seed, J. A., Dixon, R. A., McCluskey, S. E., & Young, A. H. (2000). Basal activity of the hypothalamic-pituitary-adrenal axis and cognitive function in anorexia nervosa. *European Archives of Psychiatry and Clinical Neuroscience, 250*(1), 11–15. https://doi.org/10.1007/pl00007533

Seitz, J., Trinh, S., Kogel, V., & Beyer, C. (2021). Brain volume loss, astrocyte reduction, and inflammation in anorexia nervosa. *Advances in Neurobiology, 26*, 283–313. https://doi.org/10.1007/978-3-030-77375-5_12

Serra, R., Di Nicolantonio, C., Di Febo, R., De Crescenzo, F., Vanderlinden, J., Vrieze, E., Bruffaerts, R., Loriedo, C., Pasquini, M., & Tarsitani, L. (2022). The transition from restrictive anorexia nervosa to binging and purging: A systematic review and meta-analysis. *Eating and Weight Disorders, 27*(3), 857–865. https://doi.org/10.1007/s40519-021-01226-0

Shroff, H., Reba, L., Thornton, L. M., Tozzi, F., Klump, K. L., Berrettini, W. H., Brandt, H., Crawford, S., Crow, S., Fichter, M. M., Goldman, D., Halmi, K. A., Johnson, C., Kaplan, A. S., Keel, P., LaVia, M., Mitchell, J., Rotondo, A., Strober, M., . . . Bulik, C. M. (2006). Features associated with excessive exercise in women with eating disorders. *International Journal of Eating Disorders, 39*(6), 454–461. https://doi.org/10.1002/eat.20247

Simpson, E. H., Akam, T., Patriarchi, T., Blanco-Pozo, M., Burgeno, L. M., Mohebi, A., Cragg, S. J., & Walton, M. E. (2024). Lights, fiber, action! A primer on in vivo fiber photometry. *Neuron, 112*(5), 718–739. https://doi.org/10.1016/j.neuron.2023.11.016

Smith, K. S., Bucci, D. J., Luikart, B. W., & Mahler, S. V. (2016). DREADDS: Use and application in behavioral neuroscience. *Behavioral Neuroscience, 130*(2), 137–155. https://doi.org/10.1037/bne0000135

Sodersten, P., Nergardh, R., Bergh, C., Zandian, M., & Scheurink, A. (2008). Behavioral neuroendocrinology and treatment of anorexia nervosa. *Frontiers in Neuroendocrinology, 29*(4), 445–462. https://doi.org/10.1016/j.yfrne.2008.06.001

Spadini, S., Ferro, M., Lamanna, J., & Malgaroli, A. (2021). Activity-based anorexia animal model: A review of the main neurobiological findings. *Journal of Eating Disorders, 9*(1), 123. https://doi.org/10.1186/s40337-021-00481-x

Steinglass, J. E., Walsh, B. T., & Stern, Y. (2006). Set shifting deficit in anorexia nervosa. *Journal of the International Neuropsychological Society, 12*(3), 431–435. https://doi.org/10.1017/s1355617706060528

Sternheim, L. C., van Passel, B., Dingemans, A., Cath, D., & Danner, U. N. (2022). Cognitive and experienced flexibility in patients with anorexia nervosa and obsessive compulsive disorder. *Frontiers in Psychiatry, 13*, 868921. https://doi.org/10.3389/fpsyt.2022.868921

Sun, F., Zhou, J., Dai, B., Qian, T., Zeng, J., Li, X., Zhuo, Y., Zhang, Y., Wang, Y., Qian, C., Tan, K., Feng, J., Dong, H., Lin, D., Cui, G., & Li, Y. (2020). Next-generation GRAB sensors for monitoring dopaminergic activity in vivo. *Nature Methods, 17*(11), 1156–1166. https://doi.org/10.1038/s41592-020-00981-9

Sutton Hickey, A. K., Duane, S. C., Mickelsen, L. E., Karolczak, E. O., Shamma, A. M., Skillings, A., Li, C., & Krashes, M. J. (2023). AgRP neurons coordinate the mitigation of activity-based anorexia. *Molecular Psychiatry, 28*(4), 1622–1635. https://doi.org/10.1038/s41380-022-01932-w

Tadayonnejad, R., Majid, D. A., Tsolaki, E., Rane, R., Wang, H., Moody, T. D., Pauli, W. M., Pouratian, N., Bari, A. A., Murray, S. B., O'Doherty, J. P., & Feusner, J. D. (2022). Mesolimbic neurobehavioral mechanisms of reward motivation in anorexia nervosa: A multimodal imaging study. *Frontiers in Psychiatry, 13*, 806327. https://doi.org/10.3389/fpsyt.2022.806327

Thompson, K. J., Khajehali, E., Bradley, S. J., Navarrete, J. S., Huang, X. P., Slocum, S., Jin, J., Liu, J., Xiong, Y., Olsen, R. H. J., Diberto, J. F., Boyt, K. M., Pina, M. M., Pati, D., Molloy, C., Bundgaard, C., Sexton, P. M., Kash, T. L., Krashes, M. J., . . . Tobin, A. B. (2018). DREADD agonist 21 is an effective agonist for muscarinic-based DREADDs in vitro and in vivo. *ACS Pharmacology & Translational Science Journal, 1*(1), 61–72. https://doi.org/10.1021/acsptsci.8b00012

Thorey, S., Blanchet, C., Guessoum, S. B., Moro, M. R., Ludot, M., & Carretier, E. (2023). Efficacy and tolerance of second-generation antipsychotics in anorexia nervosa: A systematic scoping review. *PLOS ONE, 18*(3), e0278189. https://doi.org/10.1371/journal.pone.0278189

Treasure, J. L., & Owen, J. B. (1997). Intriguing links between animal behavior and anorexia nervosa. *International Journal of Eating Disorders, 21*(4), 307–311. https://doi.org/10.1002/(sici)1098-108x(1997)21:4<307::aid-eat1>3.0.co;2-s

Uniacke, B., Slattery, R., Walsh, B. T., Shohamy, D., Foerde, K., & Steinglass, J. (2020). A comparison of food-based decision-making between restricting and binge-eating/purging subtypes of anorexia nervosa. *International Journal of Eating Disorders, 53*(10), 1751–1756. https://doi.org/10.1002/eat.23359

Verhagen, L. A., Egecioglu, E., Luijendijk, M. C., Hillebrand, J. J., Adan, R. A., & Dickson, S. L. (2011). Acute and chronic suppression of the central ghrelin signaling system reveals a role in food anticipatory activity. *European Neuropsychopharmacology, 21*(5), 384–392. https://doi.org/10.1016/j.euroneuro.2010.06.005

Vervaet, M., van Heeringen, C., & Audenaert, K. (2004). Personality-related characteristics in restricting versus binging and purging eating disordered patients. *Comprehensive Psychiatry, 45*(1), 37–43. https://doi.org/10.1016/j.comppsych.2003.09.008

Vincent, G. P., & Pare, W. P. (1976). Activity-stress ulcer in the rat, hamster, gerbil and guinea pig. *Physiology & Behavior, 16*(5), 557–560. https://doi.org/10.1016/0031-9384(76)90215-8

Vincent, G. P., Pare, W. P., Isom, K. E., & Reeves, J. M. (1977). Activity-stress gastric lesions in chipmunk (tamias-striatus). *Physiological Psychology, 5*(4), 449–452. https://doi.org/Doi10.3758/Bf03337853

Wang, T., Han, W., Chitre, A. S., Polesskaya, O., Solberg Woods, L. C., Palmer, A. A., & Chen, H. (2018). Social and anxiety-like behaviors contribute to nicotine self-administration in adolescent outbred rats. *Science Reports, 8*(1), 18069. https://doi.org/10.1038/s41598-018-36263-w

Warren, M. P., & Vande Wiele, R. L. (1973). Clinical and metabolic features of anorexia nervosa. *American Journal of Obstetrics & Gynecology, 117*(3), 435–449. https://doi.org/10.1016/0002-9378(73)90053-7

Watson, H. J., Yilmaz, Z., Thornton, L. M., Hubel, C., Coleman, J. R. I., Gaspar, H. A., Bryois, J., Hinney, A., Leppa, V. M., Mattheisen, M., Medland, S. E., Ripke, S., Yao, S., Giusti-Rodriguez, P., Anorexia Nervosa Genetics, I., Hanscombe, K. B., Purves, K. L., Eating Disorders Working Group of the Psychiatric Genomics, C., Adan, R. A. H., . . . Bulik, C. M. (2019). Genome-wide association study identifies eight risk loci and implicates metabo-psychiatric origins for anorexia nervosa. *Nature Genetics, 51*(8), 1207–1214. https://doi.org/10.1038/s41588-019-0439-2

Welch, A. C., Zhang, J., Lyu, J., McMurray, M. S., Javitch, J. A., Kellendonk, C., & Dulawa, S. C. (2019). Dopamine D2 receptor overexpression in the nucleus accumbens core induces robust weight loss during scheduled fasting selectively in female mice. *Molecular Psychiatry*, 26(8), 3765–3777. https://doi.org/10.1038/s41380-019-0633-8

Wierenga, C. E., Reilly, E., Bischoff-Grethe, A., Kaye, W. H., & Brown, G. G. (2022). Altered reinforcement learning from reward and punishment in anorexia nervosa: Evidence from computational modeling. *Journal of the International Neuropsychological Society, 28*(10), 1003–1015. https://doi.org/10.1017/S1355617721001326

Womperski, K., & Wozniak, J. (2021). Comorbidity of obsessive-compulsive disorder and anorexia nervosa—Diagnostic difficulties: A case study of a 14-year-old girl. Postępy Psychiatrii i Neurologii, *30*(1), 52–60. https://doi.org/10.5114/ppn.2021.106820

Yanovski, S. (2003). Sugar and fat: Cravings and aversions. *Journal of Nutrition, 133*(3), 835S–837S. https://doi.org/10.1093/jn/133.3.835S

Yasuhara, D., Naruo, T., Nagai, N., Muranaga, T., Nakahara, T., Tanaka, M., Kojima, S., Sagiyama, K., Masuda, A., & Inui, A. (2005). Glucose tolerance predicts short-term refeeding outcome in females with anorexia nervosa. *Psychosomatic Medicine, 67*(4), 669–676. https://doi.org/10.1097/01.psy.0000170332.47378.a1

Yerrapragada, S. M., & Bihl, J. C. (2022). Role of exosomes in mediating the cross-talk between adipose tissue and the brain. *Neuromolecular Medicine, 24*(2), 57–61. https://doi.org/10.1007/s12017-021-08664-0

Yoon, D. J., Zhang, J., Zapata, R. C., Ulivieri, M., Libster, A. M., McMurray, M. S., Osborn, O., & Dulawa, S. C. (2024). The attenuation of activity-based anorexia by obese adipose tissue transplant if AgRP neuron-dependent. *bioRxiv*. https://doi.org/10.1101/2024.04.23.590824

Zapata, R. C., Carretero, M., Reis, F. C. G., Chaudry, B. S., Ofrecio, J., Zhang, D., Sasik, R., Ciaraldi, T., Petrascheck, M., & Osborn, O. (2022). Adipocytes control food intake and weight regain via vacuolar-type H(+) ATPase. *Nature Communication, 13*(1), 5092. https://doi.org/10.1038/s41467-022-32764-5

Zhang, J., & Dulawa, S. C. (2021). The utility of animal models for studying the metabo-psychiatric origins of anorexia nervosa. *Frontiers in Psychiatry, 12*, 711181. https://doi.org/10.3389/fpsyt.2021.711181

Zhou, W., Zhao, L. H., Mao, Z. L., Wang, Z. H., Zhang, Z. X., & Li, M. H. (2023). Bidirectional communication between the brain and other organs: The role of extracellular vesicles. *Cellular and Molecular Neurobiology, 43*(6), 2675–2696. https://doi.org/10.1007/s10571-023-01345-5.

23

Neurobiological Model of Avoidant/Restrictive Food Intake Disorder

Jennifer J. Thomas, Laura M. Holsen, and Elizabeth A. Lawson

Brief Definitional Overview

Avoidant/restrictive food intake disorder (ARFID): A serious mental health condition characterized by severe restriction of food intake—by volume and/or variety—due to fear of aversive consequences, lack of interest in eating or food, or sensory sensitivity (American Psychiatric Association, 2013).

ARFID-fear of aversive consequences: A phenotype characterized by restriction of eating following an eating-related event perceived as traumatic, such as vomiting, choking, anaphylaxis, or acute gastrointestinal distress.

ARFID-lack of interest: A phenotype in which individuals struggle to eat enough calories overall and which is typically characterized by experiencing low hunger and satiety.

ARFID-sensory sensitivity: A phenotype characterized by strong aversions to most foods based on their taste, texture, or appearance.

Introduction

Avoidant/restrictive food intake disorder (ARFID) is a serious mental health condition that was added to the psychiatric nomenclature with the 2013 publication of the *DSM*-5 (American Psychiatric Association, 2013). Individuals with ARFID severely restrict their food intake—by volume and/or variety—due to fear of aversive consequences, lack of interest in eating or food, or sensory sensitivity. ARFID differs from other well-known eating disorders (e.g., anorexia nervosa, bulimia nervosa) because individuals with ARFID do not endorse body image concerns or purposefully diet. Nonetheless, their eating behavior leads to severe health consequences, including precipitous weight loss, nutritional deficiencies, dependence on tube feeding or nutritional supplements, and/or significant psychosocial impairment (American Psychiatric Association, 2013).

Jennifer J. Thomas, Laura M. Holsen, and Elizabeth A. Lawson, *Neurobiological Model of Avoidant/Restrictive Food Intake Disorder*. In: *The Handbook of the Neurobiology of Eating Disorders*. Edited by: Christina E. Wierenga and Joanna E. Steinglass, Oxford University Press. © Oxford University Press (2025). DOI: 10.1093/9780197675212.003.0024

The *DSM-5* describes three clinical phenotypes of ARFID, which have been empirically replicated by independent research teams (Norris et al., 2018; Reilly et al., 2019; Zickgraf et al., 2019) and can be identified through psychometrically validated interviews (e.g., Bryant-Waugh et al., 2019) and self-report questionnaires (e.g., Bryant-Waugh et al., 2022; Zickgraf et al., 2018). First, those with the ARFID fear of aversive consequences (*ARFID-fear*) phenotype restrict their eating following an eating-related event that they perceive as traumatic, such as vomiting, choking, anaphylaxis, or acute gastrointestinal distress. Second, individuals with the *ARFID-lack of interest* phenotype struggle to eat enough calories overall and typically describe themselves as experiencing low hunger and high satiety. Lastly, individuals with *ARFID-sensory sensitivity* report strong aversions to most foods based on their taste, texture, or appearance. Clinically, these phenotypes are not mutually exclusive, and they can co-occur within the same individual (Norris et al., 2018; Reilly et al., 2019; Richmond et al., 2023) across dimensions of severity (Bryant-Waugh et al., 2019).

Epidemiological studies indicate that ARFID is as common as the better-known eating disorders (e.g., anorexia nervosa, bulimia nervosa), affecting 0.3% to 15.5% of children and adolescents (Sanchez-Cerezo et al., 2023) and 0.8% (Hilbert et al., 2021) to 4% (Chua et al., 2021) of adults. Moreover, ARFID is especially common in treatment settings, where it comprises 23% of eating-disorder patients (Nicely et al., 2014) and 24% of neuro-gastroenterology patients (Murray et al., 2020). In addition to its characteristic psychosocial impairment, ARFID can be associated with serious medical consequences, including low bone density (Sella, Becker, et al., 2023), vitamin deficiencies (Nitsch et al., 2023), vision impairment (Schimansky et al., 2023), and decreased quality of life (Hay et al., 2017). Although several clinical interventions for ARFID are currently under study (e.g., Lock, 2021; Thomas & Eddy, 2019; Sharp et al., 2016), there are currently no evidence-based treatments for this common and impairing disorder.

Biological Framework

A better understanding of the neurobiology of ARFID could pave the way for understanding the etiology and maintenance of the disorder, as well as developing novel treatments. When ARFID was first described in 2013, little was known about its pathophysiology. The three-dimensional neurobiological model of ARFID (Thomas, Lawson, et al., 2017) provides testable hypotheses about ARFID development and maintenance to identify potential targets for intervention. This model was informed by the National Institute of Mental Health's Research Domain Criteria (RDoC; Insel et al., 2010). The RDoC matrix provides a structure for understanding psychopathology as emanating from neurobiological dimensions that cut across categorical diagnoses. RDoC recognizes six major domains, each divided into constructs, that can be measured across units of analysis. For example,

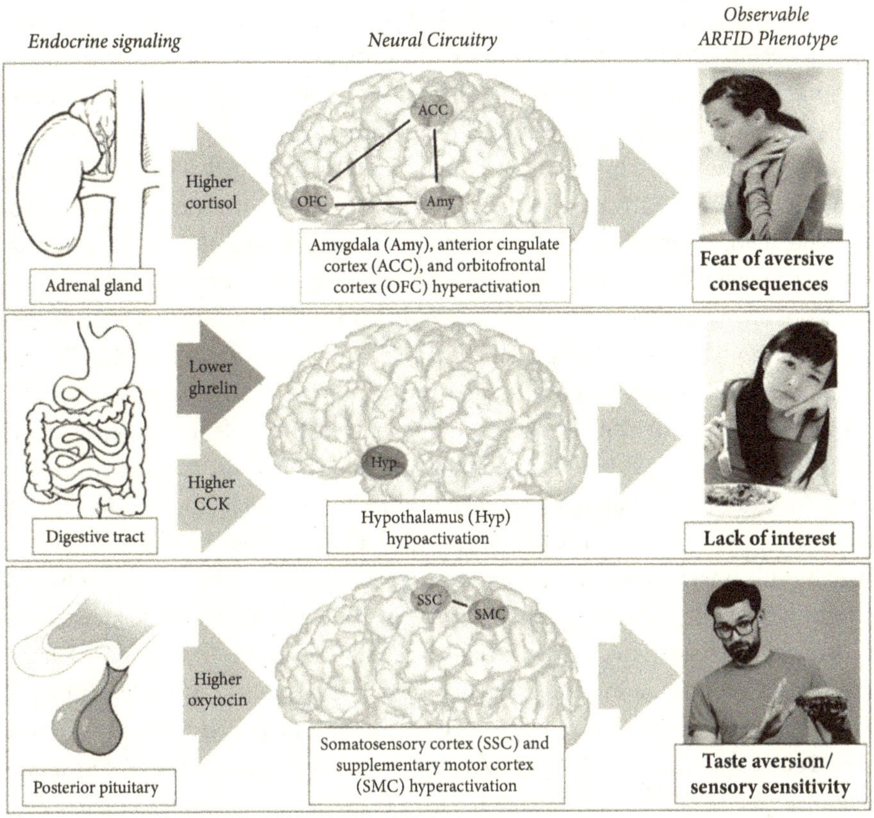

Figure 23.1 The three-dimensional neurobiological model of avoidant/restrictive food intake disorder (ARFID) suggests that endocrine signaling acts upon neural circuitry to produce observable behavioral symptoms that comprise the three ARFID phenotypes.

the first domain—Negative Valence Systems—is further made up of the constructs of acute threat (fear), potential threat (anxiety), sustained threat, loss, and frustrative non-reward, and it can be studied across many units of analysis including genes, molecules, cells, circuits, physiology, behavior, and self-report. The three-dimensional neurobiological model of ARFID posits that each of the three clinical phenotypes of ARFID—*ARFID-fear, ARFID-lack of interest, ARFID-sensory sensitivity*—is driven by a relevant construct from the RDoC framework. Figure 23.1 provides a visual schematic of the three-dimensional neurobiological model of ARFID, which is also described in detail in the following discussion.

ARFID-fear

Individuals with the *ARFID-fear* phenotype present with acute food restriction following a traumatic event. For example, an 11-year-old girl who, after choking on a pork chop, restricted her diet to just liquids and purees, resulting in precipitous weight loss, is a paradigmatic example of the *ARFID-fear* phenotype (Thomas, Brigham et al., 2017). Many people have transient episodes of choking, vomiting, anaphylaxis, or gastrointestinal distress, but few of them go on to develop ARFID. The three-dimensional model provides a possible explanation—that the *ARFID-fear* phenotype is a product of hyperactivity in Negative Valence Systems (acute threat/fear). Activation of the brain's defensive motivational system promotes behaviors that protect us from perceived danger (Lang et al., 1998). Normal fear reactions involve adaptive responses to conditioned or unconditioned threat stimuli, but hyperactivity in this domain could lead to prolonged avoidance of conditioned stimuli that are no longer harmful and explain why those with *ARFID-fear* continue to avoid feared foods even after the resolution of an acute threat.

If *ARFID-fear* is driven by hyperactivity in Negative Valence Systems (acute threat/fear), this should be observed across units of analysis, ranging from self-report to endocrine signaling to neural circuitry. For example, those with *ARFID-fear* should self-report high levels of fear and anxiety toward not just food, but other stimuli as well. At the level of endocrine signaling, they should exhibit hyperactivity of the hypothalamic–pituitary–adrenal (HPA) axis, such as greater release of cortisol, a glucocorticoid hormone which readily crosses the blood–brain barrier and enhances consolidation of fearful memories (Drexler et al., 2015). Dysfunction of the HPA axis should in turn hyperactivate the brain's fear circuitry in response to food cues. Specifically, a distinct network, including the amygdala, anterior cingulate cortex (ACC), and orbitofrontal cortex (OFC), is involved in fear encoding, maintenance of aversive conditioning, and processing of fearful stimuli. Amygdala hyperactivation to fear stimuli has been noted in posttraumatic stress (Herringa et al., 2013; Milad et al., 2009; Morey et al., 2020; Williams et al., 2006) and acute stress disorder (Reynaud et al., 2015) along with enhanced amygdala and ACC response during generalization of fear learning (Morey et al., 2020). The amygdala is connected to the ACC, hyperactivation of which is elicited during extinction recall (Milad et al., 2009), processing of angry faces (Herringa et al., 2013), and re-exposure to personalized aspects of trauma (Malejko et al., 2020) in individuals with post-traumatic stress disorder. Acute stress also alters OFC functioning, with hyperactivation to fearful and angry faces (Reynaud et al., 2015), as part of the fear network. Taken together, the three-dimensional model hypothesizes that fear circuitry should be hyperactivated among individuals with *ARFID-fear*, particularly in response to food cues.

ARFID-lack of interest

Individuals with *ARFID-lack of interest* report that they rarely feel hungry and that eating feels like a chore. Most of these individuals are underweight. For example, a 17-year-old boy with a body mass index of 14 kg/m^2 who was fed entirely by percutaneous endoscopic gastrostomy tube provides a ready example of the *ARFID-lack of interest* phenotype. When asked what got in the way of consuming solid food, he reflected that "I don't feel hungry. Ever." The three-dimensional model of ARFID suggests that *ARFID-lack of interest* is neurobiologically driven by hypoactivation in Arousal and Regulatory Systems (particularly low homeostatic appetite). Arousal/Regulatory Systems are responsible for providing homeostatic regulation of appetite and energy balance. However, homeostatic dysfunction could lead to dulling of hunger cues and intensification of satiety cues, which could explain why those with *ARFID-lack of interest* restrict their overall volume of food intake.

If *ARFID-lack of interest* is driven by Arousal and Regulatory Systems dysfunction (particularly low homeostatic appetite), this should be observed across units of analysis. At the self-report level, individuals with this ARFID presentation should self-report low pre-meal hunger and high post-meal satiety. At the level of endocrine signaling, they should also secrete abnormal levels of appetite-regulating hormones in fasted and fed states, including low levels of orexigenic hormones (such as ghrelin, an orexigenic hormone produced by the stomach that promotes food intake) and high levels of anorexigenic hormones (such as cholecystokinin [CCK], which is released by the small bowel in response to food intake and signals satiety). At the level of neural circuitry, one would also expect to see hypoactivation of the hypothalamic nuclei, which govern homeostatic appetite. Given that satiation is associated with reduced hypothalamic activity in response to glucose load (Little et al., 2014; Page et al., 2011; Page et al., 2013; Purnell et al., 2011; Smeets et al., 2005) and pure macronutrient ingestion (Li et al., 2012) among healthy individuals, the three-dimensional model posits that hypothalamic activity should be reduced among those with *ARFID-lack of interest*, particularly in response to food cues.

ARFID-sensory sensitivity

Lastly, individuals with the *ARFID-sensory sensitivity* phenotype severely limit their food variety, citing strong aversions to the taste, smell, and texture of most foods. They typically limit their diets to only a handful of foods they view as palatable—primarily dairy and grains. An adult female whose weight was in the normal range and consumed just three foods regularly (barbeque potato chips, French fries, and nutrition supplement drinks), exemplifies this phenotype. The patient's limited diet resulted in a Vitamin A deficiency which ultimately led to night blindness, and her vision returned to normal only after her Vitamin A was repleted. The three-dimensional model of ARFID proposes that heightened sensitivity in the RDoC Cognitive Systems domain (construct: sensory perception) underlies the *ARFID-sensory sensitivity* phenotype. Heightened sensitivity in sensory perception—or experiencing tastes, smells, and textures much more intensely than other people do—could explain the inability to tolerate a wide variety of food flavors and textures in the *ARFID-sensory sensitivity* phenotype.

If true, heightened sensitivity in Cognitive Systems (sensory perception) should manifest across units of analysis. For example, at the level of self-report, individuals with *ARFID-sensory sensitivity* should report that they experience sensory input more intensely than do controls, across chemosensory domains. At the level of endocrine signaling, there is preclinical evidence that the hormone oxytocin plays a key role in development of taste aversion (Panguluri et al., 2012). Circulating oxytocin is found in saliva, and receptors for oxytocin are present on taste buds (Sinclair et al., 2010). The three-dimensional model suggests that oxytocin levels should be higher in ARFID versus healthy controls. Lastly, individuals with *ARFID-sensory sensitivity* should show hyperactivation of the neural circuitry that underlies sensorimotor perception and motor planning related to food, such as the somatosensory cortex and supplementary motor cortex (SMC) (Avery et al., 2017; Small et al., 2012; Wistehube et al., 2018). For example, both actual and imagined ingestion of bitter tastants are associated with elevated somatosensory cortex and SMC connectivity (Jabbi et al., 2008). Further, multisensory responses to visual food-related cues are also observed in the somatosensory cortex, which responds specifically to visual cues of low-calorie foods (Killgore et al., 2003) and is associated with food preference ratings (Berns et al., 2001). The three-dimensional model predicts that severity of *ARFID-sensory sensitivity* should be associated with hyperactivity in this network in response to food cues.

State of the Science in Eating Disorders

When the three-dimensional neurobiological model of ARFID was first published in 2017, it was just that—a model. However, since then, evidence relevant to the model, from our team and others, has begun to emerge across units of analysis ranging from self-report to endocrine signaling to neural circuitry.

ARFID-fear and negative valence systems

There is emerging support that hyperactivation in Negative Valence Systems (particularly acute threat/fear) is associated with the *ARFID-fear* phenotype, particularly in the domain of self-report. Specifically, it is clear that individuals with the *ARFID-fear* phenotype self-report high levels of fear and anxiety and that increasing levels of *ARFID-fear* are associated with greater fear and anxiety. For example, in one study, individuals who met study criteria for *ARFID-fear* scored significantly higher on the Fear of Food Questionnaire compared to healthy controls, and the severity of *ARFID-fear* was positively associated with greater self-reported fear of food (Zickgraf et al., 2022). Importantly, consistent with the neurobiological model, Negative Valence hyperactivity appears to extend beyond food cues to include non-food stimuli as well: In one of our team's studies investigating children and adolescents with full or subthreshold ARFID, severity of fear of aversive consequences on the Pica, ARFID, and Rumination Disorder Interview was significantly positively correlated with scores on the Beck Anxiety Inventory (Cooper-Vince et al., 2022). In the same sample, severity of the *ARFID-fear* presentation was uniquely associated with the co-occurrence of anxiety, obsessive-compulsive, or trauma-related disorders on the Kiddie Schedule for Affective Disorders and Schizophrenia (KSADS) (Kambanis et al., 2020). Specifically, for every one-unit increase in *ARFID-fear* profile (scored on a 0 to 6 scale), participants showed a twofold increase in the odds of having comorbid anxiety disorder (the KSADS category that includes fear-based disorders, such as specific phobia, panic disorder, and agoraphobia) (Kambanis et al., 2020). Currently, less is known about the role of neuroendocrine signaling and neural circuitry in the *ARFID-fear* phenotype. No study to date has reported on cortisol, the specific hormone implicated in the three-dimensional model—among individuals with *ARFID-fear*. That said, our team recently examined neural responses to food cues among individuals with each profile using a validated food cue paradigm (Holsen et al., 2014). In this study, children and adults with the *ARFID-fear* phenotype showed greater activation of the amygdala when viewing images of food versus objects, compared to healthy controls.

ARFID-lack of interest and arousal and regulatory systems

There is emerging support that hypoactivation in Arousal and Regulatory Systems (particularly low homeostatic appetite) is associated with the *ARFID-lack of interest* phenotype, especially in the domains of self-report and neuroendocrine signaling. Clinically, individuals with the *ARFID-lack of interest* phenotype report low hunger and high satiety as barriers to sufficient caloric intake. Providing empirical support for clinical observations, in one study of youth with full and subthreshold ARFID, greater severity of *ARFID-lack of interest* was associated with significantly greater satiety responsiveness on the Adult Eating Behaviors Questionnaire (Cooper-Vince et al., 2022). There is also emerging evidence to support the three-dimensional model at the level of neuroendocrine signaling. In a recent study, our team found that low-weight adolescent females with ARFID (many of whom had the *ARFID-lack of interest* phenotype) had significantly lower fasting levels of ghrelin compared to similarly underweight females with anorexia nervosa (Becker et al., 2021). Given that ghrelin is known to be an appetite-regulating hormone that promotes food intake, lower levels in the ARFID group are consistent with the lower levels of hunger reported clinically in the *ARFID-lack of interest* group. In another study from our group, which examined youth of both sexes with full and subthreshold ARFID across the weight spectrum, those with ARFID had significantly higher fasting levels of cholecystokinin (CCK, a hormone that signals satiety) compared to healthy controls (Burton Murray, Becker et al., 2022).

Although this finding was not unique to individuals with the lack of interest phenotype, the higher levels of CCK observed in the ARFID group are consistent with clinical observations that some individuals with ARFID—particularly those with *ARFID-lack of interest*—experience early satiety that may contribute to food avoidance and restriction. Lastly, regarding neural circuitry, in a recent study, among children and adults with the *ARFID-lack of interest* phenotype, greater lack of interest scores were significantly associated with lower hypothalamus activation when viewing images of food versus objects (Thomas, Holsen et al., 2025).

ARFID-sensory sensitivity and cognitive systems

Third, there is mixed evidence that heightened sensitivity in Cognitive Systems (particularly sensory perception) is positively associated with the ARFID sensory sensitivity phenotype. Notably, while individuals with *ARFID-sensory sensitivity* consistently self-report that they experience a broad range of chemosensory stimuli more intensely than do healthy controls, behavioral observations at the level of chemosensory performance do not always corroborate this self-report. For example, in one study of children and adolescents with ARFID, higher sensory sensitivity scores were positively correlated with the self-reported detection of sensory input at lower thresholds on the taste/smell items of the Adolescent/Adult Sensory Profile questionnaire (Cooper-Vince et al., 2022). Similarly, in another study, individuals who self-identified as picky eaters rated bitter and sweet tastants as tasting more intense than did those who identified as non-picky eaters (Kauer et al., 2015). However, at the level of behavior, individuals with high levels of food neophobia (a potential research analogue for the *ARFID-sensory sensitivity* phenotype) have repeatedly demonstrated *poorer* olfactory performance. In one of these studies, as participants' food neophobia increased, they identified significantly fewer odors correctly on a smell identification test (Sorokowska et al., 2022). In another study, individuals who endorsed high levels of food neophobia demonstrated poorer odor discrimination ability than those who endorsed low levels of food neophobia (Menghi et al., 2020). Taken together, poorer performance on chemosensory tasks is inconsistent with the hypothesis that *ARFID-sensory sensitivity* is characterized by hypersensitivity in Cognitive Systems.

Less is known about the potential endocrine signaling and neural circuitry underpinning the *ARFID-sensory sensitivity* phenotype. In one study, individuals with full and subthreshold ARFID had significantly higher levels of oxytocin (both at fasting and in response to a test meal) compared to healthy controls (Aulinas et al., 2023). Although this finding was not specific to the *ARFID-sensory sensitivity* phenotype, higher levels of oxytocin, a hormone which plays a key role in the development of food aversion and has receptors on taste buds, are consistent with the food avoidance observed in the *ARFID-sensory sensitivity* group. The study also found that fasting levels of CCK, a hormone that may be involved in bitter taste perception (Lopez et al., 2015), were higher in ARFID than controls. Lastly, regarding neural circuitry, in a recent study, children and adults with the *ARFID-sensory sensitivity* phenotype showed hyperactivation of the somatosensory cortex and supplementary motor cortex compared to healthy controls when viewing images of food versus objects (Thomas, Holsen, et al., 2025).

Alternative Perspectives

Of course, the three-dimensional neurobiological model of ARFID is not the only lens through which the disorder could potentially be understood. Indeed, much of the evidence in support of the model comes from our own group and requires replication by others. Alternative perspectives should be considered, although most could still be contextualized within the broader framework that RDoC provides.

Alternative perspectives on ARFID-fear

The three-dimensional model focuses on the acute threat (fear) construct of the Negative Valence Systems domain, but another Negative Valence construct, of potential threat (anxiety), could also be relevant. Whereas fear is provoked by specific high imminence threats of immediate concern, anxiety is provoked by potential future harm that is more ambiguous, diffuse, and uncertain. This distinction has potential implications for the treatment of individuals with the *ARFID-fear* phenotype, as acute threat (fear) would likely be more amenable to targeted exposures (e.g., specifically to the foods the patient predicts would lead to adverse consequences), whereas potential threat (anxiety) might require additional interventions beyond food exposures (e.g., cognitive restructuring, relaxation exercises).

Alternative perspectives on ARFID-lack of interest

The three-dimensional model focuses on hypoactivation of Arousal and Regulatory Systems (homeostasis) in the *ARFID-lack of interest* presentation, but humans experience both homeostatic and hedonic motivations for food intake. Whereas homeostatic motivations focus on maintaining energy balance, hedonic motivations focus on the rewarding aspects of food. Thus, deficits in RDoC Positive Valence Systems—particularly lower reward responsiveness or reward valuation—could also potentially contribute to *ARFID-lack of interest*. Indeed, there is some evidence that individuals with *ARFID-lack of interest* have deficits in both the anticipatory and consummatory aspects of pleasure. In one study of children and adolescents with full and subthreshold ARFID, greater lack of interest was significantly associated with lower self-reported anticipatory pleasure on the

Temporal Experience of Pleasure subscale (Dolan et al., 2023). In another report on the same sample of participants, greater lack of interest was significantly associated with lower self-reported enjoyment of food (Cooper-Vince et al., 2022). The extent to which individuals with *ARFID-lack of interest* experience deficits in homeostatic versus hedonic aspects of food motivation—or both—is an important area for future research. Given that the neural circuitry associated with homeostatic and hedonic food motivation is at least partially dissociable (Holsen et al., 2012), future neuroimaging studies could provide insights into this debate.

Alternative perspectives on ARFID-sensory sensitivity

The three-dimensional model focuses on the contribution of Cognitive Systems (sensory perception) to the *ARFID-sensory sensitivity* presentation. However, as described earlier, evidence that individuals with *ARFID-sensory sensitivity* perceive tastes and smells more intensely than healthy controls is mixed, and evidence is stronger at the self-report level than the behavioral level. An alternative interpretation of these data is that individuals with high levels of food neophobia (including those with *ARFID-sensory sensitivity*) experience high levels of arousal in anticipation of chemosensory experiences, but that the intensity of the actual experiences does not differ from that of healthy controls (see Coulthard et al., 2022). This paradoxical disconnect could end up having fortuitous implications for potential interventions. Indeed, if the anticipated experience of tasting novel food were substantially worse than the actual sensory experience of tasting such foods, the expectancy violation of therapeutic food exposures would be very high. This would create an ideal opportunity for inhibitory learning, and for food exposures to have maximum efficacy in increasing food approach.

Alternative perspectives on the three-dimensional model

Finally, although the three-dimensional model emphasizes differences across ARFID phenotypes, there may be underlying neurobiological factors that cut across clinical presentations. For example, in one study, greater endorsement of fear of aversive consequences *and* greater endorsement of sensory sensitivity were *both* associated with a greater likelihood of comorbid anxiety disorders (Kambanis et al., 2020), suggesting that hyperactivation of Negative Valence Systems could be characteristic of both phenotypes. Similarly, high levels of CCK (Burton Murray, Becker et al., 2022) and oxytocin (Aulinas et al., 2023) were identified across the entire ARFID group (compared to healthy controls) and were not specific to the *ARFID-lack of interest or ARFID-sensory sensitivity* phenotypes, suggesting that hypoactivation of Arousal/Regulatory Systems and/or hypersensitivity in Cognitive Systems could cut across ARFID presentations. Similarly, the model's three dimensions may interact with one another to contribute to the overlap observed across phenotypes. For example, in one study of youth with full and subthreshold ARFID, higher levels of anxiety (a self-report unit of analysis within RDoC Negative Valence Systems) were correlated with lower levels of ghrelin (an endocrine unit of analysis within RDoC Arousal/Regulatory Systems) (Sella, Hadaway, et al., 2023), which could contribute to both the *ARFID-fear* and *ARFID-lack of interest* presentations within the same individual. Indeed, there may be shared neurobiological factors that contribute to ARFID in general, and other unique factors that give rise to specific ARFID phenotypes and/or their combinations.

Implications

Although more research is necessary, there is emerging support for the three-dimensional neurobiological model of ARFID. At the level of etiology and maintenance, emerging evidence for neurobiological correlates of ARFID phenotypes underscores that ARFID may be, in part, biologically driven. Indeed, it may be helpful for patients and families to understand that ARFID is not a choice, nor the product of individuals with the disorder being willful or stubborn. Further, if ARFID phenotypes have at least some distinct correlates across units of analyses within the RDoC matrix, treatments could be developed to intervene directly on these mechanisms. For example, at the self-report level, treatments could be tailored to target specific rationales for food refusal, as in cognitive behavioral therapy for ARFID (CBT-AR), which offers separate modules for the *ARFID-fear*, *ARFID-lack of interest*, and *ARFID-sensory sensitivity* phenotypes (Thomas & Eddy, 2019). At the level of endocrine signaling, the identification of appetite-regulating hormones that are disrupted within each ARFID phenotype could pave the way for the development of agonist medications (in the case of ghrelin) or antagonist medications (in the case of CCK) to enhance appetite and promote food intake, particularly in the *ARFID-lack of interest* phenotype. Finally, at the level of neural circuitry, if fear circuitry is hyperactivated in *ARFID-fear* and appetite circuitry is hypoactivated in *ARFID-lack of interest*, brain stimulation therapies could be developed to target these circuits directly. In summary, the first decade of research on ARFID has yielded many insights into its clinical phenotypes. Over the next decade, the field has strong potential to leverage these insights to further test the three-dimensional neurobiological model of ARFID and its alternatives, to drive new insights into etiology, maintenance, and treatment.

References

American Psychiatric Association. (2013). *Diagnostic and statistical manual of mental disorders* (5th ed.). American Psychiatric Association.

Aulinas, A., Muhammed, M., Becker, K. R., Asanza, E., Hauser, K., Stern, C., Gydus, J., Holmes, T., Burton Murray, H., Breithaupt. L., Micali, N., Misra, M., Eddy, K. T., Thomas, J. J., & Lawson, E. A. (2023). Oxytocin response to food intake in avoidant/restrictive food intake disorder. *European Journal of Endocrinology*, *189*(2), 149–155.

Avery, J. A., Gotts, S. J., Kerr, K. L., Burrows, K., Ingeholm, J. E., Bodurka, J., Martin, A., & Kyle Simmons, W. (2017). Convergent gustatory and viscerosensory processing in the human dorsal mid-insula. *Human Brain Mapping, 38*(4), 2150–2164.

Becker, K. R., Mancuso, C., Azanza, E., Breithaupt, L., Dreier, M., Slattery, M., Plessow, F., Micali, N., Thomas, J. J., Eddy, K. T., Misra, M., Lawson, E. A. (2021). Ghrelin and PYY in low-weight females with avoidant/restrictive food intake disorder compared to anorexia nervosa and healthy controls. *Psychoneuroendocrinology, 129*, 105243.

Berns, G. S., McClure, S. M., Pagnoni, G., & Montague, P. R. (2001). Predictability modulates human brain response to reward. *Journal of Neuroscience, 21*(8), 2793–2798.

Bryant-Waugh, R., Micali, N., Cooke, L., Lawson, E. A., Eddy, K. T., & Thomas, J. J. (2019). Development of the pica, ARFID, and rumination disorder interview, a multi-informant, semi-structured interview of feeding disorders across the lifespan: A pilot study for ages 10–22. *International Journal of Eating Disorders, 52*(4), 378–387.

Bryant-Waugh, R., Stern, C. M., Dreier, M. J., Micali, N., Cooke, L. J., Kuhnle, M. C., Burton Murray, H., Wang, S. B., Breithaupt, L., Becker, K. R., Misra, M., Lawson, E. A., Eddy, K. T., & Thomas, J. J. (2022). Preliminary validation of the pica, ARFID and rumination disorder interview ARFID questionnaire (PARDI-AR-Q). *Journal of Eating Disorders, 10*(1), 179.

Burton Murray, H., Becker, K. R., Harshman, S. G., Breithaupt, L., Kuhnle, M., Dreier, M. J., Hauser, K., Freizinger, M., Eddy, K. T., Misra, M., Kuo, B., Micali, N., Thomas, J. J., & Lawson, E. A. (2022). Elevated fasting satiety-promoting cholecystokinin (CCK) in avoidant/restrictive food intake disorder compared to healthy controls. *Journal of Clinical Psychiatry*, 83(5), 21m14111.

Chua, S. N., Fitzsimmons-Craft, E. E., Austin, S. B., Wilfley, D. E., & Taylor, C. B. (2021). Estimated prevalence of eating disorders in Singapore. *International Journal of Eating Disorders, 54*(1), 7–18.

Cooper-Vince, C. E., Nwaka, C., Eddy, K. T., Misra, M., Hadaway, N. A., Becker, K. R., Lawson, E. A., Cooke, L., Bryant-Waugh, R., Thomas, J. J., & Micali, N. (2022). The factor structure and validity of a diagnostic interview for avoidant/restrictive food intake disorder (ARFID) in a sample of children, adolescents, and young adults. *International Journal of Eating Disorders, 55*(11), 1575–1588.

Coulthard, H., Aldridge, V., & Fox, G. (2022). Food neophobia and the evaluation of novel foods in adults; the sensory, emotional, association (SEA) model of the decision to taste a novel food. *Appetite, 168*, 105764.

Dolan, S. C., Kambanis, P. E., Stern, C. M., Becker, K. R., Breithaupt, L., Gydus, J., Smith, S., Misra, M., Micali, N., Lawson, E. A., Eddy, K. T., & Thomas, J. J. (2023). Anticipatory and consummatory pleasure in avoidant/restrictive food intake disorder. *International Journal of Eating Disorders, 11*, 198.

Drexler, S. M., Merz, C. J., Hamacher-Dang, T. C., Tegenthoff, M., & Wolf, O. T. (2015). Effects of cortisol on reconsolidation of reactivated fear memories. *Neuropsychopharmacology, 40*(13), 3036–3043.

Hay, P., Mitchison, D., Collado, A. E. L., González-Chica, D. A., Stocks, N., & Touyz, S. (2017). Burden and health-related quality of life of eating disorders, including Avoidant/Restrictive Food Intake Disorder (ARFID), in the Australian population. *Journal of Eating Disorders, 5*(1), 1–10.

Herringa, R. J., Phillips, M. L., Fournier, J. C., Kronhaus, D. M., & Germain, A. (2013). Childhood and adult trauma both correlate with dorsal anterior cingulate activation to threat in combat veterans. *Psychological Medicine, 43*(7), 1533–1542.

Hilbert, A., Zenger, M., Eichler, J., & Brähler, E. (2021). Psychometric evaluation of the eating disorders in youth-questionnaire when used in adults: Prevalence estimates for symptoms of avoidant/restrictive food intake disorder and population norms. *International Journal of Eating Disorders, 54*(3), 399–408.

Holsen, L. M., Lawson, E. A., Blum, J., Ko, E., Makris, N., Fazeli, P. K., Pouneh, K., Klibanski, A., & Goldstein, J. M. (2012). Food motivation circuitry hypoactivation related to hedonic and nonhedonic aspects of hunger and satiety in women with active anorexia nervosa and weight-restored women with anorexia nervosa. *Journal of Psychiatry and Neuroscience, 37*(5), 322–332.

Holsen, L. M., Lawson, E. A., Christensen, K., Klibanski, A., & Goldstein, J. M. (2014). Abnormal relationships between the neural response to high- and low-calorie foods and endogenous acylated ghrelin in women with active and weight-recovered anorexia nervosa. *Psychiatry Research, 223*(2), 94–103.

Insel, T., Cuthbert, B., Garvey, M., Heinssen, R., Pine, D. S., Quinn, K., Sanislow, C., & Wang, P. (2010). Research domain criteria (RDoC): Toward a new classification framework for research on mental disorders. *American Journal of Psychiatry, 167*(7), 748–751.

Jabbi, M., Bastiaansen, J., & Keysers, C. (2008). A common anterior insula representation of disgust observation, experience and imagination shows divergent functional connectivity pathways. *PLOS ONE*, *3*(8), e2939–e2939.

Kambanis, P. E., Kuhnle, M., Wons, O. B., Keshishian, A., Hauser, K., Becker, K., Franko. D., Misra, M., Micali, N., Lawson, E. A., Eddy, K. T., & Thomas, J. J. (2020). Prevalence and correlates of psychiatric comorbidities in children and adolescents with full and subthreshold avoidant/restrictive food intake disorder. *International Journal of Eating Disorders*, *53*, 256–265. https://doi.org/10.1002/eat.23191

Kauer, J., Pelchat, M. L., Rozin, P., & Zickgraf, H. F. (2015). Adult picky eating: Phenomenology, taste sensitivity, and psychological correlates. *Appetite*, *90*, 219–228.

Killgore, W. D., Young, A. D., Femia, L. A., Bogorodzki, P., Rogowska, J., & Yurgelun-Todd, D. A. (2003). Cortical and limbic activation during viewing of high- versus low-calorie foods. *NeuroImage*, *19*(4), 1381–1394.

Lang, P. J., Bradley, M. M., & Cuthbert, B. N. (1998). Emotion, motivation, and anxiety: Brain mechanisms and psychophysiology. *Biological Psychiatry*, *44*(12), 1248–1263.

Li, J., An, R., Zhang, Y., Li, X., & Wang, S. (2012). Correlations of macronutrient-induced functional magnetic resonance imaging signal changes in human brain and gut hormone responses. *American Journal of Clinical Nutrition*, *96*(2), 275–282.

Little, T. J., McKie, S., Jones, R. B., D'Amato, M., Smith, C., Kiss, O., Thompson, D. G., & McLaughlin, J. T. (2014). Mapping glucose-mediated gut-to-brain signalling pathways in humans. *NeuroImage*, *96*, 1–11.

Lock, J. D. (2021). *Family-based treatment for avoidant/restrictive food intake disorder*. Routledge.

Loper, H. B., La Sala, M., Dotson, C., & Steinle, N. (2015). Taste perception, associated hormonal modulation, and nutrient intake. *Nutrition Reviews*, *73*(2), 83–91.

Malejko, K., Tumani, V., Rau, V., Neumann, F., Plener, P. L., Fegert, J. M., Abler, B., & Straub, J. (2020). Neural correlates of script-driven imagery in adolescents with interpersonal traumatic experiences: A pilot study. *Psychiatry Research Neuroimaging*, *303*, 111131.

Menghi, L., Khomenko, I., Pedrotti, M., Cliceri, D., Aprea, E., Endrizzi, I., Cavazzana, A., Biasioli, F., Giacalone, D., & Gasperi, F. (2020). Arousal influences olfactory abilities in adults with different degree of food neophobia. *Scientific Reports*, *10*(1), 20538.

Milad, M. R., Pitman, R. K., Ellis, C. B., Gold, A. L., Shin, L. M., Lasko, N. B., Zeidan, M. A., Handwerger, K., Orr, S. P., & Rauch, S. L. (2009). Neurobiological basis of failure to recall extinction memory in posttraumatic stress disorder. *Biological Psychiatry*, *66*(12), 1075–1082.

Morey, R. A., Haswell, C. C., Stjepanovic, D., Dunsmoor, J. E., & LaBar, K. S. (2020). Neural correlates of conceptual-level fear generalization in posttraumatic stress disorder. *Neuropsychopharmacology*, *45*(8), 1380–1389.

Murray H. B., Bailey, A. P., Keshishian, A. C., Silvernale, C. J., Staller, K., Eddy, K. T., Thomas, J. J., & Kuo, B. (2020). Prevalence and characteristics of avoidant/restrictive food intake disorder in adult neurogastroenterology patients. *Clinical Gastroenterology and Hepatology*, *18*(9), 1995–2002.

Nicely, T. A., Lane-Loney, S., Masciulli, E., Hollenbeak, C. S., & Ornstein, R. M. (2014). Prevalence and characteristics of avoidant/restrictive food intake disorder in a cohort of young patients in day treatment for eating disorders. *Journal of Eating Disorders*, *2*(1), 21.

Nitsch, A., Watters, A., Manwaring, J., Bauschka, M., Hebert, M., & Mehler, P. S. (2023). Clinical features of adult patients with avoidant/restrictive food intake disorder presenting for medical stabilization: A descriptive study. *International Journal of Eating Disorders*, 56(5), 978–990.

Norris, M. L., Spettigue, W., Hammond, N. G., Katzman, D. K., Zucker, N., Yelle, Santos, A., Gray, M., & Obeid, N. (2018). Building evidence for the use of descriptive subtypes in youth with avoidant restrictive food intake disorder. *International Journal of Eating Disorders*, *51*(2), 170–173.

Page, K. A., Chan, O., Arora, J., Belfort-DeAguiar, R., Dzuira, J., Roehmholdt, B., Cline, G. W., Naik, S., Sinha, R., Constable, R. T., & Sherwin, R. S. (2013). Effects of fructose vs glucose on regional cerebral blood flow in brain regions involved with appetite and reward pathways. *JAMA*, *309*(1), 63–70.

Page, K. A., Seo, D., Belfort-DeAguiar, R., Lacadie, C., Dzuira, J., Naik, S., Amarnath, S., Constable, R. T., Sherwin, R. S., & Sinha, R. (2011). Circulating glucose levels modulate neural control of desire for high-calorie foods in humans. *Journal of Clinical Investigation*, *121*(10), 4161–4169.

Panguluri, S. K., Kuwabara, N., Kang, Y., Cooper, N., & Lundy, R. F. (2012). Conditioned taste aversion dependent regulation of amygdala gene expression. *Physiology & Behavior*, *105*(4), 996–1006.

Purnell, J., Klopfenstein, B., Stevens, A., Havel, P., Adams, S., Dunn, T., Krisky, C., & Rooney, W. (2011). Brain functional magnetic resonance imaging response to glucose and fructose infusions in humans. *Diabetes, Obesity & Metabolism*, *13*(3), 229–234.

Richmond, T. K., Carmody, J., Freizinger, M., Milliren, C. E., Crowley, P. M., Jhe, G. B., & Bern, E. (2023). Assessment of patients with ARFID presenting to multi-disciplinary tertiary care program. *Journal of Pediatric Gastroenterology and Nutrition, 76*(6), 743–748.

Reilly, E. E., Brown, T. A., Gray, E. K., Kaye, W. H., & Menzel, J. E. (2019). Exploring the cooccurrence of behavioural phenotypes for avoidant/restrictive food intake disorder in a partial hospitalization sample. *European Eating Disorders Review, 27*(4), 429–435.

Reynaud, E., Guedj, E., Trousselard, M., El Khoury-Malhame, M., Zendjidjian, X., Fakra, E., Souville, M., Nazarian, B., Blin, O., Canini, F., & Khalfa, S. (2015). Acute stress disorder modifies cerebral activity of amygdala and prefrontal cortex. *Cognitive Neuroscience, 6*(1), 39–43.

Sanchez-Cerezo, J., Nagularaj, L., Gledhill, J., & Nicholls, D. (2023). What do we know about the epidemiology of avoidant/restrictive food intake disorder in children and adolescents? A systematic review of the literature. *European Eating Disorders Review, 31*(2), 226–246.

Schimansky, S., Jasim, H., Pope, L., Hinds, P., Fernandez, D., Choleva, P., Dev Borman, A., Sharples, P. M., Smallbone, T., & Atan, D. (2023). Nutritional blindness from avoidant-restrictive food intake disorder—Recommendations for the early diagnosis and multidisciplinary management of children at risk from restrictive eating. *Archives of Disease in Childhood, 109*(3), 181–187.

Sella, A. C., Becker, K. R., Slattery, M., Hauser, K., Asanza, E., Stern, C. M., Kuhnle, M. K., Micali, N., Eddy, K. T., Misra, M., Thomas, J. J., & Lawson, E. A. (2023). Low bone mineral density is found in low-weight female youth with avoidant/restrictive food intake disorder and associated with higher PYY levels. *Journal of Eating Disorders, 11*(1), 106.

Sella, A. C., Hadaway, N., Stern, C. M., Becker, K. R., Holsen, L., Eddy, K.T., Micali, N., Misra, M., Thomas, J. J., Lawson, & E. A. (2023). Lower ghrelin levels are associated with greater anxiety symptoms in adolescents and young adults with avoidant/restrictive food intake disorder (ARFID). *Journal of Clinical Psychiatry, 84*(3), 22m14482.

Sharp, W. G., Stubbs, K. H., Adams, H., Wells, B. M., Lesack, R. S., Criado, K. K., Simon, E. L., McCracken, C. E., West, L. L., & Scahill, L. D. (2016). Intensive, manual-based intervention for pediatric feeding disorders: Results from a randomized pilot trial. *Journal of Pediatric Gastroenterology and Nutrition, 62*(4), 658–663.

Sinclair, M. S., Perea-Martinez, I., Dvoryanchikov, G., Yoshida, M., Nishimori, K., Roper, S. D., Chaudhari, N. (2010). Oxytocin signaling in mouse taste buds. *PLOS ONE, 5*(8), e11980.

Small, D. M. (2012). Flavor is in the brain. *Physiology & Behavior, 107*(4), 540–552.

Smeets, P. A., de Graaf, C., Stafleu, A., van Osch, M. J., van der Grond, J. (2005). Functional MRI of human hypothalamic responses following glucose ingestion. *Neuroimage, 24*(2), 363–368.

Sorokowska, A., Chabin, D., Hummel, T., & Karwowski, M. (2022). Olfactory perception relates to food neophobia in adolescence. *Nutrition, 98*, 111618.

Thomas, J. J., Brigham, K. S., Sally, S. T., Hazen, E. P., & Eddy, K. T. (2017). Case records of the Massachusetts General Hospital: An 11-year-old girl with difficulty eating after a choking incident. *New England Journal of Medicine, 376*(24), 2377–2386.

Thomas, J. J., & Eddy, K. T. (2019). *Cognitive-behavioral therapy for avoidant/restrictive food intake disorder: Children, adolescents, and adults.* Cambridge University Press.

Thomas, J. J., Lawson, E. A., Micali, N., Misra, M., Deckersbach, T., & Eddy, K. T. (2017). Avoidant/restrictive food intake disorder: A three-dimensional model of neurobiology with implications for etiology and treatment. *Current Psychiatry Reports, 19*(8), 54.

Thomas, J.J., Holsen, L., Van De Water, A. L., Becker, K. R., Breithaupt, L., Burton-Murray, H., Asanza, E., Gydus, J., Palmer, L. P., Stern, C. M., Freizinger, M., Shrier, L. A., Bern, E. M., Deckersbach, T., Misra, M., Eddy, K. T., Micali, N., & Lawson, E. A. (2025). Neural response to food cues in avoidant/restrictive food intake disorder. *JAMA Network Open, 8*(2), e2460101.

Williams, L. M., Kemp, A. H., Felmingham, K., Barton, M., Olivieri, G., Peduto, A., Gordon, E., & Bryant, R. A. (2006). Trauma modulates amygdala and medial prefrontal responses to consciously attended fear. *Neuroimage, 29*(2), 347–357.

Wistehube, T., Rullmann, M., Wiacek, C., Braun, P., & Pleger, B. (2018). Fat perception in the human frontal operculum, insular and somatosensory cortex. *Scientific Reports, 8*(1), 11825–11828.

Zickgraf, H. F., & Ellis, J. M. (2018). Initial validation of the nine item avoidant/restrictive food intake disorder screen (NIAS): A measure of three restrictive eating patterns. *Appetite, 123*, 32–42.

Zickgraf, H. F., Lane-Loney, S., Essayli, J. H., & Ornstein, R. M. (2019). Further support for diagnostically meaningful ARFID symptom presentations in an adolescent medicine partial hospitalization program. *International Journal of Eating Disorders, 52*(4), 402–409.

Zickgraf, H. F., Loftus, P., Gibbons, B., Cohen, L. C., & Hunt, M. G. (2022). "If I could survive without eating, it would be a huge relief": Development and initial validation of the Fear of Food Questionnaire. *Appetite, 169*, 105808.

24

The Microbiome–Gut–Brain Axis in Anorexia Nervosa

Jochen Seitz and Stefanie Trinh

Brief Definitional Overview

Microbiome: The combined genetic material of all microorganisms living in a particular environment (skin, oral cavity, gut, etc.).

Microbiota: The sum of all the microorganisms living in a particular environment, including bacteria, archaea, fungi, viruses, and small protists (Marchesi, 2016). The terms microbiome and microbiota are often used interchangeably and often refer to (gut) bacteria as they are the largest group in terms of numbers.

Microbiome–gut–brain axis: The multiple interactions between the gut microbiome and the brain influencing subsequent behavior (Cryan et al., 2019).

Introduction

Human microbiome research has greatly accelerated since 2012 due to the development of high-throughput DNA-sequencing methods; however, microbiome research is not a new field (Walker & Hoyles, 2023). As early as the 19th century, Metchnikoff (1907) contemplated the significance of beneficial microorganisms shortly after the bacteria *Escherichia coli* was isolated for the first time in 1885 (Escherich, 1885) and *Bifidobacteria* were described in 1899 (Tissier, 1899). Conceptualization of the involvement of a gut–brain axis in health dates back even several centuries (Miller, 2018). Similarly, the impact of beneficial microbiota-associated metabolites were first described more than 40 years ago (Roediger, 1980). At the end of the 20th century, the term *gut microbiome* was introduced in the form it is used today (Prescott, 2017).

Biological Framework

Most of the biomass of the gut bacteria resides in the colon (10^{11} colony forming units), while the quantity decreases in the small intestines (10^{6}–10^{7} colony forming units) and the stomach (10^{1}–10^{3} colony forming units) (Marchesi, 2011;

Jochen Seitz and Stefanie Trinh, *The Microbiome–Gut–Brain Axis in Anorexia Nervosa*. In: *The Handbook of the Neurobiology of Eating Disorders*. Edited by: Christina E. Wierenga and Joanna E. Steinglass, Oxford University Press.
 DOI: 10.1093/9780197675212.003.0025

Turnbaugh, 2007). It is known that from about the age of six years, the microbiome has matured and is relatively stable until it changes again with aging. The number of bacteria found in the gastrointestinal tract is comparable to the number of eucaryotic cells (e.g., blood cells) in the rest of the human body. The genome of these microbiota comprises 150 times as many genes as the human genome (Sender et al., 2016). Although the total number of different microbiota varies little between individuals under physiological conditions (e.g., absence of disease), the composition is unique to each person and can be seen as a *microbial fingerprint*. The microbial fingerprint of an individual is comprised of approximately 500 different species (about 2,000 species have been identified to date) (Almeida et al., 2019; Clavel et al., 2016). The numerous species belong to seven dominant bacterial lineages (phyla), in descending order of average abundance: *Firmicutes, Bacteroidetes, Proteobacteria, Verrucomicrobia, Actinobacteria, Fusobacteria*, and *Cyanobacteria* (Lynch & Pedersen, 2016).

A newborn first encounters microbiota during birth, mostly from the mother and medical staff. The mode of birth (cesarean section or vaginal) is one of the first factors which can influence the subsequent composition of the individual bacterial population (Dominguez-Bello et al., 2010). Diet also influences the composition of the microbiome. Intestinal bacteria feed on unabsorbed components of the diet (David et al., 2014). Thus, whether an infant is breastfed or not has a stage-setting influence on future intestinal colonization. Furthermore, a change in diet (e.g., avoiding animal products) can cause a rapid and short-term alteration in the bacterial composition as bacteria grow with varying efficiency depending on the available nutrients (David et al., 2014). Additional influencing factors are personal life circumstances (e.g., age, physical activity), environmental influences (e.g., rural vs. urban environment), (epi-)genetics and general health status (e.g., medication, nicotine dependence) (Ananthakrishnan, 2015).

Host-microbiome symbiotic relationship—An evolutionary perspective

Microbiota are present in all higher developed organisms, but from a phylogenetic perspective they are significantly older than their hosts. A common coevolution functional symbiosis between the microbiota and the host has emerged leading to evolutionary advantages for the best microbiota-host match (Sender et al., 2016). The microbiota take over numerous functions that the host organism does not (or no longer) perform itself. A special ability of gut microbiota is to metabolize certain food components, such as dietary fibers, that cannot be metabolized by the human intestinal tract itself. The cleavage products (e.g., short chain fatty acids) are in turn used to generate energy for the host, which would in the absence of the microbiota not be available and are thought to account for up to 10% of the energy extracted from food.

Furthermore, due to the diversity of the microbiota and its genetic material, a flexible and relatively quick (in a matter of hours) reaction to environmental changes (e.g., changes in food availability or infections) provides an evolutionary advantage (e.g., by allowing early hunter/gatherers to change quickly from grain to mammoth and back to grain again, according to current hunting success). For a long time, the function of the gut bacteria was thought to be limited to the digestive process. More recent research indicates other important tasks are performed by these bacteria; they are part of the intestinal barrier, they are involved in the immune system and inflammatory processes through constant contact to immune cells, and they can influence complex processes such as behavior via the microbiota–gut–brain axis (Cryan et al., 2019; Möhle et al., 2016; Neuman et al., 2015). The potential mechanisms involve direct vagal nerve signaling, migration of immune cells into the brain, and changes in the secretion of cytokines, antibodies, hormones, and nutritional components (Dinan & Cryan, 2017a, 2017b).

The "microbiome–gut–brain axis"

Microbiota constantly challenge the gut immune system a little bit, thereby "training" the resident immune cells. In the case of malicious or invasive species like salmonella, they emit certain cytokines effectively alerting the gut immune system to the potential invaders and triggering an early inflammatory response. Gut microbiota also participate in regulating gut wall permeability, thus determining how much gut content can traverse the wall and, in case of bacteria or bacterial parts, can cause further inflammation. On the other hand, microbiota play a major role in limiting overflowing inflammation again, effectively regulating harmful over-excitation. These immune processes, however, also have an effect on the brain, as cytokines and certain immune cells are able to cross the blood brain barrier (e.g., via the choroid plexus). Reduced learning following antibiotic eradication of gut bacteria coincided with reduced neuroneogenesis in the hippocampus, both of which increased again after *Bifidobacteria* and *Lactobacillus* species supplementation (Möhle et al., 2016). The effects were mediated by certain lymphocytes traveling to the brain, and eliminating those lymphocytes stopped the process. Furthermore, short-chain fatty acids produced by gut bacteria not only help nourish gut enterocytes and reduce gut permeability, but they also have a direct and beneficial effect in the brain. Last, but not least, the direct nerval link between the gut and the brain, the nervus vagus, has been found to play a bidirectional role in transmitting microbiome-related information to and from the brain via electrical signaling but also antero- and retrograde transport of molecules within the axon (Sgritta et al., 2019).

Microbiota and psychiatric conditions

The gut microbiome appears to play a causal role in weight regulation as well, including obesity and underweight. Individuals with obesity appear to have a different gut microbiome than normal weight controls (Ley et al., 2005), associated with a greater ability to extract energy from the same amount of stool (Turnbaugh et al., 2006). Fecal microbiota transplantation is defined as the transfer of a fecal microbiota sample from a person with a specific disease phenotype into laboratory animals or humans. Transplantation studies into germ-free mice (gf-mice) raised without contact with bacteria consequently showed an increase in weight following stool donation by individuals with obesity (Ridaura et al., 2013). This effect was not seen any longer after fecal microbiota transplantation from individuals with obesity that had a bariatric surgery resulting in a leaner phenotype (Tremaroli et al., 2015). Inversely, a decrease in weight followed stool donation by malnourished Malawian children with Kwashiokor if the animals received typical Malawian food rich in fibers (Smith et al., 2013).

Beyond pure weight-related influences, the microbiome–gut–brain axis has been shown to causally influence complex behaviors, such as attention, learning, stress, mood, and anxiety (Dinan & Cryan, 2017a; Kleiman et al., 2015). Fecal microbiota transplantation from patients with depression, for example, resulted in a depressed phenotypes in rats that was accompanied by changes in inflammatory parameters and neurotransmitters (Kelly et al., 2016). Transplantation of stool of patients with attention deficit disorder led to a decreased structural cohesion of white matter fibers and altered gray matter regions (i.e., internal capsule, hippocampus) as well as decreased resting-state functional MRI-based connectivity and significant changes in anxious behavior (Tengeler et al., 2020). Microbiome–gut–brain axis is now implicated in several other psychiatric and neurological diseases including autism, post-traumatic stress disorder, obsessive-compulsive disorder, schizophrenia, stroke, multiple sclerosis, and Alzheimer's and Parkinsons Diseases (Cryan et al., 2019; Dinan & Cryan, 2017a).

For example, one study (Sgritta et al., 2019) showed an influence of the microbiome on three different animal models of autism and was able to alter complex social behavior in rodents using supplementation of *lactobacillus rhamnosus.* Cutting the vagal nerve prohibited such an interaction, successfully proving its causal role in transmitting the signal from the gut to the brain (Sgritta et al., 2019).

Methods of investigation

The exact definition of a healthy microbiome is not possible at the current state of our knowledge, on the one hand because of the high inter-individual variability and on the other hand because of the numerous parameters that influence microbiome composition. To understand the influence of the microbiome on diseases or, conversely, of diseases on the microbiome, group comparisons are indispensable. Due to the nature of microbiome data, it is necessary to quantify potential differences between samples/groups at two levels termed alpha (within-sample) and beta (between-sample) diversity. The α-diversity is a measure of the number of different bacterial species within a sample, and it can be determined by a simple count of species present in a sample. More complex α-diversity indices, such as the Shannon index, additionally consider the relative abundance of a species. The β-diversity is a measure of the similarity of two microbial samples, and it quantifies differences in the overall taxonomic composition between two samples as determined by the phylogenetic relationship of the identified species.

In recent years, the possibilities to investigate the gut microbiome have expanded substantially. The progress of sequencing techniques with high throughput combined with bioinformatic processing allows the complex analysis of microbial systems. One of the most frequently used methods to identify bacteria is 16S rRNA gene amplicon sequencing. The 16S complex is part of the small ribosomal subunit in prokaryotes. As sections of the 16S gene were highly conserved during evolution the 16S complex can be used to reconstruct phylogenetic relationships. In addition to evolutionarily conserved binding sites, the 16S complex also possesses hypervariable regions that are species-specific (Lagkouvardos et al., 2016, 2017). A more extensive characterization of the microbiome, with more exact taxonomic classification, intra-species genetic alterations ("gene drift"), and the actual functionality of genes, is possible using so-called shotgun metagenomic analysis (Ranjan et al., 2016). Shotgun sequencing is an untargeted ("shotgun") laboratory technique that allows one to determine the genomic DNA sequence of a sample. The described sequencing techniques allow determination of the composition (with or without functionality) and diversity within one microbial sample and to investigate differences between separate samples.

To determine active genes and their impact on the host organism, transcriptomic studies measuring mRNA and metabolomic studies measuring the different metabolites in the blood or stool can be used (Gilbert & Blaser, 2018).

State of the Science in Eating Disorders

While the involvement of the microbiome is obvious for all eating disorders, as summarized by some recent papers on bulimia nervosa and binge-eating disorder (Butler et al., 2021; Carbone et al., 2020; Fetissov & Hökfelt, 2019; Herman & Bajaka, 2021; Igudesman et al., 2023; Terry et al., 2022), we focus here on the already more extensively studied anorexia nervosa (AN) (see Figure 24.1).

More than a dozen studies on the gut microbiota of patients with AN have been published (Armougom et al., 2009; Borgo et al., 2017; Castellini et al., 2023; Di Lodovico et al., 2021; Fan et al., 2023; Fouladi et al., 2022; Kleiman et al., 2015, 2017; Mack et al., 2016; Million et al., 2013; Morita et al., 2015; Mörkl et al., 2017;

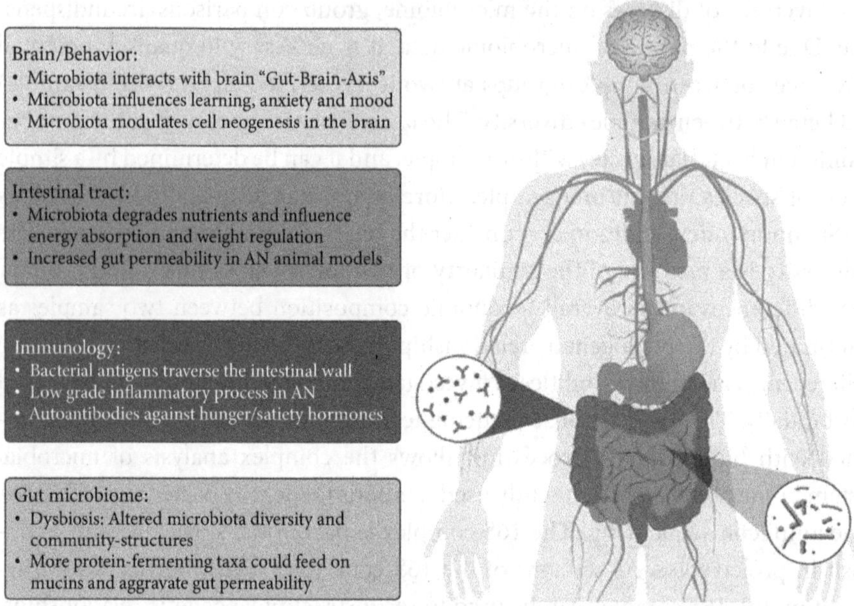

Figure 24.1 Effects of gut microbial products on brain functions and behavior in the intestinal tract and on immunological processes in patients with AN. Reproduced from Seitz et al. (2020). Gut Feelings: How Microbiota Might Impact the Development and Course of Anorexia Nervosa. *Nutrients, 12*(11), 3295. https://doi.org/10.3390/nu12113295. under a Creative Commons Attribution 4.0 International (CC BY 4.0).

Prochazkova et al., 2021; Schulz et al., 2021; Yuan et al., 2022). The results vary, as summarized in various reviews (Di Lodovico et al., 2021; Mack et al., 2018; Seitz et al., 2020). Some studies found a reduction in bacterial α-diversity in patients with acute AN (Kleiman et al., 2015; Mǫrkl et al., 2017), while others did not (Borgo et al., 2017; Mack et al., 2016; Schulz et al., 2021). Reduced bacterial diversity can be a sign of dysbiosis (Tamboli, 2004). Certain species and their functions might be lost to the bacterial community, often associated with a reduced capacity to react to pathogens or specific environmental changes. Following weight rehabilitation, several authors have found an increase in diversity (Fouladi et al., 2022; Kleiman et al., 2015; Mack et al., 2016). However, patients in Mack and colleagues' (2016) study and in our own study showed an increased absolute level of diversity after short-term weight recovery compared to healthy controls (Mack et al., 2016; Schulz et al., 2021). The reason is not yet clear, we can just speculate about short-term adaptive processes following a still unbalanced food selection, high stress levels or not-yet-normalized hormonal status, commonly observed after short-term weight recovery (Herpertz-Dahlmann, 2015).

Regarding β-diversity, the measure of similarity of whole bacterial communities, virtually all studies have found altered β-diversity in patients with acute AN (Fan et al., 2023; Fouladi et al., 2022; Kleiman et al., 2015; Mack et al., 2016; Schulz et al., 2021), which did not normalize with short-term weight recovery in either adults or adolescents (Mack et al., 2016; Schulz et al., 2021). This is in accordance with the hypothesis that microbiota composition shifts in AN are more than an epiphenomenon of low weight or altered nutritional intake. When analyzing the relative abundance of single bacterial species, the results were widely varied with some of the more commonly found differences including increased *Firmicutes* and decreased *Bacteroidetes* abundances at the phylum level compared to healthy controls (Kleiman et al., 2015; Mack et al., 2018). Furthermore, *Roseburia* and *Lactobacillus* species decreased in adults with increases in *Akkermansia, Alistipes, Parabacterioides*, and the archaea *Methanobrevibacter smithii* (Armougom et al., 2009; Borgo et al., 2017; Di Lodovico et al., 2021; Mack et al., 2016; Million et al., 2013), while *Romboutsia* and *Enterobacteriaceae* species were reduced and *Lachnospiracea* species increased in the first study with adolescent patients only (Schulz et al., 2021). Longitudinal follow-up studies exceeding short-term weight recovery are needed to understand the long-term development of gut microbiota diversity in completely recovered patients with AN.

Impact on behavior

Attempts to link bacterial taxa changes to eating disorder related behavior resulted in several possible associations with eating behavior and mental health in a large study with 77 patients with AN and 70 healthy controls (Fan et al., 2023). One group found associations of bacterial functional modules enriched in AN samples via a bioinformatic derived distinct assembly of microbiome components related to gut bacterial functional potentials (e.g., impact of a certain metabolite synthesis, etc.). They included associations with the degradation of the neurotransmitters dopamine, glutamate, and tryptophan, which have known effects on mood and appetite. Causal inference analyses implied that serum bacterial metabolites could thus mediate the impact of an altered gut microbiome on AN behavior (Fan et al., 2023).

Global microbiome alterations in patients with anorexia nervosa

Finally, gf-mice have shown several abnormalities in their brain development including reduced brain-derived neurotrophic factor (BDNF) in the blood and the brain, also known to be altered in patients with AN (Borsdorf et al., 2021; Dalton et al., 2018). They also differed in showing increased serotonin metabolites (5-hydroxyindoleacetic acid [5-HIAA] and 5 hydroxytryptamine), while the former was found to be significantly decreased in acutely ill patients with AN and increased in recovered patients (Kaye et al., 2011). GF-mice also showed reduced anxiety-like behavior which changed back to normal behavior upon transplantation of normal stool. Thus, the microbiome appears to be necessary even for normal brain development.

Gut permeability and the "leaky gut" hypothesis

Gut permeability findings in patients with AN are not conclusive as of yet. Animal studies using the activity-based anorexia model (ABA) model consistently show a reduction in gut wall thickness (Jesus et al., 2014; Trinh et al., 2023), reduced tight junctions and subsequent increase in colonic permeability (Achamrah et al., 2016; Jesus et al., 2014; L'Huillier et al., 2019) also called "leaky gut." However, findings in patients with AN are less clear and variably showed decreased small intestinal permeability (Monteleone et al., 2004), increased small intestinal permeability (Grigioni et al., 2022), and no difference in zonulin, a common gut permeability marker (Mörkl et al., 2018). Thinned intestinal walls, altered tight junctions, and increased mucin consumption leading to greater (colonic) gut permeability and increased translocation of gut material could trigger immune responses and inflammatory processes (Bambury et al., 2017; Dinan et al., 2013; Kelly et al., 2017). This is consistent with patients with AN showing a low-grade inflammatory state found in two meta-analyses (Dalton et al., 2018; Solmi et al., 2015) and increased inflammatory lymphatic patches in the ABA model (Trinh et al., 2023). Also, traversing bacterial products (through the "leaky gut") might induce auto-immune processes known to be elevated in patients with AN with increased odds ratios (ORs) especially regarding gastrointestinal diseases (OR 1.8) and endocrine diseases (OR 2.4). Crohn's disease contributed most to the risk of gastroenterological diseases (OR 1.8, 95% CI 1.4–2.5, $P<0.001$) (Raevuori et al., 2014). Interestingly, in a case study, anti-TNF-α therapy for a Crohn's disease patient comorbid with AN also improved AN symptoms (Solmi et al., 2013).

Prediction of clinical outcome

Interestingly, species belonging to the immune-modulatory *Lachnospiraceae* family helped to predict short-term clinical outcome in the form of shorter treatment duration. This was even true after correcting for other known predictors, such as illness duration and low body weight at admission (Schulz et al., 2021). *Lachnospiraceae* were also associated with increased blood glucose levels (Kameyama & Itoh, 2014) and weight gain following antibiotic treatment (Liu et al., 2019), and they could thus be linked to energy use and quicker weight gain. *Lachnospiracea* also produces butyrate (Vital et al., 2017), thus affecting the intestinal barrier.

Activity-based anorexia animal model results

The activity-based anorexia model is a widely used animal model combining food restriction and access to a running wheel. Thereby the model mimics core symptoms of anorexia nervosa such as bodyweight loss, increased physical activity, hormonal alterations, and brain volume loss. In addition, widespread changes have been found in the gut microbiota in food-restricted animals, some of which, including *Lactobacillus* and *Bifidobacterium* species, were inversely associated with serum ghrelin and positively with serum leptin concentrations (Queipo-Ortuño et al., 2013; Trinh et al., 2021, 2023). While the appetite-inducing gastric peptide ghrelin is increased in patients with AN, leptin is known to induce satiety and is severely reduced (Hebebrand et al., 2022). Starvation-induced microbiota alterations in ABA mice have been shown (Breton, 2021). Several of these altered bacteria were correlated with body weight as well as neuropeptide Y and proopiomelanocortin levels in the hypothalamus, which are known to also be involved in appetite regulation (Breton, 2021). Our own group showed similar learning deficits (e.g., object recognition) to the ones previously described (Möhle et al., 2016) following eradication of gut bacteria via antibiotics in ABA animals (Paulukat et al., 2016). Patients with AN commonly have neuropsychological deficits that can be linked to brain volume reductions measured in MRI (Seitz et al., 2015, 2018). Similarly, we found brain volume reductions in ABA animals that seem to be associated with reduced numbers of astrocytes. In recent ABA experiments we showed a link between the diversity of gut microbiota and brain volume reductions as well as an association between lower numbers of astrocytic markers in the brain and the relative abundance of the bacteria *Bifidobacterium* and *Odoribacter*. Interestingly, the higher the relative abundance of the bacteria *Lactobacillus* the lower the level of brain volume loss, rendering this bacterium as an interesting target for potential probiotic interventions (Trinh et al., 2021).

Fecal-matter transplantation

Last but not least, the maybe most intriguing data regarding the microbiome in AN comes from fecal-matter transplantation (FMT) studies (Fan et al., 2023; Hata et al., 2019). One group transplanted fresh stool from patients with AN into gf-mice and studied their offspring to at least partially offset the altered brain development in completely germ-free raised mice (see Figure 24.2) (Hata et al., 2019). They found a reduced appetite and energy-extraction rate in the AN-stool transplantation derived offspring, resulting in a significantly reduced weight gain over eight weeks. They found increased obsessive compulsive behavior in the marble-burying task as well as increased anxious behavior in the open field and reduced serotonin metabolites in the brain stem (Hata et al., 2019).

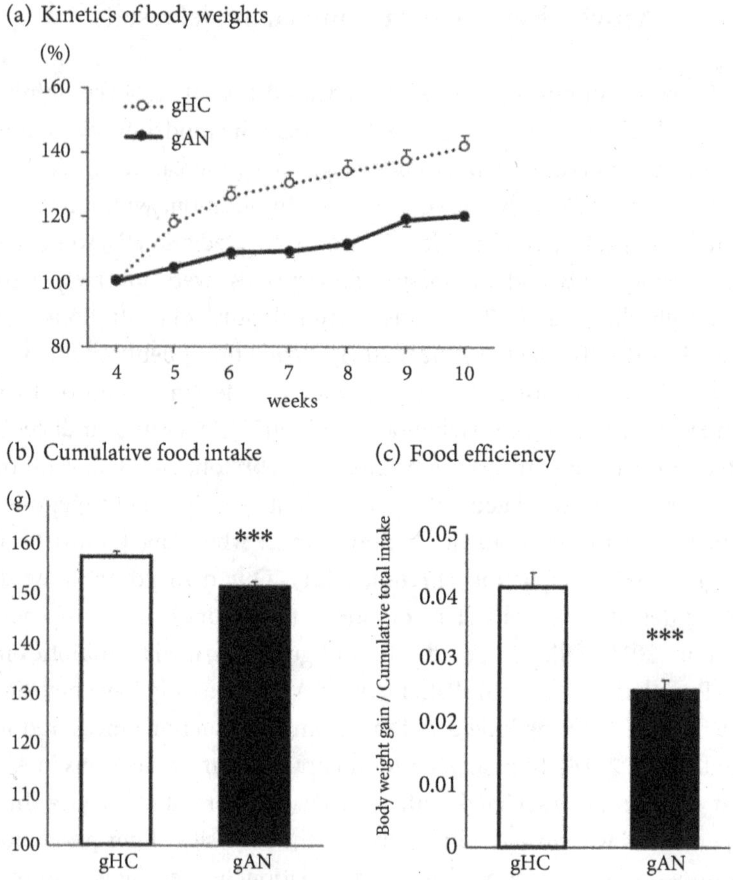

Figure 24.2 Effects of fecal transplantation from donors with AN on body weight of recipient mice. (a) The body weights of female mice reconstituted with either fecal microbiota from four patients with AN (gAN, n = 35) or those from four healthy controls (gHC, n = 37) were monitored weekly. Body weight at each time-point is expressed as a percentage of the body weight at four weeks of age (basal). A statistical difference between the two groups was evaluated by repeated measures ANOVA. (b) Cumulative food intakes in female gnotobiotic mice were calculated as a sum of daily consumption during four to 10 weeks. Differences between the gAN and gHC groups were analyzed by unpaired Student's t-tests. ***$p < 0.001$ was considered significantly different from the corresponding gHC values. (c) Food efficiency was calculated as a ratio of body weight gain during four to 10 weeks to cumulative food consumption. Differences between the gAN and gHC groups were evaluated by unpaired Student's t-tests. ***$p < 0.001$ was considered significantly different from the corresponding gHC values. Reproduced with permission from Hata et al. (2019). The Gut Microbiome Derived from Anorexia Nervosa Patients Impairs Weight Gain and Behavioral Performance in Female Mice. *Endocrinology, 160*(10), article 10. https://doi.org/10.1210/en.2019–00408

However, a second study did not find a differential effect when transplanting stool of patients with AN vs healthy controls into normally fed gf-mice (Glenny, 2021). Transplantation of stool of patients with AN resulted in weight loss and reduced subsequent weight gain when transferred into gf-mice only when they were on an energy-reduced diet but not when regularly fed (see Figure 24.3) (Fan et al., 2023). Moreover, this finding complements an early study that showed that only the combination of stool transplantation of children with Kwashiokor (protein malnutrition) with typical (less energy-dense) Malawian food leads to deleterious effect on gf-animal's weight gain (Smith et al., 2013). Several differences in mRNA-expression of hunger- and satiety-related genes in the hypothalamus of AN-FMT transplanted mice were also found, all in the direction of suppression of appetite (Fan et al., 2023). These included increases in appetite suppressors such as brain derived neurotropic factor (BDNF) and cocaine- and amphetamine-regulated transcript protein preprotein (CARTPT). Contrarily, reductions in agouti-related protein (AGRP) and ghrelin, so called hunger-hormones, were noted (Fan et al., 2023). Furthermore, the receptor for serotonin, (Htr1b) (involved in the downstream regulation of serotonin) and of Snca, which encodes the neuronal protein α-synuclein associated with several neurodegenerative diseases were increased. Together, these studies suggest a causal relationship between the stool of patients with AN (and likely the contained microbiome) at least with the perpetuation of existing AN.

Alternative Perspectives

Research regarding the microbiome–gut–brain axis in AN is still in its infancy, and there are several alternative perspectives to keep in mind. First, it all comes down to food. Nutrition is the first and foremost determining factor of the gut microbiome—simply because these microbes feed on what the host leaves over for them. Changing food to all animal or all non-animal sources for example changes the stool gut microbiome within 48 hours. Taking into account the average gut passage time of 24 hours, this implicates microbiome-adaptation within 24 hours. As patients with AN notably eat differently (and a lot less!) than healthy controls, microbiome differences could in theory result purely from this altered nutritional intake and represent an epiphenomenon instead of being involved in pathophysiology. However, longitudinal studies so far do not show a complete normalization of the gut microbiome in short-term (Mack et al., 2016; Schulz et al., 2021) or long-term weight restored individuals with a history of AN (Andreani et al., 2024), rendering this hypothesis less likely. Although these individuals do not eat exactly as their healthy counterparts, this might explain residual differences and further research is needed. As previously described, fecal microbiota transplantation studies show a causal influence of AN stool at least on appetite and bodyweight regulation. This influence thus suggests a perpetuating effect of the gut microbiome on the disease and downgrades the probability of a pure epiphenomena.

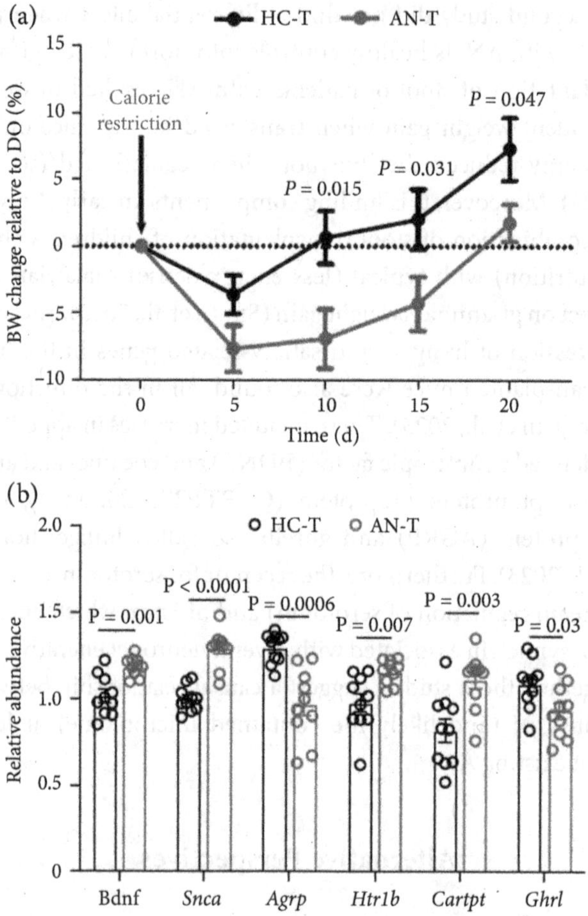

Figure 24.3 Fecal-matter transplantation using samples from donors with AN induces AN-relevant phenotypes in GF mice. (a) Body weight (BW) change compared to the body weight at day 0 after energy-restricted diet (AN-T $n = 10$, HC-T, $n = 10$ examined over three independent experiments). Significance was calculated by two-way analysis of variance (ANOVA), followed by Benjamini-Hochberg post hoc test. (b) mRNA levels of the indicated mice genes in hypothalamus: Reductions in appetite suppressors Brain Derived Neurotropic Factor (*Bdnf*), Cocaine- And Amphetamine-Regulated Transcript Protein Preprotein (*Cartpt*), the receptor for serotonin, (*Htr1b*) (involved in the downstream regulation of serotonin) and of *Snca*, which encodes the neuronal protein α-synuclein associated with several neurodegenerative diseases. Increases in Agouti-related protein (*Agrp*) and *Ghrelin*, hunger-hormones. Reproduced from Fan et al. (2023). The gut microbiota contributes to the pathogenesis of anorexia nervosa in humans and mice. *Nature Microbiology*, *8*(5), article 5. https://doi.org/10.1038/s41564-023-01355-5. Under a Creative Commons Attribution 4.0 International (CC BY 4.0).

Secondly, all the different taxa in each individual's gut interact with each other and not only with the host, so understanding each taxa's exact contribution to the microbiome–gut–brain axis is complicated. With around 500 different taxa in each individual, there are mathematically 499! (499 x 498 x 497 x . . .) possible interactions between the taxa alone (a number covering about two pages with digits). Microbiome research is thus very complex, and we might never learn all the different relations and influences amongst the different bacteria. What we can say, however, is that the microbiome as a whole does play an important part in health and disease in many psychiatric and neurologic diseases including AN, not the least proven by stool transplantations. And, with the field rapidly progressing in new methodologies and computational power, more and more scientific revelations can be expected to come—after all, we are just beginning!

Finally, the effects of microbiome-directed interventions might be small and given the complexity of the microbiome–gut–brain interactions, difficult to research as there are a lot of confounding factors difficult to control. However, in the current "crisis of care" regarding AN (Kaye & Bulik, 2021) with insufficient treatment options, even small effects may have large benefits for patients. And, if we indeed learn more about relevant underlying pathophysiological processes or important taxa, interventions are not far at hand as most involve some form of nutritional intervention that can be readily tested.

Implications

Therapeutic opportunities

As the relevance of the gut microbiome in the context of different diseases has become increasingly clear regarding the importance of extracting energy from food and the interaction with the brain, the possibility of positively influencing the microbiome is currently being studied. There are at least four possible ways to influence the microbiome directly: nutrition, prebiotics, probiotics, and stool transplantation. The World Health Organization defines probiotics as "living microorganisms that, when administered in adequate amounts, have a positive effect on health." In contrast, prebiotics are "dietary components that promote the growth of beneficial microbes in the gut" (Illiano et al., 2020; Slavin, 2013). A systematic review of 10 randomized controlled trials (RCTs) on the use of probiotics for anxiety and depression in patients found, despite methodological limitations due to the different bacterial strains applied, "preliminary evidence of psychological benefits" (Pirbaglou et al., 2016), showing their general potential. One option identified by our animal studies could be *Lactobacilli*, which already helped social deficits in intervention studies in autism animal models (Sgritta et al., 2019). A small RCT with patients with AN showed a positive effect on body weight (Žaja et al., 2021), and larger RCTs are underway (Gröbner et al., 2022). Other potential probiotics for AN include *Lachnospiracea* as previously mentioned. Their reduction is also the hallmark of gut inflammatory diseases, such as Crohn's disease and also of systemic autoimmune diseases, such as systemic lupus and multiple sclerosis (Geirnaert et al., 2017; Maukonen et al., 2015). In all of these diseases, the characteristic microbial dysbiosis is also found; thus, another mechanism of *Lachnospiracea* could be immune and inflammatory-modulatory processes (Lobionda et al., 2019). After administering butyrate-producing bacteria, Geirnaert and colleagues (2017) could, for example, modulate butyrate levels in Crohn's disease patients and increase their gut wall integrity. Further elucidating the function of these species in AN might be an interesting option for future treatment research.

In addition to supplementation with probiotic and prebiotic compounds, there is also the possibility of providing probiotic metabolites (e.g., short-chain fatty acids), as they have been shown to influence the microbiome (Constatini et al., 2019). A first small study using omega-3 fatty acids in patients with AN showed a trend toward increased energy use (Mauler et al., 2009). A large RTC supplementing omega-3 fatty acids is currently underway (Keller et al., 2022).

Fecal microbiota transplantation, the transfer of a fecal microbiota sample, can also be used therapeutically by transplanting stool from a healthy person into a diseased person for therapeutic purposes (Vindigni & Surawicz, 2017). FMT is used as guideline-therapy for *clostridium difficile* overgrowth and currently being established in treating inflammatory bowel diseases. First reports regarding autism spectrum disease are promising (Kang et al., 2017); however, these are open-label studies that need confirmation. Several FMT-RCTs in patients with AN are currently underway, however, the two only published case studies show variable results, one favorable regarding microbiome and weight increase (Prochazkova et al., 2019), one only regarding microbiome markers (de Clercq et al., 2019).

In addition, nutritional interventions, including standard refeeding therapies for patients with AN may need to be critically revised. Refeeding is usually conducted with "normal" hospital food and sometimes involves oral cow milk-based nasogastric feeding formula or oral supplementation, but little is known about the indirect and direct effects of these on the gut microbiota and their interaction with the host (Herpertz-Dahlmann et al., 2017). As changing from a non-animal-based to an animal-based diet alone already has a marked effect on the gut microbiota within one to two days, as stated previously, this could be highly relevant. This is especially true because the majority of patients with AN consume vegetarian or vegan food before being admitted to the hospital. Also, therapists must take into account that about 25% of the "regular" nonantibiotic drugs have a measurable effect on the gut microbiota (Maier et al., 2018), which has been ignored up to now. It will be important to gain more knowledge about food and drug interactions with gut microbiota to better tailor these nutritional treatments to patients' individual needs. Thus, more systematic research on refeeding and nutrition, as well as on what foods should be selected, and in what specific quantities at what times to achieve the specific desired effects, is needed.

References

Achamrah, N., Nobis, S., Breton, J., Jésus, P., Belmonte, L., Maurer, B., Legrand, R., Bôle-Feysot, C., Rego, J. L., Goichon, A., Rego, J. C. do, Déchelotte, P., Fetissov, S. O., Claeyssens, S., & Coëffier, M. (2016). Maintaining physical activity during refeeding improves body composition, intestinal hyperpermeability and behavior in anorectic mice. *Scientific Reports*, *6*, 21887. https://doi.org/10.1038/srep21887

Almeida, A., Mitchell, A. L., Boland, M., Forster, S. C., Gloor, G. B., Tarkowska, A., Lawley, T. D., & Finn, R. D. (2019). A new genomic blueprint of the human gut microbiota. *Nature*, *568*, 499–504.

Ananthakrishnan, A. N. (2015). Epidemiology and risk factors for IBD. *Nature Reviews. Gastroenterology & Hepatology*, *12*, 205–217.

Andreani, N. A., Sharma, A., Dahmen, B., Specht, H. E., Mannig, N., Ruan, V., Keller, L., Baines, J. F., Herpertz-Dahlmann, B., Dempfle, A., & Seitz, J. (2024). Longitudinal analysis of the gut microbiome in adolescent patients with anorexia nervosa: microbiome-related factors associated with clinical outcome. *Gut Microbes*, *16*(1), 2304158. https://doi.org/10.1080/19490976.2024.2304158

Armougom, F., Henry, M., Vialettes, B., Raccah, D., & Raoult, D. (2009). Monitoring bacterial community of human gut microbiota reveals an increase in Lactobacillus in obese patients and Methanogens in anorexic patients. *PLOS ONE*, *4*(9), article 9.

Bambury, A., Sandhu, K., Cryan, J. F., & Dinan, T. G. (2017). Finding the needle in the haystack: Systematic identification of psychobiotics. *British Journal of Pharmacology*, 175(24), 4430–4438. https://doi.org/10.1111/bph.14127

Borgo, F., Riva, A., Benetti, A., Casiraghi, M. C., Bertelli, S., Garbossa, S., Anselmetti, S., Scarone, S., Pontiroli, A. E., & Morace, G. (2017). Microbiota in anorexia nervosa: The triangle between bacterial species, metabolites and psychological tests. *PLOS ONE*, *12*(6), article 6.

Borsdorf, B., Dahmen, B., Buehren, K., Dempfle, A., Egberts, K., Ehrlich, S., Fleischhaker, C., Konrad, K., Schwarte, R., Timmesfeld, N., Wewetzer, C., Biemann, R., Scharke, W., Herpertz-Dahlmann, B., & Seitz, J. (2021). BDNF levels in adolescent patients with anorexia nervosa increase continuously to supranormal levels 2.5 years after first hospitalization. *Journal of Psychiatry and Neuroscience*, *46*(5), 568–578. https://doi.org/10.1503/jpn.210049

Breton, J. (2021). Gut microbiota alteration in a mouse model of anorexia nervosa. *Clinical Nutrition*, *40*, 181–189. https://doi.org/10.1016/j.clnu.2020.05.002

Butler, M. J., Perrini, A. A., & Eckel, L. A. (2021). The role of the gut microbiome, immunity, and neuroinflammation in the pathophysiology of eating disorders. *Nutrients*, *13*(2). https://doi.org/10.3390/nu13020500

Carbone, E. A., D'Amato, P., Vicchio, G., De Fazio, P., & Segura-Garcia, C. (2020). A systematic review on the role of microbiota in the pathogenesis and treatment of eating disorders. *European Psychiatry*, *64*(1), e2. https://doi.org/10.1192/j.eurpsy.2020.109

Castellini, G., Cassioli, E., Vitali, F., Rossi, E., Dani, C., Melani, G., Flaccomio, D., D'Andria, M., Mejia Monroy, M., Galli, A., Cavalieri, D., Ricca, V., Bartolucci, G. L., & De Filippo, C. (2023). Gut microbiota metabolites mediate the interplay between childhood maltreatment and psychopathology in patients with eating disorders. *Scientific Reports*, *13*(1), 11753. https://doi.org/10.1038/s41598-023-38665-x

Clavel, T., Lagkouvardos, I., & Hiergeist, A. (2016). Microbiome sequencing: Challenges and opportunities for molecular medicine. *Expert Review of Molecular Diagnostics*, *16*(7), article 7. https://doi.org/10.1080/14737159.2016.1184574

Cryan, J. F., O'Riordan, K. J., Cowan, C. S. M., Sandhu, K. V., Bastiaanssen, T. F. S., Boehme, M., Codagnone, M. G., Cussotto, S., Fulling, C., Golubeva, A. V., Guzzetta, K. E., Jaggar, M., Long-Smith, C. M., Lyte, J. M., Martin, J. A., Molinero-Perez, A., Moloney, G., Morelli, E., Morillas, E., . . . Dinan, T. G. (2019). The microbiota-gut–brain axis. *Physiological Reviews*, *99*(4), 1877–2013. https://doi.org/10.1152/physrev.00018.2018

Dalton, B., Bartholdy, S., Robinson, L., Solmi, M., Ibrahim, M. A., Breen, G., Schmidt, U., & Himmerich, H. (2018). A meta-analysis of cytokine concentrations in eating disorders. *Journal of Psychiatric Research*, 103, 252–264.

David, L. A., Maurice, C. F., Carmody, R. N., Gootenberg, D. B., Button, J. E., Wolfe, B. E., Ling, A. V., Devlin, A. S., Varma, Y., Fischbach, M. A., Biddinger, S. B., Dutton, R. J., & Turnbaugh, P. J. (2014). Diet rapidly and reproducibly alters the human gut microbiome. *Nature*, *505*(7484), article 7484. https://doi.org/10.1038/nature12820

de Clercq, N. C., Frissen, M. N., Davids, M., Groen, A. K., & Nieuwdorp, M. (2019). Weight gain after fecal microbiota transplantation in a patient with recurrent underweight following clinical recovery from anorexia nervosa. *Psychotherapy and Psychosomatics*, *88*(1), 58–60. https://doi.org/10.1159/000495044

Di Lodovico, L., Mondot, S., Doré, J., Mack, I., Hanachi, M., & Gorwood, P. (2021). Anorexia nervosa and gut microbiota: A systematic review and quantitative synthesis of pooled microbiological data. *Progress in Neuro-Psychopharmacology & Biological Psychiatry*, *106*, 110114. https://doi.org/10.1016/j.pnpbp.2020.110114

Dinan, T. G., & Cryan, J. F. (2017a). Gut instincts: Microbiota as a key regulator of brain development, ageing and neurodegeneration. *Journal of Physiology*, *595*(2), 489–503. https://doi.org/10.1113/JP273106

Dinan, T. G., & Cryan, J. F. (2017b). The microbiome–gut–brain axis in health and disease. *Gastroenterology Clinics of North America*, *46*(1), 77–89. https://doi.org/10.1016/j.gtc.2016.09.007

Dinan, T. G., Stanton, C., & Cryan, J. F. (2013). Psychobiotics: A novel class of psychotropic. *Biological Psychiatry*, *74*(10), article 10. https://doi.org/10.1016/j.biopsych.2013.05.001

Dominguez-Bello, M. G., Costello, E. K., Contreras, M., Magris, M., Hidalgo, G., Fierer, N., & Knight, R. (2010). Delivery mode shapes the acquisition and structure of the initial microbiota across multiple body habitats in newborns. *Proceedings of the National Academy of Sciences of the United States of America*, *107*, 11971–11975.

Escherich, T. (1885). Die darmbakterien des neugeborenen und säuglings. Fortschritte der Medizin, *3*, 515–522, 547–554.

Fan, Y., Støving, R. K., Berreira Ibraim, S., Hyötyläinen, T., Thirion, F., Arora, T., Lyu, L., Stankevic, E., Hansen, T. H., Déchelotte, P., Sinioja, T., Ragnarsdottir, O., Pons, N., Galleron, N., Quinquis, B., Levenez, F., Roume, H., Falony, G., Vieira-Silva, S., . . . Pedersen, O. (2023). The gut microbiota contributes to the pathogenesis of anorexia nervosa in humans and mice. *Nature Microbiology*, *8*(5), article 5. https://doi.org/10.1038/s41564-023-01355-5

Fetissov, S. O., & Hökfelt, T. (2019). On the origin of eating disorders: altered signaling between gut microbiota, adaptive immunity and the brain melanocortin system regulating feeding behavior. *Current Opinions in Pharmacology*, *48*, 82–91. doi:10.1016/j.coph.2019.07.004

Fouladi, F., Bulik-Sullivan, E. C., Glenny, E. M., Thornton, L. M., Reed, K. K., & Thomas, S. (2022). Reproducible changes in the anorexia nervosa gut microbiota following inpatient therapy remain distinct from non-eating disorder controls. *Gut Microbes*, *14*(1), 2143217.

Geirnaert, A., Calatayud, M., Grootaert, C., Laukens, D., Devriese, S., Smagghe, G., De Vos, M., Boon, N., & Van de Wiele, T. (2017). Butyrate-producing bacteria supplemented in vitro to Crohn's disease patient microbiota increased butyrate production and enhanced intestinal epithelial barrier integrity. *Scientific Reports*, *7*(1), article 1. https://doi.org/10.1038/s41598-017-11734-8

Gilbert, J. A., Blaser, M. J., Caporaso, J. G., Jansson, J. K., Lynch, S. V., & Knight, R. (2018). Current understanding of the human microbiome. *Nature Medicine*, *24*(4), 392–400. https://doi.org/10.1038/nm.4517

Glenny, E. M. (2021). Gut microbial communities from patients with anorexia nervosa do not influence body weight in recipient germ-free mice. *Gut Microbes*, *13*(1897216). https://doi.org/10.1080/19490976.2021.1897216.

Grigioni, S., Achamrah, N., Chan, P., Guérin, C., Bôle-Feysot, C., Delay, J., Colange, G., Quillard, M., Coquard, A., Bubenheim, M., Jésus, P., Tavolacci, M.-P., Déchelotte, P., & Coëffier, M. (2022). Intestinal permeability and appetite regulating peptides-reactive immunoglobulins in severely malnourished women with anorexia nervosa. *Clinical Nutrition*, *41*(8), 1752–1758. https://doi.org/10.1016/j.clnu.2022.06.036

Gröbner, E. M., Zeiler, M., Fischmeister, F. P. S., Kollndorfer, K., Schmelz, S., Schneider, A., Haid-Stecher, N., Sevecke, K., Wagner, G., Keller, L., Adan, R., Danner, U., van Elburg, A., van der Vijgh, B., Kooij, K. L., Fetissov, S., Andreani, N. A., Baines, J. F., Dempfle, A., Seitz, J., . . . Karwautz, A. (2022). The effects of probiotics administration on the gut microbiome in adolescents with anorexia nervosa—A study protocol for a longitudinal, double-blind, randomized, placebo-controlled trial. *European Eating Disorders Review*, *30*(1), 61–74. https://doi.org/10.1002/erv.2876

Hata, T., Miyata, N., Takakura, S., Yoshihara, K., Asano, Y., Kimura-Todani, T., Yamashita, M., Zhang, X.-T., Watanabe, N., Mikami, K., Koga, Y., & Sudo, N. (2019). The gut microbiome derived from anorexia nervosa patients impairs weight gain and behavioral performance in female mice. *Endocrinology*, *160*(10), article 10. https://doi.org/10.1210/en.2019-00408

Hebebrand, J., Hildebrandt, T., Schlögl, H., Seitz, J., Denecke, S., Vieira, D., Gradl-Dietsch, G., Peters, T., Antel, J., Lau, D., & Fulton, S. (2022). The role of hypoleptinemia in the psychological and behavioral adaptation to starvation: Implications for anorexia nervosa. *Neuroscience and Biobehavioral Reviews*, *141*, 104807. https://doi.org/10.1016/j.neubiorev.2022.104807

Herman, A., & Bajaka, A. (2021). The role of the intestinal microbiota in eating disorders—Bulimia nervosa and binge eating disorder. *Psychiatry Research, 300,* 113923. doi:10.1016/j.psychres.2021.113923

Herpertz-Dahlmann, B. (2015). Adolescent eating disorders: Update on definitions, symptomatology, epidemiology, and comorbidity. *Child and Adolescent Psychiatric Clinics of North America, 24*(1), article 1. https://doi.org/10.1016/j.chc.2014.08.003

Herpertz-Dahlmann, B., Seitz, J., & Baines, J. (2017). Food matters: How the microbiome and gut–brain interaction might impact the development and course of anorexia nervosa. *European Child & Adolescent Psychiatry, 26*(9), 1031–1041. https://doi.org/10.1007/s00787-017-0945-7

Igudesman, D., Abbaspour, A., Reed, K. K., Flatt, R. E., Becken, B., Thornton, L. M., Bulik, C. M., & Carroll, I. M. (2023). Laxative abuse is associated with a depleted gut microbial community structure among women and men with binge-eating disorder or bulimia nervosa: The binge eating genetics initiative. *Psychosomatic Medicine, 85*(8), 727–735. doi:10.1097/psy.0000000000001226

Jesus, P., Ouelaa, W., Francois, M., Riachy, L., Guerin, C., Aziz, M., Do Rego, J.-C., Dechelotte, P., Fetissov, S. O., & Coeffier, M. (2014). Alteration of intestinal barrier function during activity-based anorexia in mice. *Clinical Nutrition, 33*(6), article 6. https://doi.org/10.1016/j.clnu.2013.11.006

Kameyama, K., & Itoh, K. (2014). Intestinal colonization by a Lachnospiraceae bacterium contributes to the development of diabetes in obese mice. *Microbes and Environments, 29*(4), 427–430. https://doi.org/10.1264/jsme2.ME14054

Kang, D. W., Adams, J. B., Gregory, A. C., Borody, T., Chittick, L., Fasano, A., Khoruts, A., Geis, E., Maldonado, J., McDonough-Means, S., Pollard, E. L., Roux, S., Sadowsky, M. J., Lipson, K. S., Sullivan, M. B., Caporaso, J. G., & Krajmalnik-Brown, R. (2017). Microbiota Transfer Therapy alters gut ecosystem and improves gastrointestinal and autism symptoms: an open-label study. *Microbiome, 5*(1), 10. https://doi.org/10.1186/s40168-016-0225-7

Kaye, W. H., & Bulik, C. M. (2021). Treatment of patients with anorexia nervosa in the US—A Crisis in Care. *JAMA Psychiatry, 78,* 591–592. https://doi.org/10.1001/jamapsychiatry.2020.4796

Kaye, W. H., Wagner, A., Fudge, J. L., & Paulus, M. (2011). Neurocircuity of eating disorders. *Current Topics in Behavioral Neurosciences, 6,* 37–57. https://doi.org/10.1007/7854_2010_85

Keller, L., Dempfle, A., Dahmen, B., Schreiber, S., Adan, R. A. H., Andreani, N. A., Danner, U. N., Eisert, A., Fetissov, S., Fischmeister, F. P. S., Karwautz, A., Konrad, K., Kooij, K. L., Trinh, S., van der Vijgh, B., van Elburg, A. A., Zeiler, M., Baines, J., Seitz, J., & Herpertz-Dahlmann, B. (2022). The effects of polyunsaturated fatty acid (PUFA) administration on the microbiome–gut–brain axis in adolescents with anorexia nervosa (the MiGBAN study): Study protocol for a longitudinal, double-blind, randomized, placebo-controlled trial. *Trials, 23*(1), 545. https://doi.org/10.1186/s13063-022-06413-7

Kelly, J. R., Borre, Y., O'Brien, C., Patterson, E., El Aidy, S., Deane, J., Kennedy, P. J., Beers, S., Scott, K., & Moloney, G. (2016). Transferring the blues: Depression-associated gut microbiota induces neurobehavioural changes in the rat. *Journal of Psychiatric Research, 82,* 109–118.

Kelly, J. R., Minuto, C., Cryan, J. F., Clarke, G., & Dinan, T. G. (2017). Cross talk: The microbiota and neurodevelopmental disorders. *Frontiers in Neuroscience, 11,* 490. https://doi.org/10.3389/fnins.2017.00490

Kleiman, S. C., Glenny, E. M., Bulik-Sullivan, E. C., Huh, E. Y., Tsilimigras, M. C. B., Fodor, A. A., Bulik, C. M., & Carroll, I. M. (2017). Daily changes in composition and diversity of the intestinal microbiota in patients with anorexia nervosa: A series of three cases. *European Eating Disorders Review, 25*(5), Article 5. https://doi.org/10.1002/erv.2524

Kleiman, S. C., Watson, H. J., Bulik-Sullivan, E. C., Huh, E. Y., Tarantino, L. M., Bulik, C. M., & Carroll, I. M. (2015). The intestinal microbiota in acute anorexia nervosa and during renourishment: Relationship to depression, anxiety, and eating disorder psychopathology. *Psychosomatic Medicine, 77*(9), article 9.

Lagkouvardos, I., Fischer, S., Kumar, N., & Clavel, T. (2017). Rhea: A transparent and modular R pipeline for microbial profiling based on 16S rRNA gene amplicons. *PeerJ, 5,* 2836.

Lagkouvardos, I., Joseph, D., Kapfhammer, M., Giritli, S., Horn, M., Haller, D., & Clavel, T. (2016). IMNGS: A comprehensive open resource of processed 16S rRNA microbial profiles for ecology and diversity studies. *Scientific Reports, 6,* 33721.

Ley, R. E., Bäckhed, F., Turnbaugh, P., Lozupone, C. A., Knight, R. D., & Gordon, J. I. (2005). Obesity alters gut microbial ecology. *Proceedings of the National Academy of Sciences of the United States of America, 102*(31), 11070–11075. https://doi.org/10.1073/pnas.0504978102

L'Huillier, C., Jarbeau, M., Achamrah, N., Belmonte, L., Amamou, A., Nobis, S., Goichon, A., Salameh, E., Bahlouli, W., do Rego, J.-L., Déchelotte, P., & Coëffier, M. (2019). Glutamine, but not branched-chain amino acids, restores intestinal barrier function during activity-based anorexia. *Nutrients, 11*(6), 1348. https://doi.org/10.3390/nu11061348

Liu, D., Wen, B., Zhu, K., Luo, Y., Li, J., Li, Y., Lin, H., Huang, J., & Liu, Z. (2019). Antibiotics-induced perturbations in gut microbial diversity influence metabolic phenotypes in a murine model of high-fat diet-induced obesity. *Applied Microbiology and Biotechnology, 103*(13). https://doi.org/10.1007/s00253-019-09764-5

Lobionda, S., Sittipo, P., Kwon, H. Y., & Lee, Y. K. (2019). The role of gut microbiota in intestinal inflammation with respect to diet and extrinsic stressors. *Microorganisms, 7*(8), 271. https://doi.org/10.3390/microorganisms7080271

Lynch, S. V., & Pedersen, O. (2016). The human intestinal microbiome in health and disease. *New England Journal of Medicine, 375*, 2369–2379.

Mack, I., Cuntz, U., Grämer, C., Niedermaier, S., Pohl, C., Schwiertz, A., Zimmermann, K., Zipfel, S., Enck, P., & Penders, J. (2016). Weight gain in anorexia nervosa does not ameliorate the faecal microbiota, branched chain fatty acid profiles, and gastrointestinal complaints. *Scientific Reports, 6*, 26752.

Mack, I., Penders, J., Cook, J., Dugmore, J., Mazurak, N., & Enck, P. (2018). Is the impact of starvation on the gut microbiota specific or unspecific to anorexia nervosa? A narrative review based on a systematic literature search. *Current Neuropharmacology*, 16(8), 1131–1149.

Maier, L., Pruteanu, M., Kuhn, M., Zeller, G., Telzerow, A., Anderson, E. E., Brochado, A. R., Fernandez, K. C., Dose, H., Mori, H., Patil, K. R., Bork, P., & Typas, A. (2018). Extensive impact of non-antibiotic drugs on human gut bacteria. *Nature, 555*(7698), 623–628. https://doi.org/10.1038/nature25979

Marchesi, J. R. (2011). Human distal gut microbiome. *Environmental Microbiology, 13*, 3088–3102.

Marchesi, J. R., Adams, D. H., Fava, F., Hermes, G. D., Hirschfield, G. M., Hold, G., Quraishi, M. N., Kinross, J., Smidt, H., Tuohy, K. M., Thomas, L. V., Zoetendal, E. G., & Hart, A. (2016). The gut microbiota and host health: a new clinical frontier. *Gut, 65*(2), 330–339. https://doi.org/10.1136/gutjnl-2015-309990

Maukonen, J., Kolho, K. L., Paasela, M., Honkanen, J., Klemetti, P., Vaarala, O., & Saarela, M. (2015). Altered fecal microbiota in paediatric inflammatory bowel disease. *Journal of Crohn's & Colitis, 9*(12), 1088–1095. https://doi.org/10.1093/ecco-jcc/jjv147

Mauler, B., Dubben, S., Pawelzik, M., Pawelzik, D., Weigle, D. S., & Kratz, M. (2009). Hypercaloric diets differing in fat composition have similar effects on serum leptin and weight gain in female subjects with anorexia nervosa. *Nutrition Research, 29*(1), 1–7. https://doi.org/10.1016/j.nutres.2008.12.001

Metchnikoff, E. (1907). *The prolongation of life: Optimistic studies.* William Heinemann, G. P. Putnam's Sons.

Miller, I. (2018). The gut–brain axis: Historical reflections. *Microbial Ecology in Health and Disease, 29*(1), 1542921. https://doi.org/10.1080/16512235.2018.1542921

Million, M., Angelakis, E., Maraninchi, M., Henry, M., Giorgi, R., Valero, R., Vialettes, B., & Raoult, D. (2013). Correlation between body mass index and gut concentrations of Lactobacillus reuteri, Bifidobacterium animalis, Methanobrevibacter smithii and Escherichia coli. *International Journal of Obesity, 37*(11), article 11. https://doi.org/10.1038/ijo.2013.20

Möhle, L., Mattei, D., Heimesaat, M. M., Bereswill, S., Fischer, A., Alutis, M., French, T., Hambardzumyan, D., Matzinger, P., & Dunay, I. R. (2016). Ly6Chi monocytes provide a link between antibiotic-induced changes in gut microbiota and adult hippocampal neurogenesis. *Cell Reports, 15*(9), article 9.

Monteleone, P., Carratù, R., Cartenì, M., Generoso, M., Lamberti, M., Magistris, L. D., Brambilla, F., Colurcio, B., Secondulfo, M., & Maj, M. (2004). Intestinal permeability is decreased in anorexia nervosa. *Molecular Psychiatry, 9*(1), article 1. https://doi.org/10.1038/sj.mp.4001374

Morita, C., Tsuji, H., Hata, T., Gondo, M., Takakura, S., Kawai, K., Yoshihara, K., Ogata, K., Nomoto, K., Miyazaki, K., & Sudo, N. (2015). Gut dysbiosis in patients with anorexia nervosa. *PLOS ONE, 10*(12), e0145274. https://doi.org/10.1371/journal.pone.0145274

Mörkl, S., Lackner, S., Meinitzer, A., Mangge, H., Lehofer, M., Halwachs, B., Gorkiewicz, G., Kashofer, K., Painold, A., Holl, A. K., Bengesser, S. A., Müller, W., Holzer, P., & Holasek, S. J. (2018). Gut microbiota, dietary intakes and intestinal permeability reflected by serum zonulin in women. *European Journal of Nutrition*, 57(8), 2985–2997. https://doi.org/10.1007/s00394-018-1784-0

Mörkl, S., Lackner, S., Müller, W., Gorkiewicz, G., Kashofer, K., Oberascher, A., Painold, A., Holl, A., Holzer, P., & Meinitzer, A. (2017). Gut microbiota and body composition in anorexia nervosa inpatients in comparison to athletes, overweight, obese, and normal weight controls. *International Journal of Eating Disorders, 50*(12), article 12.

Neuman, H., Debelius, J. W., Knight, R., & Koren, O. (2015). Microbial endocrinology: The interplay between the microbiota and the endocrine system. *FEMS Microbiology Reviews, 39*(4), article 4. https://doi.org/10.1093/femsre/fuu010

Paulukat, L., Frintrop, L., Liesbrock, J., Heussen, N., Johann, S., Exner, C., Martien, K. J., Tolba, R., Neulen, J., & Konrad, K. (2016). Memory impairment is associated with the loss of regular oestrous cycle and plasma oestradiol levels in an activity-based anorexia animal model. *World Journal of Biological Psychiatry, 17*(4), article 4.

Pirbaglou, M., Katz, J., de Souza, R. J., Stearns, J. C., Motamed, M., & Ritvo, P. (2016). Probiotic supplementation can positively affect anxiety and depressive symptoms: A systematic review of randomized controlled trials. *Nutrition Research, 36*(9), 889–898. https://doi.org/10.1016/j.nutres.2016.06.009

Prescott, S. L. (2017). History of medicine: Origin of the term microbiome and why it matters. *Human Microbiome Journal, 4*, 24–25. https://doi.org/10.1016/j.humic.2017.05.004

Prochazkova, P., Roubalova, R., Dvorak, J., Kreisinger, J., Hill, M., Tlaskalova-Hogenova, H., Tomasova, P., Pelantova, H., Cermakova, M., Kuzma, M., Bulant, J., Bilej, M., Smitka, K., Lambertova, A., Holanova, P., & Papezova, H. (2021). The intestinal microbiota and metabolites in patients with anorexia nervosa. *Gut Microbes, 13*(1), 1–25. https://doi.org/10.1080/19490976.2021.1902771

Prochazkova, P., Roubalova, R., Dvorak, J., Tlaskalova-Hogenova, H., Cermakova, M., Tomasova, P., Sediva, B., Kuzma, M., Bulant, J., Bilej, M., Hrabak, P., Meisnerova, E., Lambertova, A., & Papezova, H. (2019). Microbiota, microbial metabolites, and barrier function in a patient with anorexia nervosa after fecal microbiota transplantation. *Microorganisms, 7*(9), 338. https://doi.org/10.3390/microorganisms7090338

Queipo-Ortuño, M. I., Seoane, L. M., Murri, M., Pardo, M., Gomez-Zumaquero, J. M., Cardona, F., Casanueva, F., & Tinahones, F. J. (2013). Gut microbiota composition in male rat models under different nutritional status and physical activity and its association with serum leptin and ghrelin levels. *PLOS ONE, 8*(5), article 5. https://doi.org/10.1371/journal.pone.0065465

Raevuori, A., Haukka, J., Vaarala, O., Suvisaari, J. M., Gissler, M., Grainger, M., Linna, M. S., & Suokas, J. T. (2014). The increased risk for autoimmune diseases in patients with eating disorders. *PLOS ONE, 9*(8), article 8. https://doi.org/10.1371/journal.pone.0104845

Ranjan, R., Rani, A., Metwally, A., McGee, H. S., & Perkins, D. L. (2016). Analysis of the microbiome: Advantages of whole genome shotgun versus 16S amplicon sequencing. *Biochemical and Biophysical Research Communications, 469*, 967–977.

Ridaura, V. K., Faith, J. J., Rey, F. E., Cheng, J., Duncan, A. E., Kau, A. L., Griffin, N. W., Lombard, V., Henrissat, B., & Bain, J. R. (2013). Gut microbiota from twins discordant for obesity modulate metabolism in mice. *Science, 341*(6150), article 6150.

Roediger, W. E. (1980). The colonic epithelium in ulcerative colitis: An energy-deficiency disease? *Lancet, 2*(8197), 712–715. https://doi.org/10.1016/s0140-6736(80)91934-0

Schulz, N., Belheouane, M., Dahmen, B., Ruan, V. A., Specht, H. E., Dempfle, A., Herpertz-Dahlmann, B., Baines, J. F., & Seitz, J. (2021). Gut microbiota alteration in adolescent anorexia nervosa does not normalize with short-term weight restoration. *The International Journal of Eating Disorders, 54*(6), 969–980. https://doi.org/10.1002/eat.23435

Seitz, J., Dahmen, B., Keller, L., & Herpertz-Dahlmann, B. (2020). Gut feelings: How microbiota might impact the development and course of anorexia nervosa. *Nutrients, 12*(11), 3295. https://doi.org/10.3390/nu12113295

Seitz, J., Konrad, K., & Herpertz-Dahlmann, B. (2018). Extend, pathomechanism and clinical consequences of brain volume changes in anorexia nervosa. *Current Neuropharmacology, 16*(8), 1164–1173. https://doi.org/10.2174/1570159X15666171109145651

Seitz, J., Walter, M., Mainz, V., Herpertz-Dahlmann, B., Konrad, K., & Polier, G. von. (2015). Brain volume reduction predicts weight development in adolescent patients with anorexia nervosa. *Journal of Psychiatric Research, 68*, 228–237. https://doi.org/10.1016/j.jpsychires.2015.06.019

Sender, R., Fuchs, S., & Milo, R. (2016). Revised estimates for the number of human and bacteria cells in the body. *PLOS Biology, 14*(8), article 8. https://doi.org/10.1371/journal.pbio.1002533

Sgritta, M., Dooling, S. W., Buffington, S. A., Momin, E. N., Francis, M. B., Britton, R. A., & Costa-Mattioli, M. (2019). Mechanisms underlying microbial-mediated changes in social behavior in mouse models of autism spectrum disorder. *Neuron, 101*, 246–259246.

Slavin, J. (2013). Fiber and prebiotics: Mechanisms and health benefits. *Nutrients, 5*, 1417–1435.

Smith, M. I., Yatsunenko, T., Manary, M. J., Trehan, I., Mkakosya, R., Cheng, J., Kau, A. L., Rich, S. S., Concannon, P., Mychaleckyj, J. C., Liu, J., Houpt, E., Li, J. V., Holmes, E., Nicholson, J., Knights, D., Ursell, L. K., Knight, R., & Gordon, J. I. (2013). Gut microbiomes of Malawian twin pairs discordant for Kwashiorkor. *Science, 339*(6119), article 6119. https://doi.org/10.1126/science.1229000

Solmi, M., Santonastaso, P., Caccaro, R., & Favaro, A. (2013). A case of anorexia nervosa with comorbid Crohn's disease: Beneficial effects of anti-TNF-α therapy? *International Journal of Eating Disorders, 46*(6), article 6. https://doi.org/10.1002/eat.22153

Solmi, M., Veronese, N., Favaro, A., Santonastaso, P., Manzato, E., Sergi, G., & Correll, C. U. (2015). Inflammatory cytokines and anorexia nervosa: A meta-analysis of cross-sectional and longitudinal studies. *Psychoneuroendocrinology, 51*, 237–252.

Tamboli, C. P. (2004). Dysbiosis in inflammatory bowel disease. *Gut, 53*, 1–4. https://doi.org/10.1136/gut.53.1.1.

Tengeler, A. C., Dam, S. A., Wiesmann, M., Naaijen, J., Bodegom, M., Belzer, C., Dederen, P. J., Verweij, V., Franke, B., Kozicz, T., Arias Vasquez, A., & Kiliaan, A. J. (2020). Gut microbiota from persons with attention-deficit/hyperactivity disorder affects the brain in mice. *Microbiome, 8*(1), 44. https://doi.org/10.1186/s40168-020-00816-x

Terry, S. M., Barnett, J. A., & Gibson, D. L. (2022). A critical analysis of eating disorders and the gut microbiome. *Journal of Eating Disorders, 10*(1), 154. https://doi.org/10.1186/s40337-022-00681-z

Tissier, M. H. (1899). La réaction chromophile d'Escherich et Bacterium Coli. *Comptes rendus hebdomadaires de la Société de biologie, 51*, 943–945.

Tremaroli, V., Karlsson, F., Werling, M., Staahlman, M., Kovatcheva-Datchary, P., Olbers, T., Fändriks, L., le Roux, C. W., Nielsen, J., & Bäckhed, F. (2015). Roux-en-Y gastric bypass and vertical banded gastroplasty induce long-term changes on the human gut microbiome contributing to fat mass regulation. *Cell Metabolism, 22*(2), article 2.

Trinh, S., Käver, L., Schlösser, A., Simon, A., Kogel, V., Voelz, C., Beyer, C., & Seitz, J. (2023). Gut-associated lymphatic tissue in food-restricted rats: Influence of refeeding and probiotic supplementation. *Microorganisms, 11*(6), 1411. https://doi.org/10.3390/microorganisms11061411

Trinh, S., Kogel, V., Voelz, C., Schlösser, A., Schwenzer, C., Kabbert, J., Heussen, N., Clavel, T., Herpertz-Dahlmann, B., Beyer, C., & Seitz, J. (2021). Gut microbiota and brain alterations in a translational anorexia nervosa rat model. *Journal of Psychiatric Research, 133*, 156–165. https://doi.org/10.1016/j.jpsychires.2020.12.030

Turnbaugh, P. J., Ley, R. E., Hamady, M., Fraser-Liggett, C. M., Knight, R., & Gordon, J. I. (2007). The human microbiome project. *Nature, 449*(7164), 804–810. https://doi.org/10.1038/nature06244

Turnbaugh, P. J., Ley, R. E., Mahowald, M. A., Magrini, V., Mardis, E. R., & Gordon, J. I. (2006). An obesity-associated gut microbiome with increased capacity for energy harvest. *Nature, 444*(7122), article 7122. https://doi.org/10.1038/nature05414

Vindigni, S. M., & Surawicz, C. M. (2017). Fecal microbiota transplantation. *Gastroenterology Clinics of North America, 46*, 171–185.

Vital, M., Karch, A., & Pieper, D. H. (2017). Colonic butyrate-producing communities in humans: An overview using omics data. *mSystems, 2*, e00130–17. https://doi.org/10.1128/mSystems.00130-17.

Walker, A. W., & Hoyles, L. (2023). Human microbiome myths and misconceptions. *Nature Microbiology, 8*(8), 1392–1396. https://doi.org/10.1038/s41564-023-01426-7

Yuan, R., Yang, L., Yao, G., Geng, S., Ge, Q., Bo, S., & Li, X. (2022). Features of gut microbiota in patients with anorexia nervosa. *Chinese Medical Journal, 135*(16), 1993–2002. https://doi.org/10.1097/CM9.0000000000002362

Žaja, O., Fiolić, M., Ćuk, M. C., & Tiljak, M. K. (2021). The role of L. reuteri DSM17938 in nutritional recovery and treatment of constipation in children and adolescents with anorexia nervosa—A randomized, double blind, placebo controlled study. *Clinical Nutrition ESPEN, 46*, 47–53. https://doi.org/10.1016/j.clnesp.2021.08.016.

25

Target Engagement and Pharmacotherapy in Eating Disorders

Guido K. W. Frank

Brief Definitional Overview

Pharmacotherapy: A medical treatment that uses one or more pharmaceutical drug to improve ongoing symptoms, treat the underlying condition, or act as a prevention for a disease.

Target engagement: Refers to the verification that the intervention has the predicted effect on a mechanism of action.

Introduction

The etiology of eating disorders is considered multifactorial across the bio-psycho-social domains. Relating eating disorder-relevant behaviors to specific brain function or developing mechanistic models to guide targeted pharmacological interventions has been difficult, and only two medications have been approved for the treatment of eating disorders: fluoxetine for bulimia nervosa (BN) and lisdexamfetamine for binge-eating disorder (BED). This chapter will review neurobiological studies in eating disorders to guide pharmacological target identification, followed by a review of the state of science of pharmacological studies. A model of eating disorder pathophysiology is proposed that can be a basis for testing medication interventions. A section on alternative views on pharmacological interventions in the eating disorder population will discuss opposing perspectives.

Biological Framework

Animal models for eating disorders have implicated the monoamine neurotransmitters dopamine and serotonin in food restriction or excessive food intake (see Chapter 22 for further discussion). The activity-based anorexia (ABA) model is the most commonly used animal model for anorexia nervosa (AN), and excessive dopaminergic activation has indicated a vulnerability and overexpression of the dopamine D2 receptor that has been associated with weight loss (Beeler et al.,

Guido K. W. Frank, *Target Engagement and Pharmacotherapy in Eating Disorders*. In: *The Handbook of the Neurobiology of Eating Disorders*. Edited by: Christina E. Wierenga and Joanna E. Steinglass, Oxford University Press. © Oxford University Press (2025). DOI: 10.1093/9780197675212.003.0026

2020; Foldi et al., 2017; Welch et al., 2019). Environmental factors, such as stress, may alter dopamine and serotonin pathways, and monoamine neurotransmission may adapt from short to long-term starvation (Beeler & Burghardt, 2021; Giunti et al., 2023; Reed et al., 2021). Animal models have furthermore suggested a change in the balance of dopamine D1 and D2 receptor neurotransmission associated with disordered eating, affecting midbrain serotonin neurotransmission and indicating state-dependent inter-relationships between neurotransmitter systems that could reinforce AN behaviors (Cai et al., 2022). There is also emerging evidence from animal models that GABA and NMDA receptors contribute to the pathophysiology of AN via altered neural plasticity (Aoki & Santiago, 2022). Animal models of binge eating behavior indicate acute elevations in dopamine neurotransmission but decreases in striatal dopamine receptor distribution after prolonged binge eating, as well as anxiety when deprived of binge eating (Avena et al., 2012; Avena, Bocarsly, et al., 2008; Johnson & Kenny, 2010). Sex hormones and neuroactive peptides are also frequently altered during the ill state of eating disorders and affect brain neurotransmission (Monteleone & Maj, 2013), as do the fat cell-derived hormones leptin or ghrelin from the gastric mucosa that may stimulate or dampen brain dopamine response and alter food approach in eating disorders (Berner et al., 2018; Monteleone et al., 2018). In summary, animal studies suggest distinct changes, especially in dopamine neurotransmission associated with food restriction or binge eating.

Human neurotransmitter receptor studies using positron emission tomography (PET) have shown higher serotonin 1A-receptor binding in individuals with AN and BN when ill and after recovery, suggesting state-independent alterations. The serotonin 2A receptor, in contrast, was normal in ill AN but lower after recovery, supporting dynamic adaptations (Frank, 2015, 2016b). One recent study found lower opioid receptor binding in AN across cortical and subcortical regions (Galusca et al., 2020), while others found lower serotonin transporter availability in the parietal cortex and dorsal raphe in ill AN (Bailer et al., 2007; Yokokura et al., 2019). Dopamine D2 receptor availability was normal in underweight AN but elevated in the striatum in individuals recovered from AN (Broft et al., 2015; Frank et al., 2005). Individuals with BN also showed no dopamine D2-receptor binding differences versus controls, but lower striatal dopamine release was associated with higher binge-eating frequency (Broft et al., 2012). One small study on the cannabinoid-1 receptor found lower regional activation in AN but normal values in BN compared to controls (Gerard et al., 2011). Another study found higher glutamate receptor binding in BN across several regions, which was related to maturity fears (Mihov et al., 2020), but, studies on GABA or glutamate using MRI spectroscopy in the eating disorder population have in general yielded inconclusive results (Mitchell et al., 2023). In another small study, mu-opioid receptor binding was lower in a group of individuals with BED, who also showed altered serotonin transporter binding that was distinctly increased or decreased depending on the brain region studied (Joutsa et al., 2018; Majuri et al., 2017). Altogether, while the literature is limited, these neuroreceptor studies indicate that serotonin receptor availability is altered in AN and BN, making those receptors potential drug intervention targets.

Task-based functional magnetic resonance imaging (fMRI) studies do not directly involve neurotransmitters, but regional activation and task specificity can yield inferences and hypotheses about neurotransmitter involvement. One of the brain circuits that has been most reliably associated with neurotransmitter function is the reward, or salience, network. Food is a natural salient stimulus, and reward pathways get activated when we desire, approach, or eat food, but also when trying to avoid salient stimuli (Kelley & Berridge, 2002; Plassmann et al., 2010). Important regions in this circuitry include the ventral striatum (receives midbrain dopaminergic input, processes motivational salience), the orbitofrontal cortex (stimulus valuation), and the anterior cingulate (error monitoring, reward expectation) (Kelley & Berridge, 2002). The primary neurotransmitters involved are dopamine (for stimulus approach and avoidance) and the opioids (for processing hedonic experiences) (Kelley et al., 2005; Puglisi-Allegra & Ventura, 2012).

Several, but not all, previous studies in AN found altered reward system responses when presented with food or body-related visual stimuli (Boehm et al., 2018; Fladung et al., 2010; Holsen et al., 2012; Horndasch et al., 2018; Lloyd & Steinglass, 2018; Sanders et al., 2015). In a study where subjects had to choose between immediate smaller or delayed larger rewards (delayed discounting), the group with AN responded faster, and lower activation in AN in cingulate and frontal regions indicated a more efficient control circuitry (King et al., 2016). In another study, youth with AN learned better in response to punishment, but associated brain activation was similar to controls (Bernardoni et al., 2018).

Receiving stimuli unexpectedly has been directly associated with brain dopamine response, and early evidence indicated heightened response to unexpected pleasant or unpleasant stimuli in AN (Cowdrey et al., 2011; Schultz, 2002). A paradigm closely associated with brain dopamine response is the prediction error model, a Pavlovian conditioning paradigm in which individuals learn to associate unconditioned taste or monetary stimuli with conditioned visual stimuli (O'Doherty et al., 2003). This paradigm tests the reward valence (processing whether expectations are violated) and motivational salience networks (processing stimuli that propel an individual's behavior *toward or away* from a particular object, perceived event, or outcome) (Puglisi-Allegra & Ventura, 2012). In two studies using monetary or sweet taste stimuli, unexpected receipt or omission was reflected in higher insula and striatal brain response in adolescents with AN versus controls. Brain activation predicted weight gain during treatment, but short-term weight restoration was associated only with some normalization of brain response (DeGuzman et al., 2017; Frank et al., 2017; Frank et al., 2022). Furthermore, weight gain and desensitization to sweet stimuli in AN supported normalization of brain response during treatment (Frank et al., 2022). Those studies suggested heightened dopamine-related brain response in AN that does not quickly normalize with weight recovery (Frank et al., 2017), among youth and adults with AN (Frank et al., 2018).

In BN, negative affect has been found to correlate positively with striatal brain response during tasting of milkshake samples (Bohon & Stice, 2012). Other studies have shown lower activation for monetary reward among individuals with BN in frontal cortical, ventral striatal, and hippocampal regions while navigating through a maze, and that activation correlated with binge/purge frequency (Cyr et al., 2016; Frank, 2013). A large transdiagnostic study indicated a strong inverse relationship between the dopamine-anchored prediction error response and body mass index (BMI) across AN, BN, and BED groups. Furthermore, that study indicated a positive relationship between the prediction error signal and activation of the food control circuitry, suggesting that responsiveness of dopamine circuits is associated in AN with higher, but in BN and BED, lower food control circuit function (Frank et al., 2021). Lower dopamine function in BN was supported by a study that suggested a desensitization of dopaminergic circuits in BN. In that study lower availability of brain dopamine altered the link between reward anticipation and effort to earn a reward in individuals recovered from BN differently comparted to controls, and the results correlated with duration of illness (Mueller et al., 2018).

In summary, reward or motivational salience related circuits showed promising results across the eating disorder spectrum and implicated the dopamine circuitry. The transdiagnostic association of dopamine-related brain response with BMI and with food control circuits makes this circuitry therefore an excellent target to manipulate or modulate using medication.

State of the Science in Eating Disorders

Anorexia nervosa

The cardinal symptom of AN is food avoidance, which has been the focus of medication interventions. Early studies investigated agents to stimulate eating, such as the antihistamine cyproheptadine or the alpha 2 adrenergic agonist clonidine, in double-blind placebo controlled trials, but did not prove successful (Casper et al., 1987). Following those studies, most psychiatric medication classes were tested in controlled or uncontrolled clinical trials.

Opiates and opiate antagonists are associated with the hedonic aspects of salient stimuli and thus could interrupt the self-reinforcing properties of food restriction and, in turn, stimulate eating in AN. The opiate antagonist naltrexone reduced binge/purge frequency in a double-blind controlled but small AN sample, but confirmatory studies are lacking (Marrazzi et al., 1995).

With the idea of targeting depressed mood and anxiety commonly occurring in AN, several studies investigated antidepressant and antianxiety medications. Tricyclic antidepressants, used for anxiety, depression, and obsessive-compulsive disorder, such as clomipramine or amitriptyline, did not show strong significant benefits in double-blind controlled studies (Biederman et al., 1985; Lacey

& Crisp, 1980; Strobel et al., 2004). The most frequently prescribed psychiatric medications, serotonin reuptake inhibitors (SSRIs), such as fluoxetine, citalopram, sertraline, or paroxetine targeting anxiety, depression, and obsessive-compulsive behaviors, have been overall similarly disappointing in double-blind or single-blind controlled or retrospective chart reviews, not revealing benefits for weight gain or weight maintenance (Barbarich, McConaha, Halmi, et al., 2004; Kaye et al., 2001; Walsh et al., 2006; Yu et al., 2011).

Benzodiazepines are fast-acting anxiolytic medications that act as positive allosteric modulators on the gamma amino butyric acid (GABA)-A receptor and allow enhanced GABA binding, inducing its calming effect (Griffin et al., 2013). Benzodiazepines over time also enhance dopamine release in the ventral striatum and attenuate neuroimmune response (Ellinwood et al., 1985; Ramirez et al., 2016; Schelp et al., 2018). The one double-blind placebo controlled study in this group using alprazolam in AN did not improve outcomes over placebo (Steinglass et al., 2014).

The perception of being fat while severely underweight can be seen as an apparent loss of touch with reality. At least in a subgroup of individuals with AN, body image misperception has a psychotic quality (Konstantakopoulos et al., 2012). Targeting a psychotic or delusional quality of body image perception has led to the use of antipsychotic medication. The results have been mixed. The early studies using pimozide, haloperidol, or sulpride in double-blind placebo controlled or one retrospective chart review study provided some support for the benefits of weight gain, body image distortion, and drive for thinness (Mauri et al., 2013; Vandereycken, 1984; Vandereycken & Pierloot, 1982). The atypical antipsychotic quetiapine, a relatively weak antagonist at the dopamine D1 and D2 and serotonin 1A and 2A receptor sites, but a strong histamine H1 receptor antagonist did not improve AN core symptoms in double-blind or open label studies (Powers et al., 2012). Similarly, risperidone, a dopamine D2, serotonin 1A, 2A, and histamine H1 receptor antagonist, did not show benefits over placebo in a double-blind, controlled study in adolescents (Hagman et al., 2011). The atypical antipsychotic most frequently studied in AN is olanzapine. It has dopamine D1 and D2 receptor antagonistic properties, and is an inverse agonist at the serotonin 2A and histamine H1 receptor, the latter which may contribute to eating stimulation and weight gain (Bymaster et al., 1996; Ninan & Kulkarni, 1999). Open-label studies suggested improved weight gain in AN (Barbarich, McConaha, Gaskill, et al., 2004; Mondraty et al., 2005), but more recent controlled studies showed mixed and small if any, benefits (Bissada et al., 2008; Brambilla, Garcia, et al., 2007; Brambilla, Monteleone, et al., 2007). One randomized controlled study found that the active drug was associated with small but significantly greater weight gain compared with placebo in an outpatient setting (Attia et al., 2011), and a multi-center follow-up study also showed a significant but small therapeutic effect of olanzapine in adult outpatients with AN, an increase in BMI in the olanzapine group of 1.2 compared to 0.4 in the control group over four months. There were no significant benefits for psychological symptoms (Attia et al., 2019) and there was no indication that olanzapine would be able to enhance the effects of psychotherapy alone (Brambilla, Garcia, et al., 2007; Brambilla, Monteleone, et al., 2007; Kafantaris et al., 2011; Norris et al., 2011).

The atypical antipsychotic aripiprazole is different from most other atypical antipsychotics, as it is a dopamine D2 and serotonin 1A receptor partial agonists while having serotonin 2A receptor antagonistic properties. No controlled studies exist. A retrospective chart review suggested improved weight gain (change from admission age-adjusted BMI percentile aripiprazole group, compared to the control group) in those individuals who were treated in inpatient or partial hospital treatment, suggesting benefits in conjunction with behavior interventions (Frank et al., 2017). In summary, olanzapine has the strongest evidence of the antipsychotics to support weight gain in AN in the outpatient setting, although the amount is modest.

AN is associated with multiple endocrinological abnormalities across the brain and gut, which could affect neurotransmitter function and behavior (Monteleone et al., 2018). The gut hormone ghrelin is produced in the stomach and pancreas to stimulate food intake. A recent controlled trial showed improved gastric emptying but only trend level weight gain benefits with the motility agent relamorelin (Fazeli et al., 2018). Sex hormone levels are low in AN, but hormone replacement had mixed results. A randomized controlled trial using estrogen showed reduced trait anxiety without specific effects on eating disorder behaviors or weight (Misra et al., 2013). The steroid hormone dehydroepiandrosterone (DHEA) did not show benefits for AN in a controlled study (DiVasta et al., 2019), neither did human growth hormone (Hill et al., 2000), and testosterone even impaired weight gain (Kimball et al., 2019). Oxytocin, a hypothalamic hormone affecting social behavior and cognition, has been shown to improve glucose homeostasis and reduce food intake by enhancing satiation during eating (Lawson, 2017; Liu et al., 2021). While counterintuitive due to the potential for weight loss, oxytocin was used in AN with the hypothesis that it could attenuate anxiety and improve social function and thus improve eating. However, double-blind controlled studies showed inconclusive results in AN for improving social relatedness (Lawson et al., 2012; Monteleone et al., 2016), and studies did not indicate weight gain or anxiety benefits (Kim et al., 2015; Kim, Kim, et al., 2014; Kim, Oh, et al., 2014; Leppanen et al., 2017a, 2017b; Russell et al., 2018).

Other pharmacological interventions targeted learning, anxiety, or neural protection. The NMDA partial agonist d-cycloserine, previously shown to augment fear extinction, was associated with greater weight gain in AN in a double-blind controlled study when paired with exposure therapy (Levinson et al., 2015). However, no confirmatory studies have been published since. Supplementation of omega-3 fatty acids, important for brain development, could not be distinguished from placebo in AN treatment (Manos et al., 2018); however, the amino acid tyrosine, a precursor for dopamine, was associated with improved depression ratings in a double-blind controlled study (Israely et al., 2017). Overall, the benefits of hormones or nutritional supplements for AN remain uncertain.

Bulimia nervosa

Tricyclic antidepressant medications tried in BN indicated improvements in mood and eating disorder behaviors in double-blind controlled studies (Agras et al., 1987; Mitchell & Groat, 1984; Pope et al., 1983), but group therapy effects were stronger than active drugs, and added drugs were not superior to psychotherapy alone for core eating disorder behaviors (Mitchell et al., 1990). Desipramine versus placebo resulted in reduced eating disorder behaviors in controlled trials, but relapse was high, as was the dropout rate, up to 50%, (Agras et al., 1992; Barlow et al., 1988; Blouin et al., 1988; McCann & Agras, 1990; Walsh et al., 1991) while the tetracyclic antidepressant mianserin did not lead to significant improvements over placebo (Sabine et al., 1983). Monoamine oxidase inhibitors (MAOIs) reduced binge-eating frequency in BN in controlled studies; however, the dropout rate across studies was high (Carruba et al., 2001; Kennedy et al., 1993; Kennedy et al., 1988; Rothschild et al., 1994; Walsh et al., 1988; Walsh et al., 1984). The norepinephrine/dopamine-reuptake inhibitor bupropion showed promise in treating BN in a controlled study; however, 7% of active drug probands suffered grand mal seizures, and bupropion is contraindicated in eating disorders associated with purging behaviors (Horne et al., 1988). The serotonin reuptake and histamine and alpha-1-adrenergic receptor blocker trazodone, compared to placebo, reduced binge eating and purging frequency in BN and improved self-control in a controlled study, but no further investigations were conducted, raising the question whether the results could be replicated (Pope et al., 1989). Controlled studies using the SSRI fluvoxamine were mixed, dropout was high, up to 75%, and potential side effects were concerning, including elevated seizure frequency and liver function test abnormalities (Brambilla et al., 1995; Fichter et al., 1996; Fichter et al., 1997; Milano, Siano, et al., 2005; Schmidt et al., 2004).

The strongest evidence for pharmacological efficacy for treating BN exists for the SSRI fluoxetine, which has FDA approval. Two large multi-center studies indicated reduced binge eating and purging behaviors over placebo but also higher side effects such as insomnia, nausea, or tremor (Anonymous, 1992; Goldstein et al., 1995). Higher fluoxetine dose provided a stronger therapeutic effect on pathologic eating attitudes, carbohydrate cravings, and depression, and the current recommendation is to quickly titrate the medication to 60 mg in adults with BN. However, a high dropout rate was concerning, with 45% in the 16-week study not completing treatment. Follow-up studies further supported the combination of medication with cognitive behavior therapy (CBT) (Goldbloom et al., 1997; Walsh et al., 1997).

On long-term follow-up, only 17% of the fluoxetine and 8% of the placebo-treated patients completed the study, suggesting that fluoxetine's effectiveness is limited, especially over time (Romano et al., 2002).

BN is associated with mood fluctuations, which may trigger binge-eating episodes; however, the mood stabilizer lithium was not superior to placebo in a controlled trial (Hsu et al., 1991). The anti-epileptic topiramate which is often used off-label for mood stabilization, reduced binge eating and purging frequency, and depression and anxiety in BN in double-blind controlled studies (Hedges et al., 2003; Hoopes et al., 2003; Nickel et al., 2005). However, its strong weight loss and potential side effects, including eye, kidney, and bone damage, are problematic.

Ondansetron, a competitive serotonin-3 receptor antagonist used to treat nausea and vomiting, showed improved binge eating and purging in a small, controlled trial (Faris et al., 2000), but no follow-up studies support ondansetron's use in BN.

The opiate naltrexone at lower dose (50 mg) did not show illness reducing effects in BN, but at higher dose (200 mg) was found to reduce binge eating and purging behaviors in double-blind controlled studies.

The high comorbidity between BN and mood disorders and the cascade from affect dysregulation to loss of control, and negative self-evaluation and binge eating and purging behaviors suggests that targeting mood dysregulation could be beneficial to reduce specific illness behavior in BN (Frank, 2020a). Lamotrigine, frequently used as a mood stabilizer showed promise in a case series with improvement in mood reactivity and instability, impulsive drives and behaviors, and eating-disorder symptoms (Trunko et al., 2014). Opioids such as naltrexone also are understudied and may hold benefits in future studies.

Binge-eating disorder

The tricyclic imipramine as an adjunct to supportive therapy and dietary counseling showed stronger effects over placebo for weight loss in BED, which may have been related to reduced depression levels (Laederach-Hofmann et al., 1999). Controlled studies on fluvoxamine showed inconsistent indications that the medication leads to reduced binge eating over placebo (Hudson et al., 1998; Pearlstein et al., 2003; Ricca et al., 2001). Studies testing fluoxetine were also inconsistent, with most controlled trials indicating improved mood but limited effects on binge eating severity, especially when comparing the drug effects with CBT, which typically had the stronger effect (Arnold et al., 2002; Devlin et al., 2005; Devlin et al., 2007; Marcus et al., 1990). Smaller controlled or open label studies using the SSRI sertraline reported significant effects of active medication over placebo in reducing binge-eating frequency (Leombruni et al., 2006; McElroy et al., 2000). A retrospective chart review suggested that the serotonin-norepinephrine reuptake inhibitor (SNRI) venlafaxine was associated with lower binge-eating frequency,

BMI, and blood pressure (Malhotra et al., 2002). The relatively new antidepressant vortioxetine, an SNRI with distinct serotonin receptor agonistic and antagonistic properties (D'Agostino et al., 2015), did not show significant group benefits over the control condition, highlighting a strong placebo effect in the BED population (Grant et al., 2019).

Topiramate reduced binge eating days and binge episodes per week and BMI compared with placebo, leading to binge eating remission in 58% (versus 29%) of patients (Claudino et al., 2007; McElroy et al., 2003; McElroy, Hudson, et al., 2007; McElroy et al., 2004; Safer et al., 2020). However, side effects included paresthesia or somnolence, raising safety concerns (Nourredine et al., 2021). Other anti-epileptic medications, zonisamide or lamotrigine, did not show promise in BED in double-blind controlled studies (Guerdjikova et al., 2009).

A relatively large number of double-blind controlled studies have investigated stimulant medications in BED. Those agents, typically prescribed for ADHD, have been associated with reducing appetite and weight loss, which could reduce binge eating drive. The d-amphetamine prodrug lisdexamfetamine has been studied in several large studies that led to FDA approval for this medication for treating moderate to severe BED in adults (Guerdjikova et al., 2016; McElroy et al., 2016; McElroy et al., 2017; McElroy, Hudson, et al., 2015). Across two large studies, 82% and 86% of lisdexamfetamine-treated patients were considered improved versus 47% and 42% of placebo-treated patients. Forty percent and 36% of patients in the active drug groups were binge episode-free for four weeks at the end of the study versus 14% and 13% of placebo-treated patients. Lisdexamfetamine was tolerated well, but elevated blood pressure and pulse rate occurred. Time to relapse was also delayed in lisdexamfetamine-treated patients versus controls (Hudson et al., 2017), but 85% of participants reported adverse events that led to treatment discontinuation in 9%, including dry mouth, headache, insomnia, and upper respiratory tract infection (Gasior et al., 2017). In contrast, methylphenidate, a norepinephrine and dopamine reuptake inhibitor, was not superior to CBT for binge eating behaviors but led to greater weight loss (Quilty et al., 2019). Dasotraline, a serotonin, norepinephrine, and dopamine reuptake inhibitor developed to treat ADHD and BED, showed promise in treating BED, but safety concerns led to a withdrawal of the medication (Grilo et al., 2020; McElroy et al., 2020).

Weight loss agents also targeted binge eating in BED. The serotonin-releasing agent D-fenfluramine was superior to placebo in reducing binge-eating episodes; however, cardiac and pulmonary side effects led to market withdrawal (Stunkard et al., 1996). The norepinephrine, serotonin, and dopamine reuptake inhibitor sibutramine was found effective over placebo in reducing binge-eating episodes and leading to more significant weight loss in several studies (Appolinario et al., 2003; Bauer et al., 2006; Milano, Petrella, et al., 2005; Wilfley et al., 2008), but sibutramine's increased risk of causing heart attack and stroke in susceptible individuals led to its discontinuation. The selective norepinephrine reuptake inhibitor atomoxetine significantly reduced binge-eating frequency, BMI, and eating disorder psychopathology but was also associated with sudden deaths, stroke, and myocardial infarction (McElroy, Guerdjikova, et al., 2007).

To target food cravings, it was hypothesized that blocking opioid receptors could reduce binge-eating episodes. The opioid receptor antagonist samidorphan did not show benefits over placebo on binge-eating pathology, though (McElroy et al., 2013). The dopamine reuptake inhibitor armodafinil showed a similar reduction in the number of days with binge-eating episodes, although the active drug resulted in a significantly lower number of binge-eating episodes and lower BMI at the end of the study (McElroy, Guerdjikova, et al., 2015).

In summary, there is an indication that serotonin-active medications can reduce binge-eating pathology, but the high placebo response is striking. Medications targeting the monamines serotonin, dopamine, and norepinephrine together can reduce binge eating but may also cause intolerable side effects. The strongest evidence for effectiveness while having an acceptable safety profile exists for the dextroamphetamine prodrug lisdexamfetamine, implicating dopaminergic and noradrenergic neurotransmission as an important target for further drug development. ADHD and BED are highly comorbid, and whether lisdexamfetamine is specific for psychopathology associated with BED or ADHD remains to be seen.

A novel indication for BED may be the glucagon-like peptide 1 (GLP-1) receptor agonists that were developed to treat type 2 diabetes mellitus and have shown benefits as treatments for obesity. One recent open label study using the GLP-1 agonist semaglutide indicated binge eating scale decreases that were superior to lisdexamfetamine or topiramate (Richards et al., 2023). Whether those types of medications can be recommended for the treatment of BED will need to be tested in controlled trials.

Avoidant/restrictive food intake disorder

No controlled medication trials exist for avoidant/restrictive food intake disorder (ARFID), but small uncontrolled studies suggested that the tetracyclic antidepressant mirtazapine could help reduce anxiety and associated bodily sensations (Gray et al., 2018; Naguy et al., 2023). Mirtazapine has been used for treating gastroparesis, and reducing nausea and vomiting (Malamood et al., 2017), which may be one of the mechanism of action in reducing distress and promoting eating in the ARFID population (Malamood et al., 2017). However, mirtazapine may have also specific anxiolytic effects that could be helpful in ARFID especially for those with fear of choking of throwing up (Garakani et al., 2020). Disentangling those mechanisms deserves further study in controlled trials.

Toward Targets for Pharmacological Interventions

The complex bio-psycho-social underpinnings of eating disorders have made it difficult to identify their underlying neurobiology. This is a problem not unique to eating disorders but common to psychiatry. For instance, genetic studies have identified gene variations that overlap across psychiatric disorders, and the genes coding specific neurotransmitter receptor functions unique to specific psychopathology are mainly elusive (Yilmaz et al., 2018).

Our lab has developed a model for psychopharmacological target engagement based on predisposing behavioral traits, precipitating events leading to altered eating, and changes in body and brain homeostasis, creating a vicious cycle reinforcing the eating disorder. Individuals with eating disorders tend to have elevated anxious traits, which may make them more susceptible to social fears and associated fears of inadequacy, a theme frequently triggered by media influences or personal social environment (Forrest et al., 2019; Marzola et al., 2020; Sternheim et al., 2017). We then postulate a triggering circumstance that leads to a change in eating. Those circumstances may vary from wanting to get better at sports or losing weight, being fearful of choking or throwing up, or not wanting to feel their body, maybe due to a traumatic experience. A person may then start changing their eating behavior, and most may initially try to eat less. Some individuals will lose weight, others will restrict for some of the time but also start binge eating and purging, or binge eating without compensatory behaviors and gain weight. Those behaviors will lead to two important changes. One, the individual will condition negatively to food and eating, a conscious behavior that may be difficult to change in the future and drives fear of eating and shape and weight concerns (Frank et al., 2023; Gorrell et al., 2023). Two, body and brain biology will adapt to under or overweight or intermittent fasting or binge-eating episodes (Figure 25.1) (Avena & Bocarsly, 2012; Bailer & Kaye, 2003; Corwin et al., 2011; Hoebel et al., 1989). Specifically, we propose that the dopamine system adapts to extremes of food intake (Avena, Rada, et al., 2008; Carr, 2007; Johnson & Kenny, 2010; Volkow, 2008), where food restriction enhances (Kelley, 2004; Oinio et al., 2017) and excessive food intake downregulates dopamine circuits (Carr et al., 2009; Carr et al., 2003; Frank et al., 2019; Johnson & Kenny, 2010; Monteleone et al., 2018).

The conditioned fear of eating that has developed will use those dopaminergic circuits to control eating. Animal research has identified a circuitry from the prefrontal cortex to the ventral striatum and hypothalamus to override hypothalamic appetitive drive by using dopamine circuits when a person is under threat (O'Connor et al., 2015; Stratford & Kelley, 1999). We postulate that in individuals with eating disorders, the conditioned fear of eating leads to a perception of threat when exposed to food, and this fear then "hijacks" this dopaminergic food control circuitry to facilitate food restriction.

Another mechanism to avoid eating also involves dopaminergic pathways in the nucleus accumbens (Faure et al., 2010). An individual may approach food when

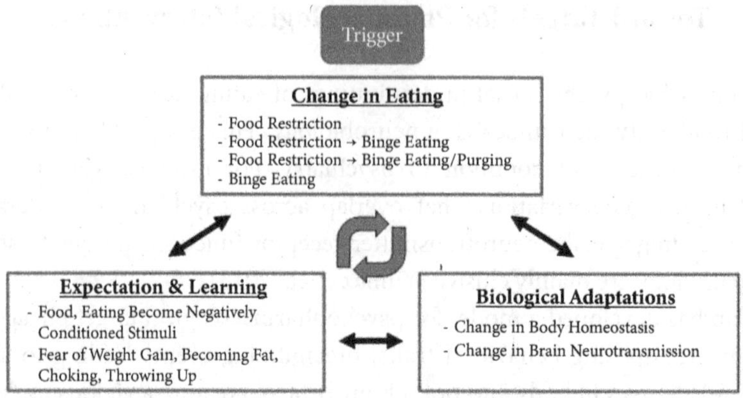

Figure 25.1 Change in eating behavior is typically preceded by a triggering circumstance and followed by negative conditioning to food and eating and biological adaptations, which will reinforce each other.

feeling safe, mediated via the rostral nucleus accumbens and dopamine D1 receptors. The same individual may express dread and avoidance toward eating when in an unsafe situation, mediated by the combination of dopamine D1 and D2 receptors in the caudal nucleus accumbens (Castro et al., 2015). Individuals with eating disorders frequently describe safe and unsafe foods reflecting those conditions. We hypothesize that negative associations with food override hypothalamic appetitive drive and trigger outward dread and avoidance toward meal situations, as frequently observed in a clinical setting. Those specific dopamine receptor-mediated circuits provide potential targeted pharmacological intervention for eating disorders.

Human brain imaging studies support this model and help separate behaviors and neurobiology across eating disorder subtypes. Recent results from our group across a transdiagnostic sample of individuals with eating disorders indicated that brain response in the dopamine-associated motivational salience brain circuitry (prediction error model, previously described) that is related to BMI is also linked to the striatal-hypothalamic food control pathways (Frank et al., 2021). That study supported the animal studies indicating that extremes of food restriction sensitize and overeating desensitizes dopamine-related brain response, and anxious conditioning (presumably facilitated by premorbid anxious traits) to food intake may recruit those circuits to engage in fearful avoidance instead of food approach (Castro et al., 2015; Frank, 2021). Specifically, the hypersensitivity of dopamine circuits in underweight eating disorders was positively related to the ventral striatal-hypothalamic food control circuitry and may thus reinforce food restriction. On the other hand, individuals with high weight eating disorders may also intermittently attempt to control food intake due to negative bias and via the same prefrontal-striatal-hypothalamic circuitry. Still, they cannot sustain this effort due to a desensitized dopamine circuit response and a weak food control circuitry. Figure 25.2 provides a graphical representation of this model.

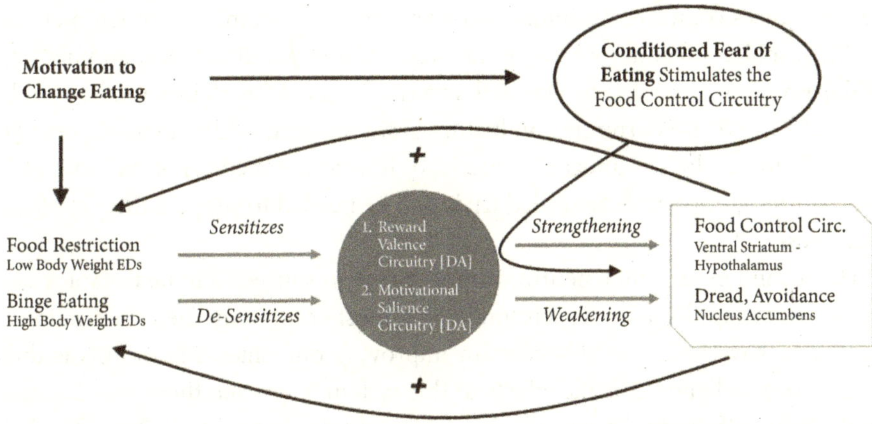

Figure 25.2 An integrative model of how conditioning to food and eating and neurobiological changes interact to lead to the vicious cycle of disordered eating behavior.

We have integrated animal and human studies to develop models for specific medication interventions in AN to reduce distress and enhance cognitive flexibility and illness insight to make psychotherapy more effective. Animal research that applied dopamine D2/3 receptor antagonists in the ABA model found an improved survival rate compared to controls. However, dopamine D2 receptor antagonists overall have not been effective in treating AN (Frank, 2020b; Klenotich et al., 2015). The dopamine D1/D2 receptor targeting medication olanzapine has shown some benefits for AN in an outpatient setting, and clinically, it is frequently used to treat acute severe anxiety or agitation in AN (Attia et al., 2019). It is possible that the combined D1 and D2 receptor action of olanzapine reduces fear and dread response via the nucleus accumbens, although it has a limited effect on appetitive food response and motivation. Second, the dopamine system adapts to the nutritional and hormonal state, and medication that can adapt to evolving neurotransmitter receptor dynamics could be specifically beneficial to target illness behaviors. A new dopamine agent category are the so-called dopamine stabilizers that adapt to the synaptic dopaminergic tone with dopamine agonistic and antagonistic properties (Ma et al., 2014). Those agents that include aripiprazole, brexpiprazole and cariprazine are dopamine stabilizers and could have a role in AN treatment across illness stages and associated neurotransmitter adaptations. The referenced retrospective chart review in adolescents with AN (Frank et al., 2017) suggests that one of those agents in this group of medications, the dopamine D2 receptor partial agonist aripiprazole, facilitates psychotherapy and thus could be beneficial to support recovery even in high-level of care settings. While the evidence is still scant, there is emerging evidence that dopamine D2 receptor partial agonism could help target illness-related preoccupations and support insight into AN (Frank, 2016a; Frank et al., 2017; Marzola et al., 2015; Tahillioglu et al., 2020; Trunko et al., 2011). Several animal studies support this hypothesis. Frontal cortex dopamine D2 receptor stimulation in the underweight state enhances cognitive flexibility and fear extinction (Frank, 2014; Jenni et al., 2017), stimulates feeding via the brain stem (Cai et al., 2022), and stimulation of dopamine neurons led to elevated survival in the ABA rodent model (Foldi et al., 2017). We are currently conducting brain imaging studies focusing on BN and BED to develop an integrative model of how to use medication in those eating disorder groups and controlled trials will be needed to support their clinical usefulness.

The second monoamine neurotransmitter system suggested in neurobiological studies in eating disorders is serotonin. The most commonly used medications, the SSRIs, have had limited success in improving outcomes. Maybe this is due to their relatively non-specific effects in this system. However, those medications might help with body dissatisfaction and mood (Holtkamp et al., 2004; Strobel et al., 2004). The latter aspect is important as those medications may not improve eating and body weight but may improve quality of life by reducing eating disorder-unrelated anxiety and depressed mood. This is an area that has been understudied but is receiving increasingly attention (Eskild-Jensen et al., 2020). A novel indication that may be emerging is the serotonin 2A receptor agonist psilocybin, a psychedelic, which shows promise in treating depression (Madsen et al., 2019). Initial small studies indicate the potential for reducing AN symptomatology (Peck et al., 2023). Whether positive results are related to improvement in mood or cognitive-emotional reset via networks involved in psychotic experiencing will require further study (see Chapter 26).

Agents that modulate the opioid system with specific ligand agonists and antagonists to the mu, delta, or kappa receptors could also be important in future AN research to engage reward experience, especially the hedonic experience around food (Browne & Lucki, 2019). Cannabinoids also stimulate appetite but caused dysphoria and sleep disturbance in an early study of AN (Gross et al., 1983), while the tetrahydrocannabinol dronabinol was associated with modest weight gain in women with longstanding AN (Andries et al., 2014). Cannabis and the hemp product cannabidiol (CBD) have been receiving increasing attention in the recent years with legalization of those substances for medical and recreational use and the growing of a multitude of novel strains, which could prove beneficial for weight gain or other behaviors relevant to AN (Piper, 2018; Szutorisz et al., 2016).

Alternative Perspectives

Pharmacological innovation in psychiatry and other medical fields has often been due to serendipity, followed by more rigorous drug development (Ban, 2006; Lopez-Munoz et al., 2012). Without a universally accepted neurobiological model for eating disorders, this field has been testing novel medications, hoping they can support recovery from an eating disorder. For some of those medications, there is preliminary evidence for how those medications could be used in the clinical setting to be further studied as described previously. However, the lack of more approved pharmacological interventions for eating disorders raises several important questions. One of them is whether we have not identified the correct targets that connect biology and behavior and that can be modulated or normalized with medication. Another alternative and most extreme view would be whether medication should have a role at all in treating eating disorders.

A whole host of factors has to come together for a person to develop an eating disorder (Frank, 2016b). Individuals who will develop an eating disorder are likely born with biological traits such as disposition to heightened anxiety (Kaye et al., 2004), increased sensitivity to salient stimuli (Jappe et al., 2011), and perhaps altered brain structure and function, which could promote stopping to eat a particular food earlier or later than maybe the physiological need would be (Frank, Shott, Hagman, & Mittal, 2013; Frank, Shott, Hagman, & Yang, 2013). The difficulty developing pharmacological interventions in psychiatry based on genetic information could argue the point that targeting behaviors using psychotherapy alone may be the more effective approach. For instance, the need for cognitive control and fear of losing control seen in eating disorders could be better treated with CBT than medication and help improve eating (Adler et al., 2021). Precipitating the onset of an eating disorder are commonly states of involuntary food restriction (travel, camp, busy schedule) or excessive food intake (holidays, frequently being exposed to buffet meals, familial habit to eat larger portions), and added life stress could have specific but different effects on eating disorder subgroups, with some rather eating less and others eating more. Preparing youth especially for those situations and adding prevention interventions could be argued to be more effective. Other factors, such as problems in family functioning, poor self-esteem, and social pressure that may drive altered food intake in response to difficult emotional situations and heightened stress could also be better targeted in psychotherapy or prevention interventions in schools (Stice et al., 2021).

Psychotherapy has been the mainstay of treatment, but its effectiveness is limited, with a high relapse rate across eating disorders and suggesting that novel interventions are needed to treat eating disorders successfully. While controversial, GLP-1 receptor agonists are effective in reducing excessive food intake and are used by many clinicians to reduce binge eating. Whether those interventions will eventually be approved for obesity or eating disorders remains to be seen. Still, they indicate that there are biological mechanisms that have often not been effectively treated using traditional interventions for obesity (McElroy et al., 2018; Pierce-Messick & Pratt, 2020). Another alternative perspective on pharmacological intervention is using ketamine alone or in conjunction with dietary interventions for eating disorders (Calabrese et al., 2022; Ragnhildstveit et al., 2022; Schwartz et al., 2021). Both ketamine and nutritional interventions affect neurotransmitter function via several mechanisms, including inflammatory processes, and the specific targets for how those interventions are best used still need to be identified.

Implications

Neurobiological research has emphasized dopamine and serotonin alterations in eating disorders, the former of which may be modulated by eating extremes and contribute to the vicious cycle of eating disorder behaviors and interfere with recovery. Medication targeting dopamine D1 and D2 receptors might normalize altered receptor and circuit function and contribute to normalizing behavior. However, this will require further study and integration with behavioral interventions, as medication may be best used to reduce distress or as a catalyst to facilitate behavior change.

In summary, medication treatment in eating disorders is still emerging. With building comprehensive neurobiological models based on empirical research followed by developing medication treatment algorithms, there is hope that we will progress toward novel interventions to improve recovery and prevent relapse.

References

Adler, L., Brown, T. A., Shott, M. E., Swindle, S., & Frank, G. K. W. (2021). I know I am not out of control, but I just cannot shake the feeling: Exploring feeling out of control in eating disorders. *Eating and Weight Disorders, 27*, 839–845. https://doi.org/10.1007/s40519-021-01211-7

Agras, W. S., Dorian, B., Kirkley, B. G., & Arnow, B. (1987). Imipramine in the treatment of bulimia: A double-blind controlled study. *International Journal of Eating Disorders, 6*(1), 29–38.

Agras, W. S., Rossiter, E. M., Arnow, B., Schneider, J. A., Telch, C. F., Raeburn, S. D., Bruce, B., Perl, M., & Koran, L. M. (1992). Pharmacologic and cognitive-behavioral treatment for bulimia nervosa: A controlled comparison. *American Journal of Psychiatry, 149*(1), 82–87. https://doi.org/10.1176/ajp.149.1.82

Andries, A., Frystyk, J., Flyvbjerg, A., & Stoving, R. K. (2014). Dronabinol in severe, enduring anorexia nervosa: A randomized controlled trial. *International Journal of Eating Disorders, 47*(1), 18–23. https://doi.org/10.1002/eat.22173

Anonymous. (1992). Fluoxetine in the treatment of bulimia nervosa. A multicenter, placebo-controlled, double-blind trial. Fluoxetine Bulimia Nervosa Collaborative Study Group. *Archives of General Psychiatry, 49*(2), 139–147.

Aoki, C., & Santiago, A. N. (2022). Pathway-specific GABAergic inhibition contributes to the gain of resilience against anorexia-like behavior of adolescent female mice. *Frontiers in Behavioral Neuroscience, 16*, 990354. https://doi.org/10.3389/fnbeh.2022.990354

Appolinario, J. C., Bacaltchuk, J., Sichieri, R., Claudino, A. M., Godoy-Matos, A., Morgan, C., Zanella, M. T., & Coutinho, W. (2003). A randomized, double-blind, placebo-controlled study of sibutramine in the treatment of binge-eating disorder. *Archives of General Psychiatry, 60*(11), 1109–1116. https://doi.org/10.1001/archpsyc.60.11.1109

Arnold, L. M., McElroy, S. L., Hudson, J. I., Welge, J. A., Bennett, A. J., & Keck, P. E. (2002). A placebo-controlled, randomized trial of fluoxetine in the treatment of binge-eating disorder. *Journal of Clinical Psychiatry, 63*(11), 1028–1033. https://doi.org/10.4088/jcp.v63n1113

Attia, E., Kaplan, A. S., Walsh, B. T., Gershkovich, M., Yilmaz, Z., Musante, D., & Wang, Y. (2011). Olanzapine versus placebo for out-patients with anorexia nervosa. *Psychological Medicine, 41*(10), 2177–2182. https://doi.org/10.1017/S0033291711000390

Attia, E., Steinglass, J. E., Walsh, B. T., Wang, Y., Wu, P., Schreyer, C., Wildes, J., Yilmaz, Z., Guarda, A. S., Kaplan, A. S., & Marcus, M. D. (2019). Olanzapine versus placebo in adult outpatients with anorexia nervosa: A randomized clinical trial. *American Journal of Psychiatry, 176*(6), 449–456. https://doi.org/10.1176/appi.ajp.2018.18101125

Avena, N. M., & Bocarsly, M. E. (2012). Dysregulation of brain reward systems in eating disorders: neurochemical information from animal models of binge eating, bulimia nervosa, and anorexia nervosa. *Neuropharmacology, 63*(1), 87–96. https://doi.org/10.1016/j.neuropharm.2011.11.010

Avena, N. M., Bocarsly, M. E., & Hoebel, B. G. (2012). Animal models of sugar and fat bingeing: Relationship to food addiction and increased body weight. *Methods in Molecular Biology, 829*, 351–365. https://doi.org/10.1007/978-1-61779-458-2_23

Avena, N. M., Bocarsly, M. E., Rada, P., Kim, A., & Hoebel, B. G. (2008). After daily bingeing on a sucrose solution, food deprivation induces anxiety and accumbens dopamine/acetylcholine imbalance. *Physiology and Behavior, 94*(3), 309–315. https://doi.org/10.1016/j.physbeh.2008.01.008

Avena, N. M., Rada, P., & Hoebel, B. G. (2008). Underweight rats have enhanced dopamine release and blunted acetylcholine response in the nucleus accumbens while bingeing on sucrose. *Neuroscience, 156*(4), 865–871. https://doi.org/10.1016/j.neuroscience.2008.08.017

Bailer, U. F., Frank, G. K., Henry, S. E., Price, J. C., Meltzer, C. C., Becker, C., Ziolko, S. K., Mathis, C. A., Wagner, A., Barbarich-Marsteller, N. C., Putnam, K., & Kaye, W. H. (2007). Serotonin transporter binding after recovery from eating disorders. *Psychopharmacology, 195*(3), 315–324. https://doi.org/10.1007/s00213-007-0896-7

Bailer, U. F., & Kaye, W. H. (2003). A review of neuropeptide and neuroendocrine dysregulation in anorexia and bulimia nervosa. *Current Drug Targets: CNS and Neurological Disorders, 2*(1), 53–59. https://www.ncbi.nlm.nih.gov/pubmed/12769812

Ban, T. A. (2006). The role of serendipity in drug discovery. *Dialogues in Clinical Neuroscience, 8*(3), 335–344. https://www.ncbi.nlm.nih.gov/pubmed/17117615

Barbarich, N. C., McConaha, C. W., Gaskill, J., La Via, M., Frank, G. K., Achenbach, S., Plotnicov, K. H., & Kaye, W. H. (2004). An open trial of olanzapine in anorexia nervosa. *Journal of Clinical Psychiatry, 65*(11), 1480–1482. https://www.ncbi.nlm.nih.gov/pubmed/15554759

Barbarich, N. C., McConaha, C. W., Halmi, K. A., Gendall, K., Sunday, S. R., Gaskill, J., La Via, M., Frank, G. K., Brooks, S., Plotnicov, K. H., & Kaye, W. H. (2004). Use of nutritional supplements to increase the efficacy of fluoxetine in the treatment of anorexia nervosa [clinical trial randomized controlled trial]. *International Journal of Eating Disorders, 35*(1), 10–15. https://doi.org/10.1002/eat.10235

Barlow, J., Blouin, J., Blouin, A., & Perez, E. (1988). Treatment of bulimia with desipramine: A double-blind crossover study. *Canadian Journal of Psychiatry, 33*(2), 129–133. http://www.ncbi.nlm.nih.gov/htbin-post/Entrez/query?db=m&form=6&dopt=r&uid=3284630

Bauer, C., Fischer, A., & Keller, U. (2006). Effect of sibutramine and of cognitive-behavioural weight loss therapy in obesity and subclinical binge eating disorder. *Diabetes, Obesity and Metabolism, 8*(3), 289–295. https://doi.org/10.1111/j.1463-1326.2005.00504.x

Beeler, J. A., & Burghardt, N. S. (2021). The rise and fall of dopamine: A two-stage model of the development and entrenchment of anorexia nervosa. *Frontiers in Psychiatry, 12*, 799548. https://doi.org/10.3389/fpsyt.2021.799548

Beeler, J. A., Mourra, D., Zanca, R. M., Kalmbach, A., Gellman, C., Klein, B. Y., Ravenelle, R., Serrano, P., Moore, H., Rayport, S., Mingote, S., & Burghardt, N. S. (2020). Vulnerable and resilient phenotypes in a mouse model of anorexia nervosa. *Biological Psychiatry*, 90(12), 829–842. https://doi.org/10.1016/j.biopsych.2020.06.030

Bernardoni, F., Geisler, D., King, J. A., Javadi, A. H., Ritschel, F., Murr, J., Reiter, A. M. F., Rossner, V., Smolka, M. N., Kiebel, S., & Ehrlich, S. (2018). Altered medial frontal feedback learning signals in anorexia nervosa. *Biological Psychiatry, 83*(3), 235–243. https://doi.org/10.1016/j.biopsych.2017.07.024

Berner, L. A., Brown, T. A., Lavender, J. M., Lopez, E., Wierenga, C. E., & Kaye, W. H. (2018). Neuroendocrinology of reward in anorexia nervosa and bulimia nervosa: Beyond leptin and ghrelin. *Molecular and Cellular Endocrinology*, 497, 110320.https://doi.org/10,1016/j.mce.2018.10.018

Biederman, J., Herzog, D. B., Rivinus, T. M., Harper, G. P., Ferber, R. A., Rosenbaum, J. F., Harmatz, J. S., Tondorf, R., Orsulak, P. J., & Schildkraut, J. J. (1985). Amitriptyline in the treatment of anorexia nervosa: A double-blind, placebo-controlled study. *Journal of Clinical Psychopharmacology, 5*(1), 10–16. https://www.ncbi.nlm.nih.gov/pubmed/3973067

Bissada, H., Tasca, G. A., Barber, A. M., & Bradwejn, J. (2008). Olanzapine in the treatment of low body weight and obsessive thinking in women with anorexia nervosa: A randomized, double-blind, placebo-controlled trial [Comparative Study Randomized Controlled Trial Research Support, Non-U.S. Gov't]. *American Journal of Psychiatry, 165*(10), 1281–1288. https://doi.org/10.1176/appi.ajp.2008.07121900

Blouin, A. G., Blouin, J. H., Perez, E. L., Bushnik, T., Zuro, C., & Mulder, E. (1988). Treatment of bulimia with fenfluramine and desipramine. *Journal of Clinical Psychopharmacology, 8*(4), 261–269.

Boehm, I., King, J. A., Bernardoni, F., Geisler, D., Seidel, M., Ritschel, F., Goschke, T., Haynes, J. D., Roessner, V., & Ehrlich, S. (2018). Subliminal and supraliminal processing of reward-related stimuli in anorexia nervosa. *Psychological Medicine, 48*(5), 790–800. https://doi.org/10.1017/S0033291717002161

Bohon, C., & Stice, E. (2012). Negative affect and neural response to palatable food intake in bulimia nervosa [Research Support, N.I.H., Extramural]. *Appetite, 58*(3), 964–970. https://doi.org/10.1016/j.appet.2012.02.051

Brambilla, F., Draisci, A., Peirone, A., & Brunetta, M. (1995). Combined cognitive-behavioral, psychopharmacological and nutritional therapy in bulimia nervosa. *Neuropsychobiology, 32*(2), 68–71.

Brambilla, F., Garcia, C. S., Fassino, S., Daga, G. A., Favaro, A., Santonastaso, P., Ramaciotti, C., Bondi, E., Mellado, C., Borriello, R., & Monteleone, P. (2007). Olanzapine therapy in anorexia nervosa: Psychobiological effects [randomized controlled trial]. *International Clinical Psychopharmacology, 22*(4), 197–204. https://doi.org/10.1097/YIC.0b013e328080ca31

Brambilla, F., Monteleone, P., & Maj, M. (2007). Olanzapine-induced weight gain in anorexia nervosa: involvement of leptin and ghrelin secretion? [Randomized Controlled Trial Research Support, Non-U.S. Gov't]. *Psychoneuroendocrinology, 32*(4), 402–406. https://doi.org/10.1016/j.psyneuen.2007.02.005

Broft, A., Shingleton, R., Kaufman, J., Liu, F., Kumar, D., Slifstein, M., Abi-Dargham, A., Schebendach, J., Van Heertum, R., Attia, E., Martinez, D., & Walsh, B. T. (2012). Striatal dopamine in bulimia nervosa: a PET imaging study. *International Journal of Eating Disorders, 45*(5), 648–656. https://doi.org/10.1002/eat.20984

Broft, A., Slifstein, M., Osborne, J., Kothari, P., Morim, S., Shingleton, R., Kenney, L., Vallabhajosula, S., Attia, E., Martinez, D., & Timothy Walsh, B. (2015). Striatal dopamine type 2 receptor availability in anorexia nervosa. *Psychiatry Research, 233*(3), 380–387. https://doi.org/10.1016/j.pscychresns.2015.06.013

Browne, C. A., & Lucki, I. (2019). Targeting opioid dysregulation in depression for the development of novel therapeutics. *Pharmacology and Therapeutics, 201*, 51–76. https://doi.org/10.1016/j.pharmthera.2019.04.009

Bymaster, F. P., Calligaro, D. O., Falcone, J. F., Marsh, R. D., Moore, N. A., Tye, N. C., Seeman, P., & Wong, D. T. (1996). Radioreceptor binding profile of the atypical antipsychotic olanzapine. *Neuropsychopharmacology, 14*(2), 87–96. https://doi.org/10.1016/0893-133X(94)00129-N

Cai, X., Liu, H., Feng, B., Yu, M., He, Y., Liu, H., Liang, C., Yang, Y., Tu, L., Zhang, N., Wang, L., Yin, N., Han, J., Yan, Z., Wang, C., Xu, P., Wu, Q., Tong, Q., He, Y., & Xu, Y. (2022). A D2 to D1 shift in dopaminergic inputs to midbrain 5-HT neurons causes anorexia in mice. *Nature Neuroscience, 25*(5), 646–658. https://doi.org/10.1038/s41593-022-01062-0

Calabrese, L., Scolnick, B., Zupec-Kania, B., Beckwith, C., Costello, K., & Frank, G. K. W. (2022). Ketogenic diet and ketamine infusion treatment to target chronic persistent eating disorder psychopathology in anorexia nervosa: A pilot study. Eat*ing and* Weight Disord*ers*, 27(8), 3751–3757. https://doi.org/10.1007/s40519-022-01455-x

Carr, K. D. (2007). Chronic food restriction: Enhancing effects on drug reward and striatal cell signaling. *Physiology and Behavior, 91*(5), 459–472. https://doi.org/10.1016/j.physbeh.2006.09.021

Carr, K. D., Cabeza de Vaca, S., Sun, Y., & Chau, L. S. (2009). Reward-potentiating effects of D-1 dopamine receptor agonist and AMPAR GluR1 antagonist in nucleus accumbens shell and their modulation by food restriction. *Psychopharmacology, 202*(4), 731–743. https://doi.org/10.1007/s00213-008-1355-9

Carr, K. D., Tsimberg, Y., Berman, Y., & Yamamoto, N. (2003). Evidence of increased dopamine receptor signaling in food-restricted rats. *Neuroscience, 119*(4), 1157–1167. https://www.ncbi.nlm.nih.gov/pubmed/12831870

Carruba, M. O., Cuzzolaro, M., Riva, L., Bosello, O., Liberti, S., Castra, R., Dalle Grave, R., Santonastaso, P., Garosi, V., & Nisoli, E. (2001). Efficacy and tolerability of moclobemide in bulimia nervosa:

a placebo-controlled trial. *International Clinical Psychopharmacology, 16*(1), 27–32. https://www.ncbi.nlm.nih.gov/pubmed/11195257

Casper, R. C., Schlemmer, R. F., Jr., & Javaid, J. I. (1987). A placebo-controlled crossover study of oral clonidine in acute anorexia nervosa. *Psychiatry Research, 20*(3), 249–260. https://www.ncbi.nlm.nih.gov/pubmed/3295935

Castro, D. C., Cole, S. L., & Berridge, K. C. (2015). Lateral hypothalamus, nucleus accumbens, and ventral pallidum roles in eating and hunger: Interactions between homeostatic and reward circuitry. *Frontiers in Systems Neuroscience, 9*, 90. https://doi.org/10.3389/fnsys.2015.00090

Claudino, A. M., de Oliveira, I. R., Appolinario, J. C., Cordas, T. A., Duchesne, M., Sichieri, R., & Bacaltchuk, J. (2007). Double-blind, randomized, placebo-controlled trial of topiramate plus cognitive-behavior therapy in binge-eating disorder. *Journal of Clinical Psychiatry, 68*(9), 1324–1332. https://doi.org/10.4088/jcp.v68n0901

Corwin, R. L., Avena, N. M., & Boggiano, M. M. (2011). Feeding and reward: Perspectives from three rat models of binge eating. *Physiology and Behavior, 104*(1), 87–97. https://doi.org/10.1016/j.physbeh.2011.04.041

Cowdrey, F. A., Park, R. J., Harmer, C. J., & McCabe, C. (2011). Increased neural processing of rewarding and aversive food stimuli in recovered anorexia nervosa. *Biological Psychiatry, 70*(8), 736–743. https://doi.org/10.1016/j.biopsych.2011.05.028

Cyr, M., Wang, Z., Tau, G. Z., Zhao, G., Friedl, E., Stefan, M., Terranova, K., & Marsh, R. (2016). Reward-based spatial learning in teens with bulimia nervosa. *Journal of the American Academy of Child and Adolescent Psychiatry, 55*(11), 962–971e963. https://doi.org/10.1016/j.jaac.2016.07.778

D'Agostino, A., English, C. D., & Rey, J. A. (2015). Vortioxetine (brintellix): A new serotonergic antidepressant. *P & T, 40*(1), 36–40. https://www.ncbi.nlm.nih.gov/pubmed/25628505

DeGuzman, M., Shott, M. E., Yang, T. T., Riederer, J., & Frank, G. K. (2017). Association of elevated reward prediction error response with weight gain in adolescent anorexia nervosa. *American Journal of Psychiatry*, 174(6), 557–565. https://doi.org/10.1176/appi.ajp.2016.16060671

Devlin, M. J., Goldfein, J. A., Petkova, E., Jiang, H., Raizman, P. S., Wolk, S., Mayer, L., Carino, J., Bellace, D., Kamenetz, C., Dobrow, I., & Walsh, B. T. (2005). Cognitive behavioral therapy and fluoxetine as adjuncts to group behavioral therapy for binge eating disorder. *Obesity Research, 13*(6), 1077–1088. https://doi.org/10.1038/oby.2005.126

Devlin, M. J., Goldfein, J. A., Petkova, E., Liu, L., & Walsh, B. T. (2007). Cognitive behavioral therapy and fluoxetine for binge eating disorder: Two-year follow-up. *Obesity, 15*(7), 1702–1709. https://doi.org/10.1038/oby.2007.203

DiVasta, A. D., Feldman, H. A., O'Donnell, J. M., Long, J., Leonard, M. B., & Gordon, C. M. (2019). Impact of adrenal hormone supplementation on bone geometry in growing teens with anorexia nervosa. *Journal of Adolescent Health, 65*(4), 462–468. https://doi.org/10.1016/j.jadohealth.2019.04.003

Ellinwood, E. H., Jr., Heatherly, D. G., Nikaido, A. M., Bjornsson, T. D., & Kilts, C. (1985). Comparative pharmacokinetics and pharmacodynamics of lorazepam, alprazolam and diazepam. *Psychopharmacology, 86*(4), 392–399. https://doi.org/10.1007/bf00427897

Eskild-Jensen, M., Stoving, R. K., Flindt, C. F., & Sjogren, M. (2020). Comorbid depression as a negative predictor of weight gain during treatment of anorexia nervosa: A systematic scoping review. *European Eating Disorders Review, 28*(6), 605–619. https://doi.org/10.1002/erv.2787

Faris, P. L., Kim, S. W., Meller, W. H., Goodale, R. L., Oakman, S. A., Hofbauer, R. D., Marshall, A. M., Daughters, R. S., Banerjee-Stevens, D., Eckert, E. D., & Hartman, B. K. (2000). Effect of decreasing afferent vagal activity with ondansetron on symptoms of bulimia nervosa: A randomised, double-blind trial. *Lancet, 355*(9206), 792–797. https://doi.org/10.1016/S0140-6736(99)09062-5

Faure, A., Richard, J. M., & Berridge, K. C. (2010). Desire and dread from the nucleus accumbens: Cortical glutamate and subcortical GABA differentially generate motivation and hedonic impact in the rat. *PLOS ONE, 5*(6), e11223. https://doi.org/10.1371/journal.pone.0011223

Fazeli, P. K., Lawson, E. A., Faje, A. T., Eddy, K. T., Lee, H., Fiedorek, F. T., Breggia, A., Gaal, I. M., DeSanti, R., & Klibanski, A. (2018). Treatment with a ghrelin agonist in outpatient women with anorexia nervosa: A randomized clinical trial. *Journal of Clinical Psychiatry, 79*(1). https://doi.org/10.4088/JCP.17m11585

Fichter, M. M., Kruger, R., Rief, W., Holland, R., & Dohne, J. (1996). Fluvoxamine in prevention of relapse in bulimia nervosa: Effects on eating-specific psychopathology. *Journal of Clinical Psychopharmacology, 16*(1), 9–18. https://doi.org/10.1097/00004714-199602000-00003

Fichter, M. M., Leibl, C., Kruger, R., & Rief, W. (1997). Effects of fluvoxamine on depression, anxiety, and other areas of general psychopathology in bulimia nervosa. *Pharmacopsychiatry, 30*(3), 85–92.

Fladung, A. K., Gron, G., Grammer, K., Herrnberger, B., Schilly, E., Grasteit, S., Wolf, R. C., Walter, H., & von Wietersheim, J. (2010). A neural signature of anorexia nervosa in the ventral striatal reward system. *American Journal of Psychiatry, 167*(2), 206–212. https://doi.org/10.1176/appi.ajp.2009.09010071

Foldi, C. J., Milton, L. K., & Oldfield, B. J. (2017). The role of mesolimbic reward neurocircuitry in prevention and rescue of the activity-based anorexia (ABA) phenotype in rats. *Neuropsychopharmacology, 42*(12), 2292–2300. https://doi.org/10.1038/npp.2017.63

Forrest, L. N., Sarfan, L. D., Ortiz, S. N., Brown, T. A., & Smith, A. R. (2019). Bridging eating disorder symptoms and trait anxiety in patients with eating disorders: A network approach. *International Journal of Eating Disorders, 52*(6), 701–711. https://doi.org/10.1002/eat.23070

Frank, G. K. (2013). Altered brain reward circuits in eating disorders: Chicken or egg? *Current Psychiatry Reports, 15*(10), 396. https://doi.org/10.1007/s11920-013-0396-x

Frank, G. K. (2014). Could dopamine agonists aid in drug development for anorexia nervosa? [hypothesis & theory]. *Frontiers in Nutrition, 1*, 19. https://doi.org/10.3389/fnut.2014.00019

Frank, G. K. (2015). Advances from neuroimaging studies in eating disorders. *CNS Spectrum*, 20(4), 391–400. https://doi.org/10.1017/S1092852915000012

Frank, G. K. (2016a). Aripiprazole, a partial dopamine agonist to improve adolescent anorexia nervosa—A case series. *International Journal of Eating Disorders, 49*(5), 529–533. https://doi.org/10.1002/eat.22485

Frank, G. K. (2016b). The perfect storm—A bio-psycho-social risk model for developing and maintaining eating disorders. *Frontiers in Behavioral Neuroscience, 10*, 44. https://doi.org/10.3389/fnbeh.2016.00044

Frank, G. K., Bailer, U. F., Henry, S. E., Drevets, W., Meltzer, C. C., Price, J. C., Mathis, C. A., Wagner, A., Hoge, J., Ziolko, S., Barbarich-Marsteller, N., Weissfeld, L., & Kaye, W. H. (2005). Increased dopamine D2/D3 receptor binding after recovery from anorexia nervosa measured by positron emission tomography and [11c]raclopride. *Biological Psychiatry, 58*(11), 908–912. https://doi.org/10.1016/j.biopsych.2005.05.003

Frank, G. K., Shott, M. E., Hagman, J. O., & Mittal, V. A. (2013). Alterations in brain structures related to taste reward circuitry in ill and recovered anorexia nervosa and in bulimia nervosa. *American Journal of Psychiatry*, 170(10), 1152–1160. https://doi.org/10.1176/appi.ajp.2013.12101294

Frank, G. K., Shott, M. E., Hagman, J. O., Schiel, M. A., DeGuzman, M. C., & Rossi, B. (2017). The partial dopamine D2 receptor agonist aripiprazole is associated with weight gain in adolescent anorexia nervosa. *International Journal of Eating Disorders, 50*(4), 447–450. https://doi.org/10.1002/eat.22704

Frank, G. K., Shott, M. E., Hagman, J. O., & Yang, T. T. (2013). Localized brain volume and white matter integrity alterations in adolescent anorexia nervosa. *Journal of the American Academy of Child and Adolescent Psychiatry, 52*(10), 1066–1075e1065. https://doi.org/10.1016/j.jaac.2013.07.007

Frank, G. K. W. (2020a). Is the pharmacological management of bulimia nervosa plausible? *Expert Opinion on Pharmacotherapy, 21*(17), 2073–2075. https://doi.org/10.1080/14656566.2020.1805434

Frank, G. K. W. (2020b). Pharmacotherapeutic strategies for the treatment of anorexia nervosa—Too much for one drug? *Expert Opinion on Pharmacotherapy*, 21(9), 1045–1058. https://doi.org/10.1080/14656566.2020.1748600

Frank, G. K. W. (2021). From desire to dread—A neurocircuitry based model for food avoidance in anorexia nervosa. *Journal of Clinical Medicine, 10*(11), 2228. https://doi.org/10.3390/jcm10112228

Frank, G. K. W., DeGuzman, M. C., & Shott, M. E. (2019). Motivation to eat and not to eat—The psycho-biological conflict in anorexia nervosa. *Physiology and Behavior, 206*, 185–190. https://doi.org/10.1016/j.physbeh.2019.04.007

Frank, G. K. W., DeGuzman, M. C., Shott, M. E., Laudenslager, M. L., Rossi, B., & Pryor, T. (2018). Association of brain reward learning response with harm avoidance, weight gain, and hypothalamic effective connectivity in adolescent anorexia nervosa. *JAMA Psychiatry, 75*(10), 1071–1080. https://doi.org/10.1001/jamapsychiatry.2018.2151

Frank, G. K. W., Shott, M. E., Pryor, T., Swindle, S., Nguyen, T., & Stoddard, J. (2023). Trait anxiety is associated with amygdala expectation and caloric taste receipt response across eating disorders. *Neuropsychopharmacology, 48*(2), 380–390. https://doi.org/10.1038/s41386-022-01440-z

Frank, G. K. W., Shott, M. E., Pryor, T., Swindle, S., & Stoddard, J. (2022). Brain reward response in adolescents and young adults with anorexia nervosa is moderated by changes in body weight and sweetness perception. *International Journal of Eating Disorders, 55*(12), 1799–1810. https://doi.org/10.1002/eat.23814

Frank, G. K. W., Shott, M. E., Stoddard, J., Swindle, S., & Pryor, T. L. (2021). Association of brain reward response with body mass index and ventral striatal-hypothalamic circuitry among young women with eating disorders. *JAMA Psychiatry, 78*(10), 1123–1133. https://doi.org/10.1001/jamapsychiatry.2021.1580

Galusca, B., Traverse, B., Costes, N., Massoubre, C., Le Bars, D., Estour, B., Germain, N., & Redoute, J. (2020). Decreased cerebral opioid receptors availability related to hormonal and psychometric profile in restrictive-type anorexia nervosa. *Psychoneuroendocrinology, 118*, 104711. https://doi.org/10.1016/j.psyneuen.2020.104711

Garakani, A., Murrough, J. W., Freire, R. C., Thom, R. P., Larkin, K., Buono, F. D., & Iosifescu, D. V. (2020). Pharmacotherapy of anxiety disorders: Current and emerging treatment options. *Frontiers in Psychiatry, 11*, 595584. https://doi.org/10.3389/fpsyt.2020.595584

Gasior, M., Hudson, J., Quintero, J., Ferreira-Cornwell, M. C., Radewonuk, J., & McElroy, S. L. (2017). A phase 3, multicenter, open-label, 12-month extension safety and tolerability trial of lisdexamfetamine dimesylate in adults with binge eating disorder. *Journal of Clinical Psychopharmacology, 37*(3), 315–322. https://doi.org/10.1097/JCP.0000000000000702

Gerard, N., Pieters, G., Goffin, K., Bormans, G., & Van Laere, K. (2011). Brain type 1 cannabinoid receptor availability in patients with anorexia and bulimia nervosa. *Biological Psychiatry, 70*(8), 777–784. https://doi.org/10.1016/j.biopsych.2011.05.010

Giunti, E., Collu, R., Dedoni, S., Castelli, M. P., Fratta, W., Scherma, M., & Fadda, P. (2023). Food restriction and hyperactivity induce changes in corticolimbic brain dopamine and serotonin levels in female rats. *Behavioural Brain Research, 444*, 114374. https://doi.org/10.1016/j.bbr.2023.114374

Goldbloom, D. S., Olmsted, M., Davis, R., Clewes, J., Heinmaa, M., Rockert, W., & Shaw, B. (1997). A randomized controlled trial of fluoxetine and cognitive behavioral therapy for bulimia nervosa: Short-term outcome. *Behaviour Research and Therapy, 35*(9), 803–811. https://www.ncbi.nlm.nih.gov/pubmed/9299800

Goldstein, D. J., Wilson, M. G., Thompson, V. L., Potvin, J. H., & Rampey, A. H., Jr. (1995). Long-term fluoxetine treatment of bulimia nervosa: Fluoxetine Bulimia Nervosa Research Group. *British Journal of Psychiatry, 166*(5), 660–666. https://www.ncbi.nlm.nih.gov/pubmed/7620754

Gorrell, S., Shott, M. E., Pryor, T., & Frank, G. K. W. (2023). Neural response to expecting a caloric sweet taste stimulus predicts body mass index longitudinally among young adult women with anorexia nervosa. *Biological Psychiatry: Cognitive Neuroscience and Neuroimaging*, 9(3), 298–304. https://doi.org/10.1016/j.bpsc.2023.07.007

Grant, J. E., Valle, S., Cavic, E., Redden, S. A., & Chamberlain, S. R. (2019). A double-blind, placebo-controlled study of vortioxetine in the treatment of binge-eating disorder. *International Journal of Eating Disorders, 52*(7), 786–794. https://doi.org/10.1002/eat.23078

Gray, E., Chen, T., Menzel, J., Schwartz, T., & Kaye, W. H. (2018). Mirtazapine and weight gain in avoidant and restrictive food intake disorder. *Journal of the American Academy of Child and Adolescent Psychiatry, 57*(4), 288–289. https://doi.org/10.1016/j.jaac.2018.01.011

Griffin, C. E., III, Kaye, A. M., Bueno, F. R., & Kaye, A. D. (2013). Benzodiazepine pharmacology and central nervous system-mediated effects. *Ochsner Journal, 13*(2), 214–223. https://www.ncbi.nlm.nih.gov/pubmed/23789008

Grilo, C. M., McElroy, S. L., Hudson, J. I., Tsai, J., Navia, B., Goldman, R., Deng, L., Kent, J., & Loebel, A. (2020). Efficacy and safety of dasotraline in adults with binge-eating disorder: A randomized, placebo-controlled, fixed-dose clinical trial. *CNS Spectrum, 26*(5), 481–490. https://doi.org/10.1017/S1092852920001406

Gross, H., Ebert, M. H., Faden, V. B., Goldberg, S. C., Kaye, W. H., Caine, E. D., Hawks, R., & Zinberg, N. (1983). A double-blind trial of delta 9-tetrahydrocannabinol in primary anorexia nervosa. *Journal of Clinical Psychopharmacology, 3*(3), 165–171. https://www.ncbi.nlm.nih.gov/pubmed/6308069

Guerdjikova, A. I., McElroy, S. L., Welge, J. A., Nelson, E., Keck, P. E., & Hudson, J. I. (2009). Lamotrigine in the treatment of binge-eating disorder with obesity: A randomized, placebo-controlled monotherapy trial. *International Clinical Psychopharmacology, 24*(3), 150–158. https://doi.org/10.1097/YIC.0b013e328329c7b5

Guerdjikova, A. I., Mori, N., Blom, T. J., Keck, P. E., Jr., Williams, S. L., Welge, J. A., & McElroy, S. L. (2016). Lisdexamfetamine dimesylate in binge eating disorder: A placebo controlled trial. *Human Psychopharmacology, 31*(5), 382–391. https://doi.org/10.1002/hup.2547

Hagman, J., Gralla, J., Sigel, E., Ellert, S., Dodge, M., Gardner, R., O'Lonergan, T., Frank, G., & Wamboldt, M. Z. (2011). A double-blind, placebo-controlled study of risperidone for the treatment of adolescents and young adults with anorexia nervosa: A pilot study [Controlled Clinical Trial Randomized Controlled Trial Research Support, N.I.H., Extramural Research Support, Non-U.S. Gov't Research Support, U.S. Gov't, P.H.S.]. *Journal of the American Academy of Child and Adolescent Psychiatry, 50*(9), 915–924. https://doi.org/10.1016/j.jaac.2011.06.009

Hedges, D. W., Reimherr, F. W., Hoopes, S. P., Rosenthal, N. R., Kamin, M., Karim, R., & Capece, J. A. (2003). Treatment of bulimia nervosa with topiramate in a randomized, double-blind, placebo-controlled trial, part 2: Improvement in psychiatric measures. *Journal of Clinical Psychiatry, 64*(12), 1449–1454. https://doi.org/10.4088/jcp.v64n1208

Hill, K., Bucuvalas, J., McClain, C., Kryscio, R., Martini, R. T., Alfaro, M. P., & Maloney, M. (2000). Pilot study of growth hormone administration during the refeeding of malnourished anorexia nervosa patients. *Journal of Child and Adolescent Psychopharmacology, 10*(1), 3–8. https://doi.org/10.1089/cap.2000.10.3

Hoebel, B. G., Hernandez, L., Schwartz, D. H., Mark, G. P., & Hunter, G. A. (1989). Microdialysis studies of brain norepinephrine, serotonin, and dopamine release during ingestive behavior. Theoretical and clinical implications. *Annals of the New York Academy of Sciences, 575*, 171–191; discussion 192–173. https://www.ncbi.nlm.nih.gov/pubmed/2699187

Holsen, L. M., Lawson, E. A., Blum, J., Ko, E., Makris, N., Fazeli, P. K., Klibanski, A., & Goldstein, J. M. (2012). Food motivation circuitry hypoactivation related to hedonic and nonhedonic aspects of hunger and satiety in women with active anorexia nervosa and weight-restored women with anorexia nervosa. *Journal of Psychiatry and Neuroscience, 37*(5), 322–332. https://doi.org/10.1503/jpn.110156

Holtkamp, K., Konrad, K., Kaiser, N., Ploenes, Y., Heussen, N., Grzella, I., & Herpertz-Dahlmann, B. (2004). A retrospective study of SSRI treatment in adolescent anorexia nervosa: insufficient evidence for efficacy. *Journal of Psychiatric Research, 39*, 303–310.

Hoopes, S. P., Reimherr, F. W., Hedges, D. W., Rosenthal, N. R., Kamin, M., Karim, R., Capece, J. A., & Karvois, D. (2003). Treatment of bulimia nervosa with topiramate in a randomized, double-blind, placebo-controlled trial, part 1: Improvement in binge and purge measures. *Journal of Clinical Psychiatry, 64*(11), 1335–1341. https://doi.org/10.4088/jcp.v64n1109

Horndasch, S., Roesch, J., Forster, C., Dorfler, A., Lindsiepe, S., Heinrich, H., Graap, H., Moll, G. H., & Kratz, O. (2018). Neural processing of food and emotional stimuli in adolescent and adult anorexia nervosa patients. *PLOS ONE, 13*(3), e0191059. https://doi.org/10.1371/journal.pone.0191059

Horne, R. L., Ferguson, J. M., Pope, H. G., Jr., Hudson, J. I., Lineberry, C. G., Ascher, J., & Cato, A. (1988). Treatment of bulimia with bupropion: A multicenter controlled trial. *Journal of Clinical Psychiatry, 49*(7), 262–266. https://www.ncbi.nlm.nih.gov/pubmed/3134343

Hsu, L. K., Clement, L., Santhouse, R., & Ju, E. S. (1991). Treatment of bulimia nervosa with lithium carbonate. A controlled study. *Journal of Nervous and Mental Disease, 179*(6), 351–355. https://www.ncbi.nlm.nih.gov/pubmed/1904908

Hudson, J. I., McElroy, S. L., Ferreira-Cornwell, M. C., Radewonuk, J., & Gasior, M. (2017). Efficacy of lisdexamfetamine in adults with moderate to severe binge-eating disorder: A randomized clinical trial. *JAMA Psychiatry, 74*(9), 903–910. https://doi.org/10.1001/jamapsychiatry.2017.1889

Hudson, J. I., McElroy, S. L., Raymond, N. C., Crow, S., Keck, P. E., Jr., Carter, W. P., Mitchell, J. E., Strakowski, S. M., Pope, H. G., Jr., Coleman, B. S., & Jonas, J. M. (1998). Fluvoxamine in the treatment of binge-eating disorder: A multicenter placebo-controlled, double-blind trial. *American Journal of Psychiatry, 155*(12), 1756–1762. https://doi.org/10.1176/ajp.155.12.1756

Israely, M., Ram, A., Brandeis, R., Alter, Z., Avraham, Y., & Berry, E. M. (2017). A double blind, randomized cross-over trial of tyrosine treatment on cognitive function and psychological parameters in severe hospitalized anorexia nervosa patients. *Israel Journal of Psychiatry and Related Sciences, 54*(3), 52–58. https://www.ncbi.nlm.nih.gov/pubmed/29735813

Jappe, L. M., Frank, G. K., Shott, M. E., Rollin, M. D., Pryor, T., Hagman, J. O., Yang, T. T., & Davis, E. (2011). Heightened sensitivity to reward and punishment in anorexia nervosa. *International Journal of Eating Disorders, 44*(4), 317–324. https://doi.org/10.1002/eat.20815

Jenni, N. L., Larkin, J. D., & Floresco, S. B. (2017). Prefrontal dopamine D1 and D2 receptors regulate dissociable aspects of decision making via distinct ventral striatal and amygdalar circuits. *Journal of Neuroscience, 37*(26), 6200–6213. https://doi.org/10.1523/JNEUROSCI.0030-17.2017

Johnson, P. M., & Kenny, P. J. (2010). Dopamine D2 receptors in addiction-like reward dysfunction and compulsive eating in obese rats. *Nature Neuroscience, 13*(5), 635–641. https://doi.org/10.1038/nn.2519

Joutsa, J., Karlsson, H. K., Majuri, J., Nuutila, P., Helin, S., Kaasinen, V., & Nummenmaa, L. (2018). Binge eating disorder and morbid obesity are associated with lowered mu-opioid receptor availability in the brain. *Psychiatry Research: Neuroimaging, 276*, 41–45. https://doi.org/10.1016/j.pscychresns.2018.03.006

Kafantaris, V., Leigh, E., Hertz, S., Berest, A., Schebendach, J., Sterling, W. M., Saito, E., Sunday, S., Higdon, C., Golden, N. H., & Malhotra, A. K. (2011). A placebo-controlled pilot study of adjunctive olanzapine for adolescents with anorexia nervosa. *Journal of Child and Adolescent Psychopharmacology, 21*(3), 207–212. https://doi.org/10.1089/cap.2010.0139

Kaye, W. H., Bulik, C. M., Thornton, L., Barbarich, N., & Masters, K. (2004). Comorbidity of anxiety disorders with anorexia and bulimia nervosa. *American Journal of Psychiatry, 161*(12), 2215–2221. https://doi.org/10.1176/appi.ajp.161.12.2215

Kaye, W. H., Nagata, T., Weltzin, T. E., Hsu, L. K., Sokol, M. S., McConaha, C., Plotnicov, K. H., Weise, J., & Deep, D. (2001). Double-blind placebo-controlled administration of fluoxetine in restricting- and restricting-purging-type anorexia nervosa. *Biological Psychiatry, 49*(7), 644–652. https://www.ncbi.nlm.nih.gov/pubmed/11297722

Kelley, A. E. (2004). Ventral striatal control of appetitive motivation: Role in ingestive behavior and reward-related learning. *Neuroscience and Biobehavioral Reviews, 27*(8), 765–776. https://doi.org/10.1016/j.neubiorev.2003.11.015

Kelley, A. E., Baldo, B. A., Pratt, W. E., & Will, M. J. (2005). Corticostriatal-hypothalamic circuitry and food motivation: Integration of energy, action and reward. *Physiology and Behavior, 86*(5), 773–795. https://doi.org/10.1016/j.physbeh.2005.08.066

Kelley, A. E., & Berridge, K. C. (2002). The neuroscience of natural rewards: Relevance to addictive drugs. *Journal of Neuroscience, 22*(9), 3306–3311. https://doi.org/20026361

Kennedy, S. H., Goldbloom, D. S., Ralevski, E., Davis, C., D'Souza, J. D., & Lofchy, J. (1993). Is there a role for selective monoamine oxidase inhibitor therapy in bulimia nervosa? A placebo-controlled trial of brofaromine. *Journal of Clinical Psychopharmacology, 13*(6), 415–422. https://www.ncbi.nlm.nih.gov/pubmed/8120155

Kennedy, S. H., Piran, N., Warsh, J. J., Prendergast, P., Mainprize, E., Whynot, C., & Garfinkel, P. E. (1988). A trial of isocarboxazid in the treatment of bulimia nervosa. *Journal of Clinical Psychopharmacology, 8*(6), 391–396. https://www.ncbi.nlm.nih.gov/pubmed/3069879

Kim, Y. R., Eom, J. S., Yang, J. W., Kang, J., & Treasure, J. (2015). The impact of oxytocin on food intake and emotion recognition in patients with eating disorders: A double blind single dose within-subject cross-over design. *PLOS ONE, 10*(9), e0137514. https://doi.org/10.1371/journal.pone.0137514

Kim, Y. R., Kim, C. H., Cardi, V., Eom, J. S., Seong, Y., & Treasure, J. (2014). Intranasal oxytocin attenuates attentional bias for eating and fat shape stimuli in patients with anorexia nervosa. *Psychoneuroendocrinology, 44*, 133–142. https://doi.org/10.1016/j.psyneuen.2014.02.019

Kim, Y. R., Oh, S. M., Corfield, F., Jeong, D. W., Jang, E. Y., & Treasure, J. (2014). Intranasal oxytocin lessens the attentional bias to adult negative faces: A double blind within-subject experiment. *Psychiatry Investigation, 11*(2), 160–166. https://doi.org/10.4306/pi.2014.11.2.160

Kimball, A., Schorr, M., Meenaghan, E., Bachmann, K. N., Eddy, K. T., Misra, M., Lawson, E. A., Kreiger-Benson, E., Herzog, D. B., Koman, S., Keane, R. J., Ebrahimi, S., Schoenfeld, D., Klibanski, A., & Miller, K. K. (2019). A randomized placebo-controlled trial of low-dose testosterone therapy in women with anorexia nervosa. *Journal of Clinical Endocrinology and Metabolism, 104*(10), 4347–4355. https://doi.org/10.1210/jc.2019-00828

King, J. A., Geisler, D., Bernardoni, F., Ritschel, F., Bohm, I., Seidel, M., Mennigen, E., Ripke, S., Smolka, M. N., Roessner, V., & Ehrlich, S. (2016). Altered neural efficiency of decision making during temporal reward discounting in anorexia nervosa. *Journal of the American Academy of Child and Adolescent Psychiatry, 55*(11), 972–979. https://doi.org/10.1016/j.jaac.2016.08.005

Klenotich, S. J., Ho, E. V., McMurray, M. S., Server, C. H., & Dulawa, S. C. (2015). Dopamine D2/3 receptor antagonism reduces activity-based anorexia. *Translational Psychiatry, 5*, e613. https://doi.org/10.1038/tp.2015.109

Konstantakopoulos, G., Varsou, E., Dikeos, D., Ioannidi, N., Gonidakis, F., Papadimitriou, G., & Oulis, P. (2012). Delusionality of body image beliefs in eating disorders. *Psychiatry Research, 200*(2–3), 482–488. https://doi.org/10.1016/j.psychres.2012.03.023

Lacey, J. H., & Crisp, A. H. (1980). Hunger, food intake and weight: The impact of clomipramine on a refeeding anorexia nervosa population. *Postgraduate Medical Journal, 56* (Suppl 1), 79–85. https://www.ncbi.nlm.nih.gov/pubmed/6994086

Laederach-Hofmann, K., Graf, C., Horber, F., Lippuner, K., Lederer, S., Michel, R., & Schneider, M. (1999). Imipramine and diet counseling with psychological support in the treatment of obese binge eaters: A randomized, placebo-controlled double-blind study. *International Journal of Eating Disorders, 26*(3), 231–244. https://doi.org/10.1002/(sici)1098-108x(199911)26:3<231::aid-eat1>3.0.co;2-6

Lawson, E. A. (2017). The effects of oxytocin on eating behaviour and metabolism in humans. *Nature Reviews: Endocrinology, 13*(12), 700–709. https://doi.org/10.1038/nrendo.2017.115

Lawson, E. A., Holsen, L. M., Santin, M., Meenaghan, E., Eddy, K. T., Becker, A. E., Herzog, D. B., Goldstein, J. M., & Klibanski, A. (2012). Oxytocin secretion is associated with severity of disordered eating psychopathology and insular cortex hypoactivation in anorexia nervosa. *Journal of Clinical Endocrinology and Metabolism, 97*(10), E1898–1908. https://doi.org/10.1210/jc.2012-1702

Leombruni, P., Piero, A., Brustolin, A., Mondelli, V., Levi, M., Campisi, S., Marozio, S., Abbate-Daga, G., & Fassino, S. (2006). A 12 to 24 weeks pilot study of sertraline treatment in obese women binge eaters. *Human Psychopharmacology, 21*(3), 181–188. https://doi.org/10.1002/hup.758

Leppanen, J., Cardi, V., Ng, K. W., Paloyelis, Y., Stein, D., Tchanturia, K., & Treasure, J. (2017a). The effects of intranasal oxytocin on smoothie intake, cortisol and attentional bias in anorexia nervosa. *Psychoneuroendocrinology, 79*, 167–174. https://doi.org/10.1016/j.psyneuen.2017.01.017

Leppanen, J., Cardi, V., Ng, K. W., Paloyelis, Y., Stein, D., Tchanturia, K., & Treasure, J. (2017b). Effects of intranasal oxytocin on the interpretation and expression of emotions in anorexia nervosa. *Journal of Neuroendocrinology, 29*(3). https://doi.org/10.1111/jne.12458

Levinson, C. A., Rodebaugh, T. L., Fewell, L., Kass, A. E., Riley, E. N., Stark, L., McCallum, K., & Lenze, E. J. (2015). D-Cycloserine facilitation of exposure therapy improves weight regain in patients with anorexia nervosa: A pilot randomized controlled trial. *Journal of Clinical Psychiatry, 76*(6), e787–793. https://doi.org/10.4088/JCP.14m09299

Liu, C. M., Spaulding, M. O., Rea, J. J., Noble, E. E., & Kanoski, S. E. (2021). Oxytocin and food intake control: Neural, behavioral, and signaling mechanisms. *International Journal of Molecular Science, 22*(19). https://doi.org/10.3390/ijms221910859

Lloyd, E. C., & Steinglass, J. E. (2018). What can food-image tasks teach us about anorexia nervosa? A systematic review. *Journal of Eating Disorders, 6*, 31. https://doi.org/10.1186/s40337-018-0217-z

Lopez-Munoz, F., Baumeister, A. A., Hawkins, M. F., & Alamo, C. (2012). The role of serendipity in the discovery of the clinical effects of psychotropic drugs: Beyond of the myth. *Actas Españolas de Psiquiatría: Acepsi, 40*(1), 34–42. https://www.ncbi.nlm.nih.gov/pubmed/22344494

Ma, G. F., Raivio, N., Sabria, J., & Ortiz, J. (2014). Agonist and antagonist effects of aripiprazole on D(2)-like receptors controlling rat brain dopamine synthesis depend on the dopaminergic tone. *International Journal of Neuropsychopharmacology, 18*(4). https://doi.org/10.1093/ijnp/pyu046

Madsen, M. K., Fisher, P. M., Burmester, D., Dyssegaard, A., Stenbaek, D. S., Kristiansen, S., Johansen, S. S., Lehel, S., Linnet, K., Svarer, C., Erritzoe, D., Ozenne, B., & Knudsen, G. M. (2019). Psychedelic effects of psilocybin correlate with serotonin 2A receptor occupancy and plasma psilocin levels. *Neuropsychopharmacology, 44*(7), 1328–1334. https://doi.org/10.1038/s41386-019-0324-9

Majuri, J., Joutsa, J., Johansson, J., Voon, V., Parkkola, R., Alho, H., Arponen, E., & Kaasinen, V. (2017). Serotonin transporter density in binge eating disorder and pathological gambling: A PET study with [(11)C]MADAM. *European Neuropsychopharmacology, 27*(12), 1281–1288. https://doi.org/10.1016/j.euroneuro.2017.09.007

Malamood, M., Roberts, A., Kataria, R., Parkman, H. P., & Schey, R. (2017). Mirtazapine for symptom control in refractory gastroparesis. *Drug Design, Development and Therapy, 11*, 1035–1041. https://doi.org/10.2147/DDDT.S125743

Malhotra, S., King, K. H., Welge, J. A., Brusman-Lovins, L., & McElroy, S. L. (2002). Venlafaxine treatment of binge-eating disorder associated with obesity: A series of 35 patients. *Journal of Clinical Psychiatry, 63*(9), 802–806. https://doi.org/10.4088/jcp.v63n0909

Manos, B. E., Bravender, T. D., Harrison, T. M., Lange, H. L. H., Cottrill, C. B., Abdel-Rasoul, M., & Bonny, A. E. (2018). A pilot randomized controlled trial of omega-3 fatty acid supplementation for the treatment of anxiety in adolescents with anorexia nervosa. *International Journal of Eating Disorders, 51*(12), 1367–1372. https://doi.org/10.1002/eat.22964

Marcus, M. D., Wing, R. R., Ewing, L., Kern, E., McDermott, M., & Gooding, W. (1990). A double-blind, placebo-controlled trial of fluoxetine plus behavior modification in the treatment of obese binge-eaters and non-binge-eaters. *American Journal of Psychiatry, 147*(7), 876–881. https://doi.org/10.1176/ajp.147.7.876

Marrazzi, M. A., Bacon, J. P., Kinzie, J., & Luby, E. D. (1995). Naltrexone use in the treatment of anorexia nervosa and bulimia nervosa. *International Clinical Psychopharmacology, 10*(3), 163–172. https://www.ncbi.nlm.nih.gov/pubmed/8675969

Marzola, E., Desedime, N., Giovannone, C., Amianto, F., Fassino, S., & Abbate-Daga, G. (2015). Atypical antipsychotics as augmentation therapy in anorexia nervosa. *PLOS ONE, 10*(4), e0125569. https://doi.org/10.1371/journal.pone.0125569

Marzola, E., Porliod, A., Panero, M., De-Bacco, C., & Abbate-Daga, G. (2020). Affective temperaments and eating psychopathology in anorexia nervosa: Which role for anxious and depressive traits? *Journal of Affective Disorders, 266*, 374–380. https://doi.org/10.1016/j.jad.2020.01.142

Mauri, M., Miniati, M., Mariani, M. G., Ciberti, A., & Dell'Osso, L. (2013). Haloperidol for severe anorexia nervosa restricting type with delusional body image disturbance: A nine-case chart review. *Eating and Weight Disorders, 18*(3), 329–332. https://doi.org/10.1007/s40519-013-0052-9

McCann, U. D., & Agras, W. S. (1990). Successful treatment of nonpurging bulimia nervosa with desipramine: A double-blind, placebo-controlled study. *American Journal of Psychiatry, 147*(11), 1509–1513. https://doi.org/10.1176/ajp.147.11.1509

McElroy, S. L., Arnold, L. M., Shapira, N. A., Keck, P. E., Jr., Rosenthal, N. R., Karim, M. R., Kamin, M., & Hudson, J. I. (2003). Topiramate in the treatment of binge eating disorder associated with obesity: A randomized, placebo-controlled trial. *American Journal of Psychiatry, 160*(2), 255–261. https://doi.org/10.1176/appi.ajp.160.2.255

McElroy, S. L., Casuto, L. S., Nelson, E. B., Lake, K. A., Soutullo, C. A., Keck, P. E., Jr., & Hudson, J. I. (2000). Placebo-controlled trial of sertraline in the treatment of binge eating disorder. *American Journal of Psychiatry, 157*(6), 1004–1006. https://doi.org/10.1176/appi.ajp.157.6.1004

McElroy, S. L., Guerdjikova, A., Kotwal, R., Welge, J. A., Nelson, E. B., Lake, K. A., Keck, P. E., Jr., & Hudson, J. I. (2007). Atomoxetine in the treatment of binge-eating disorder: A randomized placebo-controlled trial. *Journal of Clinical Psychiatry, 68*(3), 390–398. https://doi.org/10.4088/jcp.v68n0306

McElroy, S. L., Guerdjikova, A. I., Blom, T. J., Crow, S. J., Memisoglu, A., Silverman, B. L., & Ehrich, E. W. (2013). A placebo-controlled pilot study of the novel opioid receptor antagonist ALKS-33 in binge eating disorder. *International Journal of Eating Disorders, 46*(3), 239–245. https://doi.org/10.1002/eat.22114

McElroy, S. L., Guerdjikova, A. I., Mori, N., Blom, T. J., Williams, S., Casuto, L. S., & Keck, P. E., Jr. (2015). Armodafinil in binge eating disorder: A randomized, placebo-controlled trial. *International Clinical Psychopharmacology, 30*(4), 209–215. https://doi.org/10.1097/YIC.0000000000000079

McElroy, S. L., Hudson, J., Ferreira-Cornwell, M. C., Radewonuk, J., Whitaker, T., & Gasior, M. (2016). Lisdexamfetamine dimesylate for adults with moderate to severe binge eating disorder: results of two pivotal phase 3 randomized controlled trials. *Neuropsychopharmacology, 41*(5), 1251–1260. https://doi.org/10.1038/npp.2015.275

McElroy, S. L., Hudson, J. I., Capece, J. A., Beyers, K., Fisher, A. C., Rosenthal, N. R., & Topiramate Binge Eating Disorder Research Group. (2007). Topiramate for the treatment of binge eating disorder associated with obesity: A placebo-controlled study. *Biological Psychiatry, 61*(9), 1039–1048. https://doi.org/10.1016/j.biopsych.2006.08.008

McElroy, S. L., Hudson, J. I., Gasior, M., Herman, B. K., Radewonuk, J., Wilfley, D., & Busner, J. (2017). Time course of the effects of lisdexamfetamine dimesylate in two phase 3, randomized, double-blind, placebo-controlled trials in adults with binge-eating disorder. *International Journal of Eating Disorders, 50*(8), 884–892. https://doi.org/10.1002/eat.22722

McElroy, S. L., Hudson, J. I., Grilo, C. M., Guerdjikova, A. I., Deng, L., Koblan, K. S., Goldman, R., Navia, B., Hopkins, S., & Loebel, A. (2020). Efficacy and safety of dasotraline in adults with binge-eating disorder: A randomized, placebo-controlled, flexible-dose clinical trial. *Journal of Clinical Psychiatry, 81*(5). https://doi.org/10.4088/JCP.19m13068

McElroy, S. L., Hudson, J. I., Mitchell, J. E., Wilfley, D., Ferreira-Cornwell, M. C., Gao, J., Wang, J., Whitaker, T., Jonas, J., & Gasior, M. (2015). Efficacy and safety of lisdexamfetamine for treatment of adults with moderate to severe binge-eating disorder: a randomized clinical trial. *JAMA Psychiatry, 72*(3), 235–246. https://doi.org/10.1001/jamapsychiatry.2014.2162

McElroy, S. L., Mori, N., Guerdjikova, A. I., & Keck, P. E., Jr. (2018). Would glucagon-like peptide-1 receptor agonists have efficacy in binge eating disorder and bulimia nervosa? A review of the current literature. *Medical Hypotheses*, *111*, 90–93. https://doi.org/10.1016/j.mehy.2017.12.029

McElroy, S. L., Shapira, N. A., Arnold, L. M., Keck, P. E., Rosenthal, N. R., Wu, S. C., Capece, J. A., Fazzio, L., & Hudson, J. I. (2004). Topiramate in the long-term treatment of binge-eating disorder associated with obesity. *Journal of Clinical Psychiatry*, *65*(11), 1463–1469. https://doi.org/10.4088/jcp.v65n1104

Mihov, Y., Treyer, V., Akkus, F., Toman, E., Milos, G., Ametamey, S. M., Johayem, A., & Hasler, G. (2020). Metabotropic glutamate receptor 5 in bulimia nervosa. *Scientific Reports*, *10*(1), 6374. https://doi.org/10.1038/s41598-020-63389-7

Milano, W., Petrella, C., Casella, A., Capasso, A., Carrino, S., & Milano, L. (2005). Use of sibutramine, an inhibitor of the reuptake of serotonin and noradrenaline, in the treatment of binge eating disorder: A placebo-controlled study. *Advances in Therapy*, *22*(1), 25–31. https://doi.org/10.1007/BF02850181

Milano, W., Siano, C., Putrella, C., & Capasso, A. (2005). Treatment of bulimia nervosa with fluvoxamine: A randomized controlled trial. *Advances in Therapy*, *22*(3), 278–283. https://doi.org/10.1007/BF02849936

Misra, M., Katzman, D. K., Estella, N. M., Eddy, K. T., Weigel, T., Goldstein, M. A., Miller, K. K., & Klibanski, A. (2013). Impact of physiologic estrogen replacement on anxiety symptoms, body shape perception, and eating attitudes in adolescent girls with anorexia nervosa: data from a randomized controlled trial. *Journal of Clinical Psychiatry*, *74*(8), e765–771. https://doi.org/10.4088/JCP.13m08365

Mitchell, J. E., & Groat, R. (1984). A placebo-controlled, double-blind trial of amitriptyline in bulimia. *Journal of Clinical Psychopharmacology*, *4*(4), 186–193.

Mitchell, J. E., Pyle, R. L., Eckert, E. D., Hatsukami, D., Pomeroy, C., & Zimmerman, R. (1990). A comparison study of antidepressants and structured intensive group psychotherapy in the treatment of bulimia nervosa. *Archives of General Psychiatry*, *47*(2), 149–157. https://www.ncbi.nlm.nih.gov/pubmed/2405806

Mitchell, J. S., Anijarv, T. E., Levenstein, J. L., Hermens, D. F., & Lagopoulos, J. (2023). Excitatory and inhibitory neurometabolites in anorexia nervosa: A systematic review of proton magnetic resonance spectroscopy studies. *Neuroscience and Biobehavioral Reviews*, *152*, 105279. https://doi.org/10.1016/j.neubiorev.2023.105279

Mondraty, N., Birmingham, C. L., Touyz, S., Sundakov, V., Chapman, L., & Beumont, P. (2005). Randomized controlled trial of olanzapine in the treatment of cognitions in anorexia nervosa. *Australasian Psychiatry*, *13*(1), 72–75. https://doi.org/10.1080/j.1440-1665.2004.02154.x

Monteleone, A. M., Castellini, G., Volpe, U., Ricca, V., Lelli, L., Monteleone, P., & Maj, M. (2018). Neuroendocrinology and brain imaging of reward in eating disorders: A possible key to the treatment of anorexia nervosa and bulimia nervosa. *Progress in Neuro-Psychopharmacology and Biological Psychiatry*, *80*(Pt B), 132–142. https://doi.org/10.1016/j.pnpbp.2017.02.020

Monteleone, A. M., Scognamiglio, P., Volpe, U., Di Maso, V., & Monteleone, P. (2016). Investigation of oxytocin secretion in anorexia nervosa and bulimia nervosa: Relationships to temperament personality dimensions. *European Eating Disorders Review*, *24*(1), 52–56. https://doi.org/10.1002/erv.2391

Monteleone, P., & Maj, M. (2013). Dysfunctions of leptin, ghrelin, BDNF and endocannabinoids in eating disorders: Beyond the homeostatic control of food intake. *Psychoneuroendocrinology*, *38*(3), 312–330. https://doi.org/10.1016/j.psyneuen.2012.10.021

Mueller, S. V., Morishima, Y., Schwab, S., Wiest, R., Federspiel, A., & Hasler, G. (2018). Neural correlates of impaired reward-effort integration in remitted bulimia nervosa. *Neuropsychopharmacology*, *43*(4), 868–876. https://doi.org/10.1038/npp.2017.277

Naguy, A., Roshdy, R., Al-Mutairi, A., Alwetayan, S., & Alamiri, B. (2023). Mirtazapine improved eating patterns in avoidant/restrictive food intake disorder. *American Journal of Therapeutics*, *30*(2), 173–175. https://doi.org/10.1097/MJT.0000000000001338

Nickel, C., Tritt, K., Muehlbacher, M., Pedrosa Gil, F., Mitterlehner, F. O., Kaplan, P., Lahmann, C., Leiberich, P. K., Krawczyk, J., Kettler, C., Rother, W. K., Loew, T. H., & Nickel, M. K. (2005). Topiramate treatment in bulimia nervosa patients: A randomized, double-blind, placebo-controlled trial. *International Journal of Eating Disorders*, *38*(4), 295–300. https://doi.org/10.1002/eat.20202

Ninan, I., & Kulkarni, S. K. (1999). Differential effects of olanzapine at dopamine D1 and D2 receptors in dopamine depleted animals. *Psychopharmacology*, *142*(2), 175–181. https://doi.org/10.1007/s002130050877

Norris, M. L., Spettigue, W., Buchholz, A., Henderson, K. A., Gomez, R., Maras, D., Gaboury, I., & Ni, A. (2011). Olanzapine use for the adjunctive treatment of adolescents with anorexia nervosa. *Journal of Child and Adolescent Psychopharmacology, 21*(3), 213–220. https://doi.org/10.1089/cap.2010.0131

Nourredine, M., Jurek, L., Auffret, M., Iceta, S., Grenet, G., Kassai, B., Cucherat, M., & Rolland, B. (2021). Efficacy and safety of topiramate in binge eating disorder: A systematic review and meta-analysis. *CNS Spectrum, 26*(5), 459–467. https://doi.org/10.1017/S1092852920001613

O'Connor, E. C., Kremer, Y., Lefort, S., Harada, M., Pascoli, V., Rohner, C., & Luscher, C. (2015). Accumbal D1R neurons projecting to lateral hypothalamus authorize feeding. *Neuron, 88*(3), 553–564. https://doi.org/10.1016/j.neuron.2015.09.038

O'Doherty, J. P., Dayan, P., Friston, K., Critchley, H., & Dolan, R. J. (2003). Temporal difference models and reward-related learning in the human brain. *Neuron, 38*(2), 329–337. https://www.ncbi.nlm.nih.gov/pubmed/12718865

Oinio, V., Backstrom, P., Uhari-Vaananen, J., Raasmaja, A., Piepponen, P., & Kiianmaa, K. (2017). Dopaminergic modulation of reward-guided decision making in alcohol-preferring AA rats. *Behavioural Brain Research, 326*, 87–95. https://doi.org/10.1016/j.bbr.2017.03.007

Pearlstein, T., Spurell, E., Hohlstein, L. A., Gurney, V., Read, J., Fuchs, C., & Keller, M. B. (2003). A double-blind, placebo-controlled trial of fluvoxamine in binge eating disorder: A high placebo response. *Archives of Women's Mental Health, 6*(2), 147–151. https://doi.org/10.1007/s00737-003-0172-8

Peck, S. K., Shao, S., Gruen, T., Yang, K., Babakanian, A., Trim, J., Finn, D. M., & Kaye, W. H. (2023). Psilocybin therapy for females with anorexia nervosa: A phase 1, open-label feasibility study. *Nature Medicine, 29*(8), 1947–1953. https://doi.org/10.1038/s41591-023-02455-9

Pierce-Messick, Z., & Pratt, W. E. (2020). Glucagon-like peptide-1 receptors modulate the binge-like feeding induced by micro-opioid receptor stimulation of the nucleus accumbens in the rat. *NeuroReport, 31*(18), 1283–1288. https://doi.org/10.1097/WNR.0000000000001545

Piper, B. J. (2018). Mother of berries, ACDC, or chocolope: Examination of the strains used by medical cannabis patients in New England. *Journal of Psychoactive Drugs, 50*(2), 95–104. https://doi.org/10.1080/02791072.2017.1390179

Plassmann, H., O'Doherty, J. P., & Rangel, A. (2010). Appetitive and aversive goal values are encoded in the medial orbitofrontal cortex at the time of decision making [Research Support, Non-U.S. Gov'tResearch Support, U.S. Gov't, Non-P.H.S.]. *Journal of Neuroscience, 30*(32), 10799–10808. https://doi.org/10.1523/JNEUROSCI.0788-10.2010

Pope, H. G., Jr., Hudson, J. I., Jonas, J. M., & Yurgelun-Todd, D. (1983). Bulimia treated with imipramine: A placebo-controlled, double-blind study. *American Journal of Psychiatry, 140*(5), 554–558. https://doi.org/10.1176/ajp.140.5.554

Pope, H. G., Jr., Keck, P. E., Jr., McElroy, S. L., & Hudson, J. I. (1989). A placebo-controlled study of trazodone in bulimia nervosa. *Journal of Clinical Psychopharmacology, 9*(4), 254–259. https://www.ncbi.nlm.nih.gov/pubmed/2671058

Powers, P. S., Klabunde, M., & Kaye, W. (2012). Double-blind placebo-controlled trial of quetiapine in anorexia nervosa. *European Eating Disorders Review, 20*(4), 331–334. https://doi.org/10.1002/erv.2169

Puglisi-Allegra, S., & Ventura, R. (2012). Prefrontal/accumbal catecholamine system processes emotionally driven attribution of motivational salience. *Reviews in the Neurosciences, 23*(5–6), 509–526. https://doi.org/10.1515/revneuro-2012-0076

Quilty, L. C., Allen, T. A., Davis, C., Knyahnytska, Y., & Kaplan, A. S. (2019). A randomized comparison of long acting methylphenidate and cognitive behavioral therapy in the treatment of binge eating disorder. *Psychiatry Research, 273*, 467–474. https://doi.org/10.1016/j.psychres.2019.01.066

Ragnhildstveit, A., Slayton, M., Jackson, L. K., Brendle, M., Ahuja, S., Holle, W., Moore, C., Sollars, K., Seli, P., & Robison, R. (2022). Ketamine as a novel psychopharmacotherapy for eating disorders: Evidence and future directions. *Brain Sciences, 12*(3). https://doi.org/10.3390/brainsci12030382

Ramirez, K., Niraula, A., & Sheridan, J. F. (2016). GABAergic modulation with classical benzodiazepines prevent stress-induced neuro-immune dysregulation and behavioral alterations. *Brain, Behavior, and Immunity, 51*, 154–168. https://doi.org/10.1016/j.bbi.2015.08.011

Reed, C. H., Bauer, E. E., Shoeman, A., Buhr, T. J., & Clark, P. J. (2021). Acute stress exposure alters food-related brain monoaminergic profiles in a rat model of anorexia. *Journal of Nutrition, 151*(12), 3617–3627. https://doi.org/10.1093/jn/nxab298

Ricca, V., Mannucci, E., Mezzani, B., Moretti, S., Di Bernardo, M., Bertelli, M., Rotella, C. M., & Faravelli, C. (2001). Fluoxetine and fluvoxamine combined with individual cognitive-behaviour therapy in binge eating disorder: A one-year follow-up study. *Psychotherapy and Psychosomatics, 70*(6), 298–306. https://doi.org/10.1159/000056270

Richards, J., Bang, N., Ratliff, E. L., Paszkowiak, M. A., Khorgami, Z., Khalsa, S. S., & Simmons, W. K. (2023). Successful treatment of binge eating disorder with the GLP-1 agonist semaglutide: A retrospective cohort study. *Obesity Pillars, 7*, 100080. https://doi.org/10.1016/j.obpill.2023.100080

Romano, S. J., Halmi, K. A., Sarkar, N. P., Koke, S. C., & Lee, J. S. (2002). A placebo-controlled study of fluoxetine in continued treatment of bulimia nervosa after successful acute fluoxetine treatment. *American Journal of Psychiatry, 159*(1), 96–102. https://doi.org/10.1176/appi.ajp.159.1.96

Rothschild, R., Quitkin, H. M., Quitkin, F. M., Stewart, J. W., Ocepek-Welikson, K., McGrath, P. J., & Tricamo, E. (1994). A double-blind placebo-controlled comparison of phenelzine and imipramine in the treatment of bulimia in atypical depressives. *International Journal of Eating Disorders, 15*(1), 1–9. https://www.ncbi.nlm.nih.gov/pubmed/8124322

Russell, J., Maguire, S., Hunt, G. E., Kesby, A., Suraev, A., Stuart, J., Booth, J., & McGregor, I. S. (2018). Intranasal oxytocin in the treatment of anorexia nervosa: Randomized controlled trial during re-feeding. *Psychoneuroendocrinology, 87*, 83–92. https://doi.org/10.1016/j.psyneuen.2017.10.014

Sabine, E. J., Yonace, A., Farrington, A. J., Barratt, K. H., & Wakeling, A. (1983). Bulimia nervosa: A placebo controlled double-blind therapeutic trial of mianserin. *British Journal of Clinical Pharmacology*, 15 Suppl 2(Suppl 2), 195S–202S. https://www.ncbi.nlm.nih.gov/pubmed/6337607

Safer, D. L., Adler, S., Dalai, S. S., Bentley, J. P., Toyama, H., Pajarito, S., & Najarian, T. (2020). A randomized, placebo-controlled crossover trial of phentermine-topiramate ER in patients with binge-eating disorder and bulimia nervosa. *International Journal of Eating Disorders, 53*(2), 266–277. https://doi.org/10.1002/eat.23192

Sanders, N., Smeets, P. A., van Elburg, A. A., Danner, U. N., van Meer, F., Hoek, H. W., & Adan, R. A. (2015). Altered food-cue processing in chronically ill and recovered women with anorexia nervosa. *Frontiers in Behavioral Neuroscience, 9*, 46. https://doi.org/10.3389/fnbeh.2015.00046

Schelp, S. A., Brodnik, Z. D., Rakowski, D. R., Pultorak, K. J., Sambells, A. T., Espana, R. A., & Oleson, E. B. (2018). Diazepam concurrently increases the frequency and decreases the amplitude of transient dopamine release events in the nucleus accumbens. *Journal of Pharmacology and Experimental Therapeutics, 364*(1), 145–155. https://doi.org/10.1124/jpet.117.241802

Schmidt, U., Cooper, P. J., Essers, H., Freeman, C. P., Holland, R. L., Palmer, R. L., Shur, E., Russell, G. F., Bowler, C., Coker, S., Geddes, J. R., Mackenzie, F., Munro, J., Newton, R., Tiller, J., Tattersall, M. L., Vize, C., & Webster, J. (2004). Fluvoxamine and graded psychotherapy in the treatment of bulimia nervosa: A randomized, double-blind, placebo-controlled, multicenter study of short-term and long-term pharmacotherapy combined with a stepped care approach to psychotherapy. *Journal of Clinical Psychopharmacology, 24*(5), 549–552. https://doi.org/10.1097/01.jcp.0000138776.32891.3e

Schultz, W. (2002). Getting formal with dopamine and reward. *Neuron, 36*(2), 241–263. https://www.ncbi.nlm.nih.gov/pubmed/12383780

Schwartz, T., Trunko, M. E., Feifel, D., Lopez, E., Peterson, D., Frank, G. K. W., & Kaye, W. (2021). A longitudinal case series of IM ketamine for patients with severe and enduring eating disorders and comorbid treatment-resistant depression. *Clinical Case Reports, 9*(5), e03869. https://doi.org/10.1002/ccr3.3869

Steinglass, J. E., Kaplan, S. C., Liu, Y., Wang, Y., & Walsh, B. T. (2014). The (lack of) effect of alprazolam on eating behavior in anorexia nervosa: A preliminary report. *International Journal of Eating Disorders, 47*(8), 901–904. https://doi.org/10.1002/eat.22343

Sternheim, L. C., Fisher, M., Harrison, A., & Watling, R. (2017). Predicting intolerance of uncertainty in individuals with eating disorder symptoms. *Journal of Eating Disorders, 5*, 26. https://doi.org/10.1186/s40337-017-0152-4

Stice, E., Onipede, Z. A., & Marti, C. N. (2021). A meta-analytic review of trials that tested whether eating disorder prevention programs prevent eating disorder onset. *Clinical Psychology Review, 87*, 102046. https://doi.org/10.1016/j.cpr.2021.102046

Stratford, T. R., & Kelley, A. E. (1999). Evidence of a functional relationship between the nucleus accumbens shell and lateral hypothalamus subserving the control of feeding behavior. *Journal of Neuroscience, 19*(24), 11040–11048. https://www.ncbi.nlm.nih.gov/pubmed/10594084

Strobel, M., Warnke, A., Roth, M., & Schulze, U. (2004). [Paroxetine versus clomipramine in female adolescents suffering from anorexia nervosa and depressive episode—a retrospective study on tolerability, reasons for discontinuing the antidepressive treatment and different outcome measurements]. *Zeitschrift für Kinder- und Jugendpsychiatrie und Psychotherapie, 32*(4), 279–289. https://

doi.org/10.1024/1422-4917.32.4.279 (Psychopharmakotherapie mit Clomipramin und Paroxetin bei jugendlichen Patientinnen mit "Anorexia nervosa" und "Depressiver Episode"—eine Pilotstudie zu Vertraglichkeit, Absetzquote und therapeutischen Verlaufskriterien.)

Stunkard, A., Berkowitz, R., Tanrikut, C., Reiss, E., & Young, L. (1996). d-Fenfluramine treatment of binge eating disorder. *American Journal of Psychiatry, 153*(11), 1455–1459.

Szutorisz, H., Egervari, G., Sperry, J., Carter, J. M., & Hurd, Y. L. (2016). Cross-generational THC exposure alters the developmental sensitivity of ventral and dorsal striatal gene expression in male and female offspring. *Neurotoxicology and Teratology, 58*, 107–114. https://doi.org/10.1016/j.ntt.2016.05.005

Tahillioglu, A., Ozcan, T., Yuksel, G., Majroh, N., Kose, S., & Ozbaran, B. (2020). Is aripiprazole a key to unlock anorexia nervosa?: A case series. *Clinical Case Reports, 8*(12), 2827–2834. https://doi.org/10.1002/ccr3.3271

Trunko, M. E., Schwartz, T. A., Duvvuri, V., & Kaye, W. H. (2011). Aripiprazole in anorexia nervosa and low-weight bulimia nervosa: case reports [case reports]. *International Journal of Eating Disorders, 44*(3), 269–275. https://doi.org/10.1002/eat.20807

Trunko, M. E., Schwartz, T. A., Marzola, E., Klein, A. S., & Kaye, W. H. (2014). Lamotrigine use in patients with binge eating and purging, significant affect dysregulation, and poor impulse control. *International Journal of Eating Disorders, 47*(3), 329–334. https://doi.org/10.1002/eat.22234

Vandereycken, W. (1984). Neuroleptics in the short-term treatment of anorexia nervosa: A double-blind placebo-controlled study with sulpiride. *British Journal of Psychiatry, 144*, 288–292. https://www.ncbi.nlm.nih.gov/pubmed/6367876

Vandereycken, W., & Pierloot, R. (1982). Pimozide combined with behavior therapy in the short-term treatment of anorexia nervosa. A double-blind placebo-controlled cross-over study. *Acta Psychiatrica Scandinavica, 66*(6), 445–450. https://www.ncbi.nlm.nih.gov/pubmed/6758492

Volkow, N. D. (2008). Addiction reviews: Introduction. *Annals of the New York Academy of Sciences, 1141*, xi–xii. https://doi.org/10.1196/annals.1441.034

Walsh, B. T., Gladis, M., Roose, S. P., Stewart, J. W., Stetner, F., & Glassman, A. H. (1988). Phenelzine vs placebo in 50 patients with bulimia. *Archives of General Psychiatry, 45*(5), 471–475. https://www.ncbi.nlm.nih.gov/pubmed/3282482

Walsh, B. T., Hadigan, C. M., Devlin, M. J., Gladis, M., & Roose, S. P. (1991). Long-term outcome of antidepressant treatment for bulimia nervosa. *American Journal of Psychiatry, 148*(9), 1206–1212. https://doi.org/10.1176/ajp.148.9.1206

Walsh, B. T., Kaplan, A. S., Attia, E., Olmsted, M., Parides, M., Carter, J. C., Pike, K. M., Devlin, M. J., Woodside, B., Roberto, C. A., & Rockert, W. (2006). Fluoxetine after weight restoration in anorexia nervosa: A randomized controlled trial. *JAMA, 295*(22), 2605–2612. https://doi.org/10.1001/jama.295.22.2605

Walsh, B. T., Stewart, J. W., Roose, S. P., Gladis, M., & Glassman, A. H. (1984). Treatment of bulimia with phenelzine: A double-blind, placebo-controlled study. *Archives of General Psychiatry, 41*(11), 1105–1109. https://www.ncbi.nlm.nih.gov/pubmed/6388524

Walsh, B. T., Wilson, G. T., Loeb, K. L., Devlin, M. J., Pike, K. M., Roose, S. P., Fleiss, J., & Waternaux, C. (1997). Medication and psychotherapy in the treatment of bulimia nervosa. *American Journal of Psychiatry, 154*(4), 523–531. https://doi.org/10.1176/ajp.154.4.523

Welch, A. C., Zhang, J., Lyu, J., McMurray, M. S., Javitch, J. A., Kellendonk, C., & Dulawa, S. C. (2019). Dopamine D2 receptor overexpression in the nucleus accumbens core induces robust weight loss during scheduled fasting selectively in female mice. *Molecular Psychiatry*, 26(8), 3765–3777. https://doi.org/10.1038/s41380-019-0633-8

Wilfley, D. E., Crow, S. J., Hudson, J. I., Mitchell, J. E., Berkowitz, R. I., Blakesley, V., Walsh, B. T., & Sibutramine Binge Eating Disorder Research Group. (2008). Efficacy of sibutramine for the treatment of binge eating disorder: A randomized multicenter placebo-controlled double-blind study. *American Journal of Psychiatry, 165*(1), 51–58. https://doi.org/10.1176/appi.ajp.2007.06121970

Yilmaz, Z., Halvorsen, M., Bryois, J., Yu, D., Thornton, L. M., Zerwas, S., Micali, N., Moessner, R., Burton, C. L., Zai, G., Erdman, L., Kas, M. J., Arnold, P. D., Davis, L. K., Knowles, J. A., Breen, G., Scharf, J. M., Nestadt, G., Mathews, C. A., Bulik, C. M., Eating Disorders Working Group of the Psychiatric Genomics Consortium, Tourette Syndrome/Obsessive–Compulsive Disorder Working Group of the Psychiatric Genomics Consortium. (2018). Examination of the shared genetic basis of anorexia nervosa and obsessive-compulsive disorder. *Molecular Psychiatry*, 25(9), 2036–2046. https://doi.org/10.1038/s41380-018-0115-4

Yokokura, M., Terada, T., Bunai, T., Nakaizumi, K., Kato, Y., Yoshikawa, E., Futatsubashi, M., Suzuki, K., Yamasue, H., & Ouchi, Y. (2019). Alterations in serotonin transporter and body image-related cognition in anorexia nervosa. *NeuroImage: Clinical*, *23*, 101928. https://doi.org/10.1016/j.nicl.2019.101928

Yu, J., Stewart Agras, W., Halmi, K. A., Crow, S., Mitchell, J., & Bryson, S. W. (2011). A 1-year follow-up of a multi-center treatment trial of adults with anorexia nervosa. *Eating and Weight Disorders*, *16*(3), e177–181. https://www.ncbi.nlm.nih.gov/pubmed/22290033.

26

The Potential of Psychedelics in the Treatment of Eating Disorders

Natalie Gukasyan, Samantha Hilbert, and Angela S. Guarda

Brief Definitional Overview

Psychedelic: A somewhat disputed term that comprises drugs known to produce acute perceptual, cognitive, and mood changes. The term was coined by psychiatrist Humphrey Osmond in the 1950s (Osmond, 1957), from the Greek *psyche* and *delos*, meaning "mind-manifesting." "Classic" psychedelics are those drugs that exert effects primarily through serotonin 2A ($5\text{-}HT_{2A}$) receptor agonism, such as psilocybin or LSD. However, drugs functioning via other primary mechanisms but sharing some subjective effects (e.g., ketamine, ibogaine, MDMA, and others) are often described as psychedelic.

Psychedelic-assisted therapy (PAT): The provision of a few moderate to high doses of a psychedelic drug provided in a supportive psychotherapeutic setting. This usually includes some preparatory visits, as well as follow-up or "integration" visits.

Psilocybin: A classic psychedelic drug that occurs naturally in some species of fungi. In moderate to high doses, it produces an altered state lasting four to six hours. A synthetic formulation of psilocybin is being investigated for the treatment of major depressive disorder and other conditions.

Set and setting: A term commonly used to describe extrapharmacologic factors that may influence the contents or outcome of a psychedelic experience. Set refers to the psychological factors of the individual taking the drug, such as their mindset, temperament, expectations, and mood going into the experience. Setting refers to elements of the physical and social environment, such as the immediate surroundings, presence of others during the drug effects, and cultural environment, among other factors. Both set and setting are key considerations in PAT.

Microdosing: The use of a very low and often sub-perceptual dose of a psychedelic drug. This has been a practice that is increasing in popularity reportedly for its mood- or creativity-enhancing effects. Typically, the drug is taken on a regular schedule (e.g., three times a week for several

Natalie Gukasyan, Samantha Hilbert, and Angela S. Guarda, *The Potential of Psychedelics in the Treatment of Eating Disorders*. In: *The Handbook of the Neurobiology of Eating Disorders*. Edited by: Christina E. Wierenga and Joanna E. Steinglass, Oxford University Press. © Oxford University Press (2025). DOI: 10.1093/9780197675212.003.0027 weeks or longer). Survey studies of individuals who report microdosing often show self-reported benefit. However, there is relatively little high-quality research on this practice, and the few laboratory studies published to date have failed to demonstrate clear benefits.

Introduction

The past 20 years have witnessed a significant revival in scientific and public interest in psychedelics following a multi-decade lull in research. A growing body of literature suggests the potential for rapid and substantial therapeutic efficacy covering a growing list of indications including depressive disorders, addiction, anxiety disorders, and recently, eating disorders. Promising preliminary results are typically achieved via the provision of a few moderate to high doses of a drug provided in a supportive psychotherapeutic setting, often described as psychedelic-assisted therapy (PAT). While this "second wave" of PAT clinical trials is still in its infancy, the promising findings have sparked substantial public and commercial attention.

The US Food and Drug Administration (FDA) has acknowledged this potential, granting the "Breakthrough Therapy" designation to several companies for their efforts to bring psilocybin, lysergic acid diethylamide (LSD), and 3,4-methylenedioxymethamphetamine (MDMA) to market, targeting major depressive disorder (MDD), generalized anxiety disorder, and post-traumatic stress disorder (PTSD) respectively. While many phase III trials are yet to be completed and the majority of psychedelics are categorized as illegal under the United Nations Convention on Psychotropic Substances, commercial entities are proactively positioning themselves for the potential regulatory approval of these substances for clinical use in both the United States and international markets (Phelps et al., 2022). Concurrently, state and local governments are making efforts toward the decriminalization and legalization of classic psychedelics and related substances (Smith & Appelbaum, 2021), and private establishments offering psychedelics in retreat settings are already proliferating, both domestically and abroad (Flaherty et al., 2017).

Yet, amidst this burgeoning interest, there is tangible risk. The surge in enthusiasm for psychedelic treatments risks outpacing the current progress of scientific understanding, particularly in complex conditions like anorexia nervosa (AN), which poses high treatment nonresponse, significant disease burden, and mortality. This chapter aims to review the current landscape of psychedelic-assisted therapies specifically for eating disorders. While there is reason for cautious optimism, further research is still needed to better understand the precise conditions under which these treatments can be effective, identify potential risks, and ascertain any adverse reactions, ensuring the best outcomes for those seeking help.

Types of psychedelics

"Classic" psychedelics comprise those drugs that exert effects primarily through serotonin 2A (5-HT_{2A}) receptor agonism and can be further subdivided into tryptamine and phenethylamine compounds. Tryptamines are characterized by an indole ring, with structural similarity to tryptophan, the precursor for serotonin. They include *N, N*-dimethyltryptamine (*N, N*-DMT, a chief psychoactive component of the psychedelic plant admixture ayahuasca), 5-methoxy-*N, N*-dimethyltryptamine (5-MeO-DMT), psilocybin, and LSD. The basic structure of phenethylamine drugs includes a benzene ring with a two-carbon ethyl group. Phenethylamine drugs as a broader category also include some compounds not typically thought of as having psychedelic effects, such as amphetamine. Classic phenethylamine psychedelics include mescaline, the chief psychoactive drug found in the peyote cactus. Among contemporary classic psychedelic clinical trials, psilocybin has been the most studied for eating disorders. Psilocybin is the chief psychoactive compound found in "magic" mushrooms, with an onset of action of 15 to 60 minutes, and a duration of action of about four to six hours at moderate to high doses (about 0.3 to 0.4 mg/kg). Psilocybin has good oral availability but it is not able to cross the blood–brain barrier; upon ingestion, it is hepatically dephosphorylated to its active metabolite, psilocin.

Other compounds, the non-classic psychedelics, can produce similar subjective and somatic effects to the classic psychedelics but function via alternative primary mechanisms. These include the phenethylamine amphetamine derivative MDMA, the N-methyl-D-aspartate (NDMA) receptor antagonist ketamine, and plant alkaloids, such as ibogaine, among others. Many drugs spanning both broad categories have been classified as Schedule 1 substances under the United States Controlled Substances Act and similar other programs internationally. The exception, at present, is ketamine, a dissociative anesthetic increasingly used off-label at non-anesthetic doses (often approximately 0.5 mg/kg) to treat depressive disorders due to its rapid antidepressant effects (Berman et al., 2000; Dakwar et al., 2019; Fond et al., 2014). An intranasal preparation of the S-enantiomer is FDA-approved for treatment resistant depression. Other potential indications of interest for ketamine are addictive and anxiety disorders.

Psychedelic use

The PAT model, which uses a limited number of moderate to high doses of a psychedelic with supportive therapy, is the most commonly used approach in contemporary clinical research with psychedelics. A similar model has been adopted among some community practitioners using ketamine, although ketamine-assisted psychotherapy has been less well represented among clinical research to date. Importantly, both racemic ketamine and the S-enantiomer appear to be able to produce clinical improvement without the use of significant psychotherapeutic support (Hock et al., 2022; K. Freind et al., 2023; Price et al., 2022). Broadly, the PAT model typical of psilocybin studies includes a significant amount of contact between patients and clinicians (also called facilitators or monitors) over three treatment phases spanning a period of days to weeks. An initial preparatory phase usually occurs over at least several hours, during which the patient meets with study staff, usually a team of two clinicians. The focus of this stage is on history taking, role induction, and establishment of therapeutic rapport. This is followed by the drug administration phase, in which both facilitators are present with the patient for the duration of drug effects to provide psychological support and to monitor for safety (about six hours for both MDMA and psilocybin, about two hours for ketamine). The number of drug administrations for psilocybin and MDMA is usually limited to one to three sessions spaced a few weeks apart, although the number and frequency is often higher for ketamine. Patients then undergo follow-up or "integration" visits during which the patient and facilitators review the events of dosing days and explore the meaning and after-effects of the experience relative to illness recovery. Given this amount of concomitant therapy focused on the set and setting and patient–practitioner interaction (up to 15 hours for the acute phase of treatment), a common criticism of research on this treatment is that it is difficult to disentangle independent contributions of the drug from that of the adjunctive psychotherapy (Gukasyan & Nayak, 2022).

Another notable practice is that of microdosing, the use of sub-perceptual doses of a psychedelic substance, often about one-tenth of a large dose, with the intended goal of improving cognitive function, emotional well-being, or creativity without causing a significantly altered state. Despite growing enthusiasm and anecdotal evidence of possible benefits among naturalistic users, most laboratory studies of microdosing have failed to show significant positive impact on mood or cognition (Bershad et al., 2019, 2020; Hutten et al., 2020; Murphy et al., 2023; Yanakieva et al., 2019). Furthermore, there are concerns about the safety of this practice due to the 5-HT_{2B} receptor agonism of many classic psychedelics, which may carry risk of cardiac valvulopathy with frequent repeated dosing (Tagen et al., 2023). As of this writing, there remains an open question on whether this practice offers legitimate, measurable advantages or if the observed benefits are largely placebo-driven (Bershad, 2023). Indeed, a recent survey study suggested that improvements in mental health outcomes were driven by expectancy effects (Kaertner et al., 2021).

Biological Framework

It is crucial to note that due to the emergent state of research in this field, the wide range of drug classes, and incomplete understanding of the underlying pathophysiology of eating disorders, discussion on the mechanisms of action will inherently be tentative and incomplete. Nonetheless, this chapter aims to provide a well-informed, although speculative, overview based on the most current evidence available. The discussion will concentrate on AN given that this has been a primary focus of research in this area to date, and the substances psilocybin, MDMA, and ketamine, as these are similarly best represented among existing research.

The role of serotonergic signaling, specifically through 5-HT_{2A} receptor agonism, is pivotal in generating the subjective and behavioral effects associated with classic psychedelics. Activation of the 5-HT_{2A} receptor induces a series of cellular responses, including desensitization and down-regulation of these receptors (Darmon et al., 2015; Hanley & Hensler, 2002). The relationship between serotonergic signaling and the pathophysiology of eating disorders, including AN, remains unclear, but it cannot be dismissed given serotonin's key role in regulating various aspects of feeding behavior, mood, and anxiety (Bonhomme, 1998; De Vry & Schreiber, 2017; Stockmeier, 1997). Increased 5-HT signaling, or a hyper-serotonergic state, has been suggested as a risk factor for AN that is suppressed by dieting behavior via the depletion of tryptophan for 5-HT synthesis (Steding et al., 2023). Underweight patients with AN have been found to have lower levels of serotonin in cerebrospinal fluid than healthy controls, with levels normalizing or increasing with weight restoration relative to those of women without history of AN (Kaye et al., 1988). Additionally, women in recovery from AN have altered 5-HT_{2A} binding patterns in the mesial temporal lobe and the pre- and subgenual cingulate cortex, brain regions involved in aversive conditioning, obsessive-compulsive disorder (OCD), and affective symptoms, when compared to healthy control women (Frank et al., 2002). Differences in allele frequencies of the 5-HT_{2A} promoter polymorphism −1438G/A, a finding associated with OCD has also been described in individuals with AN (Yan et al., 2021). Although only one small pilot study of psilocybin in nine patients examined PAT for OCD to date, there was a reduction in obsessions and compulsions in the acute setting after treatment (Moreno et al., 2006). At the time of this writing, a second, larger study is underway (NCT03356483). Despite limited existing evidence, there is biological plausibility to the idea that modulating serotonin neurotransmission could have therapeutic benefits in the treatment of AN. As regards bulimia nervosa (BN) and binge-eating disorder (BED), selective serotonin reuptake inhibitors have shown efficacy in decreasing binge eating and vomiting behaviors (Davis & Attia, 2017) and studies of 5-HT biomarkers in blood consistently reveal differences between individuals with BN and healthy controls supporting involvement of the serotoninergic system in the psychopathology of BN (Sjögren et al., 2019).

Preclinical research has identified at least several other biological mechanisms of note. Downstream effects of serotonergic psychedelics include glutamatergic signaling via mGluR2/3 receptors (Moreno et al., 2011, 2013). The NMDA receptor antagonist ketamine is also known to increase glutamate neurotransmission

(Ragnhildstveit et al., 2022). Both ketamine and classic psychedelics are known to promote synaptogenesis and neuroplasticity via modulation of brain-derived neurotrophic factor (BDNF) release (Ly et al., 2018; Ragnhildstveit et al., 2022). Some classic psychedelics may also have anti-inflammatory effects, mediated by changes in TNF-alpha (Nau Jr. et al., 2013). Clinical research in patients with AN has found that despite low BMI, inflammatory markers such as TNF-alpha tend to be elevated in the acute illness and to correct with recovery (Solmi et al., 2015).

Functional imaging studies in humans have also highlighted the potential role of network-level brain changes in the therapeutic potential of psychedelics. One area of research focus has been the default mode network (DMN), a network of brain regions active during unfocused awareness that is thought to be involved in a variety of functions including self-referential thought and sense of self. In healthy participants, both psilocybin and *N, N*-DMT in the form of ayahuasca acutely decrease resting state functional connectivity (rsFC) in the DMN (Carhart-Harris et al., 2012, 2014; Palhano-Fontes et al., 2015). This is of interest given that patients with AN have increased rsFC between the DMN and angular gyrus, which has been correlated with self-reported problems in interoceptive awareness (Lee et al., 2014). Increased rsFC between the DMN and frontoparietal network has also been observed in AN, is associated with self-reported measures of persistence, and appears to partially correct after recovery (Boehm et al., 2014, 2016). Similarly, increased rsFC within the DMN has also been reported in women with BN relative to healthy controls (Stopyra et al., 2019). Other notable findings in the psychedelic functional imaging literature include both acute and subacute decreases in amygdala reactivity in response to emotional stimuli after psilocybin administration in healthy volunteers (Barrett et al., 2020; Kraehenmann et al., 2015). This may be relevant in addressing the heightened emotional response to food and body-related signals seen in individuals with AN (Simon et al., 2019; Zhu et al., 2012).

Individuals with AN have been shown to have impaired set shifting and cognitive rigidity (Sternheim et al., 2022) and PAT has been associated with increases in cognitive and psychological flexibility in individuals with depression (Davis et al., 2020; Doss et al., 2021), which may have pertinence for facilitating behavior change. Preclinical work in rodents suggests improvements in cognitive flexibility following psilocybin treatment, supporting the biological plausibility of changes in cognitive flexibility as a mechanism underlying the effects of psilocybin in enhancing psychotherapy in PAT (Torrado Pacheco et al., 2023). Of particular relevance to AN, preliminary data from a study using the activity-based anorexia (ABA) model of AN in rats found that psilocybin improved reversal learning, reduced compulsive wheel running and increased food intake (Milton et al., 2022). Similarly, data in mice found that ketamine has potential to attenuate vulnerability to ABA (Chen et al., 2018; Goodwin-Groen et al., 2023; Li et al., 2023). Finally, a study in mice examining social-reward conditioned place preference in response to treatment with a range of psychedelic compounds suggests that psychedelics may reopen critical periods in brain development during which the central nervous system is more sensitive to relevant stimuli and more malleable in terms of synaptic and circuitry modulation (Nardou et al., 2023). This increased plasticity, in turn, may be reflected in increased psychological flexibility and potential for cognitive reappraisal and associated behavior change.

Other psychological changes documented after PAT in hallucinogen-naïve heathy controls which are of potential relevance to AN include increases in trait openness, an outcome more common among those individuals who experienced mystical-type effects during drug administration (MacLean et al., 2011). Mystical experiences induced by psychedelics are often rated by participants as among the most meaningful experiences of their lives, and they have been associated with long-term improvements in mood and positive behavior change (Griffiths et al., 2006, 2008). Psychologically insightful experiences may also occur, and are associated with improved longer-term outcomes for people with mood and substance use disorders (Garcia-Romeu et al., 2019; Roseman et al., 2018).

Finally, disorders shown to respond to PAT in preliminary trials are commonly comorbid in people with AN, and improvement in these co-occurring conditions may contribute to benefits in quality of life and well-being. Up to 45% of patients with AN have a comorbid anxiety disorder, up to 33% have a comorbid mood disorder, and about 7% to 19% have comorbid OCD (Mandelli et al., 2020; Ulfvebrand et al., 2015). Substance use disorders are also commonly comorbid (Ulfvebrand et al., 2015). Inpatients undergoing treatment showed that reduced levels of depression and worry, coupled with enhanced psychosocial functioning, were indicators of improved eating disorder symptoms and decreased psychological distress after one year (Fewell et al., 2017). PAT therefore has potential to increase self-rated well-being across multiple domains, including mood and anxiety, in both short and long-term follow-up (Griffiths et al., 2008; Gukasyan et al., 2022).

State of the Science in Eating Disorders

A brief overview of the history of the use of classic psychedelics and MDMA for other psychiatric indications is helpful. At the time of this writing, evidence to support the efficacy and safety of psychedelics in people with eating disorders is limited. With respect to the classic psychedelics and MDMA, results from only one small, open-label clinical trial of psilocybin have been published (Peck et al., 2023). Several others are planned or underway. Other contemporary research has included qualitative studies of naturalistic users, a secondary analysis of a clinical trial focused on another indication, and survey studies. With respect to the PAT model as applied to ketamine in people with eating disorders, the literature is similarly limited and includes few case reports and small, open-label clinical trials.

Evidence for efficacy of psychedelics in humans

Classic psychedelics

The "first wave" of psychedelic clinical research spanned the 1940s to the 1970s. Most treatment studies during this time were done with individuals with addictive and mood (neurotic) disorders, with very few published findings on the effects of these drugs in people with eating disorders. While reports hinted at possible therapeutic benefits, the studies were often compromised by methodological shortcomings, including the absence of standardized treatment protocols and consistent outcome measures. The most substantive publication from this period on eating disorders was a case report of a 35-year-old French woman with AN, likely binge/purge (AN-BP) subtype, treated with intravenous (IV) psilocybin and described as having a "definitive recovery" (Delay et al., 1959). Unfortunately, as was typical of publications from this time, characterization of illness severity and symptoms, dose used, and other details concerning treatment and eating disorder symptom improvement were omitted. A few subsequent published case series made brief mention of the use of LSD in patients with AN but these, too, were lacking in detail (Johnsen, 1964; Larsen, 2016).

The second wave of psychedelic clinical research, spanning the late 1990s to the present, has benefited from more rigorous study design; however, most of this work has focused on mood and addictive disorders, with eating disorders being a relatively recent indication of interest. Among contemporary studies, psilocybin PAT has shown substantial efficacy for MDD, with very large effect sizes (up to a Cohen *d* 2.2–2.5) and rates of treatment response and remission as high as 71% and 58% respectively (Carhart-Harris et al., 2018; Davis et al., 2021). Antidepressant effects are typically observed within one day to one week of treatment and may be durable through one year or longer in some patients (Gukasyan et al., 2022; Ross et al., 2016). Similarly, phase I–II studies have shown high rates of efficacy for tobacco and alcohol use disorders (Bogenschutz et al., 2022; Johnson et al., 2014). MDMA PAT has also been examined for a variety of conditions, and efficacy data for PTSD appear promising (Mitchell et al., 2021a). At present, several pharmaceutical companies have completed or are preparing to run phase III studies to evaluate safety and efficacy of psilocybin and MDMA for MDD and PTSD respectively (NCT03775200, NCT03866174, NCT03537014).

At the time of this writing, three small, open-label pilot studies of psilocybin PAT for AN have completed recruitment (NCT04052568, NCT04505189, NCT04661514), with results from the first of these recently published (Peck et al., 2023). A phase II study with psilocybin is underway, and one study with MDMA is planned. There are additionally two recently published case reports and an older case series on the use of ketamine to treat individuals with AN (Mills et al., 1998; Scolnick et al., 2020; Schwartz et al., 2021). Peck and colleagues (2023) reported results from 10 patients, of whom nine had the restricting subtype of AN (AN-R). Half of participants met the criteria for AN in partial remission at study entry and mean enrollment body mass index (BMI) for the group was in the normal range (19.7 kg/m^2). Exclusion criteria included a BMI less than 16 kg/m^2, medical instability, substance use disorder, history of a psychotic disorder, suicide risk, or a positive screen for borderline personality disorder. Primary outcomes included safety, feasibility, and tolerability. The study found that the acute effects of psilocybin at a single dose of 25 mg administered in a supportive setting in patients with mild to moderate AN were well-tolerated, with no serious acute adverse events reported. Two participants experienced transient asymptomatic hypoglycemia, which resolved without intervention. One participant with a history of MDD reported an increase in suicidal ideation at the three-month follow-up, which was deemed unrelated to the study. The most common adverse events were mild and transient, including headache, nausea, and fatigue. Secondary outcome measures included eating disorder symptom severity as measured by the Eating Disorder Examination (EDE), changes in BMI, and mood scales. These were mixed and varied greatly between participants; however, the authors found a significant improvement in mean scores of the weight and shape concern subscales of the EDE with medium to large effect sizes at one month (Cohen's d = 0.78 and 0.62 respectively). Weight concerns remained significantly improved at three months, although improvement in shape concerns lost significance at this later timepoint. Changes in eating concern and dietary restraint were not significant, although four of the 10 participants were judged to have experienced a clinically significant result, as indicated by global EDE scores decreasing to within one standard deviation of community norms at three months. Of these four, two had an increase in BMI, one was unchanged, and one had a significant drop. Overall mean BMI was not significantly different, although numerically higher in half of participants at the three-month follow up. Results from the ongoing two additional open-label trials that recently completed recruitment are pending (NCT04052568, NCT04505189).

Other studies of interest on classic psychedelics include those presenting qualitative evidence for the utility of ayahuasca in reducing symptoms of eating disorders (Lafrance et al., 2017). Sixteen North American individuals with self-reported history of eating disorders, including AN and BN, underwent semi-structured interviews on experiences with ceremonial ayahuasca drinking. Themes included reduction or cessation of disordered eating behaviors and shifts in body image perception. Eleven participants (69%) reported some decrease in symptom severity and half reported reductions in co-morbid anxiety, depression, or substance use. One person reported brief symptom exacerbation shortly after ayahuasca use, but this was followed by improvement. Limitations of this study included sparse information about participant diagnoses and treatment histories.

Spriggs and colleagues (2021) reported relevant findings from a secondary analysis of a large online survey in which participants completed a battery of questionnaires before and after planned independent use of psychedelics. Among 28 participants with a self-reported lifetime history of an eating disorder, there were significant improvements in depression and well-being scores two weeks after use of psychedelics compared to baseline. Study limitations included a self-reported lifetime history of an eating disorder, and neither current nor past specific diagnostic criteria were assessed.

Non-classic psychedelics

The literature on ketamine for individuals with eating disorders is similarly sparse. A 1998 paper describes a series of 15 individuals with either AN or BN treated with a variable number of IV ketamine infusions (Mills et al., 1998). Specifics of illness severity and assessment are missing so interpretation of findings is limited. Researchers defined nine participants as responders following an average of four ketamine infusions, whereas the six non-responders received a mean of eight infusions. Response was categorized based on "a marked and sustained clinical response . . . return to normal eating behavior and the acceptance of normal weight relative to height." Of the nine responders, five had AN-R and were partially weight restored as inpatients prior to ketamine treatment but had been resisting further weight gain. All five gained significant weight during the treatment with ketamine. The remaining responders included two with BN, one with restrictive eating and psychogenic polydipsia and one with AN-BP and alcohol use disorder. Of note, the non-responder group appeared to include the three most severely ill cases: the lowest weight case with AN and a very significant trauma history, the case with the highest depression score, and a case with type 1 diabetes and AN-BP. A second, more recent ketamine case series describes effects of repeated dosing in four female patients with chronic eating disorders and comorbid depression (Schwartz et al., 2021). All patients had eating disorder symptoms for greater than seven years along with treatment-resistant depression and had recently completed a partial hospitalization program but remained symptomatic. Two cases had AN-R and the other two had DSM-IV eating disorder not otherwise specified (EDNOS) consistent with the DSM-5 criteria for other specified feeding or eating disorder (OSFED). Additional comorbid diagnoses present in one or more cases included PTSD, borderline personality disorder, substance use, and suicidality. All four participants received a mix of IV and intramuscular (IM) ketamine treatments, starting at a dose of 0.5 mg/kg and had significant reduction in depressive symptoms as assessed by the Beck Depression Inventory and clinical assessment of symptoms. Improvement in eating disorder symptoms on the EDE-Q was, however, reported as more modest. Both cases with AN-R achieved weight restoration, although starting BMI for one case was already 19 kg/m^2 prior to treatment. Results from these small, open-label case series of ketamine treatment for eating disorders should be taken lightly although they suggest the potential for improvement in weight and eating disorder symptoms and reduction in depressive and anxiety symptoms in patients with a co-occurring depressive and eating disorder. The relationship between reduction in mood symptoms and the less significant reduction in eating disorders symptoms is notable and warrants further exploration.

A third, small (n = 5), open-label pilot study recently investigated the effects of a ketogenic diet in combination with six infusions of IV ketamine at a dose of 0.75 to 1.2 mg/kg in individuals with largely weight-restored AN and BMI greater than 18.5 kg/m^2 (Calabrese et al., 2022). The authors indicated interest in this combined intervention due to a hypothesized synergistic effects on dopamine signaling, as well as success with a previous patient (Scolnick et al., 2020). Treatment started with a two-day intensive "immersive" retreat during which participants, their support person (a family member or friend), a peer support member—the index case from the prior single case study—and the research team, which included a nutritionist, prepared ketogenic meals, and lived and ate together. Following this immersion program and four weeks on the ketogenic diet, six ketamine infusions were administered over a 17-day period. The investigators found significant improvements on measures of eating disorder symptom severity as assessed by the EDE-Q but not in BMI over six-month follow-up. One participant gradually lost weight after treatment and required admission to a residential treatment program.

Among other non-classic psychedelics, MDMA has also been suggested as a compound of interest. A trial looking at the effects of MDMA in people with AN-R or BED is planned (NCT04454684). Among contemporary clinical trials with MDMA, the most commonly studied indication has been for PTSD (Mitchell et al., 2021b). A secondary analysis of eating disorder symptoms was conducted among participants in a placebo-controlled study of MDMA-assisted therapy (PAT) for PTSD, analyzing change in EAT-26 scores from baseline to follow-up (Brewerton et al., 2022). Of the 89 participants, 13 (15%) had EAT-26 scores in the clinical range (≥ 20), and 28 (31%) had scores in the high-risk range (≥ 11). Fifteen met criteria for a current eating disorder (BED or OSFED), and 13 additional patients met criteria for a lifetime history of an eating disorder (BN, AN-BP, or OSFED) based on clinical interview. Among participants with EAT-26 scores in the clinical range (≥ 20), there were no significant differences between mean changes in MDMA versus placebo groups (−14.80 [SD = 8.96] vs. −13.50 [SD = 12.53], p =0.074) although improvement in EAT-26 scores for participants in the high-risk range (≥ 11) was significantly higher in the MDMA than the placebo group (−9.58 (7.59) vs −5.58 (14.29), p = 0.0058).

Alternative Perspectives

It is important to acknowledge that there are a variety of perspectives on psychedelics and their potential uses. Since the passage of the Controlled Substances Act in the United States, most psychedelics have been classified as Schedule I substances, a category reserved for drugs considered to have a high potential for abuse and no recognized medical value. Their common use for recreation often casts doubt on their therapeutic potential relative to potential risks. Moreover, with the recent revival of interest in psychedelic research, some critics have voiced concerns regarding possible risks in vulnerable populations, such as substance misuse and dependence, among other possible adverse effects. Rates of psychedelic use have risen significantly in recent years, with rates of increase being particularly high in young adults with depression (Walsh et al., 2024).

Beyond their recreational use in the contemporary Western context, psychedelics have a rich history among indigenous cultures, where they have been integral to spiritual, medicinal, and social practices for millennia. In contrast to the often-recreational consumption in modern societies, these substances have traditionally been used with great reverence, typically within the framework of ritualistic ceremonies aimed at healing, transcending the self, or connecting with the spiritual world. In recent critiques of the Western psychedelic movement, there is a growing concern regarding the cultural appropriation and commodification of these sacred practices. Many argue that current research, training programs, and guided psychedelic sessions often strip away the cultural context and significance of these rituals, repurposing them without proper acknowledgment or permission from the indigenous communities that have been their stewards since time immemorial (Celidwen et al., 2023). The critics point out a profound disconnect in how scientists and clinicians approach the study and application of psychedelics, often overlooking the need for acknowledgment, reciprocity, and the ethical sharing of benefits with the indigenous groups. This disregard, they argue, reflects a broader issue of cultural insensitivity and exploitation. On the other hand, not all substances, nor accompanying practices being explored in Western contexts have historical roots in indigenous practices. For instance, the therapeutic use of MDMA, a synthetic compound, represents a departure from the natural psychedelics traditionally used by indigenous communities.

On a practical level, it is important for clinicians and researchers to understand that the rise in hype has been accompanied by increases in alternative avenues for access, both legal and illegal. A growing number of state and local governments in the United States are considering or implementing legalization or decriminalization, most notably Oregon. Oregon voters approved a 2020 ballot initiative calling for creation of a board to oversee the development of "supported adult use" of psilocybin. Treatment and referral by a health care provider is not required and screening appears minimal, existing in the form of a self-report checklist asking about previous and current psychiatric diagnoses. Requirements for prospective facilitators are minimal and include a high school diploma, criminal background check, completion of a 120+ hour facilitator training program, and passing a licensure exam. As more individuals resort to self-medication or seek unregulated treatments without medical or psychiatric oversight, the likelihood of such programs encountering those at greater risk for complications rises.

Despite state and local changes in the law, psychedelics will likely remain federally illegal until sufficient evidence is produced to warrant rescheduling, which will likely only apply to highly controlled or synthetic preparations of these drugs. This has uncertain implications for state-level legislation. Patients may also seek treatment at the growing number of international retreat centers offering psychedelics. It is thus crucial for healthcare providers to stay abreast of the latest research and developments in this field and be prepared to engage in well-informed dialogues.

With respect to notable debates within the research community, concerns have been raised about the validity of many clinical trials due to difficulty with blinding. During a six- to eight-hour drug administration session, the subjective experiences induced by moderate to high doses of psychedelics are often easily distinguishable from those of a true (inert) placebo and may amplify the expectancy effect or positive expectations of improvement. Expectancy effects may also give rise to nocebo effects among participants who believe they have received an inactive placebo rather than a much-hyped novel intervention with potential to exacerbate demoralization or hopelessness (Gukasyan & Nayak, 2022). Problems with blinding can also result in allegiance effects among the research staff. Team members who hold strong convictions regarding the comparative efficacy of psychedelics over placebos may unwittingly alter their behavior toward the participants they believe received active drug versus placebo in ways that enhance or hinder response respectively. All these phenomena may inflate effect sizes.

Researchers have attempted a variety of alternative designs involving active placebo conditions, including both psychoactive (e.g., amphetamine, methylphenidate, dextromethorphan), and non-psychoactive drugs (niacin, sham ayahuasca), in an effort to mimic aspects of the psychedelic drug experience (Nayak et al., 2023). However, non-psychoactive controls have a considerable problem with unblinding. In one study of psilocybin-assisted therapy for people with alcohol use disorder using a diphenhydramine control condition, 93.6% of study participants and 92.4% of study staff accurately guessed their treatment assignment in the first drug session (Bogenschutz et al., 2022). Psychoactive controls present similar problems. In a study of psilocybin that used a methylphenidate control, 77% of participants correctly guessed their treatment arm (Griffiths et al., 2006). A further complicating factor is that many of the psychoactive medications used in control conditions, such as stimulants or dissociative agents, may have a therapeutic effect on the condition studied. Some have argued that expectancy effects and unblinding are inevitable in psychedelic research and that well-designed unblinded trials of psychedelics should still be considered if the drugs have potential in disorders for which we have limited treatment options available (Butler et al., 2022). Others have offered further suggestions on how researchers may more faithfully design randomized controlled trials (RCTs) or efficacy trials and advocate for the use of independent blinded external raters, videotaping dosing sessions, or supervision by external PAT experts (Muthukumaraswamy et al., 2022).

A further question of high relevance to eating disorders is how to optimally support patients who receive PAT. While this is a general concern in the realm of PAT—where the most effective style, timing, and quantity of accompanying psychotherapy remain undetermined—individuals suffering from eating disorders may benefit from other supplementary interventions, such as nutritional rehabilitation or more intensive or specially tailored psychotherapies, although superiority of any one psychotherapeutic approach for adults with anorexia remains debatable (Atwood & Friedman, 2020). Unlike the efficacy of psychedelic agents for depressive disorders, where a drug administration session may have immediately observable effects on primary outcomes with direct impact on diagnosis, recovery from an eating disorder is typically protracted and requires sustained commitment to behavior change. Even if a person should experience significant increases in motivation or readiness to change with psychedelic assisted therapy, a lack of sustained subsequent change in eating and weight control behaviors precludes recovery. Given that prolonged malnutrition can lead to diminished serotonin receptor density, those with AN who are malnourished may have reduced responses to PAT. Therefore, it may be most effective to administer PAT during or just after the nutritional and behavioral recovery phases. This approach may enhance the prevention of relapse by reinforcing the physical, behavioral, and psychological progress achieved.

In people with eating disorders, the use of PAT may carry heightened risks due to the serious physiological repercussions of these conditions. Common medical complications in this patient group include electrolyte imbalances, hypoglycemia, and arrhythmias, which can escalate the chances of life-threatening reactions from drug interactions. Furthermore, individuals with AN who are more severely ill can experience liver and kidney dysfunction that may affect drug metabolism. Recent preliminary studies on PAT for AN set a minimum BMI threshold of greater than or equal to 15 or 16 kg/m^2 to screen out the most vulnerable individuals. These studies also incorporated initial medical and psychiatric evaluation to manage potential immediate medical issues during PAT. Still, a more comprehensive exploration of these safety considerations is essential.

Finally, there are other ethical concerns. For example, in the case of extreme AN there is the question of whether some individuals have the capacity to consent to an experimental and potentially risky treatment given that the capacity for consent to treatment can be impaired by the illness itself. Positive hype around psychedelics in the popular media may influence patients to favor PAT over more established interventions, including inpatient behavioral treatment and weight restoration. Caution is warranted, especially for those who may be most vulnerable to harm, including those with severe and chronic eating disorders or serious medical or psychiatric comorbidity. Additionally, PAT involves many hours of supportive care, usually with one to two trained therapists and, as such, is highly resource-intensive, raising questions about its scalability and equity of access (Muthukumaraswamy et al., 2022).

Implications

At present, the use of psychedelics in the treatment of eating disorders remains a nascent area of clinical research. Understanding of the neurobiology underlying the mechanism of action of psychedelics or the pathophysiology of eating disorders are both limited. Nonetheless putative mechanisms of action by which psychedelics may facilitate active treatments of eating disorders have some face validity. These include biological effects on modulating serotonergic neurotransmission or enhancing functional brain connectivity and neuroplasticity which, in turn, may help modulate characteristics that impair behavior change in eating disorders, such as cognitive rigidity and low openness. No classic psychedelic has been approved for any clinical indication, let alone any eating disorder. The scarcity of approved therapeutic applications underscores the need for rigorous, controlled studies to better understand the safety and efficacy of these substances in clinical settings, especially in more vulnerable populations, such as those with severe or extreme eating disorders who may be more likely to seek out these approaches. Those with eating disorders may need to be especially cautious due to high levels of physical and psychiatric comorbidity that may place them at increased risk. Studies to date remain underpowered and preliminary. This gap in the literature signifies a considerable opportunity for future research aimed at elucidating the potential therapeutic benefits and limitations of psychedelics; however, study designs for RCTs are challenging due to expectancy effects, blinding concerns, and the confounds of psychotherapeutic effects related to PAT and adjunctive therapies. There is a need for rigorous, thoughtful research in this area, as well as a system for open and transparent data collection with respect to the reporting of adverse events. Study designs should pay attention to individual and situational factors likely to influence outcomes, including illness severity, comorbid diagnoses, timing of the intervention, dosing, type of psychological support or treatment used, and expectations of both patient and interventionist.

References

Atwood, M. E., & Friedman, A. (2020). A systematic review of enhanced cognitive behavioral therapy (CBT-E) for eating disorders. *International Journal of Eating Disorders*, *53*(3), 311–330. https://doi.org/10.1002/eat.23206

Barrett, F. S., Doss, M. K., Sepeda, N. D., Pekar, J. J., & Griffiths, R. R. (2020). Emotions and brain function are altered up to one month after a single high dose of psilocybin. *Scientific Reports*, *10*(1), Article 1.

Berman, R. M., Cappiello, A., Anand, A., Oren, D. A., Heninger, G. R., Charney, D. S., & Krystal, J. H. (2000). Antidepressant effects of ketamine in depressed patients. *Biological Psychiatry*, *47*(4), 351–354.

Bershad, A. K. (2023). Psychedelic microdosing: What is it good for? *Biological Psychiatry*, *94*(6), e23–e24.

Bershad, A. K., Preller, K. H., Lee, R., Keedy, S., Wren-Jarvis, J., Bremmer, M. P., & de Wit, H. (2020). Preliminary report on the effects of a low dose of LSD on resting-state amygdala functional connectivity. *Biological Psychiatry: Cognitive Neuroscience and Neuroimaging*, *5*(4), Article 4.

Bershad, A. K., Schepers, S. T., Bremmer, M. P., Lee, R., & de Wit, H. (2019). Acute subjective and behavioral effects of microdoses of lysergic acid diethylamide in healthy human volunteers. *Biological Psychiatry*, *86*(10), article 10.

Boehm, I., Geisler, D., King, J. A., Ritschel, F., Seidel, M., Araujo, Y. D., Petermann, J., Lohmeier, H., Weiss, J., Walter, M., Roessner, V., & Ehrlich, S. (2014). Increased resting state functional connectivity in the fronto-parietal and default mode network in anorexia nervosa. *Frontiers in Behavioral Neuroscience*, *8*, 346. https://doi.org/10.3389/fnbeh.2014.00346

Boehm, I., Geisler, D., Tam, F., King, J. A., Ritschel, F., Seidel, M., Bernardoni, F., Murr, J., Goschke, T., Calhoun, V. D., Roessner, V., & Ehrlich, S. (2016). Partially restored resting-state functional connectivity in women recovered from anorexia nervosa. *Journal of Psychiatry & Neuroscience*, *41*(6), article 6. https://doi.org/10.1503/jpn.150259

Bogenschutz, M. P., Ross, S., Bhatt, S., Baron, T., Forcehimes, A. A., Laska, E., Mennenga, S. E., O'Donnell, K., Owens, L. T., Podrebarac, S., Rotrosen, J., Tonigan, J. S., & Worth, L. (2022). Percentage of heavy drinking days following psilocybin-assisted psychotherapy vs placebo in the treatment of adult patients with alcohol use disorder: A randomized clinical trial. *JAMA Psychiatry*, *79*(10), 953–962. https://doi.org/10.1001/jamapsychiatry.2022.2096

Bonhomme, N. (1998). Involvement of serotonin and dopamine in the mechanism of action of novel antidepressant drugs: A review. *Journal of Clinical Psychopharmacology*, *18*(6), article 6. https://doi.org/10.1097/00004714-199812000-00005

Brewerton, T. D., Wang, J. B., Lafrance, A., Pamplin, C., Mithoefer, M., Yazar-Klosinki, B., Emerson, A., & Doblin, R. (2022). MDMA-assisted therapy significantly reduces eating disorder symptoms in a randomized placebo-controlled trial of adults with severe PTSD. *Journal of Psychiatric Research*, *149*, 128–135. https://doi.org/10.1016/j.jpsychires.2022.03.008

Butler, M., Jelen, L., & Rucker, J. (2022). Expectancy in placebo-controlled trials of psychedelics: If so, so what? *Psychopharmacology*, *239*(10), article 10.

Calabrese, L., Scolnick, B., Zupec-Kania, B., Beckwith, C., Costello, K., & Frank, G. K. (2022). Ketogenic diet and ketamine infusion treatment to target chronic persistent eating disorder psychopathology in anorexia nervosa: A pilot study. *Eating and Weight Disorders*, *27*(8), 3751–3757.

Carhart-Harris, R. L., Bolstridge, M., Day, C. M. J., Rucker, J., Watts, R., Erritzoe, D. E., Kaelen, M., Giribaldi, B., Bloomfield, M., & Pilling, S. (2018). Psilocybin with psychological support for treatment-resistant depression: Six-month follow-up. *Psychopharmacology*, *235*(2), Article 2.

Carhart-Harris, R. L., Erritzoe, D., Williams, T., Stone, J. M., Reed, L. J., Colasanti, A., Tyacke, R. J., Leech, R., Malizia, A. L., Murphy, K., Hobden, P., Evans, J., Feilding, A., Wise, R. G., & Nutt, D. J. (2012). Neural correlates of the psychedelic state as determined by fMRI studies with psilocybin. *Proceedings of the National Academy of Sciences*, *109*(6), article 6. https://doi.org/10.1073/pnas.1119598109

Carhart-Harris, R. L., Leech, R., Hellyer, P. J., Shanahan, M., Feilding, A., Tagliazucchi, E., Chialvo, D. R., & Nutt, D. (2014). The entropic brain: A theory of conscious states informed by neuroimaging research with psychedelic drugs. *Frontiers in Human Neuroscience*, 8. https://doi.org/10.3389/fnhum.2014.00020

Celidwen, Y., Redvers, N., Githaiga, C., Calambás, J., Añaños, K., Chindoy, M. E., Vitale, R., Rojas, J. N., Mondragón, D., & Rosalío, Y. V. (2023). Ethical principles of traditional Indigenous medicine to guide western psychedelic research and practice. *The Lancet Regional Health—Americas*, *18*, 100410.

Chen, Y., Sherpa, A. D., & Aoki, C. (2018). Single injection of ketamine during mid-adolescence promotes long-lasting resilience to activity-based anorexia of female mice by increasing food intake and attenuating hyperactivity as well as anxiety-like behavior. *International Journal of Eating Disorders*, *51*(8), 1020–1025. https://doi.org/10.1002/eat.22937

Dakwar, E., Nunes, E. V., Hart, C. L., Foltin, R. W., Mathew, S. J., Carpenter, K. M., Choi, C. J. J., Basaraba, C. N., Pavlicova, M., & Levin, F. R. (2019). A single ketamine infusion combined with mindfulness-based behavioral modification to treat cocaine dependence: A randomized clinical trial. *American Journal of Psychiatry*, *176*(11), 923–930.

Darmon, M., Awabdh, S. A., Emerit, M. B., & Masson, J. (2015). Insights into serotonin receptor trafficking: Cell membrane targeting and internalization. *Progress in Molecular Biology and Translational Science*, *132*, 97. https://doi.org/10.1016/bs.pmbts.2015.02.009

Davis, A. K., Barrett, F. S., & Griffiths, R. R. (2020). Psychological flexibility mediates the relations between acute psychedelic effects and subjective decreases in depression and anxiety. *Journal of Contextual Behavioral Science*, *15*, 39–45.

Davis, A. K., Barrett, F. S., May, D. G., Cosimano, M. P., Sepeda, N. D., Johnson, M. W., Finan, P. H., & Griffiths, R. R. (2021). Effects of psilocybin-assisted therapy on major depressive disorder: A randomized clinical trial. *JAMA Psychiatry, 78*(5), article 5.

Davis, H., & Attia, E. (2017). Pharmacotherapy of eating disorders. *Current Opinion in Psychiatry, 30*(6), 452.

De Vry, J., & Schreiber, R. (2017). Effects of selected serotonin 5-HT 1 and 5-HT 2 receptor agonists on feeding behavior: Possible mechanisms of action. Neuroscience and Biobehavioral Reviews, 24(3), 341–353. https://doi.org/10.1016/s0149-7634(99)00083-4

Delay, J., Pichot, P., Lempérière, T., & Quetin, A. (1959). Effets thérapeutiques de la psilocybine sur une névrose convulsive. *Annales Médico-Psychologiques, 117*, 509–515.

Doss, M. K., Považan, M., Rosenberg, M. D., Sepeda, N. D., Davis, A. K., Finan, P. H., Smith, G. S., Pekar, J. J., Barker, P. B., & Griffiths, R. R. (2021). Psilocybin therapy increases cognitive and neural flexibility in patients with major depressive disorder. *Translational Psychiatry, 11*(1), 1–10.

Fewell, L. K., Levinson, C. A., & Stark, L. (2017). Depression, worry, and psychosocial functioning predict eating disorder treatment outcomes in a residential and partial hospitalization setting. *Eating and Weight Disorders, 22*(2), article 2. https://doi.org/10.1007/s40519-016-0357-6

Flaherty, G. T., Maxemous, K. K., Nossier, R. E., & Bui, Y.-G. (2017). The highs and lows of drug tourism: A travel medicine perspective. *Journal of Travel Medicine, 24*(6). https://doi.org/10.1093/jtm/tax068

Fond, G., Loundou, A., Rabu, C., Macgregor, A., Lançon, C., Brittner, M., Micoulaud-Franchi, J.-A., Richieri, R., Courtet, P., & Abbar, M. (2014). Ketamine administration in depressive disorders: A systematic review and meta-analysis. *Psychopharmacology, 231*, 3663–3676.

Frank, G. K., Kaye, W. H., Meltzer, C. C., Price, J. C., Greer, P., McConaha, C., & Skovira, K. (2002). Reduced 5-HT2A receptor binding after recovery from anorexia nervosa. *Biological Psychiatry, 52*(9), article 9. https://doi.org/10.1016/S0006-3223(02)01378-1

Garcia-Romeu, A., Davis, A. K., Erowid, F., Erowid, E., Griffiths, R. R., & Johnson, M. W. (2019). Cessation and reduction in alcohol consumption and misuse after psychedelic use. *Journal of Psychopharmacology*, 33(9), 1088–1101.

Goodwin-Groen, S., Dong, Y., & Aoki, C. (2023). Three daily intraperitoneal injections of subanesthetic ketamine ameliorate activity-based anorexia vulnerability of adult female mice. *International Journal of Eating Disorders, 57*(7), 1447–1464. https://doi.org/10.1002/eat.24036

Griffiths, R. R., Richards, W. A., Johnson, M. W., McCann, U. D., & Jesse, R. (2008). Mystical-type experiences occasioned by psilocybin mediate the attribution of personal meaning and spiritual significance 14 months later. *Journal of Psychopharmacology, 22*(6), article 6. https://doi.org/10.1177/0269881108094300

Griffiths, R. R., Richards, W. A., McCann, U., & Jesse, R. (2006). Psilocybin can occasion mystical-type experiences having substantial and sustained personal meaning and spiritual significance. *Psychopharmacology, 187*(3), article 3. https://doi.org/10.1007/s00213-006-0457-5

Gukasyan, N., Davis, A. K., Barrett, F. S., Cosimano, M. P., Sepeda, N. D., Johnson, M. W., & Griffiths, R. R. (2022). Efficacy and safety of psilocybin-assisted treatment for major depressive disorder: Prospective 12-month follow-up. *Journal of Psychopharmacology, 36*(2), 151–158.

Gukasyan, N., & Nayak, S. M. (2022). Psychedelics, placebo effects, and set and setting: Insights from common factors theory of psychotherapy. *Transcultural Psychiatry, 59*(5), article 5. https://doi.org/10.1177/1363461520983684

Hanley, N. R., & Hensler, J. G. (2002). Mechanisms of ligand-induced desensitization of the 5-hydroxytryptamine(2A) receptor. *Journal of Pharmacology and Experimental Therapeutics, 300*(2), article 2.

Hock, R. S., Feeney, A., Iovieno, N., Murrough, J. W., Mathew, S. J., Iosifescu, D. V., Fava, M., Jha, M. K., & Papakostas, G. I. (2022). Rapidity of symptom improvement with intranasal esketamine for major depressive disorder: A systematic review and meta-analysis. *Journal of Clinical Psychiatry, 84*(1), 44591.

Hutten, N. R. P. W., Mason, N. L., Dolder, P. C., Theunissen, E. L., Holze, F., Liechti, M. E., Feilding, A., Ramaekers, J. G., & Kuypers, K. P. C. (2020). Mood and cognition after administration of low LSD doses in healthy volunteers: A placebo controlled dose-effect finding study. *European Neuropsychopharmacology*, 41, 81–91. https://doi.org/10.1016/j.euroneuro.2020.10.002

Johnsen, G. (1964). Three years experience with the use of LSD as an aid in psychotherapy. *Acta Psychiatrica Scandinavica, 39*(S180), article S180.

Johnson, M. W., Garcia-Romeu, A., Cosimano, M. P., & Griffiths, R. R. (2014). Pilot study of the 5-HT2AR agonist psilocybin in the treatment of tobacco addiction. *Journal of Psychopharmacology, 28*(11), article 11. https://doi.org/10.1177/0269881114548296

K. Freind, J. M., Beserra, F. R., Menezes, B. S., & Mograbi, D. C. (2023). Therapeutic protocols using ketamine and esketamine for depressive disorders: A systematic review. *Journal of Psychoactive Drugs, 56*(4), 496–512. https://doi.org/10.1080/02791072.2023.2248989

Kaertner, L. S., Steinborn, M. B., Kettner, H., Spriggs, M. J., Roseman, L., Buchborn, T., Balaet, M., Timmermann, C., Erritzoe, D., & Carhart-Harris, R. L. (2021). Positive expectations predict improved mental-health outcomes linked to psychedelic microdosing. *Scientific Reports, 11*(1), 1941.

Kaye, W. H., Gwirtsman, H. E., George, D. T., Jimerson, D. C., & Ebert, M. H. (1988). CSF 5-HIAA concentrations in anorexia nervosa: Reduced values in underweight subjects normalize after weight gain. *Biological Psychiatry, 23*(1), article 1. https://doi.org/10.1016/0006-3223(88)90113-8

Kraehenmann, R., Preller, K. H., Scheidegger, M., Pokorny, T., Bosch, O. G., Seifritz, E., & Vollenweider, F. X. (2015). Psilocybin-induced decrease in amygdala reactivity correlates with enhanced positive mood in healthy volunteers. *Biological Psychiatry, 78*(8), article 8. https://doi.org/10.1016/j.biopsych.2014.04.010

Lafrance, A., Loizaga-Velder, A., Fletcher, J., Renelli, M., Files, N., & Tupper, K. W. (2017). Nourishing the spirit: Exploratory research on ayahuasca experiences along the continuum of recovery from eating disorders. *Journal of Psychoactive Drugs, 49*(5), article 5. https://doi.org/10.1080/02791072.2017.1361559

Larsen, J. K. (2016). Neurotoxicity and LSD treatment: A follow-up study of 151 patients in Denmark. *History of Psychiatry, 27*(2), article 2.

Lee, S., Kim, K. R., Ku, J., Lee, J.-H., Namkoong, K., & Jung, Y.-C. (2014). Resting-state synchrony between anterior cingulate cortex and precuneus relates to body shape concern in anorexia nervosa and bulimia nervosa. *Psychiatry Research: Neuroimaging, 221*(1), article 1. https://doi.org/10.1016/j.pscychresns.2013.11.004

Li, J., Chen, Y.-W., & Aoki, C. (2023). Ketamine ameliorates activity-based anorexia of adolescent female mice through changes in the prevalence of NR2B-containing NMDA receptors at excitatory synapses that are in opposite directions for of pyramidal neurons versus GABA interneurons in medial prefrontal cortex. Research Square, rs.3.rs-2514157. https://doi.org/10.21203/rs.3.rs-2514157/

Ly, C., Greb, A. C., Cameron, L. P., Wong, J. M., Barragan, E. V., Wilson, P. C., Burbach, K. F., Zarandi, S. S., Sood, A., & Paddy, M. R. (2018). Psychedelics promote structural and functional neural plasticity. *Cell Reports, 23*(11), article 11.

MacLean, K. A., Johnson, M. W., & Griffiths, R. R. (2011). Mystical experiences occasioned by the hallucinogen psilocybin lead to increases in the personality domain of openness. *Journal of Psychopharmacology, 25*(11), article 11. https://doi.org/10.1177/0269881111420188

Mandelli, L., Draghetti, S., Albert, U., De Ronchi, D., & Atti, A.-R. (2020). Rates of comorbid obsessive-compulsive disorder in eating disorders: A meta-analysis of the literature. *Journal of Affective Disorders, 277*, 927–939.

Mills, I. H., Park, G. R., Manara, A. R., & Merriman, R. J. (1998). Treatment of compulsive behaviour in eating disorders with intermittent ketamine infusions. *QJM: Monthly Journal of the Association of Physicians, 91*(7), article 7.

Milton, L. K., Farrell, G. A., Oldfield, B. J., & Foldi, C. J. (2022, July 14). Effects of psilocybin on activity-based anorexia and cognitive flexibility in female rats. Society for the Study of Ingestive Behavior 29th Annual Meeting, Porto, Portugal.

Mitchell, J. M., Bogenschutz, M., Lilienstein, A., Harrison, C., Kleiman, S., Parker-Guilbert, K., Ot'alora G, M., Garas, W., Paleos, C., & Gorman, I. (2021a). MDMA-assisted therapy for severe PTSD: A randomized, double-blind, placebo-controlled phase 3 study. *Nature Medicine, 27*(6), 1025–1033.

Mitchell, J. M., Bogenschutz, M., Lilienstein, A., Harrison, C., Kleiman, S., Parker-Guilbert, K., Ot'alora G, M., Garas, W., Paleos, C., & Gorman, I. (2021b). MDMA-assisted therapy for severe PTSD: A randomized, double-blind, placebo-controlled phase 3 study. *Nature Medicine, 27*(6), article 6.

Moreno, F. A., Wiegand, C. B., Taitano, E. K., & Delgado, P. L. (2006). Safety, tolerability, and efficacy of psilocybin in 9 patients with obsessive-compulsive disorder. *Journal of Clinical Psychiatry, 67*(11), article 11. https://doi.org/10.4088/JCP.v67n1110

Moreno, J. L., Holloway, T., Albizu, L., Sealfon, S. C., & González-Maeso, J. (2011). Metabotropic glutamate mGlu2 receptor is necessary for the pharmacological and behavioral effects induced by hallucinogenic 5-HT2A receptor agonists. *Neuroscience Letters, 493*(3), article 3.

Moreno, J. L., Holloway, T., Rayannavar, V., Sealfon, S. C., & González-Maeso, J. (2013). Chronic treatment with LY341495 decreases 5-HT2A receptor binding and hallucinogenic effects of LSD in mice. *Neuroscience Letters, 536*, 69–73.

Murphy, R. J., Sumner, R., Evans, W., Ponton, R., Ram, S., Godfrey, K., Forsyth, A., Cavadino, A., Naga, V. K., & Smith, T. (2023). Acute mood-elevating properties of microdosed lysergic acid diethylamide in healthy volunteers: A home-administered randomized controlled trial. *Biological Psychiatry, 94*(6), 511–521.

Muthukumaraswamy, S., Forsyth, A., & Sumner, R. L. (2022). The challenges ahead for psychedelic "medicine." *Australian & New Zealand Journal of Psychiatry, 56*(11), 1378–1383. https://doi.org/10.1177/00048674221081763

Nardou, R., Sawyer, E., Song, Y. J., Wilkinson, M., Padovan-Hernandez, Y., de Deus, J. L., Wright, N., Lama, C., Faltin, S., & Goff, L. A. (2023). Psychedelics reopen the social reward learning critical period. *Nature, 618*(7966), 790–798.

Nau Jr, F., Yu, B., Martin, D., & Nichols, C. D. (2013). Serotonin 5-HT2A receptor activation blocks TNF-α mediated inflammation in vivo. *PLOS ONE, 8*(10), e75426.

Nayak, S. M., Bradley, M. K., Kleykamp, B. A., Strain, E. C., Dworkin, R. H., & Johnson, M. W. (2023). Control conditions in randomized trials of psychedelics: An ACTTION systematic review. *Journal of Clinical Psychiatry, 84*(3), 47000.

Osmond, H. (1957). A review of the clinical effects of psychotomimetic agents. *Annals of the New York Academy of Sciences, 66*(3), article 3.

Palhano-Fontes, F., Andrade, K. C., Tofoli, L. F., Santos, A. C., Crippa, J. A. S., Hallak, J. E. C., Ribeiro, S., & de Araujo, D. B. (2015). The psychedelic state induced by ayahuasca modulates the activity and connectivity of the default mode network. *PLOS ONE, 10*(2), article 2. https://doi.org/10.1371/journal.pone.0118143

Peck, S. K., Shao, S., Gruen, T., Yang, K., Babakanian, A., Trim, J., Finn, D. M., & Kaye, W. H. (2023). Psilocybin therapy for females with anorexia nervosa: A phase 1, open-label feasibility study. *Nature Medicine, 29*(8), 1947–1953.

Phelps, J., Shah, R. N., & Lieberman, J. A. (2022). The rapid rise in investment in psychedelics—Cart before the horse. *JAMA Psychiatry, 79*(3), 189–190.

Price, R. B., Kissel, N., Baumeister, A., Rohac, R., Woody, M. L., Ballard, E. D., Zarate Jr, C. A., Deakin, W., Abdallah, C. G., & Feder, A. (2022). International pooled patient-level meta-analysis of ketamine infusion for depression: In search of clinical moderators. *Molecular Psychiatry, 27*(12), 5096–5112.

Ragnhildstveit, A., Slayton, M., Jackson, L. K., Brendle, M., Ahuja, S., Holle, W., Moore, C., Sollars, K., Seli, P., & Robison, R. (2022). Ketamine as a novel psychopharmacotherapy for eating disorders: evidence and future directions. *Brain Sciences, 12*(3), article 3.

Roseman, L., Nutt, D. J., & Carhart-Harris, R. L. (2018). Quality of acute psychedelic experience predicts therapeutic efficacy of psilocybin for treatment-resistant depression. *Frontiers in Pharmacology, 8*, 974.

Ross, S., Bossis, A., Guss, J., Agin-Liebes, G., Malone, T., Cohen, B., Mennenga, S. E., Belser, A., Kalliontzi, K., Babb, J., Su, Z., Corby, P., & Schmidt, B. L. (2016). Rapid and sustained symptom reduction following psilocybin treatment for anxiety and depression in patients with life-threatening cancer: A randomized controlled trial. *Journal of Psychopharmacology, 30*(12), article 12. https://doi.org/10.1177/0269881116675512

Schwartz, T., Trunko, M. E., Feifel, D., Lopez, E., Peterson, D., Frank, G. K. W., & Kaye, W. (2021). A longitudinal case series of IM ketamine for patients with severe and enduring eating disorders and comorbid treatment-resistant depression. *Clinical Case Reports, 9*(5), e03869. https://doi.org/10.1002/ccr3.3869

Scolnick, B., Zupec-Kania, B., Calabrese, L., Aoki, C., & Hildebrandt, T. (2020). Remission from chronic anorexia nervosa with ketogenic diet and ketamine: Case report. *Frontiers in Psychiatry, 11*. https://doi.org/10.3389/fpsyt.2020.00763

Simon, J. J., Stopyra, M. A., & Friederich, H.-C. (2019). Neural processing of disorder-related stimuli in patients with anorexia nervosa: A narrative review of brain imaging studies. *Journal of Clinical Medicine, 8*(7), 1047.

Sjögren, M., Nielsen, A. S. M., Hasselbalch, K. C., Wøllo, M., & Hansen, J. S. (2019). A systematic review of blood-based serotonergic biomarkers in bulimia nervosa. *Psychiatry Research, 279*, 155–171.

Smith, W. R., & Appelbaum, P. S. (2021). Two models of legalization of psychedelic substances: reasons for concern. *JAMA, 326*(8), 697–698.

Solmi, M., Veronese, N., Favaro, A., Santonastaso, P., Manzato, E., Sergi, G., & Correll, C. U. (2015). Inflammatory cytokines and anorexia nervosa: A meta-analysis of cross-sectional and longitudinal studies. *Psychoneuroendocrinology, 51*, 237–252.

Spriggs, M. J., Kettner, H., & Carhart-Harris, R. L. (2021). Positive effects of psychedelics on depression and wellbeing scores in individuals reporting an eating disorder. *Eating and Weight Disorders*, *26*(4), 1265–1270.

Steding, J., Ritschel, F., Boehm, I., Geisler, D., King, J. A., Roessner, V., Smolka, M. N., Zepf, F. D., & Ehrlich, S. (2023). The effects of acute tryptophan depletion on instrumental reward learning in anorexia nervosa—An fMRI study. *Psychological Medicine*, *53*(8), 3426–3436.

Sternheim, L. C., van Passel, B., Dingemans, A., Cath, D., & Danner, U. N. (2022). Cognitive and experienced flexibility in patients with anorexia nervosa and obsessive compulsive disorder. *Frontiers in Psychiatry*, *13*, 868921.

Stockmeier, C. A. (1997). Neurobiology of serotonin in depression and suicide. Annals of the New York Academy of Sciences, 836, 220–232.

Stopyra, M. A., Simon, J. J., Skunde, M., Walther, S., Bendszus, M., Herzog, W., & Friederich, H.-C. (2019). Altered functional connectivity in binge eating disorder and bulimia nervosa. *Brain and Behavior*, 9(2), e01207. https://doi.org/10.1002/brb3.1207

Tagen, M., Mantuani, D., van Heerden, L., Holstein, A., Klumpers, L. E., & Knowles, R. (2023). The risk of chronic psychedelic and MDMA microdosing for valvular heart disease. *Journal of Psychopharmacology*, *37*(9), 876–890.

Torrado Pacheco, A., Olson, R. J., Garza, G., & Moghaddam, B. (2023). Acute psilocybin enhances cognitive flexibility in rats. *Neuropsychopharmacology*, 48(7), 1011–1020. https://doi.org/10.1038/s41386-023-01545-z

Ulfvebrand, S., Birgegård, A., Norring, C., Högdahl, L., & von Hausswolff-juhlin, Y. (2015). Psychiatric comorbidity in women and men with eating disorders results from a large clinical database. *Psychiatry Research*, *230*(2), article 2. https://doi.org/10.1016/j.psychres.2015.09.008

Walsh, C. A., Gorfinkel, L., Shmulewitz, D., Stohl, M., & Hasin, D. S. (2024). Use of lysergic acid diethylamide by major depression status. *JAMA Psychiatry*, *81*(1), 89–96.

Yan, P., Gao, B., Wang, S., Wang, S., Li, J., & Song, M. (2021). Association of 5-HTR2A-1438A/G polymorphism with anorexia nervosa and bulimia nervosa: A meta-analysis. *Neuroscience Letters*, *755*, 135918.

Yanakieva, S., Polychroni, N., Family, N., Williams, L. T., Luke, D. P., & Terhune, D. B. (2019). The effects of microdose LSD on time perception: A randomised, double-blind, placebo-controlled trial. *Psychopharmacology*, *236*(4), article 4.

Zhu, Y., Hu, X., Wang, J., Chen, J., Guo, Q., Li, C., & Enck, P. (2012). Processing of food, body and emotional stimuli in anorexia nervosa: A systematic review and meta-analysis of functional magnetic resonance imaging studies. *European Eating Disorders Review*, *20*(6), 439–450.

Afterword

This book began as a concept more than two years before it came to fruition, and the journey has been profoundly stimulating for both of us. When we first started reading and talking about *Think Again*, we envisioned creating a work that would distinguish itself from other compilations, and we had lofty aspirations to challenge our colleagues to present their own research within a broader context. Our colleagues exceeded our expectations.

This project was not a typical chapter-writing exercise. In addition to summarizing the familiar information, each group was asked to explore and articulate the other "parts of the elephant." The contributors fully rose to the challenge. One author shared that she used the opportunity to involve her trainees by seeking their ideas about what might be challenges to the existing formulations, which resulted in truly refreshing perspectives. Another group took an unconventional approach by summarizing the current science and then identifying that their perspective actually presented an alternative to the standard approach.

At the conclusion of this process, it is the alternative perspectives sections that stand out most for us. Having read all these inspiring contributions, we find ourselves more receptive to challenges to our own models. We hope others have a similar experience and will find it as rewarding. We are excited to continue the discourse.

Index

For the benefit of digital users, indexed terms that span two pages (e.g., 52–53) may, on occasion, appear on only one of those pages.